Paediatric Intensive Care Nursing

Edited by

Michaela Dixon
Clinical Development Nurse
Paediatric Intensive Care Unit
Bristol Royal Hospital for Children
University Hospitals Bristol NHS Foundation Trust
Bristol
UK

Doreen Crawford
Chair of Royal College of Nursing Children and Young People Acute Care Forum
Senior Lecturer – Neonatal and Child Programmes
School of Nursing and Midwifery
Faculty of Health and Life Sciences
De Montfort University
Leicester
UK

WILEY-BLACKWELL
A John Wiley & Sons, Ltd., Publication

This edition first published 2012
© 2012 by John Wiley and Sons, Ltd

Wiley-Blackwell is an imprint of John Wiley & Sons, formed by the merger of Wiley's global Scientific, Technical and Medical business with Blackwell Publishing.

Registered office: John Wiley & Sons, Ltd, The Atrium, Southern Gate, Chichester, West Sussex, PO19 8SQ, UK

Editorial offices: 9600 Garsington Road, Oxford, OX4 2DQ, UK
                     The Atrium, Southern Gate, Chichester, West Sussex, PO19 8SQ, UK
                     2121 State Avenue, Ames, Iowa 50014-8300, USA

For details of our global editorial offices, for customer services and for information about how to apply for permission to reuse the copyright material in this book please see our website at www.wiley.com/wiley-blackwell.

Library of Congress Cataloging-in-Publication Data
Paediatric intensive care nursing / edited by Michaela Dixon, Doreen Crawford.
       p. ; cm.
   Includes bibliographical references and index.
   ISBN 978-1-4051-9936-0 (pbk. : alk. paper)
   I. Dixon, Michaela.   II. Crawford, Doreen.
   [DNLM: 1. Intensive Care–methods.   2. Pediatric Nursing–methods. WY 159]
   618.92'0028–dc23
                                            2012011411

A catalogue record for this book is available from the British Library.

Wiley also publishes its books in a variety of electronic formats. Some content that appears in print may not be available in electronic books.

Cover images: main image – iStockphoto/Fertnig; top left – iStockphoto/lovleah; top middle – Fotolia/Blend Images; top right – Fotolia/Gert Very
Cover design by Meaden Creative

Set in 9.5/12 pt Times by Toppan Best-set Premedia Limited, Hong Kong
Printed in Singapore by Ho Printing Singapore Pte Ltd

1   2012

CONTENTS

LIST OF CONTRIBUTORS

Editors

Michaela Dixon
Clinical Development Nurse
Paediatric Intensive Care Unit
Bristol Royal Hospital for Children
University Hospitals Bristol NHS Foundation Trust
Bristol, UK

Doreen Crawford
Chair of Royal College of Nursing Children and Young
People Acute Care Forum
Senior Lecturer, Child Health
School of Nursing and Midwifery
Faculty of Health and Life Sciences
De Montfort University
Leicester, UK

Contributors

Sandra Batcheler
Sister
Paediatric Intensive Care Unit
Bristol Royal Hospital for Children
University Hospitals Bristol NHS Foundation Trust
Bristol, UK

Dave Clarke
Lecturer, Children and Young People
Cardiff School of Nursing and Midwifery Studies
Cardiff University
Cardiff, UK

Gillian Earl
Independent Nurse Consultant (Child Protection)
CCJJ, Child Protection Training and Consultancy
Services
Lincolnshire, UK

Mark Fores
Senior Clinical Skills Facilitator
Clinical Skills Unit
Leicester Royal Hospital
University Hospitals of Leicester NHS Trust
Leicester, UK

Ben Harvey
Advanced Nurse Practitioner
Paediatric Intensive Care Unit
Sheffield Children's Hospital
Sheffield, UK

Caroline Langford
Advanced Nurse Practitioner
Oncology Services
Alder Hey Children's Hospital
Royal Liverpool Children's NHS Trust
Liverpool, UK

Jane Leaver
Senior Lecturer/Practitioner
School of Nursing and Midwifery
Faculty of Health
Birmingham City University
Birmingham, UK

Peter McNee
Senior Lecturer
Cardiff School of Nursing and Midwifery Studies
Cardiff University
Cardiff, UK

Alison Oliver
Regional Training and Development Nurse
Paediatric Intensive Care
University Hospital of Wales
Cardiff, UK

Karen Selwood
Advanced Nurse Practitioner
Oncology Services
Alder Hey Children's Hospital
Royal Liverpool Children's NHS Trust
Liverpool, UK

Debra Teasdale
Head of Department
Health, Wellbeing and the Family
Canterbury Christ Church University
Canterbury, UK

Clare Thomas
Lead Nurse in Paediatric Burns
Burns Centre
Birmingham Children's Hospital
Birmingham, UK

Michelle Wright
Advanced Nurse Practitioner
Oncology Services
Alder Hey Children's Hospital
Royal Liverpool Children's NHS Trust
Liverpool, UK

ACKNOWLEDGEMENTS

We would like to acknowledge all the infants, children and their families who have taught us more about children's critical care nursing than any book ever could. Our thanks go to the publishing team at Wiley-Blackwell, Magenta Styles and Sarah Claridge, for their tenacity and patience. Finally, a huge thank you to our friends and family for the sacrifice of free time that ought to have been theirs.

Section 1
INTRODUCTION TO PAEDIATRIC INTENSIVE CARE NURSING

Chapter 1
INTRODUCTION TO CHILDREN'S INTENSIVE CARE

Dave Clarke

Cardiff School of Nursing and Midwifery Studies, Cardiff University, Cardiff, UK

Introduction and background

It is widely accepted that paediatric intensive care (PIC) is a service for children and young people with potentially recoverable diseases, who can benefit from more detailed observation and treatment than is generally available in the ward environment (DH 1997). While this describes the nature of the care on the unit, the paediatric intensive care unit (PICU) is much more complex, and many elements contribute to the intensive care environment. Children's nurses and their medical colleagues are experienced and educated to a high standard in very specific and advanced care practices. The physical environment is dominated by advanced technology, which plays an ever-increasing role in monitoring, treating and supporting children and young people who are critically unwell. However, the core of the ethos of care in the PICU are the children, young people and their families, for whom this experience will be one of the most stressful events of their lives.

The criticality of the situation for many of the children and young people admitted to the PICU is immense, however the most recent audit of PIC services in the United Kingdom (UK) demonstrates that the large majority (>95%) survive beyond their admission to the PICU (PICANet 2010). In the period 2006–8 there were 47 125 PIC admissions to 28 NHS hospitals in the UK, with children under 1 year of age comprising 47% of all admissions, and an overall excess of boys (56%) over girls (44%). The majority of admissions (57%) were unplanned and 78% of children who are retrieved are done so by specialist PIC teams (PICANet 2009). It is clear that PIC makes a large contribution to the care of children and young people in the UK, offering specialist skills, care and knowledge, alongside ever-advancing treatment.

The organisation of PICU care

PICUs, like paediatric high dependency units, historically have been organised in an ad hoc manner. They were often located in specialist children's hospitals or supported specialist services, such as cardiology and neurosurgery. During the early 1980s the Paediatric Intensive Care Society and the British Paediatric Association started to raise concerns about the patchy organisation and lack of standards for children and young people requiring intensive care.

In 1993 a multidisciplinary working party published a report, based on a retrospective survey of 12 882 children identified as having received intensive care in 1991, which highlighted issues facing the provision of paediatric intensive care (British Paediatric Association 1993).Their findings indicated that 29% of children were cared for in

Paediatric Intensive Care Nursing, First Edition. Edited by Michaela Dixon and Doreen Crawford.

children's wards, 20% in adult intensive care units and only 51% in PICUs. Of the 2 627 children cared for in adult units, 23% were <1 year and almost 5% were <1 month old. In adult units fewer than 2% of nurses had a children's nursing qualification. Only 36% of PICUs provided a transport service for retrieving critically ill children. The working party expressed particular concern about facilities where medical and nursing staff had not received specific training and where the staffing levels were too low for managing critically ill children, for example in children's wards.

While the findings were shocking when compared to the high standard of care and organisation associated with the modern PICU service, the report was largely ignored until the death of a young person (NG) in 1995. NG died in a PICU as the result of a cerebral haemorrhage. Before reaching the unit he had been moved from the admitting hospital to another hospital for computed tomography (CT) scanning and only then to an intensive care unit (in another region) for management. After the publication of the resulting inquiry (Ashworth 1996), the Secretary of State commissioned a report on the development of paediatric intensive care services and the Department of Health (DH) set up a national coordinating group to develop a policy framework.

The evidence gathered and documentation recognised that the national PIC service was disorganised, having developed over a 20-year period in a makeshift manner. They recognised that the service was a low-volume but high-cost provision and identified that there were no national standards or evidence base. Ten of the 29 PICUs identified had three beds or fewer, placing in question their ability to offer services to the most critically ill children. *Paediatric Intensive Care: A Framework for the Future* (DH 1997) set out a strategy for developing and integrating the service for critically ill children within a geographical area. During the following three years lead centres for PICU care were identified, and within each region one, or at most two, lead centres were designated, to serve a population of at least 500 000 children. Lead centres had to be based in hospitals with a full range of tertiary paediatric services, run a 24-hour transport service for the region and have sufficient throughput to maintain staff expertise and act as educational and training centres. Lead centres were also responsible for the provision of retrieval training to referring hospitals and compiling audit and quality data for their regional service.

While this hub-and-spoke arrangement generally worked well, some areas (e.g. the London region, the Midlands and Scotland) had more than one large PICU within a geo-graphical locality. The introduction in 2001 of Managed Clinical Networks (MCNs – partnerships of healthcare professionals and organisations involved in the commissioning, planning and provision of a health service in a specific geographical area) has furthered the development of paediatric intensive care services, offering more opportunities for joint working and service coordination, especially where duplicated services existed. MCNs were recommended for neonatal intensive care services in 2003 following a service review (DH 2003) and the National Service Framework for Children and Maternity Services (DH and DfES 2004) recommends MCNs for all children and young people's services. Their aim is to provide quality of care by dismantling the barriers between primary, secondary, tertiary and social care. They require multidisciplinary management and ensure that all staff working with a particular patient adhere to the same protocols and policies (DH and DfES 2005). For paediatric intensive care services in particular, MCNs enable the development of core training, treatment pathways and standards. They include referring hospitals, local lead PICUs, Accident and Emergency Departments as members, with the aim of ensuring high quality and safe paediatric intensive care services. The largest MCN for PICU services is the Pan Thames Consortium, which includes nine core hospitals and two retrieval services (see www.picupt.nhs.uk for further information).

Differentiating paediatric intensive care

Paediatric intensive care can be distinguished from other forms of care by the severity of illness the child or young person is experiencing, the standard level of care being that available on a ward, with high dependency care being an intermediate level, followed by intensive care. Within intensive care it is important to recognise the level of dependency a child or young person presents with, as this will have an impact on the nurse staffing levels required to ensure safe and appropriate care. The DH (1997) report identified one level of high dependency care, two main levels of intensive care, while alluding to a fourth level, which includes treatment with Extra Corporeal Membrane Oxygenation (ECMO). The Paediatric Intensive Care Society (2010) has developed the criteria further (Table 1.1).

Commissioning auditing and costing

The DH utilises a non-clinical system to assess levels of care and dependency for audit and costing purposes. Health care Resource Groups (HRGs) have been used to cost care since 2007, based on seven levels:

Table 1.1 Differentiating paediatric intensive care

Level/recommended staffing ratio	Descriptor
Level 1 High dependency care requiring a nurse-to-patient ratio of 0.5:1	Close monitoring and observation required, but not acute mechanical ventilation. Examples include the recently extubated child who is stable and awaiting transfer to a general ward; the child undergoing close postoperative observation with ECG and pulse oximetry, receiving intravenous fluids or parenteral nutrition. Children requiring long-term chronic ventilation with tracheostomy are included in this category.
Level 2 Intensive care requiring a nurse-to-patient ratio of 1:1	The child requires continuous nursing supervision and is usually intubated and ventilated (including CPAP). Also included is the unstable, non-intubated child, for example, some cases with acute upper airway obstruction who may be receiving nebulised adrenaline. The recently extubated child. The dependency of a Level 1 patient increases to Level 2 if the child is nursed in a cubicle.
Level 3 Intensive care requiring a nurse-to-patient ratio of 1.5:1	The child requires intensive supervision at all times and needs additional complex therapeutic procedures and nursing, for example, unstable ventilated children on vasoactive drugs and inotropic support or with multiple organ failure. The dependency of a Level 2 patient increases to Level 3 if the child is nursed in a cubicle.
Level 4 Intensive care requiring a nurse-to-patient ratio of 2:1	Children requiring the most intensive interventions such as particularly unstable patients, Level 3 patients managed in a cubicle, those on ECMO or other extracorporeal support and children undergoing renal replacement therapy.

- HRG1 – High Dependency (HD1)
- HRG2 – High Dependency Advanced (HD2)
- HRG3 – Intensive Care Basic (IC1)
- HRG4 – Intensive Care Basic Enhanced (IC2)
- HRG5 – Intensive Care Advanced (IC3)
- HRG6 – Intensive Care Advanced Enhanced (IC4)
- HRG7 – Intensive Care – ECMO/ECLS (IC5)

While this further division of dependency may be more sensitive, it is widely regarded as too cumbersome and complex for clinical use and takes no account of the individual and holistic care needs for the child's parents or carers and siblings.

Standards for staffing and skill mix

A fundamental issue in the commissioning and management of paediatric intensive care services is the number of nurses required to ensure safe, high quality care, bearing in mind the unpredictable dependency of patients and rate of bed occupancy. Murphy and Morris (2008) performed an audit of 10 PICUs and found that 83% of costs were staff-related, with the largest being nursing. Workforce planning is also affected by the number of beds, the layout of the unit and the number of single rooms. The recent introduction of Agenda for Change has also increased the whole-time equivalent (WTE) from the traditional benchmark of 6.4 WTE per bed to 6.7 WTE on an average unit due to the increased annual leave entitlement for experienced nurses (Paediatric Intensive Care Society 2010).

Commissioners of paediatric intensive care services have had to take into consideration the seasonal fluctuation many units experience and the effect this has on bed capacity. Many commissioners plan nursing staff levels based on an average bed capacity of 80%, however this can be problematic at times of peak capacity when it may be necessary to ask staff who are already working to their full capacity to undertake extra shifts or employ bank and agency staff, which can both impact on quality of care and be costly. Some units have used annualised hours for part-time staff, enabling them to undertake more planned shifts in busy periods and more leave in the summer.

In addition to annual leave, workforce planning needs to take into consideration additional burdens on staffing. Associated with the levels of patient dependency in paediatric intensive care are minimum recommended nurse-to-patient ratios, Level 2 being 1:1; Level 3 1.5:1 and Level 4 2:1. Furthermore, the need for a nurse in charge who has no direct responsibility for a particular patient, the need for a runner, staffing of retrieval teams, calculations for sickness (thought to be 5% of a WTE) and study leave for mandatory training need to be considered. The calculation of 6.7 WTE per bed the Paediatric Intensive Care Society recommend PICUs work towards does not include factors that can increase the WTE considerably, for example maternity leave which is difficult to anticipate and has to be incorporated into workforce planning on a case-by-case basis, as does study leave to undertake specialist paediatric intensive care courses and the level of supervision and induction new staff require and for how long. Table 1.2 summarises the Paediatric Intensive Care Society's calculations.

A worked example – A PICU with 15 beds with nurses working a two-shift/day roster (each nurse working 3–4 days a week). The mean dependency on the unit is a 1.0 nurse per patient per shift ratio and the average occupancy is 80%. The unit uses nurse runners, that is nurses with no allocated patient who check drugs and infusions, help set up equipment, assist with more dependent patients and cover meal-breaks.

The unit requires 4.65 WTE bedside nurses per bed for 80% occupancy. When one includes the runners and the nurse in charge (who should not be providing bedside care or meal-break cover) this rises to 5.38 WTE per bed. Commissioners must decide whether they want to staff to capacity (6.7 WTE/bed) to allow for peak demand (Paediatric Intensive Care Society 2010).

Consideration of the skill mix alongside minimum staffing levels is essential. However, it is difficult to match skill mix on a shift-by-shift basis, when the severity of illness of patients presenting may vary enormously. Current standards for nursing skill mix from the Paediatric Intensive Care Society recommend 'that all PICUs should have a senior and experienced practitioner to coordinate and supervise less experienced nurses to ensure high quality care over the 24-hour period with a Registered Children's Nurse at Band 7 or above and that all units should be managed overall by a Senior Nurse/Matron, Band 8a or above' (Paediatric Intensive Care Society 2010, p. 44).

The most recent report of the UK PICU Staffing Survey (Tucker et al. 2009) indicates that the PICU workforce is highly qualified and highly skilled: 93% of nurses hold a children's nursing registration, a third are senior nurses at Grade F or higher (pre-Agenda for Change) and identified in the skill mix for some units were advanced practitioners and nurse consultants. However, the survey did find that staffing, education and skill mix were increasingly problematic areas for some units, specifically in managing long-term sickness, difficulties in recruitment and retention, cuts in training budgets and increased pressure on beds. Furthermore, the reduction in junior doctors' hours

Table 1.2 Summary of the Paediatric Intensive Care Society's calculations

Row	Category	Formula	Column B
1	Mean dependency		1.0
2	Number of nursing shifts per day		2
3	Number of days worked per nurse per week		3.12
4	Allowance for sickness/annual leave/training	26% Deficit – Factor = 1.26	1.26
5	Number of beds in unit		15
6	Number of beds per runner		8
7	Number of WTE bedside nurses/bed	B1 × B2 × (7/B3) × B4	5.65
8	Total number of nurses (includes 1 in charge per shift and runners)	(B7 × B5) + B7 + ((B5/B6) × B7)	101
9	Total number of bedside nurses	B7 × B5	85
10	WTE of bedside nurses per bed at capacity	B9/B5	5.7
11	Overall number WTE per bed at capacity (includes one in charge per shift and runners)	B8/B5	6.7

resulting from the European Working Time Directive seems to have had an impact, and the survey identified the substitution of junior medical staff with advanced nursing posts in some units.

Developing roles in PICU

The current developments in nursing roles are underpinned by the policy document *Modernising Nursing Careers* (DH 2006) and the subsequent *Towards a Framework for Post-Registration Nursing Careers: Consultation response report* (DH 2008). The 2010 government review of nursing may also influence the development of specialist roles as well as guiding the profession as a whole. Currently, there are three levels of practitioner in paediatric intensive care: Specialist Practitioner, Advanced Practitioner and Nurse Consultant. The recent reviews of nursing career frameworks emphasised the need to move away from traditional careers pathways which removed aspiring practitioners from clinical care, to education and management posts. The roles of Advanced Practitioner and Nurse Consultant are designed to enable nurses to remain in clinical practice while developing skills in areas such as advanced clinical skills, leadership, education and research. The roles of Advanced Nurse Practitioners are currently developed at a local level and there are few common roles or standards. Llewellyn and Day (2008) found that a survey of staff attitudes to advanced practice revealed multiple interpretations of the role. The Nursing and Midwifery Council (NMC) have for some time been discussing the Advanced Practitioner role, but have failed to incorporate it into the current system of professional regulation by recording educational achievement to this standard on the register.

The UK PICU Staffing Survey (Srivastava et al. 2008; Tucker et al. 2009) found that many advanced tasks are undertaken in PICUs: taking blood samples, processing blood samples, altering oxygen levels; adjusting ventilator settings, chest assessment, broncho-alveolar lavage, setting up CPAP (continuous positive airway pressure), initiation of non-invasive ventilation, planned nurse-led extubation, end-of-life extubation, intubation, venepuncture, arterial cannulation, titration of analgesia, weaning of analgesia, titration of inotropes, setting up CFAM (cerebral function analysis monitor); advanced life support skills, nurse-led retrieval and haemodialysis.

Of 27 eligible PICANet units, 26 completed the survey. Of these, only four reported having a designated advanced post of Nurse Consultant or Advanced Nurse Practitioner. Further analysis of these tasks identified that some advanced skills (e.g. blood sampling and processing, setting up CPAP drivers, titration and weaning off analgesia) were routinely

reported as undertaken by specified grades of trained nurses in nearly all units. Clearly, the role of Advanced Nurse Practitioner cannot be defined purely by the tasks undertaken; the role also includes professional autonomy and accountability for one's caseload, diagnostic skills and the authority to initiate investigations/referrals, clinical and professional leadership (McGee 2009). According to the Department of Health (2006), Advanced Practitioners can provide 'high productivity and value for money'. Thus far the role of Advanced Nurse Practitioner in PICU remains relatively new (unlike in neonatal nursing where the role has flourished). Advanced nursing practice is complex, concerned with the development of nursing with greater inter-professional collaboration, not necessarily with the amalgamation of nursing into medical roles (Heward 2009).

Nurse Consultants within paediatric intensive care services are few. Even though the role was introduced in 1999, it was not utilised widely until the last four years. The role is centred on improving the quality of patient care. McGee (2009) identifies the main facets of the role as: working at least half their time in clinical practice; being experts in the field; working directly with patients and acting as focal points for professional advice; undertaking research activities; and being involved in education of staff across the multidisciplinary team. Nurse Consultants currently found within paediatric intensive care services also contribute at a national level, influencing policy decisions within the Department of Health, the Royal College of Nursing and the Paediatric Intensive Care Forum. Nurse Consultants are often affiliated to a local university department (either a nursing or medical school).

The role nurses fulfil within paediatric intensive care services at all levels is vital to the care of children and young people, and their families, in order to provide high quality care. The contribution of children's nurses to the development of paediatric intensive care services is significant and their role is expanding to include counselling, family liaison (e.g. in Birmingham Children's Hospital) and post-PICU inter-hospital transfer (Solomon and Clarke 2009).

Education in PICU

The education of nurses within paediatric intensive care is currently provided by in-house education programmes or BA/BSc, MA/MSc and PhD programmes. The links between Benner's levels of clinical practice (Benner 1984), current role alignment and educational attainment are outlined in Table 1.3.

All PICUs have an induction and training programme for new nursing staff to ensure that all nurses achieve

Table 1.3 From novice to expert

Benner's level	Role	Professional/educational level
Novice	Staff nurse new to PICU	Registered plus Diploma/Degree undertaking preceptorship period
Advanced beginner	Staff Nurse	Registered plus diploma/degree completed in-house education programmes
Competent	Specialist Practitioner	Degree specialist practice
Proficient	Advanced Practitioner	MA
Expert	Nurse Consultant	PhD

Source: modified from Benner 1984.

a basic level of intensive care competence and can offer safe and effective care to the majority of ventilated children and young people on the unit. These courses are usually facilitated by the PICU lead nurse for training and development, and in some units are linked to the local university's Specialist Practitioner PICU course. Standards for in-service programmes have been developed by the PICS-E (2002), although there is little evidence to indicate widespread adoption of these. Education within PICU is essential to ensure regular updating and the achievement of mandatory and statutory training.

A number of issues can influence the ability to deliver effective training and development opportunities within PICU.

- Unpredictable dependency of patients, leading to an inability to release staff for in-service training.
- Formalising training and development activities through the development of reflective journals and competency-based documents are time-consuming.
- Limited training equipment and teaching space.
- Limited funding for external courses and the need to prioritise Specialist Practitioner courses and Paediatric Advanced Life Support Courses.

The role of the training and development lead within PICU is essential and multifaceted. It includes:

- Developing and facilitating in-service induction, orientation and competency-based programmes to ensure the competence of all nurses in intensive nursing care.
- Monitoring and facilitating opportunities for mandatory and statutory training on the unit.
- Leading the educational component of new clinical developments and inter-professional learning opportunities.
- Developing and documenting the unit's training needs analysis in conjunction with the unit's matron.
- Liaising with university education providers in relation to mentorship of pre-registration nursing students, mentorship of students on Specialist Practice programmes and procedures for nurses wishing to access higher education courses.
- Supporting the education component of capability programmes associated with fitness-to-practice issues in conjunction with the unit's matron.

Higher education and professional body partnerships

Specialist Practitioner programmes for paediatric intensive care nurses are undertaken in universities and are usually delivered at degree level. The NMC monitors these courses as they can currently lead to a recordable qualification on the register. However, the Paediatric Intensive Care Society Education Group has identified some concerns and has called for validation of a national paediatric intensive care course. Their concerns are:

- The number of 'taught' hours in these programmes is being reduced by higher education institutions. This is justified by the HE institutions as the programmes are expensive to run for a small number of students.
- The pressure of time on the clinical staff makes it increasingly difficult to allow them time off to attend programmes and learn.

The lack of basic knowledge in clinical sciences, and anatomy and physiology on the part of holders of nursing diplomas or degrees makes revision of these topics essential to equip them to function effectively in an intensive care environment. This reduces the amount of time that can be spent delivering PIC content even further. The regulations of HE place restrictions on the educators when working within academic institutions, for example, the assessment times may be set or there may be limits on the course leader's ability or authority to change and modify the programme's assessment processes. There are general difficulties in marrying the academic and service demands of these programmes – for example, should clinical assessment be graded or not? If yes, there are issues of parity across the assessment opportunity afforded to students and of parity among assessors.

There are recommendations for a national course at degree level of 6–9 months with three main aims:

- At the end of the course the student should be a competent PICU nurse and be able to manage without support a Level 2 intensive care patient and Level 3 or 4 ICU patients with senior supervision and support.
- Graduates will be able to deliver evidence-based care to the child and family and be able to communicate effectively with the patient, family and health care team.
- Graduates will understand the organisational and political context of paediatric critical care.
  (Paediatric Intensive Care Society Education Group 2010).

While the aim of these recommendations is useful in guiding the development of paediatric intensive care courses, the NMC is reluctant to include specific content in addition to the existing generic Specialist Practitioner outcomes, which will limit the implementation of any national guidance.

New ways of learning in PICU

In recent years the technological ability to simulate the sick baby and child has developed tremendously, and the traditional 'resuscianne' used for teaching basic life support has been superseded by a number of high-fidelity patient manikins. These include one neonatal simulator (SimNewB©, Laerdal Medical), two infant simulators (SimBaby©, Laerdal Medical; and BabySim©, METI: Medical Education Technologies) and one child simulator (PediaSim©, METI: Medical Education Technologies). These simulators are capable of simulating advanced airway procedures, lung, heart and bowel sounds, vital signs and advanced monitoring, palpable pulses and pneumothorax procedures and are constantly developing. They are used in complex, scenario-based education which includes, but is not exclusive to, resuscitation. A number of PICUs have purchased these simulators, the average cost of which is £25 000, and they are utilised in pre-retrieval training at referring hospitals (Cardiff and Nottingham are examples), and in multi-environment simulations such as Accident and Emergency/Children's Ward to PICU (for example Bristol Children's Hospital and St. Mary's in London.)

Simulations using high-fidelity simulators are ideal for developing the clinical decision-making and team working skills of the multi-professional team, who include those working as paramedics, in children's wards, Emergency Departments and PICU staff. Gabba (2004) suggests that simulation enhances patient safety by focusing on the education of teams rather than of individuals, offering a structured approach and the ability regularly and systematically to mirror reality. While there is some evidence of simulation being integrated into university programmes (Clarke and Davies 2009), much of the discussion continues to take place in the United States. In the United Kingdom it is recognised that while simulation is beneficial, planning, enacting and debriefing can be labour-intensive (Summers and Kingsland 2009); however, the benefits in relation to patient safety in high-risk areas, such as intensive care, outweigh the effort required.

Conclusion

Paediatric intensive care is a highly complex environment and is dependent on adequate and planned staffing, clear patient assessment and educational programmes based on competency and the attainment of clinical skills. Within the last 10 years there have been significant advances in the development of paediatric intensive care standards and services, supported by an increasing number of roles which are breaking down traditional boundaries. This chapter has outlined the fundamental elements of ensuring that paediatric intensive care services and nurses are fit for purpose and ready to deliver high standards of care.

References

Ashworth W. 1996. Inquiry into the Care and Treatment of Nicholas Geldard. Manchester: North West Regional Health Authority.

Benner P. 1984. From Novice to Expert: Excellence and power in clinical nursing practice. Menlo Park, CA: Addison-Wesley.

British Paediatric Association. 1993. The Care of Critically Ill Children: Report of a multidisciplinary working party on intensive care. London: BPA.

Clarke D, Davies J. 2009. Learning to practise: 20 years of change in children's nursing education. Paediatric Nursing, 21(2):15–17.

Department of Health. 1997. Paediatric Intensive Care: A Framework for the Future. July. London: DH.

Department of Health. 2003. Intensive Care Services – Report of the Department of Health Expert Working Group. London: DH.

Department of Health. 2006. Modernising Nursing Careers – Setting the direction. London: DH.

Department of Health. 2008. Towards a Framework for Post-registration Nursing Careers: Consultation response report. www.dh.gov.uk/cno.

Department of Health and Department for Education and Skills. 2004. National Service Framework for Children, Young People and Maternity Services. London: DH and DfES.

Department of Health and Department for Education and Skills. 2005. Guide to Promote a Shared Understanding of the Benefits of Managed Local Networks. London: DH and DfES.

Gabba DM. 2004. The future of simulation in health care. Quality and Safety in Health Care, 13:i2–i10.

Heward Y. 2009. Advanced practice in paediatric intensive care: a review. Paediatric Nursing, 21(1):18–21.

Llewellyn LE, Day HL. 2008. Advanced nursing practice in paediatric critical care. Paediatric Nursing, 20(1):30–3.

McGee P. (Ed). 2009. Advanced Practice in Nursing and the Allied Professions, 3rd edition. Chichester: Wiley-Blackwell.

Murphy J, Morris K. 2008. Accounting for care: health care resource groups for paediatric critical care. Paediatric Nursing, 20(1):37–9.

Paediatric Intensive Care Audit Network (PICANet). 2009. Annual report. www.picanet.org.uk.

Paediatric Intensive Care Audit Network (PICANet). 2010. Annual report. www.picanet.org.uk.

Paediatric Intensive Care Society. 2010. Standards for the Care of Critically Ill Children (4th edition, version 2). London: PICS.

Paediatric Intensive Care Society Educators Group (PICS-E). 2002. National Standards for Orientation / Development Programmes for Nurses in PICU. London: Paediatric Intensive Care Society.

Paediatric Intensive Care Society Educators Group (PICS-E). 2010. Recommendations for a Nationally Consistent Paediatric Intensive Care Education Programme for Nurses – Appendix 14: Standards for the Care of Critically Ill Children (4th edition, Version 2). London: Paediatric Intensive Care Society.

Solomon J, Clarke D. 2009. Safe transport from a specialist paediatric intensive care unit to a referral hospital. Paediatric Nursing, 21(1):30–4.

Srivastava NJ, Draper E, Milner M, on behalf of the UK PICU Staffing Study. 2008. A literature review of principles, policies and practice in extended nursing roles relating to UK intensive care settings. Journal of Clinical Nursing, 17: 2671–80.

Summers K, Kingsland S. 2009. Simulation: issues and challenges. Paediatric Nursing, 21(3):33.

Tucker JS, Parry G et al. 2009. The Impact of Changing Workforce Patterns in UK Paediatric Intensive Care Services on Staff Practice and Patient Outcomes. Report for the National Institute for Health Research Service Delivery and Organisation programme. London: HMSO.

Chapter 2
ASSESSMENT AND MANAGEMENT OF THE CRITICALLY ILL CHILD/ RESUSCITATION

Mark Fores[1] and Doreen Crawford[2]

[1] Clinical Skills Unit, Leicester Royal Hospital, University Hospitals of Leicester NHS Trust, Leicester, UK
[2] School of Nursing and Midwifery, Faculty of Health and Life Sciences, De Montfort University, Leicester, UK

Introduction

This chapter is presented in three sections. The first focuses on the assessment and essential care of the child who has a complex and multi-system dysfunction (the more specialist assessment required, for example, following skeletal trauma will be considered in the relevant chapters). The second section reviews the resuscitation procedure and ongoing recovery, maintenance and essential care. The third and final section concentrates on some of the associated challenges which require attention when caring for these children, such as not for resuscitation orders, withholding or withdrawing further intervention considerations and the care of the parents.

The priority

Rapid, thorough multidisciplinary team assessment of a new admission is vital as children have fewer functional reserves and can decompensate quickly. The immediate priorities are to assess the airway, breathing and circulation and to obtain access to the circulatory system; these need to be done within minutes. Once the child has a secure airway, a means of effective ventilation and has had their circulation stabilised, the next level of priority can be addressed with the aim of sustaining this stability (Table 2.1). A top-to-toe examination and a plan for the management of fluids, therapeutic agents and so on should be done during the first hour. After this, a more extensive review can be undertaken to ascertain the child's health history, usual health status, their family structure and any relevant developmental/psychosocial issues which will impact on the child's future.

Second-level priorities

These can be linked to major body systems and include (in no order of priority as the homeostasis of systems are so interlinked):

- Fluids and drugs – renal.
- Nutrition – gastrointestinal.
- Potential impact on development and disability – neurological.
- Essential nursing care – potential to affect all body systems.

Fluids and drugs

Management of fluids and electrolytes is important because most children in critical care units will require intravenous fluids (IVFs) and may have shifts of fluids between

Table 2.1 The A, B, C and D

Assessment	Ask these questions	Observations and action
Assessment of the airway	Is the airway clear? Can patency be maintained? What strategies are required to protect the airway?	Obstructions? Presence of foreign body, risk of loose teeth, blood, etc. Secretions – suction with care to remove. Ability to respond; cough, gag and swallow reflexes. The reaction to suction can give good indication of these factors. Check position of endotracheal tube if intubated. If not and required, arrange for intubation, support process and secure endotracheal tube.
Breathing	How efficient is breathing/ventilation? Is the effort the child can make sustainable?	Respiratory rate, rhythm, character, e.g. level of chest expansion, symmetrical movement, bilateral air entry, presence of intercostal recession, sternal tug, use of accessory muscles. Listen to lungs for any unusual sounds (wheeze, crepitations, rales, rhonchi, stridor. etc.). Check ventilator settings to ensure they are optimal.
Circulation	How efficient is the child's cardiac and circulatory system?	Gain access to the circulation and secure this. Assess perfusion – temperature of extremities, capillary refill time, presence of pulses and character of these, such as volume, rate. Attach saturations probe, note wave form. Colour of child. Listen to apex rate, rhythm and any unusual characteristics such as murmurs. Linked to the stability of a child's circulation is the assessment and management of pain and the need for sedation (see Chapter 13).
Document the baseline assessment	Is this documentation factually accurate, clear and concise? Is it a contemporaneous record?	Important points to document include signs of neglect, the presence of any unexplained physical features or any unusual behaviour from the parents/carers. Take care when expressing opinion.
Dignity	Is the child's name known? Is their dignity being respected?	The child might be critically ill and may have to be exposed for thorough examination, however they should never be exposed and left uncovered unnecessarily and every effort should be taken to ensure that the child is referred to by name and is not exposed to inappropriate comments with regards to their condition which might cause them distress and anxiety. This is very important as the sense of hearing can become very acute when other senses, such as sight, are diminished. The child may be sedated and their eyes closed, but this does not mean they cannot hear and possibly misunderstand what is going on.

intracellular, extracellular and vascular compartments. For the calculation and management of a child's fluids and therapy an approximate weight is required. The laminated and colour-coded Broselow tape is one means of determining the weight of the child.

Place the tape alongside the child who is lying in a supine position and extend the legs so the knees are not bent. Adjust the foot so the toes are pointing straight up. To measure ensure the red arrow is positioned and aligned with the top of the child's head – red to head. Look at the subdivision of the coloured areas directly under the sole of the foot. Decide which of the subdivisions the child belongs in for weight classification. The Broselow tape works best for infants and when the child is within normal/average

Table 2.2 At-a-glance fluid calculator

Weight of child (kg)	Fluid maintenance required ml/24 hour
<2 kg 2–10 kg 10–20 kg 20 kg to maximum	Best calculated on individual basis depending on renal function and weight increases 100 ml/kg 1000 ml + 50 ml for each 1 kg above 10 kg 1500 ml + 20 ml for each 1 kg above 20 kg Maximum daily amount: girls 2000 ml Maximum daily amount: boys 2500 ml

Adjustments and increases	Examples of need to increase:
	Hypovolaemia – may require a bolus of 10–20 ml/kg of 0.9% sodium chloride which may be repeated. This is in excess of their daily calculations.
	Severely dehydrated state where there are multiple physical signs present, cold pale peripheries with prolonged capillary return time, decreased skin tone, loss of ocular tension, when the infant has a fontanel this may be sunken +/− acidosis and hypotension.
	Anticipated massive fluid loss such as burns.
	Pyrexia.
	If unable to concentrate urine or where there has been excessive secretion of antidiuretic hormone (ADH), e.g. pneumonia, head injury, meningitis.
	When having phototherapy or under a radiant heater.
	Examples of need to decrease:
	    Waterlogged and oedematous children.
	    When they are mechanically ventilated and are having heavily humidified gas.
	    Renal impairment.
	    Major head injury.

size for their age. If the child is obese, there is a potential risk of under-resuscitation (Nieman et al. 2006).

Alternatively, if the child's age is known, one of the following formulae can be used to calculate a working weight in kg (Advanced Life Support Group 2011):

- 0–12 months – (0.5 × age in months) + 4
- 1–5 years – (2 × age in years) + 8
- 6–12 years – (3 × age in years) + 7

This can be used to calculate their maintenance fluids as shown in Table 2.2.

Children admitted to critical care need to have their urea, electrolytes and serum glucose checked on admission and 3–4 hours after commencing IVs, with subsequent tests according to the results and their clinical situation until they are stable. Once stable the U&Es need to be checked at least daily.

Acceptable fluids

In the newborn and during infancy 10% dextrose may be used with sodium and potassium additives as prescribed, titrated to individual requirement.

Other suitable maintenance fluids include 0.9% sodium chloride (NaCl), 0.9% NaCl with 5% dextrose and 0.45% NaCl with 5% dextrose. Additional electrolytes are added as prescribed. Nurses need to be cautious as to the concentration of these, as strong solutions increase the risk of extravasation injury. Some electrolytes (e.g. calcium) need to be given centrally.

It is advisable that the administration of the maintenance fluids is not interrupted so a second cannula should be inserted for the administration of drugs. The fluid volume of medications and the administration of flushes between IV medications need to be recorded on the fluid balance chart.

Calorie requirement and nutrition

Children admitted to a critical care area are usually in a hypercatabolic state and will not recover unless their need for calories is addressed. A referral to the dietician should be made. Where it is not possible to commence an enteral feed owing to the condition of the child, consideration should be given to total parenteral nutrition (TPN) (see Chapter 12).

Potential impact on development and disability

The reasons for admission can have a profound impact of the future development of the child and even a positive outcome may include some level of disability. There are no guarantees for recovery in children who have been this sick and, even when recovering, a view towards cautious optimism is recommended until the outcome is certain. The neurological examination is one of the most difficult to perform in children who are sick, in pain and uncooperative, or are unconscious or sedated. The initial examination can only ever be a crude indicator until more sophisticated investigations can inform or confirm any concerns. The Alert, Voice, Pain, Unresponsive (AVPU) scale is simple as it has only four possible outcomes for recording, unlike the assessment outcomes of the Pinderfield, Adelaide or modified Glasgow Coma Scale. The various coma scales continue to be adapted for use with immature children and to meet the challenges of assessing children who are heavily sedated (Tatman et al. 1997). Any scale is only as good as its users and there is evidence to support the assertion that the more complex the tool the less reliable it can be, thereby increasing the risk of inaccurate results (Barrett-Goode 2000). It is important that nurses are familiar with their use and regularly check their scores with colleagues to ensure inter-rater reliability.

Despite the difficulties of assessment and the high risk of morbidity and mortality it is important to attempt a thorough assessment as prompt, specialist neuro-critical care is associated with improved outcome (Moppett 2007) as there is less risk of secondary brain injury.

Indicators of brain injury

Thermal instability with hypothermia, a complication of a brain injury which disturbs hypothalamic activity and hyperpyrexia, may result from dysautonomias (a broad term which describes a dysfunction of the autonomic nervous system).

Circulatory dysautonomia may result in tachycardia, syncope and hypotension caused by autonomic instability. (For assessment of a catastrophic neurological event and assessment of brain stem functioning see Chapter 7.)

An eye examination for reflexes and anomalies is a pivotal indicator of neurological function (see Table 2.3).

Once the child is stable with a secure airway, adequately ventilated, pink, warm and well perfused with fluid management planned it is time to take a small step back and

Table 2.3 Eye examination

Structure	Assessment
Ocular appearance and response	Open the eyes with care if there is no spontaneous eye opening or in response to request in cognisant children, and note the position of the pupils at rest. Document any spontaneous eye movements, any apparent nystagmus and any dysconjugate or conjugate eye position. When catastrophic brain injury is suspected the medical team may carry out an assessment of the oculocephalic reflex 'doll's eye' where a rapid rotation of the child's head right and left should result in movement of the pupils where the neural pathway is intact. In an abnormal response the pupils stay fixed in the position they were in when the manoeuvre was commenced and do not deviate.
Corneal reflex	The level of inhibited corneal reflex is proportional to the level of coma.
Pupil size and reaction	Pupil reaction and size are variable signs and can be indicative of a problem, but may not be a conclusive finding. The pupils in health and under normal circumstances should react and constrict when exposed to light. Asymmetrical pupils need further investigation. A fixed dilated pupil needs urgent attention. Pinpoint pupils may be a feature of opiate sedation and analgesia.
Fundus	This can be distressing for the child so is best left until last; the child can then rest and recover from the examination. Infants and small children may need mydriatrics to facilitate a good view. Papilloedema is an accurate indicator of raised intracranial pressure. It usually takes time to build up so in cases where there could be raised intracranial pressure this investigation ought to be checked again as the child's condition dictates. Papillitis may be a feature of encephalitis. The presence of retinal haemorrhages might also indicate bleeding elsewhere.

review in order to plan ongoing management, formulate a plan of care and take a more thorough history. This will help to inform essential nursing care.

Essential nursing care

Skin assessment

The sicker the child the more their skin integrity is at risk for a number of reasons: poorly perfused tissues leading to hypoxia, poor availability of nutrients and prolonged periods of immobility. Urinary and faecal incontinence can damage the skin; the use of pads can create a moist, warm micro-environment that can macerate the perianal and sacral areas (for more consideration of skin at risk, see Chapter 14). Intubation and airway/respiratory management and indwelling lines can restrict the positions of rest for nursing these children. It is important to assess and document the state of the child's skin using a validated and reliable assessment tool (Willcock et al. 2008). Using the tool to inform an individualised plan of care in which the parents can participate can reduce the risk of developing sores, which is vitally important as the impact of skin breakdown has a considerable cost both economically and in the child's suffering. The true incidence of this complication in this population is unknown (Schindler et al. 2007). However, the condition is preventable with scrupulous attention to the areas at risk and by anticipating iatrogenic risks such as name-bands being applied too tightly or a poorly fixed endotracheal tube.

Bowel and bladder care in the PICU

Children are at risk of constipation in the PICU as a result of reduced mobility, reduced enteral intake, dehydration through fever or their pathology, and opiate analgesics. Even for children who have attained conscious control over their bowel movement, the altered level of consciousness because of illness or sedation, not to mention their circumstances, may make it impossible to communicate their need to evacuate their bowels. Owing to the function of the bowel wall in absorbing water, any retained faeces will get harder and be more difficult to pass. This may manifest itself by the child seeming to be less settled or more irritable. The ability to override the defecation reflex can only be maintained for a short period and the child will eventually defecate. The nurse needs to ensure the continence pad is the appropriate size, not creased and the child's skin is cared for following reflex evacuation and their dignity maintained.

Initially, the level of bowel care is conservative and the child will be allowed 24–48 hours before intervention. The Bristol stool chart (Lewis and Heaton 1997) can be used to support the nurse in making an assessment of the need for intervention as it demonstrates a range of stool characteristics. The characteristic of the child's stools will dictate the further need for intervention in the form of stool softening agents, small enema or suppository.

Diarrhoea can be problematic in the PICU from both a practical management perspective and its challenge to accurate fluid measurement. For the infant and young child nappies and pads can be used. These need to be changed frequently and weighed as part of a fluid management strategy. For the adolescent or young person a range of temporary containment devices can be used. These are ideal for bed-bound and incontinent patients who have liquid or semi-liquid stools. They are designed to safely and effectively contain and divert faeces and help prevent complications such as wound contamination and skin breakdown (Ousey et al. 2010).

Because of the need to monitor fluid balance the majority of children in PICU will have an indwelling urinary catheter. Short-term use of an indwelling urethral catheter is a safe and effective means to ensure bladder health and assess renal function; however catheterisation of the bladder is thought to be the most common risk factor for acquired urinary tract infection (Bray and Sanders 2006). Meatal cleansing is an integral part of good catheter care. Evidence indicates that normal genital hygiene is sufficient to achieve good meatal hygiene and that a strict regimen using antiseptics can be detrimental as it can compromise the normal skin flora (Leaver 2007).

To minimise the risk of ascending infection the breaking of the closed system should be kept to a minimum, the nurse should wear gloves and, before emptying the collecting bag, the tap should be cleaned with 70% isopropyl alcohol.

Oral hygiene

This is an essential nursing procedure and should be considered an integral part in maintaining the general hygiene of the patient; it is performed to maintain oral health (Whiteing and Hunter 2008). Oral health is more than just cleaning teeth or preventing dental caries; it involves consideration of the lips, teeth, gums, tongue, palate and surrounding soft tissues. There needs to be a comprehensive assessment of the mouth and a plan of care formulated (Huskinson and Lloyd 2009). When teeth and gums are not brushed regularly, dental plaque, a biofilm of organisms comprising approximately 70% microorganisms and 30%

inter-bacterial substances, accumulates (Huskinson and Lloyd 2009). Plaque left undisturbed produces acid which can lead to demineralisation of the tooth surface. Plaque can harden and result in the formation of calculus which is difficult to remove. In essence poor oral hygiene provides a source of bacterial infection (Huskinson and Lloyd 2009) and can be associated with ventilator-associated infection (Koeman et al. 2006), although the decision to use of chlorhexidine mouthwash in young children needs to be assessed on an individual basis. Use of an assessment tool can identify the children most at risk and children's intensive care nurses can be creative when aiming to encourage salivation to keep the mouth moist; for example, when dealing with a nasally intubated child or a child on nasal CPAP a pacifier can be offered (McDougall 2011) which also helps keep a good seal. Some children are more at risk from poor or incomplete oral hygiene than others (for additional consideration of oncology children, see Chapter 11).

Eye care

Infants and children who are heavily sedated can lose their blink reflex which can put the eye at considerable risk when turning and handling. When this is combined with impairment of the normally closing eyelid it can lead to the drying of the surface membrane and corneal tissue (Douglas and Berry 2011).

There is considerable variation in the way eye care is performed and what can be used to maintain eye health. The use of a lubricant with a hydrogel dressing to promote eyelid closure is highly endorsed in much of the literature (Sorce et al. 2009). Douglas and Berry (2011) have developed an eye assessment tool and a care pathway recommending levels of intervention depending on the condition of the child's eyes and the level of assessed risk.

Passive limb physiotherapy

The sedated infant or child is at risk of limb stiffness, muscle wastage, foot drop and (occasionally) contractures. The longer the period of sedation the more the child is at risk. There is considerable variation in practice with regard to positioning and passive limb movement (Wiles and Stiller 2009) and there are cost implications in using a highly skilled physiotherapist to perform these activities (Stiller 2000). Safety issues will need to be considered when mobilising and moving the critically ill child (Stiller 2007), however these risks need to be set against the risk of providing care which is detrimental to the child's future functioning.

Children's nurses, with the help and support of the parents, are ideally placed to maintain or improve the child's range of motion, soft tissue length, muscle strength and function by careful positioning, the use of splints and supports as appropriate, and when moving the child or performing other planned interventions by putting the child's limbs through repeated sequences of natural movements. In addition, enhancing the circulatory return will decrease the risk of thromboembolism.

Resuscitation in the PICU

The outcome from cardiopulmonary arrests in children remains poor and identification of the preceding stages of respiratory failure or cardiac compromise is a priority as early intervention may be life-saving (UKRC 2010). In children, cardiopulmonary arrest is usually secondary and caused by respiratory or circulatory failure. Secondary arrest is much more frequent (and preventable) than primary arrest caused by arrhythmias. The platform of resuscitation for children who are in the PICU remains the basic life support (Figure 2.1): ABC with airway management and manoeuvres, the delivery of rescue breaths and compressions performed to the ratio of 15:2 as recommended by the UKRC (2010).

Uninterrupted, good quality CPR is vital (Figure 2.2). Chest compressions and ventilation should only be interrupted for defibrillation. Chest compressions are tiring for those delivering them; therefore to sustain the quality of the compressions the coordinator should continuously assess and give feedback. Those who are delivering the compressions need to change every 2 minutes.

Children should continue to be ventilated with high-concentration oxygen at a rate of 10–12 breaths/min. The ratio of breaths to compressions should be 2:15 and the aim should be to sustain a compression rate of 100–20/min. As the child is intubated the chest compressions can be continuous providing they do not interfere with satisfactory ventilation.

Drugs used in resuscitation

Adrenaline

Adrenaline is a catecholamine with a powerful vasoconstriction action. It increases coronary perfusion, enhances the contractile state of the heart, stimulates spontaneous contractions and increases the intensity of ventricular fibrillation so enhancing the possibility of successful defibrillation (UKRC 2010).

The recommended IV/IO dose of adrenaline in children is 10 mcg/kg. Subsequent doses can be given every 3–5 minutes, but higher doses of intravascular adrenaline

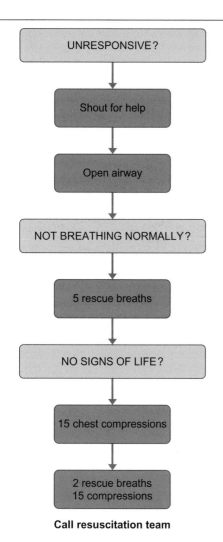

Call resuscitation team

Figure 2.1 Paediatric basic life support (healthcare professionals with a duty to respond). Reproduced with the kind permission of the Resuscitation Council (UK).

should not be used routinely in children because this may worsen the outcome (UKRC 2010).

Amiodarone

Amiodarone is a membrane-stabilising anti-arrhythmic drug that increases the duration of the action potential and refractory period in atrial and ventricular myocardium. It also slows atrioventricular conduction. It has a mildly negative inotropic action which causes peripheral vasodilation and can cause hypotension. In shockable rhythms, an initial IV bolus dose (5 mg/kg) can be given after the

third shock; if the child is still in VF/VT, the dose can be repeated after the fifth shock. If the defibrillation was successful but VF/VT recurs, amiodarone can be repeated (unless two doses have already been injected) and an infusion of amiodarone can be commenced preferably using a central line (UKRC 2010).

Atropine

Atropine is effective in increasing the heart rate when the bradycardia has been caused by excessive vagal stimulation. The dose is 20 mcg/kg and a minimum dose of 100 mcg should be given to avoid the risk of a paradoxical effect. There is no evidence that atropine has any benefit in asphyxia bradycardia or asystole and its routine use has been removed from the ALS algorithms (UKRC 2010).

Sodium bicarbonate

Cardiac arrest can result in combined respiratory and metabolic acidosis, caused by the loss of gas exchange and the development of anaerobic cellular metabolism. The best treatment for acidaemia in cardiac arrest is prevention by effective chest compression and ventilation. The administration of sodium bicarbonate generates carbon dioxide, which diffuses rapidly into the cells, exacerbating intracellular acidosis if it is not rapidly cleared through the lungs. In addition, it produces a negative inotropic effect on an ischaemic myocardium, causes a large, osmotically active sodium load to an already compromised circulation and brain, and produces a shift to the left in the oxygen dissociation curve, which decreases the level of oxygen available to the tissues. The routine use of sodium bicarbonate in cardiac arrest is not recommended (UKRC 2010).

Dextrose

Hypoglycaemia is associated with poor outcome. After cardiopulmonary arrest blood glucose concentrations should be monitored closely, and also during and after cardiac arrest, and dextrose administered only for treatment of hypoglycaemia and not routinely.

Electrolytes (magnesium and calcium)

Magnesium is a major intracellular cation and serves as a cofactor in many enzymatic reactions. Magnesium treatment is indicated for children with hypomagnesaemia (UKRC 2010).

Calcium plays a vital role in the cellular mechanisms underlying myocardial contraction, but high plasma concentrations achieved after injection may be harmful to the ischaemic myocardium and may also impair cerebral recovery. The routine administration of calcium during

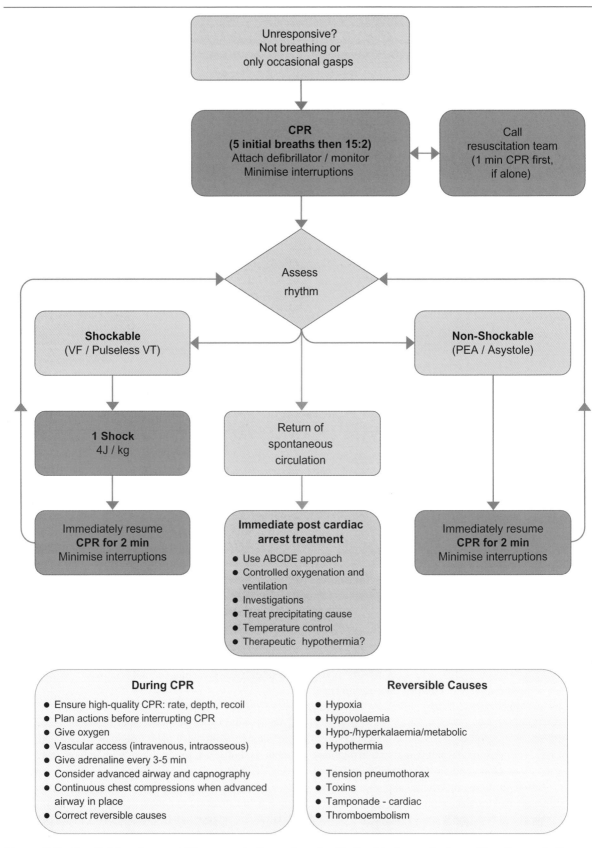

Figure 2.2 Paediatric advanced life support. Reproduced with the kind permission of the Resuscitation Council (UK).

cardiac arrest has been associated with increased mortality and it should be given only when specifically indicated, for example in hyperkalaemia, hypocalcaemia, and overdose of calcium-channel-blocking drugs (UKRC 2010).

Parents present during resuscitation

The presence of parents during resuscitation of their child is controversial (Moore 2009) and certainly one set of guidelines could never be produced to inform all possible scenarios, however many parents ask to be present during a resuscitation attempt so that they can be reassured that everything possible was done for their child and that the child was treated with kindness and given every possible consideration to their dignity.

Parents' reports suggest that being present was comforting and helped them to gain a realistic view of the attempted resuscitation and the child's death. Families who have been present in the resuscitation room grieve more successfully and experience less anxiety and depression. Managing this aspect of the resuscitation is as important as any other, and a dedicated and experienced member of staff should be present in order to explain what is happening and provide emotional support (Perry 2009).

If the parents interfere with the resuscitation process or distract the resuscitation team, they need to be sensitively guided or be asked to leave. Evolving good practice would include the parents being part of the decision-making process on when to stop, although the final decision should rest with the resuscitation team leader.

Advance directives, personal resuscitation plans, end-of-life instructions

The Association for Children's Palliative Care (ACT) endorsed the Wishes Document as a template for end-of-life discussions and instructions for actions when caring for children with life-limiting conditions (Fraser et al. 2010). The Wishes Document is a comprehensive set of considerations which could greatly enhance end-of-life care and sets out:

- Plans for management during life.
- Plans for when the child becomes more unwell.
- Plans for care during an acute life-threatening event.
- Wishes for after death.

However, personal resuscitation plans or any other of these documents are not legal contracts; they inform not dictate a nursing and medical care plan to be instigated in the event of deterioration or in an emergency. They should be agreed by the multidisciplinary team and the parents; they ought to be signed by the lead consultant and by the parents (or the child's legal guardian). They are not fixed, but can be reviewed or overturned. They are important as one study (Tuffrey et al. 2007) indicated that 54% of children die on a hospital ward or intensive care unit, many of whom had pre-existing conditions and death in a PICU could have been an inappropriate ending. Only 20% of children who had life-limiting conditions and were in a PICU had a documented end-of-life plan (Fraser et al. 2010).

There are more and more children with severe and complex conditions who are often dependent on technological support, such as gastrostomy, tracheostomy, oxygen and respiratory support suction facilities. Many enjoy good quality lives with the support of children's community nurses, special school staff and the devoted love and attention of their parents and carers. However, some children, particularly those with neurodegenerative conditions, are progressively deteriorating towards inevitable death and others (e.g. those who have a severe spinal cord injury) are at risk of life-threatening events. Although predicting the progress and time frame of a child's condition is problematic and these are difficult issues to raise, they should be seen positively as they can be used to prevent prolonging possible distress and suffering.

To instigate an end-of-life care plan the child's lead paediatrician could consider initiating sensitive discussions with the child (when possible) and their parents about the appropriate level of intervention during a life-threatening event regarding the withholding or withdrawing of life-prolonging management (Wolff et al. 2011). Not every child at risk of dying in the PICU is going to have a set of instructions to help inform care and there are always going to be difficult cases where parents and staff are faced with very hard decisions and make not for resuscitation orders or withdrawal/withholding of treatment plans.

Not for resuscitation

There are no national guidelines. Generally, not for resuscitation forms are placed in the child's notes which are often unavailable in an emergency, especially if it occurs outside the hospital. In any case, some do not attempt resuscitation (DNAR) forms are not very helpful for children and their families as many are adapted from the adult form, are complex and contain legal and medical phrases (Wolff et al. 2011). The words used are also very negative and this may influence the staff. 'Allow natural death' has been suggested as an improvement in wording (Jones et al. 2008).

Not for resuscitation can be regarded as an all-or-nothing system and families might find the concept easier if there were some supportive management and interventions such as some airway manoeuvres and a trial of bag and mask ventilation (Wolff et al. 2011). At the very least parents need the reassurance that staff will respond in the best interests of the child and provide dignity and comfort during a terminal event.

Withdrawing and withholding intervention

Children's nurses are committed to promoting the health of children, relieving their suffering, enhancing their development, helping them to achieve a sense of worth and confidence in their future. Supporting parents and medical colleagues while the decision is made to withdraw or withhold life-sustaining treatment is one of the most difficult aspects of children's nursing practice. Current guidelines support the withholding or withdrawing of life-sustaining treatment from children in brain death, permanent vegetative state, and no chance, no purpose or unbearable situations (RCPCH 2004). Societal and professional attitudes to euthanasia and assisted suicide are changing and this could lead to changes in legislation and guidelines. However, nurses must be clear about the differences as currently any measure, practice or treatment administered with the primary intention to cause death is illegal. However, this is not the same as any measure, practice or treatment administered with the intent to relieve suffering and promote comfort, which may incidentally cause or hasten death (Crawford and Way 2009).

Conclusion

This chapter has briefly considered the admission of a child to PICU and reviewed some of the holistic aspects of care, although each of these elements on its own could be the basis of a chapter. This chapter has presented current resuscitation guidelines and overviewed some of the difficult medico-legal challenges which can present at the end of life. In this book there are chapters designed to provide a holistic perspective to caring for these challenging children (see Chapters 16–18).

References

Advanced Life Support Group. 2011. Advanced Paediatric Life Support: The Practical Approach (5th edition). Chichester: Wiley-Blackwell / BMJ Books.

Barrett-Goode P. 2000. Reliability of the Adelaide Coma Scale. Paediatric Nursing, 12(8):32–8.

Bray L, Sanders C. 2006. Nursing management of paediatric urethral catheterisation. Nursing Standard, 20(24):51–60.

Crawford D, Way C. 2009. Just because we can, should we? A discussion of treatment withdrawal. Paediatric Nurse, 21(1):22–5.

Douglas L, Berry S. 2011. Developing clinical guidelines in eye care for intensive care units. Nursing Children and Young People, 23(5):14–20.

Fraser J, Harris N et al. 2010. Advanced care planning in children with life-limiting conditions – the Wishes Document. Archives of Disease in Childhood, 95(2):79–82.

Huskinson W, Lloyd H. 2009. Oral health in hospitalised patients: assessment and hygiene. Nursing Standard, 23(36):43–7.

Jones B, Parker-Raley J et al. 2008. Finding the right words: using the terms allow natural death (AND) and do not resuscitate (DNR) in pediatric palliative care. Journal for Healthcare Quality, 30(5):55–63.

Koeman M, Van der Ven A et al. 2006. Oral decontamination with chlorhexidine reduces the incidence of ventilator-associated pneumonia. American Journal of Respiratory and Critical Care Medicine, 10(2):242–5.

Leaver R. 2007. The evidence for urethral meatal cleansing. Nursing Standard, 21(41):39–42.

Lewis S, Heaton K. 1997. Stool form scale as a useful guide to intestinal transit time. Scandinavian Journal of Gastroenterology, 32(9):920–4.

McDougall P. 2011. Caring for bronchiolitic infants needing continuous positive airway pressure. Paediatric Nursing, 23(1):30–5.

Moore H. 2009. Witnessed resuscitation: staff issues and benefits to parents. Paediatric Nursing, 21(6):22–5.

Moppett K. 2007. Traumatic brain injury: assessment, resuscitation and early management. British Journal of Anaesthesia, 99(1):18–31.

Nieman C, Manacci C et al. 2006. Use of the Broselow tape may result in the under-resuscitation of children. Academy Emergency Medicine, 13(10):1011–19.

Perry S. 2009. Support for parents witnessing resuscitation: nurse perspectives. Paediatric Nursing, 21(6):26–31.

Ousey K, Gillibrand W, Lui S. 2010. Effective management of acute faecal incontinence in hospital: a review of continence management systems. Frontline Gastroenterology, 1(2):94–7.

RCPCH. 2004. Withholding or Withdrawing Life Sustaining Treatment in Children: A Framework for Practice (2nd edition). www.rcpch.ac.uk/publications/recentpublications/witholding.pdf.

Schindler C, Mikhailov T et al. 2007. Skin integrity in critically ill and injured children. American Journal of Critical Care, 16(6):568–74.

Sorce L, Hamilton SM et al. 2009. Preventing corneal abrasions in critically ill children receiving neuromuscular blockade: a randomized controlled trial. Pediatric Critical Care Medicine, 10(2):171–5.

Stiller K. 2000. Physiotherapy in intensive care: towards an evidence-based practice. Chest, 118(6):1801–13.

Stiller K. 2007. Safety issues that should be considered when mobilizing critically ill patients. Critical Care Clinics, 23(1):35–53.

Tatman A, Warrena A, Williams A. 1997, Development of a modified paediatric coma scale in intensive care clinical practice. Archives of Disease in Childhood, 27(6):519–21.

Tuffrey C, Finlay F, Lewis M. 2007. The needs of children and their families at end of life: an analysis of community nursing practice. International Journal of Palliative Nursing, 13(2):64–71.

UK Resuscitation Council (UKRC) (2010) Guidelines. www.resus.org.uk.

Whiteing N, Hunter J. 2008. Nursing management of patients who are nil by mouth. Nursing Standard, 22(26):40–5.

Wiles L, Stiller K. 2009. Passive limb movements for patients in an intensive care unit: a survey of physiotherapy practice in Australia. Journal of Critical Care, 25(3):501–8.

Willcock J, Anthony D, Richardson J. 2008. Inter-rater reliability of the Glamorgan Paediatric Pressure Ulcer Risk Assessment Scale. Paediatric Nursing, 20(7):14–19.

Wolff A, Browne J, Whitehouse P. 2011. Personal resuscitation plans and end of life planning for children with disability and life-limiting/life-threatening conditions. Archives of Disease in Childhood, 96(2):42–8.

Resources

Royal Children's Hospital Melbourne Clinical Paediatric Guidelines www.rch.org.au/emplibrary/clinicalguide/IVFLUIDCHART.pdf.

Royal College of Nursing. 2011. Standards for Assessing, Measuring and Monitoring Vital Signs in Infants, Children and Young People. www.rcn.org.uk/_data/assets/pdf_file/0004/114484/003196.pdf.

Spotting the sick child. spottingthesickchild.com

The recognition and assessment of acute pain in children. www.rcn.org.uk/data/assets/pdf_file/0004/269185/003542.pdf.

Chapter 3
PHYSIOLOGICAL MONITORING OF INFANTS AND CHILDREN IN THE INTENSIVE CARE UNIT

Michaela Dixon[1] and Debra Teasdale[2]

[1] Paediatric Intensive Care Unit, Bristol Royal Hospital for Children,
University Hospitals Bristol NHS Foundation Trust, Bristol, UK
[2] Health, Wellbeing and the Family, Canterbury Christ Church University, Canterbury, UK

Introduction

Paediatric intensive care is a relatively young speciality and as such has developed and continues to develop at a rapid pace. Alongside this technology have come ever more complex and invasive methods of monitoring a child's physiological parameters. The correct use of this technology to support constant physiological monitoring allows for rapid detection of changes in the clinical picture and an instant overview of the child's response to pre-scribed therapies or medications.

The safe and efficient delivery of critical care can be greatly enhanced by adequate preparation of both equip-ment and staff. As part of the induction to the clinical area the competence of staff in the use of the local equipment must be established. As new equipment becomes available and using it is added to the repertoire of nursing skills, additional training will be required for all staff who may need to use it. This is a joint responsibility as employers must provide training and nurses must actively seek out training for any deficits expected within their scope of practice (Nursing and Midwifery Council 2008). As equip-ment may be used intermittently it is good practice to ensure that instruction manuals are accessible, that training updates are organised and that a mechanism for technical support is established. There are many monitoring systems in use in different units, so this chapter will only provide an overview of the principles involved; it remains the responsibility of the individual practitioner to become familiar with and competent in the use of equipment pro-vided in the unit in which they practise.

Physiological monitoring can be divided into invasive and non-invasive categories and this chapter will primarily examine the monitoring that facilitates the assessment and monitoring of cardiac and respiratory function. General principles of clinical assessment for each body system are detailed in the relevant chapters to this volume.

General safety and preparation before use

It is the responsibility of the individual putting a piece of monitoring equipment into use to ensure that it is clean and in a serviceable condition. This means that before moving equipment to the child's bedspace it should be thoroughly checked, paying particular attention to electrical cables and plugs. Any cables that are split or have exposed wires should not be used but sent for immediate repair.

Electrocardiographic (ECG) monitoring

Standard continuous monitoring in the ICU is usually three-electrode bipolar lead monitoring. This generates a

Paediatric Intensive Care Nursing, First Edition. Edited by Michaela Dixon and Doreen Crawford.
© 2012 John Wiley & Sons, Ltd. Published 2012 by John Wiley & Sons, Ltd.

single-channel ECG recording and provides general information about electrical activity within the heart. (See Chapter 5 for further detail.)

Electrode placement for the three-lead ECG follows the colour of the leads. Standard placement is:

- Red – positive electrode placed in V1 location around the 4th intercostal space on the right side.
- Yellow – negative electrode placed in the left infraclavicular fossa.
- Green/black – reference electrode placed below the diaphragm on the left side.

Five-electrode limb leads plus one precordial lead combination

This lead system is often used in adult critical care practice, and five electrodes are used. The four limb electrodes are placed in the LA, RA, LL and RL positions so that any of the six limb leads can be obtained (leads I, II, III, aVR, aVL or aVF). A fifth chest electrode can be placed in any of the standard V1 to V6 locations, but in general V1 is selected because of its value in arrhythmia monitoring. Cardiac monitors with this lead system often have two channels displayed so that one limb lead and one precordial lead can be displayed simultaneously (Drew et al. 2004).

Troubleshooting ECG monitoring (Table 3.1)

The ECG monitor will determine the rate according to the number of complexes measured on the continuous waveform. Inaccuracies can occur when the complexes are too large, being double-counted as part of the results; or the complexes are too small and so are not picked up at all.

Twelve-lead ECG recording (Figure 3.1)

The twelve-lead ECG is used to gain a three-dimensional picture of the electrical activity of the heart from right to left, superior to inferior and anterior to posterior. A total of 10 electrodes are required to record the standard ECG: one on each wrist and ankle and six across the precordium (Drew et al. 2004) (see Table 3.2).

Atrial wire ECG recordings

In certain conditions following cardiac surgery it is of use to record an atrial wire ECG. This is achieved by connecting one of the temporary atrial pacing wires to the V1 lead and running a recording. This is most useful when the child is tachycardic and there is a need to analyse the relationship between the P wave and the QRS complex.

Invasive pressure monitoring

Haemodynamic monitoring has two distinct components: electronic equipment, and a fluid-filled tubing system (McGhee and Bridges 2002).

Table 3.1 Troubleshooting ECGs

Problem	Potential reason	Actions
Flat line or poor quality trace	Child has no cardiac activity	Check pulse.
	The complex size is too small	Adjust size/gain, reposition electrodes, change to lead II.
	Poor connection	Check electrode connections to leads, check lead connection in monitor.
	Poor electrode contact	Replace the electrodes.
Interference/ artefact appearing in the trace	Poor electrode contact	Move electrodes over bone rather than muscle (normally the reverse applies).
	Electrical interference from patient movement, infusion pumps or other equipment (e.g. HFOV)	Ensure the lower electrode is placed well below the lower ribs to prevent respiratory interference.
		Ensure that the filter mode is selected.
Incorrect heart rate displayed	Complex too small – rate displayed is low	Increase the size/gain.
		Check lead II selected.
	Complex too large – rate displayed is too high	Observe for T-wave size and for artefact which will lead to elevated rates due to increased pick-up of 'complex'.
		Alter lead selection until normal complex seen.
		Decrease the size/gain.

Source: adapted and extended from Jevon and Ewens 2005; Laight et al. 2005.

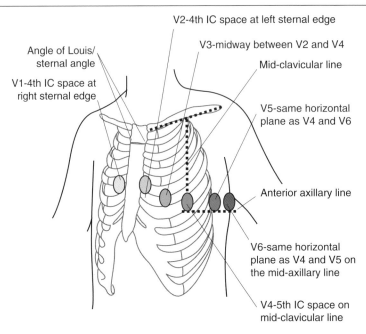

Figure 3.1   Correct lead placement for 12 lead ECG recording. Adapted from SCTS 2005.

Table 3.2   Lead placement for a twelve-lead ECG recording

Chest leads	Limb leads
There are six chest leads to site:	There are four limb leads, one of which is neutral:
V1: right 4th intercostal space, two spaces below the angle of Louis	aVR: A bony point between heart and right hand; around the wrist joint is ideal (red)
V2: left 4th intercostal space, two spaces below the angle of Louis	aVL: A bony point between heart and left hand; around the wrist joint is ideal (yellow)
V3: this is found between V2 and V4	aVF: A bony point between heart and left foot; the ankle/anterior superior iliac spine is ideal (green)
V4: left 5th intercostal space, in the mid-clavicular line	
V5: found between V4 and V6	Neutral: A bony point between heart and left foot; the ankle/anterior superior iliac spine is ideal (black)
V6: left 5th intercostal space, in the mid-axillary line	

The electronic equipment has three elements (Scales 2010):

1. a transducer to detect physiological activity
2. an amplifier to increase the size of the signal
3. a recording device to display the information (e.g. a monitor screen).

Connecting either an arterial catheter or central venous catheter to a fluid-filled tubing system allows the pressure in the vessel to be transmitted through the tubing to a transducer. The transducer links the tubing to the electrical system and converts the mechanical pressure wave from the blood into an electrical signal (McGhee and Bridges 2002). The signal is transmitted along a pressure cable to the monitor where the signal is amplified and displayed as a waveform (Scales 2008).

To ensure that accurate monitoring data is displayed the transducer must be calibrated to zero pressure. This is performed as follows:

1. Ensure the transducers are level with the right atrium (use a spirit level).
2. Cancel monitor alarms temporarily – ensure that the child is clinically stable.
3. Open the transducer three-way tap off to the patient and open to air (Figure 3.2).

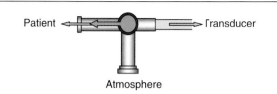

Figure 3.2 The three-way tap position for zero calibration. Adapted from Garretson 2005.

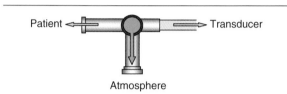

Figure 3.3 The three-way tap position for patient monitoring. Adapted from Garretson 2005.

4. Press the zero key on the monitor and allow the calibration to complete – visually the waveform will fall to the zero level on the monitor display.
5. Close the transducer three-way tap to air and open it again to the patient (Figure 3.3) – at this point a waveform should be visible on the screen; set the waveform scale so the entire pressure wave is visible and input appropriate limits.
6. Record the zero calibration on nursing documentation.

Maintaining line patency

There is considerable discussion regarding the use of heparin to maintain the patency of invasive monitoring lines, and studies in adults have identified that there is no difference in line patency when comparing the use of heparin infusions with plain 0.9% sodium chloride infusions (Hall et al. 2006; Kannan 2008; Tuncali et al. 2005). Ultimately, local policy will determine its use or non-use. The mechanism for continuously infusing through invasive monitoring lines is usually through the use of a 50 ml syringe and an infusion pump. Infusion rates tend to be adjusted according to age (an important consideration in the fluid-restricted neonate or young child) with rates from 0.5 ml/hr for the neonate to 3 ml/hr for the adolescent. If there are concerns regarding line patency, the volume of the infusate may be increased, however, this increase must be accounted for in the child's fluid intake.

Arterial lines and monitoring

Arteries have a similar structure to veins and consist of three layers:

- Inner coat: the tunica interna (intima) is composed of a lining of endothelium which is in contact with the blood, a basement membrane and a layer of elastic tissue called the internal elastic lamina.
- Middle coat: the tunica media is usually the thickest layer and consists of elastic fibres and smooth muscle.
- Outer coat: the tunica externa (adventitia) consists of mainly elastic and collagenous fibres.

Thanks to the structure of the middle layer, arteries have two major properties: elasticity and contractility. When the ventricles of the heart contract and eject blood into the large arteries they have the capacity to expand and accommodate the extra blood volume. When the ventricles relax, the elastic recoil of the arteries forces the blood on through the systemic and pulmonary circuits respectively.

The contractility of the artery arises from its smooth muscle which is arranged both longitudinally and circumferentially around the lumen. Sympathetic branches of the autonomic nervous system innervate this muscle.

When there is sympathetic stimulation the smooth muscle contracts, squeezing the wall around the lumen, which narrows the vessel causing vasoconstriction. Conversely, when sympathetic stimulation is removed the smooth muscle fibres relax, allowing the size of vessels lumen to increase causing vasodilation. Vasodilation is usually a consequence of the inhibition of vasoconstriction. The contractility of arteries also occurs as a protective mechanism to reduce bleeding, a process known as vascular spasm.

Key difference between veins and arteries

- Arteries lie deep in the tissue and are protected by muscle.
- Veins have valves to prevent the back flow of blood; arteries do not.
- The muscular arterial wall maintains patency of the lumen even when blood pressure is low.
- There may be an occasional aberrant artery, which is located superficially in an unusual place. This should not be mistaken for a vein. A common place for this to occur is in the antecubital fossa region.

Types of artery

- Elastic (conducting) arteries.
- Muscular (distributing) arteries.

- Arterioles.
- Anastomoses.

Elastic arteries

Large arteries are referred to as elastic or conducting arteries. Examples include:

- Aorta.
- Brachiocephalic.
- Common carotid.
- Subclavian.
- Vertebral.
- Common iliac.

The walls of elastic arteries are relatively thin in proportion to the diameter, and the tunica media contains more elastic fibres and less smooth muscle. As the heart contracts and relaxes, so the rate of blood flow tends to be intermittent. When the heart contracts (systole) and forces blood into the aorta the walls of the elastic arteries stretch to accommodate the surge of blood and store the pressure energy. During relaxation of the heart (diastole) the walls of the elastic arteries recoil to create pressure, moving blood forward in a more continuous flow.

Muscular arteries

Medium-sized arteries are called muscular or distributing arteries. Examples include:

- Axillary.
- Brachial.
- Radial.
- Intercostal.
- Splenic.
- Mesenteric.
- Femoral, popliteal, tibial.

In these vessels the tunica media contains more smooth muscle than elastic fibres. These arteries are capable of greater vasoconstriction/vasodilation, allowing adaptation of the volume of blood to suit the needs of the structure being supplied. The walls of these arteries are relatively thick, mainly due to the large amounts of smooth muscle fibres.

Arterioles

Arterioles are very small, almost microscopic arteries which deliver blood to the capillaries. The structure of the arterioles varies according to how close they are to the arteries from which they branch. Those closest to the feed

artery have a tunica interna similar to of the main arteries, a tunica media composed of smooth muscle with very few elastic fibres and a tunica externa composed of mostly elastic and collagenous fibres. Conversely, arterioles nearest to the capillaries consist of little more than a layer of endothelium surrounded by a few scattered muscle fibres. Changes in the diameter of arterioles can significantly affect blood pressure.

Anastomoses

Most areas of the body receive arterial supply from the branches of more than one artery. In such areas the distal ends of the vessel unite. The junction of these vessels is known as an anastomosis. This allows for an alternative blood supply to continue after damage to one of the supplying vessels, termed collateral circulation. (Arteries that do not anastomose are known as end arteries. Occlusion to an end artery will cause damage to the organ being supplied.)

Sites for arterial line placement

The site chosen for arterial line insertion will depend on the clinical condition of the child and the experience of the practitioner undertaking the procedure. Commonly used sites are detailed in Table 3.3.

Physiology of the arterial pressure-pulse wave (arterial waveform) (Figure 3.4)

Left ventricular ejection results in the creation of a pressure wave and blood flow into the systemic arterial system. Pressure waves move at a rate of 10 m/s while blood flows at a rate of 0.5 m/s, therefore the pressure wave is transmitted to the peripheral arteries more rapidly and precedes actual blood flow. The waveform displayed on the monitor is relative to the phases of the cardiac cycle (see Chapter 4).

Phase one (A)

This occurs in early systole when the opening of the aortic valve transfers the tremendous energy generated by the contracting left ventricle to the aorta. This creates the pressure wave that moves rapidly down the arterial tree. At the same time the first portion of stroke volume is delivered into the aortic root. This initial steep upstroke seen on the waveform is known as the anacrotic rise and is a reflection of left ventricular contractility.

- A decreased inotropic component (demonstrated by a sloping upstroke) is indicative of poor contractility and

Table 3.3 Common sites for arterial line insertion

Site	Advantages	Disadvantages
Radial artery	Easy to identify and cannulate due to superficial location. Accessible during most surgery. Dual circulation to the hand. Easy to immobilise.	High complication rate. Small artery requiring small catheter. Higher rate of occlusion due to thrombus formation. Nerve trauma during insertion. Increased artefact due to small catheter size.
Brachial artery	Large accessible vessel. Collateral circulation present. Less incidence of artefact.	Difficult to immobilise. Nerve damage from haematoma formation/traumatic insertion.
Femoral artery	Useful in shocked patient when unable to palpate other peripheral pulses. Large vessel – larger catheter may be used. Can be used for prolonged periods of time.	Difficult to immobilise. Difficult to keep site clean. Haematoma formation during insertion.
Axillary artery	Large vessel – larger catheter may be used. Collateral circulation present. Useful in patients with peripheral vascular disease. Reduced incidence of artefact. Accurate reflection of blood pressure.	Cerebral air embolism. Difficult to cannulate. Difficult to immobilise or secure site. Nerve damage.
Dorsalis pedis artery	Useful when other vessels unavailable. Dual circulation present.	Poor vessel for haemodynamic monitoring. Difficult to immobilise or secure site. Small vessel – small catheter. Greater risk of thrombosis formation.

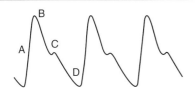

Figure 3.4 A simple arterial waveform. From Teasdale, D (2009) Physiological Monitoring in Dixon et al (2009) *Nursing the Highly Dependent Child or Infant: A Manual of Care*. Reproduced with permission from John Wiley and Sons, Ltd.

may be seen in patients with cardiomyopathy, ischaemic heart disease and with some drug therapies.

- An increased inotropic component (demonstrated by a near-vertical upstroke) is indicative of hyperdynamic circulation and may be seen in patients with compensated moderate to severe aortic regurgitation.

Phase two (A–C) volume displacement component (ejection period)

This fills out and sustains the pressure pulse. The rounded appearance is produced by the continued ejection of stroke volume from the left ventricle, displacement of blood and the distension of the arterial walls. The volume displacement component is narrow in patients with low stroke volume. An anacrotic notch may be noted and is thought to mark the change from phase one to phase two.

Phase three (C–D) late systole and diastole

This is associated with a sloping decline as the rate of peripheral runoff exceeds volume input into the arterial circulation. Aortic valve closure heralds the onset of diastole and is indicated by the dicrotic notch on the waveform (C). Following the dicrotic notch there is a continuous downstroke seen in the waveform until the next systole. There may be small undulations seen on the downstroke after the dicrotic notch; these represent reflections of the pressure waves from the distal arterioles.

Factors affecting arterial waveforms

- Size of artery cannulated or size of the arterial catheter used.
- Age of patient.
- Transducer height in relation to zero reference point.
- Waveform scale used on monitor.
- Length of time in situ.
- Ventricular function.
- Hypotension.
- Hypertension.
- Dysrhythmias or arrhythmias.

Considerations for practice

Care of the child with intra-arterial access is detailed in Table 3.4.

Complications of indwelling arterial lines

- Arterial embolisation.
- Systemic embolisation.
- Vascular insufficiency.
- Ischaemic necrosis of overlying skin.
- Infection.
- Haemorrhage.
- Accidental injection of drugs through arterial access.
- Poor perfusion to limb distal to line insertion site.
- Nerve damage.

Troubleshooting arterial lines

There are a number of problems which may be encountered when caring for the child with an arterial line; some are detailed in the complications of arterial lines. Others include:

Table 3.4 Care considerations for the child with intra-arterial access

Action	Rationale
Children who have continuous arterial pressure monitoring must also have ECG monitoring. Occasionally there will be a child for whom this is not possible (e.g. a child with significant burns involving the chest area) but for all other children ECG monitoring is required.	Any child's clinical condition that warrants invasive pressure monitoring should already be receiving the minimum PICU monitoring: ECG/SpO$_2$ / NIBP. Invasive monitoring should be regarded as more intensive than standard monitoring. It should be discontinued first when de-intensifying a child within PICU before discharge to the ward.
Arterial lines must be clearly identified and the line site should be visible at all times.	To prevent the line being mistaken for peripheral venous access and early identification of bleeding due to disconnection or dislodgement of catheter.
Bandages should not be used to assist with splinting if through their use the line site is not visible.	To observe for signs of inadequate skin or limb perfusion.
Splints must be removed at the beginning of each shift to allow a thorough examination.	To allow a thorough visual examination of the skin surrounding the line observing for signs of infection (redness) or blanching of the skin which may indicate altered perfusion due to the line's presence.
Injectable T-pieces must not be used for arterial lines.	To avoid accidental injection of bolus medications.
The perfusion to limb distal to the arterial line must be assessed hourly throughout each shift.	To detect changes in the colour and/or warmth of the limb distal to the line which may indicate inadequate circulation.
Arterial lines must be calibrated (zeroed) at the beginning of every shift as a minimum and then at any time indicated.	To ensure accurate data are provided relating to the child's haemodynamic status.
Universal precautions must be used when accessing or sampling from an arterial line (e.g. gloves must be worn).	Prevention of potential cross-infection between child and practitioner.
Syringes and waste must be discarded into the appropriate bins after use.	Safe and effective disposal of waste and effective use of waste disposal resources according to local policy.

- Dampened trace/waveform – may be caused by occlusion of the catheter tip, either by a clot or the tip being pushed up against the artery wall or because of clots or bubbles being present in the transducer or pressure tubing.
- Waveform not visible or is a straight line – this is usually caused by an incorrect scale being used for the values being determined by the system. Alternatively, it may be caused by a loose connection between the pressure transducer and the monitor cable.
- Blanching (whitening of the skin) when flushing the line – this is normally evident when the child has a radial or brachial arterial line in situ and may be caused by excessive pressure being used to flush the line, however it is essential that perfusion to the limb distal to the line is assessed and if there is any suggestion of compromise, the line should be removed after discussion with medical staff.

Central venous pressure (CVP) monitoring

CVP monitoring provides information about the pressure in the right atrium and as such provides information relating to the child's volume status, venous return (cardiac output) and right ventricular/pulmonary pressures.

The systems used to transduce a CVP are identical to those used for intra-arterial pressure monitoring. The waveform displayed from a CVP line is very different from the waveform displayed from the arterial line as the CVP waveform represents a low pressure waveform (Figure 3.5).

As with the arterial waveform, the CVP waveform seen on the monitor reflects the events of cardiac cycle. There are three positive waves (*a*, *c* and *v*) and two negative waves (*x* and *y*), and these correlate with different phases of the cardiac cycle and ECG (Magder 2005, 2006; Scales 2010):

- The *a* wave point is due to the increased atrial pressure during right atrial contraction. It correlates with the P-wave on the ECG.

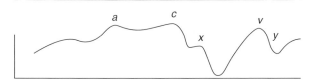

Figure 3.5 A single simple CVP waveform.

- The *c* wave point is caused by a slight elevation of the tricuspid valve into the right atrium during early ventricular contraction. It correlates with the end of the QRS segment on the ECG.
- The *x* wave point is thought to be caused by the downward movement of the ventricle during systolic contraction. It occurs just before the T-wave on the ECG.
- The *v* wave point arises from the pressure produced when the blood filling the right atrium comes up against a closed tricuspid valve. It occurs as the T-wave is ending on the ECG.
- The *y* descent point is produced by the tricuspid valve opening in diastole with blood flowing into the right ventricle. It occurs before the P-wave on the ECG.

Changes in waveform

Certain clinical conditions may elicit changes in the waveform demonstrated on the monitor:

- Atrial fibrillation will cause the loss of the *a* wave and the *c* wave to become larger than normal as atrial volume is larger at the beginning of systole due to atria not emptying.
- A junctional rhythm will cause a bigger than usual *a* wave as the atria are contracting in systole (when the tricuspid valve is closed) causing an increase in right atrial pressure. Cannon *a* waves, as they are known, also occur in any condition where there is atrioventricular dissociation (e.g. complete heart block or ventricular tachycardias).
- Tricuspid regurgitation will cause elevated *c* and *v* waves as the right atrium gains volume during systole.

Central venous catheter placement

The ideal site for a central venous catheter that will be most accurate for CVP monitoring is one where the tip sits at the junction of the superior vena cava and the right atrium. If the catheter is advanced too far into the right atrium, there is a risk of causing dysrhythmias, therefore the line placement should be confirmed by chest X-ray before use. Most central venous catheters are now inserted using ultrasound guidance to avoid misplacement and the potential complications associated with this (NICE 2002). The guide wire used for insertion may also cause a very transient dysrhythmia when it enters the right atrium. Femoral central venous catheters do not provide such accurate data in terms of waveform or pressure but may still be used to monitor trends in the CVP.

Left atrial pressure (LAP) lines

These lines are only placed in children post-open cardiac surgical procedures or those receiving ECLS and are useful for monitoring the left ventricular function in a child with the potential for significant left-sided dysfunction. The waveform demonstrated on the monitor should mimic the CVP waveform as the left atrium is also a low-pressure waveform. Changes in the LAP waveform may be indicative of left ventricular dysfunction such as mitral valve regurgitation. The use of these lines will depend on the surgeon's preference and individual centres will have their own protocols for the management of the lines. There is no difference in the setup of an LA line to that of the arterial or CVP line, however great care must be taken to ensure that no air enters the LA line or circuit as an air embolism through this line will travel directly to the cerebral circulation with potentially catastrophic effects for the child.

Cardiac output measurements

Invasive methods of measuring cardiac output, such as thermodilution using a pulmonary artery catheter, are not widely used in paediatric critical care due in part to the lack of data supporting their use. Further studies are advocated (Proulx et al. 2011). Non-invasive approaches, such as oesophageal Doppler monitoring (ODM), are currently more widely used for monitoring cardiac output in critically ill patients (Mathews and Singh 2008) and ODM was recommended by the National Institute for Health and Clinical Evidence (NICE) in 2011. It is based on measurement of blood velocity in the descending thoracic aorta by means of Doppler transducer from a probe inserted into the oesophagus. By applying the Doppler principle, the reflected signal can be used to determine flow velocity. A validated nomogram is used to derive volumetric data such as stoke volume and cardiac output (Mathews and Singh 2008; NICE 2011).

Pulse oximetry

Pulse oximetry has become a standard part of intensive care monitoring and provides non-invasive continuous monitoring of the child's oxygen saturation levels. The estimation of arterial haemoglobin oxygen saturation through pulse oximetry works because oxygenated and deoxygenated blood have different characteristics in terms of light absorption within the red and infrared spectra (Fouzas et al. 2011): oxyhaemoglobin has a higher absorption in the infrared spectrum; deoxyhaemoglobin has a higher absorption in the red spectrum.

The probe is two-sided; one side is a light-emitting diode (LED) which emits light at 660 nm (red light) and 940 nm (infrared light) wavelengths across the tissue bed. The other side, which is located underneath the digit/appendage, uses a photo-detector to measure the amount of light transmitted across the tissue bed. The software algorithm within the monitor removes the non-pulsatile component/background artefact then processes the measured changes in light absorption to produce numerical values for the heart rate and local arterial oxygen saturation (SpO_2) (Fouzas et al. 2011; Severinghaus and Aoyagi 2007).

Advances in technology have enhanced the removal of motion artefact and improved the clinical performance of new-generation monitors (Sahni et al. 2003), however, the key to reliable and accurate pulse oximetry is dependent on a number of variables, and external factors may affect the value elicited (Table 3.5).

Considerations for practice

- Respiratory failure may occur as a consequence of ventilation failure (indicated by an increasing $PaCO_2$ and respiratory acidosis), a failure of oxygenation (indicated by low PaO_2 and corresponding low SpO_2 values) or a combination of these. Pulse oximetry is a useful adjunct for detecting hypoxia, but it cannot determine ventilation failure. Blood gas sampling is required to determine this.
- There is a delay between the calculation of the value by the sensor and the value displayed on the monitor. Although this has been significantly reduced in the new-generation monitors there is still the potential for up to 15 seconds delay for an episode of desaturation to become apparent on the monitor.

Capnography and ETCO$_2$ monitoring

The measurement of carbon dioxide in the gas mix at the end of expiration is known as capnography when presented as a wave form or capnometry when presented as numerical data. Capnography was originally developed as an anaesthetic tool and has since been taken up in the wider environment (Galvagno and Kodali 2011). There are two types available:

- Disposable colorimetric device – Generally used to confirm immediate correct ETT placement after intubation. These devices are widely used in emergency care settings. Each colorimetric CO_2 detector has a pH-sensitive chemical indicator that undergoes colour change with each inspiration and expiration, thus reflecting the change in CO_2 concentration and are safe for use

Table 3.5 Limitations of pulse oximetry

Poor peripheral perfusion	Decreased signal secondary to decreased pulsatile component of the light absorption will lead to lower or inaccurate readings.
Abnormal haemoglobin molecules	Carboxyhaemoglobin mimics the red light absorption of oxyhaemoglobin, which means that even if the child has significant hypoxia this is not reflected in the value displayed. Methaemoglobinaemia absorbs equal amounts of energy in the red and infrared light spectra, therefore inaccurate readings will result. If there is any suspicion of the presence of abnormal haemoglobin molecules pulse co-oximetry is necessary and is usually performed via arterial blood gas sampling.
Ambient light	Intense external lighting such as phototherapy lights may flood the photo-sensor and provide inaccurate readings (usually lower than actual value).
Inappropriate probe size	The use of probes that are too big for the child's digit or too small will provide inaccurate data. It is the responsibility of the practitioner to select the correct-sized probe based on the manufacturer's size and weight guidance.
Nail polish and/or artificial nails	Dark nail polish (e.g. black, blue, purple or green) may interfere with the quality of the signal and produce an inaccurate value.

in all patient age groups including the pre-term infant (Garey et al. 2008). False negative readings, defined as a failure to detect CO_2 despite confirmed endotracheal tube placement in the trachea, may occur during cardiac arrest. In the low-flow hypodynamic state of cardiac arrest, delivery of CO_2 back to the lungs may be significantly decreased and colour changes may not be apparent (Galvagno and Kodali 2011).

- A portable electronic capnograph – This will use infrared, photo-acoustic or mass spectrometry technology to sample exhaled air providing a snapshot of the end tidal CO_2 (ETCO$_2$) which correlates well with the blood CO_2 levels (McArthur 2003). Sampling and analysis use a mainstream or a sidestream analyser:

  – Mainstream sampling – the analyser head is attached directly to the airway and the gas is analysed within the respiratory circuit through a clear window or cuvette. In the intensive care setting where inspired gases are actively humidified, mainstream may be more reliable than sidestream capnography.

  – Sidestream sampling is more common and describes the technique of continually aspirating a sample of gas from the respiratory circuit, which is then fed through the analyser. The gas is either returned to the respiratory circuit or scavenged. Sidestream capnography is favoured during anaesthesia owing to the convenience of a lightweight attachment to the airway, but may be troublesome due to sampling line blockage by water vapour following protracted use.

Considerations for practice

- Measurements may become erratic with no other obvious changes in the child's clinical state. This is often be caused by condensation or secretions in the sampling line or by intermittent kinking of the sample line when the patient moves. Replacement of the sampling line should remedy this.
- Capnography provides information about trends in the level of CO_2 – changes in the values and/or waveform should always be investigated and a clinical assessment of the child's respiratory status should be undertaken.
- Capnography should be used when transferring the child from the PICU for a CT or MRI scan or to theatre, and is always indicated in transport medicine for the ventilated child as most portable ventilators have limited alarm capacity.

Near-infrared spectroscopy

Tissue oximetry has been suggested as a non-invasive tool to continuously monitor and detect states of low body perfusion (Mittnacht 2010). Near-infrared spectroscopy (NIRS) is a non-invasive, continuous form of cerebral oximetry, which provides information relating to the assessment of brain oxygen delivery and utilisation (Kasman and Brady 2011). NIRS-based cerebral oximeters quantitate a venous-weighted ratio of oxygenated and deoxygenated haemoglobin in the region of cerebral cortex underlying the sensors, which are usually placed on the forehead. These sensors may also be placed on the abdomen and used for somatic sensing of perfusion (Mittnacht 2010). The use of NIRS is well established in cardiac anaesthesia and postoperative management, however there remains considerable discussion within the literature about the wider application of NIRS monitoring in the intensive care setting.

Conclusion

This chapter has reviewed key aspects of monitoring and considered equipment currently in use in the PICU. No monitor has been designed to replace diligent and constant observation of a sick child by an experienced children's nurse. They are supportive aspects of technological advancement and should enhance the nurses role in the PICU, not replace or detract from it.

References

Drew BJ, Califf RM et al. 2004. Practice standards for electrocardiographic monitoring in hospital settings. Circulation, 110:2721–46.

Fouzas S, Priftis KN, Anthracopoulos MB. 2011 Pulse oximetry in pediatric practice. Pediatrics, 128:740–52.

Galvagno Jr, SM, Kodali BS. 2011. Capnography in Intensive Care Unit. Available from Capnography – A Comprehensive Educational Website at www.capnography.com

Garey DM, Ward R et al. 2008. Tidal volume threshold for colorimetric carbon dioxide detectors available for use in neonates. Pediatrics, 121(6):1524–7.

Garretson S. 2005. Haemodynamic monitoring: arterial catheters. Nursing Standard, 19(31):55–64.

Hall KF, Bennetts TM et al. 2006. Effect of heparin in arterial line flushing solutions on platelet count: a randomised double-blind study. Critical Care and Resuscitation, 8(4): 294–6.

Jevon P, Ewens, B. 2005. Monitoring the Critically Ill Patient. Oxford: Blackwell Science.

Kannan A. 2008. Heparinised saline or normal saline. Journal of Perioperative Practice, 18(10):440–1.

Kasman N, Brady K. 2011. Cerebral oximetry for pediatric anesthesia: why do intelligent clinicians disagree? Pediatric Anesthesia, 21(5):473–8.

Laight S, Currie M, Davis N. 2005. Cardiac care. In M Sheppard, M Wright, Principle and Practice of High Dependency Nursing (2nd edition). London: Baillière Tindall/Elsevier.

Magder S. 2005. How to use central venous pressure measurements. Current Opinion in Critical Care, 11(3):264–70.

Magder S. 2006. Central venous pressure monitoring. Current Opinion in Critical Care, 12(3):219–27.

Mathews L, Singh KR. 2008. Cardiac output monitoring. Annals of Cardiac Anaesthesia, 11(1):56–68.

McArthur C. 2003. Clinical practice guideline. Capnography/capnometry during mechanical ventilation. Revision and update. Respiratory Care, 48(5):534–9.

McGhee BH, Bridges EJ. 2002. Monitoring arterial blood pressure – what you may not know. Critical Care Nurse, 22(2):60–79.

Mittnacht AJ. 2010. Near infrared spectroscopy in children at high risk of low perfusion. Current Opinion in Anaesthesiology, 23(3):342–7.

National Institute for Health and Clinical Excellence. 2002. Guidance on the use of ultrasound locating devices for placing central venous catheters. TA49 Central venous catheters – ultrasound locating devices: guidance. www.nice.org.uk.

National Institute for Health and Clinical Excellence. 2011. CardioQ-ODM oesophageal doppler monitor – NICE medical technology guidance 3. www.nice.org.uk.

Nursing and Midwifery Council (NMC). 2008. The Code: Standards of conduct, performance and ethics for nurses and midwives. www.nmc-uk.org/Publications-/Standards1.

Proulx F, Lemson J et al. 2011. Hemodynamic monitoring by transpulmonary thermodilution and pulse contour analysis in critically ill children. Pediatric Critical Care Medicine, 12(4):459–66.

Sahni R, Gupta A et al. 2003. Motion resistant pulse oximetry in neonates. Archives of Diseases in Childhood (Fetal Neonatal edition), 88(6):F505–8.

Scales K. 2008. Vascular access in the acute care setting. In L Dougherty, J Lamb (Eds). Intravenous Therapy in Nursing Practice (2nd edition). Oxford: Blackwell.

Scales K. 2010. Central venous pressure monitoring in clinical practice. Nursing Standard, 24(29):49–55.

Severinghaus JW, Aoyagi T. 2007. Discovery of pulse oximetry. Anesthesia and Analgesia, 105(6 supplement):S1–S4.

Society for Cardiological Science and Technology (SCST). 2005. Clinical Guidelines by Consensus. Number 1 Recording the 12 lead electrocardiogram. Available from http://scst.org.uk/docs

Teasdale, D. 2009. Physiological Monitoring in Dixon, Crawford, Teasdale and Murphy (Eds) Nursing the Highly Dependent Child or Infant. Oxford: Wiley Blackwell.

Tuncali BE, Kuvaki B et al. 2005. A comparison of the efficacy of heparinized and nonheparinized solutions for maintenance of perioperative radial arterial catheter patency and subsequent occlusion. Anesthesia and Analgesia, 100(4):1117–21.

Section 2
SYSTEMS APPROACH

Chapter 4
CARE OF AN INFANT OR CHILD WITH A RESPIRATORY ILLNESS AND/OR THE NEED FOR RESPIRATORY SUPPORT

Michaela Dixon

Paediatric Intensive Care Unit, Bristol Royal Hospital for Children, University Hospitals Bristol NHS Foundation Trust, Bristol, UK

Introduction

This chapter reviews the development of the respiratory tract and considers the care of a child admitted to PICU with a disorder of the respiratory system or who is in need of airway management and respiratory support strategies. Intensive care is a balance between doing enough to support the child and not causing iatrogenic damage to the lungs. The common pharmaceutical agents used in the respiratory support of children in PICU are briefly considered.

The primary role of the respiratory system, in conjunction with the cardiovascular system, is to supply oxygen to the cells of the body and remove a by-product of cellular metabolism, carbon dioxide. The lungs also play a major role in maintaining homeostasis and mounting a host defence response to potentially threatening organisms. To achieve this, the respiratory system has a number of anatomical and physiological attributes, some of which develop at key points during foetal growth; however full maturation of the respiratory system is not complete until around 8 years of age and possibly beyond that, into early adolescence. Indeed, throughout embryonic and foetal development the respiratory system does not carry out its primary role: gas exchange. This lack of maturity, both anatomically and physiologically, contributes significantly to the high incidence of respiratory illness and respiratory failure seen in the newborn, infant and young child. It also has significance when considering the nursing care of the child with respiratory illness in the critical care setting.

Embryology

The development of the respiratory tract takes place in five distinct phases, although there is an overlap between the phases and some variability in the timing of the phases in the literature.

During the embryonic period, which takes place between 4 and 9 weeks of gestational age, the respiratory tract starts to develop in the form of a respiratory diverticulum from the primitive foregut. The foregut later divides into two – the ventral portion, which will form the trachea, and the lung buds and the distal portion, which will form the oesophagus. Failed or incomplete separation of the foregut leads to the development of congenital conditions such as tracheoesophageal fistula and or oesophageal atresia (OA). The primary lung bud develops into a left and right bronchial bud, which in turn continue to divide into the main bronchi and the lung lobes – the right bronchial bud forms three main bronchi and three lobes, while the left forms two main bronchi and two lobes. The blood supply for these structures is delivered by the primitive pulmonary artery.

From week 8 onwards the term foetal development is usually applied for the remaining four phases.

During the pseudoglandular period (day 56 to week 16 gestation) all the major conducting airways develop. These include the terminal bronchioles, which are the last component of the airway before air reaches the alveoli. The arterial blood supply increases as more and more structures are defined and vascularisation begins. The diaphragm is derived from the fusion of pleuro-peritoneal fields (normally between weeks 8 and 10) and failure of this process will lead to congenital diaphragmatic hernia and possible lung hypoplasia. The canalicular period (weeks 17 to 26) sees the development of the respiratory bronchioles, each of which ends in a small dilated bulge – the primitive alveoli. There is also continued development of the pulmonary vascular beds. The following saccular period (weeks 24 to 38) sees the development of the elastic fibres which provide support to the structures of the respiratory tract. True alveoli are present by week 34; however gas exchange, while suboptimal, is possible throughout this period. The relationship between the alveoli and pulmonary capillaries is optimised and close contact between air spaces and capillaries develops. The final period, known as the alveolar period, occurs from week 36 onwards and, as the name suggests, sees the final refinement of the developing alveoli in preparation for birth and the transition to extra-uterine circulation and gas exchange. The columnar cells of the alveolar walls differentiate into two types, each of which has a specific role:

• Type one cells – alveolar surface area and gas exchange.
• Type two cells – surfactant production.

Transition to extra-uterine respiratory function

During foetal development the lungs are fluid-filled with no air–fluid interface present. In addition, the pulmonary vascular resistance is high due to the presence of a relatively hypoxic foetal circulation causing persistent pulmonary vasoconstriction. At birth a number of changes take place which facilitate the transition from foetal circulation to extra-uterine respiratory function. These are identified in Figure 4.1.

Brief overview of respiratory physiology

The role of surfactant

Pulmonary surfactant is a mixture of phospholipids produced by type 2 alveolar pneumocytes from around week 36 of gestational age. The primary function of surfactant is to lower surface tension in the alveolar air–liquid interface which helps to stabilise the expanded alveolus at the end of inspiration, prevent collapse at the end of expiration and increase compliance. There is a fluid film which coats the inner wall of the alveolus containing water molecules. Water molecules have a weak mutual physical attraction and the presence of surfactant reduces this physical attraction, preventing the walls of the alveoli collapsing in towards each other. In turn, it reduces the pressure required for subsequent re-inflation of the alveoli. Surfactant also contributes to the innate defence system and has been shown to possess anti-inflammatory properties.

Gas exchange

All organ systems rely to a greater or lesser degree on the delivery of oxygen to maintain normal cellular metabolic function. The primary function of the respiratory system is to move O_2 from the air to the blood and CO_2 from the blood to the air.

This process of gas exchange involves three stages:

• Pulmonary ventilation – the movement of air between the atmosphere and the lungs which is dependent on the existence of a pressure gradient (Boyle's law) and lung compliance.
• External respiration – the exchange of O_2 and CO_2 between the alveoli and the blood in the pulmonary capillaries and the conversion of deoxygenated blood to oxygenated blood. The exchange of gases occurs through diffusion and Fick's law applies here. Several anatomical features assist with this process, including:
  – the total thickness of the alveolar–capillary membrane, which is only 0.5 micrometres;
  – multiple capillaries lying over each alveolus allow 100 ml of blood to participate in gas exchange at any one time;
  – the structure of the pulmonary capillaries is designed to give maximum exposure to facilitate gas exchange.
• Internal respiration – oxygenated blood (transported by the circulatory system) leaves the lungs and is delivered to the tissue cells. The exchange of O_2 and CO_2 occurs again at this point through diffusion and the presence of a concentration gradient. At rest only 25%% of available O_2 is extracted by the cells to meet metabolic demand.

Gas transport

Partial pressures of gases

The total pressure of a gas is the sum of all the partial pressures of the gases within the mixture. Normal atmospheric air consists of two main gases – oxygen (O_2) and

(Initiation of breathing)

Change from placental to pulmonary oxygenation

Pressures in pulmonary circulation and right side of heart fall as foetal lung fluid is replaced by air

Lung expansion decreases the pressure transmitted to the pulmonary vascular beds

Lung inflation causes increase in alveolar oxygen tension (pressure)

↓

Reversal of hypoxia induced vasoconstriction in lungs

Cord clamping and removal of low resistance placental circulation produces an increase in systemic vascular resistance (SVR) and increased pressure in the left ventricle

Fall in right atrial (RA) pressure and rise in left atrial (LA) pressure produces functional closure of the foramen ovale (persistent high PVR may delay this closure)

Constriction of ductal smooth muscle leads to a gradual closure of ductus arteriosus over 3–14 days of life

Figure 4.1   Transition to extra-uterine respiratory function.

nitrogen (N_2) – with the remaining very small percentage being made up from carbon dioxide (CO_2) along with argon and helium, and water. When considering respiratory physiology it is the two main gases that are significant. Normal atmospheric pressure is 760 mmHg (101 kPa). Of this, nitrogen provides the greatest quantity (78%), oxygen 21%, while carbon dioxide accounts for a mere 0.03%. Therefore, the partial pressures of the gases in dry air at sea level are:

- PN_2 = 592.8 mmHg
- PO_2 = 159.6 mmHg
- PCO_2 = 0.2 mmHg
- P other = 7.4 mmHg

Almost all (≈ 98.5%) of the oxygen transported in systemic arterial blood is chemically bound to haemoglobin found in red blood cells with the remaining 1.5% being dissolved in plasma. The normal haemoglobin molecule is composed of four polypeptide chains: two alpha (α) globin chains and two beta (β) globin chains. Attached to each of the polypeptide chains is an iron-containing molecule called haem, therefore each haemoglobin molecule has four binding sites for oxygen to be transported around the body.

Because so much of the body's oxygen is transported in this manner there are a number of factors which influence the ease with which it either binds to or dissociates from haemoglobin.

Partial pressure of oxygen

The most important factor influencing how much oxygen binds to haemoglobin is the partial pressure of oxygen (PO_2). When the PO_2 is high, haemoglobin binds with large

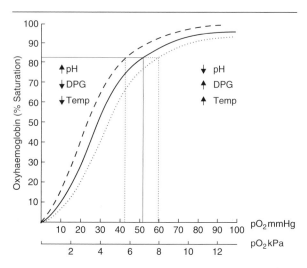

Figure 4.2 The oxyhaemoglobin dissociation curve. From Dixon et al. (2009) *Nursing the Highly Dependent Child or Infant: A Manual of Care.* Reproduced with permission from John Wiley and Sons, Ltd.

amounts of oxygen and is almost 100% saturated. Therefore, in the pulmonary capillaries where the PO_2 is high (because the PO_2 in atmospheric air is higher) a lot of oxygen binds with haemoglobin. In the tissue capillaries where the PO_2 is lower, haemoglobin does not hold as much oxygen; therefore oxygen is released for use by the tissues through diffusion. The relationship between the PO_2 and haemoglobin binding is demonstrated by the oxyhaemoglobin dissociation curve (OHDC). This curve describes the relationship between the percentage saturation of O_2 (shown on the y axis) to partial pressure of oxygen (shown on the x axis) (Figure 4.2). The curve can move to the left or the right depending on the environment and the influence of the factors noted in Table 4.1. At any given PO_2 when the curve shifts to the right haemoglobin will be less well saturated with O_2 (the Bohr effect), while if the curve shifts to the left haemoglobin will be more saturated with O_2.

Control of respiration

Breathing is essentially an involuntary process which is controlled by the medulla and pons of the brain stem. The

Table 4.1 Factors affecting haemoglobin and oxygen binding

Factors	Effects
Acidity (blood pH)	Haemoglobin can act as a buffer for H^+ ions in the blood to maintain blood pH within normal limits. In an acidosis, H^+ can bind to the amino acids in haemoglobin causing a slight change in the structure of haemoglobin, decreasing its O_2 carrying capacity. This causes a right shift on the curve and will facilitate increased oxygen release to the tissues in times of greater demand.
Carbon dioxide	This can affect the curve in two ways: 1. Most (80–90%) of the CO_2 is transported as bicarbonate ions. The formation of a bicarbonate ion will release a proton into the plasma. Elevated CO_2 levels create a respiratory acidosis and shift the oxygen–haemoglobin dissociation curve to the right as the CO_2 accumulates. 2. Carbamino compounds are generated through chemical interactions, resulting in carbaminohaemoglobin. Low levels of carbamino compounds have the effect of shifting the curve to the right, while high levels cause a shift to the left.
Temperature	As body temperature increases the OHDC moves to the right and more oxygen is released to the tissues. This occurs because heat is a by-product of the metabolic activity in the cells and metabolically active cells require more O_2 to maintain aerobic metabolism. In addition, a by-product of increased metabolism is the production of acids which in turn will decrease the pH.
BPG (2,3 bisphosphoglycerate)	Decreases the affinity of haemoglobin for O_2 making it more available to the tissues. BPG is produced by the red cells when they metabolise glucose to produce energy in the form of ATP. Increased energy demands from cells cause an increase in BPG levels and so an increase in oxygen available for the tissues as the OHDC shifts to the right. (This is also referred to as 2,3 diphosphoglycerate or 2,3 DPG)

frequency of normal, involuntary breathing is controlled by three groups of neurons or brain stem centres: the medullary respiratory centre, the apneustic centre and the pneumotaxic centre. The cerebral cortex provides voluntary control of respiration, although this can be overridden by the responses generated by the chemoreceptors. An individual's emotional state can effect changes in respiratory rate via the limbic system.

Central chemoreceptors

These are located in the brainstem and are the most important for the minute-by-minute control of respiration. These chemoreceptors are located on the ventral surface of the medulla near the point of exit for the glossopharyngeal and vagus nerves and are only a short distance from the medullary inspiratory centre. Central chemoreceptors communicate directly with the inspiratory centre. The brain stem chemoreceptors are exquisitely sensitive to changes in the pH of cerebrospinal fluid (CSF). Decreases in the pH of CSF produce an increase in the respiratory rate, while an increase in the pH of CSF produce a decrease in the respiratory rate.

Peripheral chemoreceptors

These are peripheral chemoreceptors for O_2, CO_2 and H^+ in the carotid bodies, located at the bifurcation of the common carotid arteries and in the aortic bodies above and below the aortic arch. Information about $PaO_2/PaCO_2$ and pH is relayed to the medullary inspiratory centre, which orchestrates an appropriate change in respiratory rate. Decreases in PaO_2 are the most important responsibility of the peripheral chemoreceptors but they are relatively insensitive to changes until PaO_2 reaches 60 mmHg (8 kPa) or less. Once in this range the chemoreceptors are exceptionally sensitive to further changes. Decreases in arterial pH cause an increase in respiration mediated by the peripheral chemoreceptors based on their sensitivity to H^+. This effect is independent of changes in the $PaCO_2$ and is mediated only by the chemoreceptors in the carotid bodies, not by those in the aortic bodies. In a metabolic acidosis, therefore, where there is a decreased arterial pH but not an elevated $PaCO_2$ level, the peripheral chemoreceptors are stimulated directly to increase the respiratory rate. The peripheral chemoreceptors also detect increases in $PaCO_2$ but the effect is less important than their response to decreases in PaO_2. Detection of changes in $PaCO_2$ by the peripheral chemoreceptors is also less important than the detection of changes in $PaCO_2$ by the central chemoreceptors.

Lung stretch receptors

Mechanoreceptors are present in the smooth muscle of the airways. When stimulated by distension of the lungs and airways, mechanoreceptors initiate a reflex decrease in the respiratory rate: this is called the Hering–Breuer reflex. The reflex decreases the respiratory rate by prolonging the expiratory time.

Joint and muscle receptors

Mechanoreceptors located in the joints and muscles detect the movement of limbs and instruct the inspiratory centre to increase the respiratory rate. Information from the joints and muscles is important in the early (anticipatory) ventilatory response to exercise.

Irritant receptors

Receptors for noxious chemicals and particles are located between the epithelial cells lining the airways. Information from these receptors is relayed to the medulla and causes a reflex constriction of the bronchial smooth muscles in response with an associated increase in the respiratory rate.

J receptors (juxtacapillary receptors)

These are found in the walls of each of the alveoli and, as the name suggests, are near the pulmonary capillaries. Increases in the presence of interstitial fluid volume may activate these receptors as well as increased pulmonary capillary blood flow. The response produced is an increase in respiratory rate.

Ventilation perfusion ratio and mismatch

Gas exchange becomes optimal when both ventilation and pulmonary blood flow are equal. Even under normal conditions in fit healthy individuals, the ventilation/perfusion ratio (V/Q) is < 1.0. Gravitational forces create regional differences in intra-pleural and pulmonary pressures, which results in a mismatch between areas of the lung being ventilated and pulmonary blood flow. Conditions that affect either the ventilation component or the perfusion component will significantly increase the mismatch.

Intra-pulmonary shunting is a major cause of hypoxaemia. A shunt here refers to venous blood that travels from the right to left side of the circulation without coming into contact with ventilated lung. Shunts can be identified as anatomic or physiologic (capillary).

An anatomic shunt occurs when blood bypasses the lungs through an anatomic channel, such as from the right to the left ventricle through a ventricular septal defect or

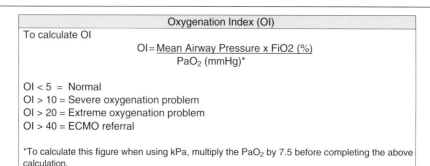

Figure 4.3 Summary of the Oxygenation Index.

from a branch of the pulmonary artery directly to a pulmonary vein.

A physiologic (capillary) shunt occurs when a portion of the cardiac output goes through the regular pulmonary vasculature without coming into any contact with alveolar air for gas exchange. There is no abnormal connection between the blood vessels; rather, there is a redistribution of pulmonary blood flow. Physiologic shunting is often seen in pulmonary oedema, pneumonia and lobar atelectasis.

Venous blood passing non-functioning alveoli creates an admixture of venous and arterial blood which decreases the PaO_2 and therefore increases the degree of hypoxaemia. This venous admixture can be described as the ratio of shunted blood (Qs) to total pulmonary blood flow (Qt). The normal Qs/Qt is 3–7% and changes of more than 5% are considered significant in terms of respiratory performance. From a clinical perspective, the work of breathing is markedly increased when the Qs/Qt > 15%, however measuring this in the clinical setting is extremely difficult.

Calculating the Oxygenation Index (OI) (Figure 4.3) provides readily available information about the ability of the lungs to diffuse oxygen across the alveolar capillary membrane. It represents the ratio between the level of oxygen being delivered to the lungs and the amount diffusing into the blood and can be used as an assessment tool for the efficacy of interventions, such as the introduction of high frequency oscillation ventilation (HFOV) and/or nitric oxide therapy. It is also used as an index of the severity of underlying lung damage and as one of the referral criteria for the provision of extracorporeal membrane oxygenation (ECMO).

Pulmonary volumes and capacities

There are a number of important volumes or capacities which influence normal respiratory function. These are detailed in Table 4.2 and Figure 4.4.

Respiratory assessment

Within the critical care setting, respiratory assessment utilises a number of approaches to create a complete picture. Sound knowledge of anatomy and physiology, including the ability to identify thoracic landmarks (Figure 4.5 and Table 4.3), is the main underpinning requirement to an effective assessment. The key components of assessment include:

• General physical inspection, including palpation and percussion and assessment of respiratory pattern and rate.
• Auscultation.
• Chest X-ray (CXR) review.
• Blood gas analysis.

Physical inspection

Good visual inspection before disturbing the child can provide the practitioner with a wealth of information about the child's general wellbeing as well as previous and current medical history, which may or may not be relevant to the current illness episode. Areas to consider include:

• General nutritional status of the child – may be demonstrated by rib prominence or the presence of large amounts of fatty tissue.
• General colour of the child – presence of peripheral or central cyanosis. Look for signs of finger clubbing (indicative of chronic hypoxaemia) or prominent superficial venous patterns across the chest and abdominal walls, which can be a sign of increased right-sided heart pressure/vascular obstruction.
• The size and shape of the child's chest and the presence of any skeletal abnormalities such as scoliosis, which may affect the child's respiratory performance.

Table 4.2   Summary of pulmonary volumes and capacities

	Definition and notes
Tidal volume (TV or V_t)	The volume of air entering and leaving the lungs in a single breath in the resting state. Tidal volume is constant between 6 and 8 ml/kg throughout life. Infant of 3 kg: TV = 18–24 ml (6/8 × 3) Adult of 70 kg: TV = 420–560 ml (6/8 × 70)
Inspiratory reserve volume (IRV)	The amount of air that can be inspired over and above the resting tidal volume.
Expiratory reserve volume (ERV)	The volume of air remaining in the lungs at the end of normal expiration, which can be exhaled by active contraction of the expiratory muscles.
Residual volume (RV)	The amount of air remaining in the lungs after maximal expiration; the presence of this prevents the lungs from emptying completely.
Vital capacity (VC)	The sum of normal tidal volume, inspiratory reserve volume and expiratory reserve volume. Infants: 33–40 ml/kg Adults: 52 ml/kg
Functional residual capacity (FRC)	The amount of air remaining in the lungs at the end of normal expiration. In the presence of atelectasis FRC falls as the number of alveoli participating in gas exchange decreases. Any pulmonary disease which affects the relationship between tidal volume, FRC and closing capacity will contribute significantly to ventilation – perfusion mismatching and hypoxia such as chronic lung disease (infants), cystic fibrosis, asthma, bronchiolitis and pneumonia.
Closing volume/capacity	Airway closure (complete collapse) occurs in areas of the lungs that have low volumes – this is known as the closing volume or capacity: • In adults closing capacity is usually at residual volume (amount of air remaining in the lungs after maximal expiration). • In infants closing capacity is at FRC due to the reduced elasticity of lung tissue, therefore closing capacity may be present during normal tidal breathing.
Dead space ventilation	Anatomic dead space – the volume of conducting air that fills the nose, mouth, pharynx, larynx, trachea, bronchi and distal bronchial branches which does not participate in gas exchange. Normal anatomic dead space is 2 ml/kg. Alveolar dead space – the volume of gas which fills alveoli, the perfusion of which is either reduced or absent. Contributing factors include hypotension, compression of the alveolar capillary bed and, rarely in children, pulmonary embolism. Physiologic dead space – the sum of both anatomic and alveolar dead space. Dead space ventilation – the amount of gas ventilating physiologic dead space per minute. It is expressed as a fraction of TV and the normal ratio is 0.3 (30%), which means that 30% of the volume of each breath does not participate in gas exchange.

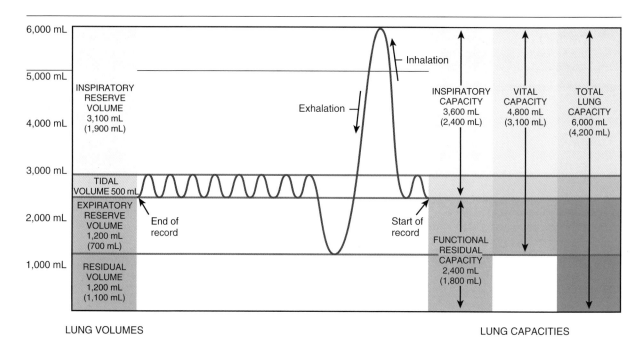

Figure 4.4 Lung volumes and capacities. From Tortora, G.J. and Derrickson, B.H. (2009) *Principles of Anatomy and Physiology*, 12th edn. Reproduced with permission from John Wiley and Sons, Inc.

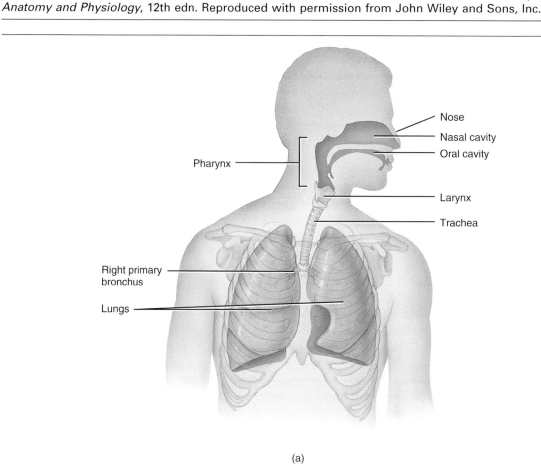

(a)

Figure 4.5 Anatomy of the respiratory system. (a) Anterior view showing the organs of respiration. (b) Branching of airways from the trachea. From Tortora, G.J. and Derrickson, B.H. (2009) *Principles of Anatomy and Physiology*, 12th edn. Reproduced with permission from John Wiley and Sons, Inc.

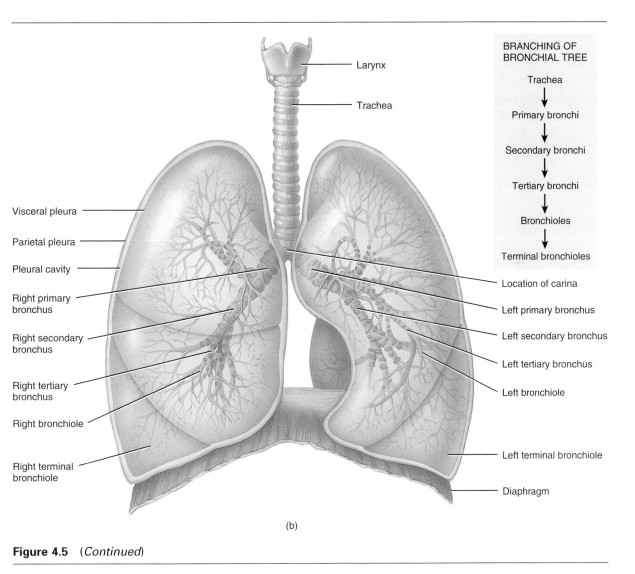

(b)

Figure 4.5 (*Continued*)

Table 4.3 Thoracic landmarks and their anatomical position for documentation of clinical assessment findings

Landmark	Position
Midsternal (MS) line	Vertical down the midline of the sternum.
R/L midclavicular (MC) lines	Parallel to the MS line – begins at mid-clavicle.
	The inferior borders of lungs cross the 6th rib at the MC line.
R/L anterior axillary lines	Parallel to the MS line – begins at anterior axillary folds.
R/L mid-axillary (MA) lines	Parallel to the MS line – begins at mid-axilla.
R/L posterior axillary lines	Parallel to the MS line – begins at posterior axillary folds.
Vertebral line	Vertical down the spinal processes.
R/L scapular lines	Parallel to the vertebral line – through the inferior angle of the scapula if patient is sitting up.

- The presence of scars from previous surgical interventions (e.g. sternotomy, thoracotomy or chest drain sites).
- The presence of new surgical incisions (front and back), chest drains and/or pacing wires in the postoperative cardiac patient.

Considerations for practice – newborns

Cyanosis of hands and feet (acrocyanosis) is common in the newborn and may persist for several days in a cool environment. Infants are obligate nose breathers (up to 6 months of age) and nasal flaring is a common finding without clinical significance in the absence of any other signs of respiratory distress. Infants born prematurely have a greater incidence of irregularity of respiratory pattern which is not clinically significant unless the infant is compromised by periods of apnoea. Coughing in newborns is rare and is normally pathological in origin, whereas sneezing is frequent and to be expected without underlying pathology. Hiccups in newborns are common, usually silent and associated with feeds. Frequent non-feed-associated hiccups maybe suggestive of seizures, drug withdrawal or encephalopathy in the newborn.

Cyanosis

Central cyanosis may be evident in a child with hypoxia, but may not be apparent in an anaemic child, even in the presence of profound hypoxia. The presence of cyanosis is therefore not a reliable or early indicator of hypoxia. If present, it should be considered a late and pre-terminal sign, unless the child has known underlying cyanotic heart disease. However, even in this scenario further investigation is necessary to rule out deterioration in the child's condition from baseline.

Palpation

Palpation is useful to assess for:

- Pulsations.
- Areas of tenderness.

- Bulges.
- Depressions.
- Unusual movement of the chest wall during inspiration and/or expiration.

Normal palpation should reveal bilateral symmetry of movement of the chest wall, with a degree of elasticity of the rib cage. The sternum should be relatively inflexible, however consideration should be given to the child post-sternotomy and particular care must be taken in the child whose chest remains open post-cardiac surgery. The trachea should be positioned in the midline directly above the suprasternal notch (a very slight deviation to the right is a relatively common, non-symptomatic finding). Abnormal findings from palpation usually require further investigation and intervention.

Crepitus

This is a crackly/crinkly sensation which can be both palpated and heard, and is indicative of air in the subcutaneous tissues, either from an air leak or, much more rarely, from the presence of a gas-producing organism (*Clostridium welchii*). The cause will determine whether further intervention is necessary.

Pleural friction rub

This is a palpable, coarse, grating vibration felt on both inspiration and expiration, which may be compared to the feel of leather rubbing on leather. It may be indicative of a pleural friction rub caused by inflammation of the pleural surfaces. It is a rare finding in the under-5 age group.

Percussion

This is a valuable skill which enables the practitioner to assess whether underlying tissue is air-filled, fluid-filled or solid. Different percussive notes are gained accordingly and a description of the differences is detailed in Table 4.4. Percussion is underutilised in nursing assessment but the

Table 4.4 Classification of percussive notes

Tone	Intensity	Pitch	Duration	Quality	Example
Tympanic	Loud	High	Moderate	Drum-like	Gastric bubble
Resonant	Loud	Low	Long	Hollow	Healthy lungs
Hyperresonant	Very loud	Low	Long	Boom-like	Air-filled spaces
Dull	Soft	Mid–high	Moderate	Thudding	Solid organs, e.g. liver
Flat	Soft	High	Short	Very dull	Muscle

Source: adapted from *Mosby's Guide to Clinical Examination Skills*, 5th edition, 2003.

skill should be developed under the supervision of a member of the medical staff or a physiotherapist until practitioners feel confident in its use.

Considerations for practice

The round shape of the infant's chest gives rise to a hyper-resonant percussive note, which is considered an abnormal finding in the older child. By the age of 6 years normal percussive notes should have a resonant pitch, therefore hyperresonance in this age group is indicative of underlying pathology such as pneumothorax.

The respiratory rate and rhythm

The respiratory rate (Table 4.5) and pattern (Table 4.6) are important indicators of underlying respiratory pathology

Table 4.5 Normal respiratory rates by age

Age of child	Respiratory rate (range)
Newborn	<60 breaths/min
<1 year	30–40 breaths/min
1–2 years	25–35 breaths/min
2–5 years	25–30 breaths/min
5–12 years	20–25 breaths/min
>12 years	15–20 breaths/min

and also considerations for instituting or increasing respiratory support. The first step is to determine the rate and pattern appropriate for the age of the child, taking into consideration any pre-existing clinical conditions which may affect the child's normal rate and pattern.

Auscultation

This should be a symmetrical assessment allowing for side-by-side comparison, moving from top to bottom, anteriorly and posteriorly, remembering to auscultate into the axillary spaces on each side. The purpose of auscultation is to assess for:

- The presence and location of normal breath sounds.
- The presence of normal breath sounds in abnormal locations.
- The presence of adventitious breath sounds.

There are three types of normal breath sounds heard in the healthy infant and child:

- Bronchial – heard over the trachea, loud and high-pitched (large airways).
- Bronchovesicular – heard over the main bronchi, moderate in pitch and intensity.

Table 4.6 A summary of terminology and descriptors of abnormal respiratory rates and/or patterns

Term used	Description
Tachypnoea	Rate is faster than the highest anticipated rate for age.
Bradypnoea	Rate is less than the lowest anticipated rate for age.
Apnoea	Absence of respirations.
Hyperpnoea	Rate is usually faster than anticipated for age and the breath taken is deeper.
Dyspnoea	Laboured or difficult respiration.
Orthopnoea	Dyspnoea at rest; difficulty in lying supine due to respiratory rate.
Hypoventilation	Slow, shallow breaths generating very small tidal volumes.
Sighing breaths	Frequently interspersed deeper breath.
Air trapping	Increasing difficulty in getting air out during expiration, usually associated with the presence of a wheeze.
Kussmaul respirations (also known as acidotic breathing)	Rapid, deep breaths with an additional effort at the end of expiration; this pattern is associated with the presence of a metabolic acidosis.
Biot respirations	Irregular, interspersed periods of apnoea in a disorganised sequence of breaths; usually indicative of pontine damage.
Ataxic respirations	Significant disorganisation with irregular and varying depth of respiration – an extreme form of biot respirations.
Cheyne–Stokes 'periodic breathing'	Varying periods of increasing depth of respiration interspersed with apnoea; this is often, although not always, a terminal respiratory pattern.

Table 4.7 Descriptors of adventitious breath sounds

	Definition and notes
Crackles	Discrete, non-continuous sounds, which can be divided into three types: • Fine – High-pitched, dry sounds, heard during the end of inspiration, which are not cleared by coughing (caused by the reopening of collapsed alveoli). • Medium – Lower-pitched, moister sounds heard during inspiration, which are not cleared by coughing. • Coarse – Loud, bubbly noises heard during inspiration, which are not cleared by coughing.
Wheezes	'Musical' sounds produced by the rapid or forced movement of air through narrowed airways. These sounds are common in the infant due to their narrower airways and are typically heard in expiration, although may also be present during inspiration. In normal, spontaneous ventilation, the intra-thoracic airways widen during inspiration and narrow on exhalation, while the opposite is true of the extra-thoracic airways. Maximum resistance to airflow occurs in expiration in the intra-thoracic airways and during inspiration in the extra-thoracic airways. Expiratory wheezes are indicative of a lower airway problem, while inspiratory wheezes indicate upper airway problems. The sudden disappearance of a wheeze in a child with asthma is usually indicative of impending respiratory failure.
Stridor	A high-pitched, piercing sound which is heard most often on inspiration. It is indicative of an obstruction in the upper respiratory tract and may be mechanical (e.g. due to tracheomalacia), due to infective processes (e.g. croup) or as a consequence of foreign body inhalation.

• Vesicular – heard over smaller bronchi, bronchioles and healthy lung tissue, low in pitch and intensity.

Abnormal or adventitious breath sounds have a number of different descriptors in the literature and the terms used have changed over the years. Currently, the terms widely recognised are crackles, wheezes and stridors (Table 4.7).

Less common abnormal sounds found on auscultation are pleural rubs and mediastinal crunch (Hamman's sign). As noted previously, a pleural rub is indicative of inflammation of the pleural membranes which may be heard in both inspiration and expiration. It is usually best heard over the lower lateral anterior surface of the chest wall. A mediastinal crunch is usually heard in the presence of mediastinal emphysema and is best described as a loud, clicking sound which is synchronous with the heart beat rather than with respiration, although it is sometimes louder towards the end of expiration.

Considerations for practice
• Breath sounds from right middle and left lingular lobe are best heard in respective axillae, hence the need to auscultate into the axillary spaces.
• Breath sounds are usually louder in infants and young children due to their thinner chest wall.

• Bronchovesicular sounds may be heard right to lung edges.
• Referred breath sounds are common in infants and young children due to their small thoracic cavity. Therefore, even in the presence of significant pneumothorax breath sounds may be heard over collapsed areas.

The chest X-ray

The chest X-ray remains a useful tool in assessing pulmonary health and function. A chest X-ray review should be approached in a logical, step-by-step manner to ensure that all areas are reviewed and small, sometime subtle changes are detected in a timely manner. A systematic approach is suggested in Table 4.8, however most practitioners will develop their own system.

Blood gas analysis

Blood gas analysis is undertaken for two reasons: to monitor the child's respiratory performance in terms of effective oxygenation and carbon dioxide removal; and, to provide information about the child's blood acid base environment related to primary non-respiratory causes of imbalance (e.g. metabolic acidosis).

Blood gases may be taken from venous stabs/lines, arterial stabs/lines or from a capillary stab, however the choice of sample for assessment of respiratory performance is an

Table 4.8   Systematic approach to CXR interpretation

Review process	Comments
Name, date, time	Ensure the most recent film is being reviewed, plus previous film for comparison.
Film view	Check whether film is AP or PA. Consider changes in heart size accordingly.
Patient position	Check whether film is erect or supine view.
Exposure, penetration	Identify whether film is too light or too dark – good exposure and presentation will allow visualisation of the spinal processes and the disc spaces below the diaphragm.
Inspiratory/ expiratory film	Inspiratory film – use anterior ribs and count down. A good film will have the 7th rib transecting the right hemi-diaphragm. Always use the right and not the left side (the right diaphragm sits higher than the left due to position of liver). Hyperinflation – expansion down to 9th anterior rib.
Rotation	The clavicle ends should be equidistant from the middle of the vertebral column.
Soft tissues and bones	Presence of chest wall oedema or fat. Signs of previous fractures (calcifications). Surgical emphysema – air striations in muscle fibres.
Additions	Endotracheal tube – check chin position halfway between clavicle and carina (remember – nose up tube up/nose down tube down). • Presence of central venous lines/pacing wires/sternal wires/LA and or PA lines post-cardiac surgery. • Presence/position of naso-/orogastric tube and/or naso-jejunal tube. • Clips from PDA ligations, etc. • Chest drains – pleural/mediastinal/pericardial.
Borders – heart and diaphragm	• Borders should be clearly evident. • Left diaphragm should be visible under heart shadow. • Clear, crisp costophrenic angles.
Lung fields	Tracheal position – midline or deviated. Consider: Fluid – mediastinum moves to opposite side Collapse – loss of volume with mediastinal shift towards area. Consolidation – no loss of volume, no real mediastinal movement, presence of air bronchograms, usually non- segmental. R/LLL: loss of diaphragm. LUL: shadowing only (veil sign). RML: loss of heart border. RUL: movement of horizontal fissure upwards. L lingular: loss of heart border. Pneumo-pericardium – air right around and under heart. Pneumo-mediastinum – air pockets but not under heart. Pneumothorax – absence of visible lungs markings. Increased vascular markings – increased/excessive pulmonary blood flow.

arterial sample through established arterial access. The use of single arterial stabs is not common practice in paediatric intensive care.

Considerations for practice

Arterial blood gases provide the most information from the measured parameters when assessing respiratory or metabolic function, while venous blood gases are more useful in providing an indication of metabolic function such as cardiac output and tissue perfusion rather than respiratory function per se. Capillary blood gases are useful for monitoring pH and PCO_2 but are not particularly helpful for oxygenation levels. Additionally, a capillary sample needs to be obtained without applying too much squeeze to the area being sampled (if it is, the results will be inaccurate). Therefore, assessment of the child's peripheral perfusion is essential before undertaking the procedure. The age of the child must also be considered when selecting the site to be used for sampling. As with any monitoring intervention, results should not be used in isolation; the goal is always to treat the child not the numbers.

Monitoring the acid base balance (an acid is a potential hydrogen (H^+) ion donor while a base is a potential hydrogen ion acceptor) is important because the body systems will only operate effectively if the internal environment is conducive, which depends on an arterial pH of 7.35–7.45. Normal aerobic metabolism results in the production of acids mainly in the form of CO_2, while anaerobic metabolism produces not only CO_2 but other metabolic acids, such as lactic acid. The majority of acids produced are buffered and therefore not in free form. The measurement of those in free form (and therefore potentially immediately harmful) found in the extracellular fluid is quantified by the use of the term pH. The normal concentration of free H^+ is very small, approximately 40 nanomilliequivalents (nmeq) per litre. The term pH is an expression of the negative logarithm of free H^+ concentration and the relationship

is inversely proportional. Therefore, as the free H^+ concentration increases so the pH decreases, and vice versa.

The systemic effects of acid base imbalance are detailed in Table 4.9.

If pH is to be maintained within the normal range and prevent potentially harmful effects occurring, the level of these acids needs to be regulated. There are three discrete but interrelated pathways that work to maintain the acid base balance.

Buffering system

The buffering response is activated in seconds and is considered the first line of defence against changes in pH. Buffers in the blood include bicarbonate, proteins such as haemoglobin and other substances such as phosphate. The most important pair in this system is the bicarbonate–carbonic acid pairing, which is responsible for buffering the extracellular fluid (ECF). If the pH of the ECF is threatened by the presence of a strong acid, then the weak HCO_3^- base becomes active, whereas if the ECF is threatened by the presence of a strong base, the weak H_2CO_3 acid becomes active (Figure 4.6).

As CO_2 is formed and diffuses into the capillary blood it enters the erythrocytes and reacts with water to form carbonic acid (H_2CO_3). Carbonic acid dissociates to form H^+ and H_2O (this occurs rapidly in the presence of carbonic anhydrase, but less so in its absence). The H^+ ions bind to reduced haemoglobin to form HHb. Bicarbonate ions (HCO_3^-) generated by this process pass back into the plasma in exchange for chloride ions (Cl^-), a process known as chloride shift, which ensures there is no net loss or gain of negative ions by the red cells. In the lungs, this process is reversed – the H^+ ions bound to haemoglobin in the form of HHb recombine with HCO_3^- to form carbonic acid, which in turn dissociates into CO_2 and H_2O. The CO_2 diffuses into the alveoli to be excreted through ventilation. In addition, reduced HHb re-forms to return to the tissues

Table 4.9 The systemic effects of acid base imbalance

Arterial pH < 7.35 (acidosis)	Arterial pH > 7.45 (alkalosis)
Increased pulmonary vascular resistance (PVR)	Decreased vascular resistance and tone
Right shift of the oxyhaemoglobin dissociation curve	Left shift of the oxyhaemoglobin dissociation curve
Decreased insulin secretion/binding to receptors	Increased response to catecholamines
Decreased pulmonary macrophage function	Decreased Krebs cycle oxidations in muscles and renal cortex
Lower threshold for ventricular fibrillation	Increased insulin glycolysis
Decreased response to catecholamines	
Decreased immune responses	
Decreased mesenteric blood flow	

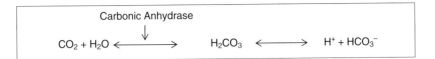

Figure 4.6 The bicarbonate–carbonic acid pairing.

Excessive acid load bicarbonate / carbonic acid (CA) pair is activated to buffer the acid
↓
Net increase in the presence of CA
↓
Dissociation into CO_2 and H_2O – excess CO_2 is excreted by the lungs
↓
Excessive H^+ concentration stimulates the respiratory centre in the medulla increasing respiratory rate to clear CO_2

Conversely elevated pH due to an increase in HCO_3^- causes inhibition of the respiratory centre and respiratory rate falls
↓
CO_2 retention occurs – allows formation of CA to buffer excessive HCO_3 thus returning pH to normal

Figure 4.7 The role of the respiratory system in the regulation of the acid base balance.

carrying oxygen once more. This system does not work in isolation and the respiratory system plays a major role in maintaining pH balance.

While the buffering system works within seconds, the respiratory system activates changes in pH within minutes. The balance is achieved through the conservation or elimination of CO_2 as the respiratory system cannot achieve any loss or gain of hydrogen ions (Figure 4.7).

The respiratory system is able to compensate for changes in pH relating to metabolic disorders where there is a build-up of fixed or non-titratable acids (e.g. ketoacids in diabetic ketoacidosis or lactic acid in sepsis).

The final pathway in the regulation of the acid base environment is the renal system which is discussed in Chapter 6.

Compensatory mechanisms

The body will seek ways in which it can compensate for acid base imbalances and for every acidosis or alkalosis will create the opposing acid base environment to maintain equilibrium.

Primary disorder	Compensation
Respiratory acidosis	Metabolic alkalosis
Respiratory alkalosis	Metabolic acidosis
Metabolic acidosis	Respiratory alkalosis
Metabolic alkalosis	Respiratory acidosis

Electrolytes and acid base balance

Potassium interacts with hydrogen. When the H^+ concentration is elevated in the ECF (e.g. metabolic acidosis), hydrogen moves into the cell and potassium moves out. This allows the H^+ access to the intracellular protein buffers, which can minimise changes in pH. However, the shift in potassium from the intracellular to extracellular fluids can result in relative hyperkalaemia. When H^+ concentration is reduced (e.g. metabolic alkalosis), H^+ moves out of the cell and potassium moves in, which can result in relative hypokalaemia.

Calcium is vital for neuromuscular and cardiac function. When pH is normal, 45% of calcium is bound to protein (mostly albumin) and is biologically inert. Fifty per cent is free or ionised calcium and is metabolically active, while 5% is bound to other organic anions such as citrate. Changes in pH alter the split and an acidosis will produce a reduction in the free (ionised) calcium available to the body. The presence of $NaHCO_3^-$ restores or maintains normal calcium reabsorption.

Normal blood gas values

Some units use hydrogen ion values to determine acidity when reviewing blood gases, therefore it is essential that practitioners are familiar with their institution's preferred method. Table 4.10 shows the blood gas values associated with standard pH measurements and a guide to hydrogen ions concentration matched to pH.

Blood gas interpretation

Developing a systematic approach to blood gas interpretation is essential to ensure that nothing is overlooked. There are different ways in which this can be done, which will depend on the individual practitioner. A commonly used approach using five main questions is outlined in Table 4.11.

There are two primary imbalances of the acid base environment which can be attributed to the respiratory system (Table 4.12). Primary metabolic imbalances are addressed in Chapter 5, although children may also present with a mixed imbalance, for example, in sepsis, children can often

Table 4.10   Standard blood gas values

Values	Arterial	Mixed venous	Capillary	H^+ = pH
pH	7.35–7.45	7.33–7.44	7.35–7.45	20 = 7.7
PCO_2	35–45 mmHg 4.6–6.0 kPa	40–50 mmHg 5.3–6.6 kPa	35–45 mmHg 4.6–6.0 kPa	31 = 7.5
PO_2	80–100 mmHg 10.6–13.3 kPa	35–40 mmHg 4.6–5.3 kPa	Variable	40 = 7.4
HCO_3^-	22–27 mEq/L	20–27 mEq/L	20–27 mEq/L	50 = 7.3
Base excess/deficit (BE)	$^-2$–$^+2$	$^-2$–$^+2$	$^-2$–$^+2$	80 = 7.1
Saturations	>95	72–75	Variable	100 = 7.0
Lactate	<2	<2	<2	180 = 6.8

Note: A child with cyanotic heart disease will have a lower PaO_2 even when well. In these instances it is important to be cognisant of the child's usual or expected PaO_2 range and saturations before implementing treatment.

Table 4.11   Systematic approach to blood gas interpretation

Main question	Further questions
1. What is the pH?	Is the primary disorder an acidosis? pH < 7.35 Is the primary disorder an alkalosis? pH > 7.45
2. What is $PaCO_2$?	Is there agreement with the pH? Respiratory acidosis ($PaCO_2$ > 45 mmHg/6.0 kPa) Respiratory alkalosis ($PaCO_2$ < 35 mmHg/4/6 kPa) If there is no agreement, then the primary disorder is not respiratory in origin
3. What is PaO_2?	Is patient hypoxic? (PaO_2 < 80 mmHg/10.6 kPa)
4. What is HCO_3^-?	Is level raised? (HCO_3^- > 27 mEq/l) Is level low? (HCO_3^- < 22 mEq/l) Does this agree with pH?
5. What is the base excess/deficit?	Is level raised/high? (BE > $^+2$, e.g. $^+8$ or a base excess) Is level low? BE < $^-2$, e.g. $^-12$ or a base deficit) Does this agree with HCO_3^- and pH?

Finally, put all the answers together and it should be possible to describe the patient's clinical status in terms of acid base balance and whether the result indicates a primary respiratory or metabolic acidosis/alkalosis or a mixed picture (i.e. the imbalance has both a respiratory and a metabolic component).

Lactate is an important indicator of tissue perfusion – high lactates are indicative of abnormal tissue metabolism secondary to inadequate delivery of the essential nutrients and oxygen required for normal metabolic processes. Rising lactate levels should always be investigated further.

Table 4.12 Primary respiratory acid base imbalances

	Respiratory acidosis	Respiratory alkalosis
Definition	pH < 7.35 PCO_2 > 45 mmHg/6.1 kPa HCO_3^- – normal or elevated	pH > 7.45 PCO_2 < 35 mmHg/4.5 kPa
Causes	Results from an accumulation of CO_2 due to inadequate respiration/ventilation • Chronic/acute obstructive airways disease • Pulmonary restrictive disease • Neuromuscular disorders • CNS depressants • Iatrogenic causes, such as inadequate ventilator rate/inspiratory peak pressure • Circulatory disorders	Results from an excessive loss of CO_2 • Hyperventilation secondary to pain or anxiety • Ventilator rate/pressures set too high
Management	1. Respiratory support – invasive or non-invasive based on assessment of need 2. Adjustment to mechanical ventilation 3. Treat underlying cause	1. Reduce ventilatory support by reducing rate/pressures 2. Encourage slow breathing and use a paper bag to allow for rebreathing of CO_2 in a self-ventilating child 3. Assess and treat pain/anxiety

present with a primary respiratory and a primary metabolic acidosis from inadequate respiratory performance and inadequate tissue perfusion. In this instance the practitioner must address both problems as a matter of urgency.

Systemic effects of a respiratory acidosis

Cardiovascular

• Tachycardia
• Increased cardiac output
• Increased blood pressure

Occurs due to sympathetic nervous system (SNS) stimulation and release of adrenaline from the adrenal medulla (the mechanism is stimulated by hypercapnia and low pH). While receptor response to inotropes/catecholamines is decreased in acidosis, this is overcome in the initial phase by an increase in the level of endogenous catecholamine released.

Pulmonary vasculature

Increased $PaCO_2$ can precipitate pulmonary vasospasm, which increases pulmonary vascular resistance (PVR) and decreases pulmonary blood flow. The underlying disorder responsible for the acidosis will be made worse by the increased PVR.

Cerebral vasculature

The pH of CSF changes in relation to blood pH, but CSF contains far fewer buffers so that the pH of CSF will decrease markedly in response to a relatively small change in the blood pH. Increased $PaCO_2$ leads to decreased cerebral vascular resistance and increased cerebral blood flow (CBF), which if unresolved may lead to cerebral oedema.

Peripheral vasculature

There is a combination of vasoconstriction due to catecholamine release and vasodilation due to action of CO_2 on smooth muscle.

Clinical signs of a respiratory acidosis

• Altered respiratory pattern.
• Dyspnoea.
• Tachycardia.
• Headache.
• Fatigue or weakness.
• Decreased level of consciousness, with agitation and restlessness.
• Decreased reflexes.
• Seizures.
• Nausea and vomiting.

Assessment of the non-intubated child or the child with a tracheostomy

- General appearance.
- Position adopted.
- Level of activity and responsiveness.
- Assessment of respiratory rate, pattern and mechanics (use of accessory muscles).
- Assessment of vital signs – heart rate, blood pressure and saturations.
- Auscultation of breath sounds.
- Chest X-ray review (if available).
- Blood gas analysis (as necessary).

In addition, for children with a tracheostomy:

- Cleanliness and security of tracheostomy tapes and dressings.
- Assessment of type of secretions yielded with suction.
- Integrity of the skin surrounding stoma and the neck.

Assessment of the intubated child or child with a tracheostomy receiving mechanical ventilation

In addition to all the assessment points identified above, consideration must be given to the following when assessing a child who is intubated or child with a tracheostomy who is receiving mechanical ventilation:

- Assess for synchronicity with the ventilator.
- Is rate appropriate for age of infant/child?
- Note inspiratory/expiratory time.
- Tidal volumes of each breath.
- Adequate chest expansion with each breath.
- Appropriate alarm parameters set.
- Humidification provided.
- Assessment of level of sedation using an appropriate scoring tool (e.g. COMFORT score).

Respiratory support and airway protection

Oxygen is required by all the cells of the body for effective cellular metabolism. The effects of even short episodes of inadequate oxygenation can be serious, while periods of prolonged hypoxia have potentially irreversible consequences.

The simplest form of respiratory support which can be delivered is oxygen therapy, however oxygen is a very potent medication and is not without complications in certain age groups or in children with chronic lung diseases or with single ventricle anatomy. Changes in the pulmonary parenchyma can occur as a consequence of the toxic effects of oxygen, such as damage to the capillary endothelium, destruction of type I alveolar cells and interstitial oedema. Preterm infants, in particular those born before 37 weeks of gestation, are deemed to be especially vulnerable to the harmful effects of supplementary oxygen therapy (Levene et al. 2008).

Consideration needs to be given to the age and size of the child, in addition to the amount of oxygen required, before deciding on the best method of delivery (Table 4.13).

All supplementary gases should be warmed and humidified prior to delivery to the child. Humidification prevents drying of the airways, potential cilial dysfunction and reduced airway defence (Fassassi et al. 2007), while warming supplementary gases reduces or prevents heat loss, which is especially important in the neonate, and increases the volume of the gas delivered to the lungs. According to Charles' law, when a gas is heated, the molecules move faster and the force exerted by the molecules causes an expansion of the gas volume as the volume of a gas is directly proportional to temperature, assuming pressure is constant. In addition, it is thought that receptors in the nasal mucosa respond to cold and dry gas to elicit a protective bronchoconstrictor response (Fontanari et al. 1996).

Table 4.13 Methods of supplementary oxygen delivery

Method	Age group	Oxygen available (approximate values)
Nasal cannula	Available in sizes for all age groups	30–50%
Simple face mask	Available in sizes for all age ranges	40–50%
Non-rebreathe mask	1 year upwards	98–100%
Head box	<8 months but need to consider size and weight of infant	50–60%
Bucket mask	3 years upwards	30–60%
Vapotherm™	Available in sizes for all age ranges	21–100%

Source: Haines (2009) from Dixon et al. (2009) *Nursing the Highly Dependent Child or Infant: A Manual of Care.* Reproduced with permission from John Wiley and Sons, Ltd.

Non-invasive respiratory support – continuous positive airway pressure (CPAP)

CPAP is usually delivered non-invasively, although it can also be delivered to children with tracheostomies and those who are intubated. Like any intervention there are advantages and disadvantages (Table 4.14) with the therapy and it ultimately does not provide adequate respiratory support to the tiring infant or child. The use of nasal CPAP in infants with bronchiolitis has been shown to decrease respiratory muscle overload and improve symptoms of respiratory distress (Cambonie et al. 2008).

There are a number of CPAP systems available and the therapy is usually delivered through the use of soft silicone nasal prongs or nasal mask in the infant or nasal or face mask in the older child. It is also possible to provide 'long prong' CPAP, making use of a shortened endotracheal tube, measured in the same way as measuring for a nasopharyngeal airway (measure from tip of nose to tragus of the ear) and a simple flow-driven, pressure-cycled ventilator.

Considerations for practice

Careful positioning of the infant may reduce their work of breathing – ensure that the head of the bed is elevated to approximately 30° and the infant is well supported to maintain this position. This will reduce the pressure effects that the intra-abdominal contents may exert on the diaphragm, thus allowing better diaphragmatic expansion during inspiration. If there are no contraindications, then turning the infant prone will also reduce the effects of the compliant chest wall, again reducing the work of breathing. This positioning strategy also helps to reduce the effects of any gastro-oesophageal reflux and has been shown to reduce the infant's energy expenditure (Pryor and Prasad 2002).

It is important to ensure that the calorific needs of the infant are augmented to meet their increased energy demands. Small frequent feeds (e.g. 2-hourly bolus feeds) help to reduce the splinting effects of a full stomach against the diaphragm and should enable the infant to carry on receiving enteral feeds via a naso/orogastric tube. Sometimes, smaller volume feeds are not adequate to satisfy the infant and 3-hourly feeds of larger volumes may be necessary. The decision about feeding strategy should always be based on clinical assessment prior to the infant receiving the feed, assessment of the infant's tolerance during the feed and response at the end of the feed.

The use of sedative agents may be considered to facilitate the provision of CPAP, but their use should only be instituted when non-pharmacological methods, such as swaddling or the use of other comfort measures, have been tried. A small dose of an oral sedative agent such as chloral hydrate may be necessary to reduce distress or intolerance of the CPAP prongs/mask, however it is important that practitioners are familiar with the possible effects of any medications they are administering. Chloral hydrate is particularly effective in the younger patient population (<3 years of age), but its duration is unpredictable and it does have the potential to engender a degree of respiratory depression (Buck 2005).

Although the nasal prongs are made of a soft silicone material the constant pressure they exert can cause mild to severe trauma to the nares and nasal septum. While this is not a common finding in the infant population receiving short-term therapy (<48 hours), reddening of the skin and/ or blanching may be seen even in this patient group if the mask/prongs are poorly fitting or inadequately applied (McCoskey 2008).

Table 4.14 Advantages and disadvantages of CPAP

Advantages	Disadvantages
Non-invasive	Over-distension of alveoli if CPAP > 10 cm
Splints the upper airway, therefore can help manage conditions which cause stridor	Barotrauma
	Increases ventilation–perfusion mismatching
Splints the lower airways and promotes smoother airflow through the bronchioles (e.g. bronchiolitis)	Increases work of breathing if CPAP moves the lung onto flat upper part of the compliance curve
Recruits collapsed alveoli and small airways	Possible increase in air trapping
Decreases intrapulmonary shunting	Increases ICP in children with intracranial hypertension
Decreases $PaCO_2$ and improves PaO_2	Constant increased positive pressure in the thoracic cavity can decrease venous return
Improves lung compliance and decreases work of breathing	Decreases cardiac output
Sedative agents should not be required	Fluid retention secondary to inappropriate anti-diuretic hormone (ADH) release

Airway adjuncts

Oropharyngeal airway

These are commonly known as a Guedel airway and can be used to maintain a patent airway in an emergency, prior to intubation and to facilitate effective bag–valve–mask ventilation after the administration of medications for intubation. As these are rigid plastic airways they should not be used for prolonged periods and should only be used in children or infants with absent gag reflexes. Correct sizing is determined by measuring from the centre of the incisors (or their anticipated position in infants lacking dentition) to the angle of the jaw. Care must be taken when inserting the airway as the rigid plastic structure can cause trauma to the soft oropharynx if significant force is used or the airway is inserted incorrectly.

Nasopharyngeal (NP) airways

These can also be used to maintain a patent airway and are usually well tolerated by infants/children who are awake and have intact cough and gag reflexes. Shortened endotracheal tubes (ETT) or specialised soft silk tubes can be used and should be considered if the NP airway is to be used for a prolonged period. Correct length is determined by measuring from the tip of the nose to the tragus of the ear. If a shortened ETT is being used, then the correct size can be determined by calculating the size of ETT the child would normally require and then measuring as above for the length. Caution must be applied as the insertion of the airway may cause trauma to the friable tissues of the nasopharynx and consequent haemorrhage. Regular assessment of skin integrity around and under any securing tapes, along with inspection of the nares for signs of blanching/redness, as well as assessment of the patency of the airway must be undertaken. The clinical indication for use will determine how often the NP airway is changed. In infants and children with potential airway compromise, tube change should only be undertaken in the presence of a practitioner competent in advanced airway management in case the child decompensates after the indwelling NP airway has been removed.

Laryngeal mask airway

The laryngeal mask is a device for supporting and maintaining the airway without tracheal intubation. It can be used for the administration of inhalation anaesthesia, to help maintain the airway during difficult intubations or for the emergency management of the airway after unsuccessful intubation attempts. Sizing of the LMA is different

Table 4.15 Size guide for laryngeal masks

Calculated size of ETT	Laryngeal mask size
3.5	1
4.5	2
5.0	3
6.0 (cuffed)	4
7.5 (cuffed)	5

from the conventional ETT sizing, but an approximate sizing guide can be used (Table 4.15).

Intubation

Endotracheal intubation may be undertaken for a number of reasons, including elective (e.g. for the provision of general anaesthesia during surgery), but in the PICU the majority are urgent or emergencies. Some of the clinical conditions seen in children necessitating intubation are detailed in Table 4.16.

Clinical indications for intubation regardless of the underlying aetiology include:

- A silent chest.
- Respiratory exhaustion.
- Persistent or worsening acidosis with a pH < 7.2 (not usually indicated in diabetic ketoacidosis).
- Glasgow Coma Scale (GCS) score < 8.
- Poor cardiac output.
- Safe transportation.

Preparation for intubation

Wherever possible, intubation should be undertaken in a controlled manner and if effective bag–valve–mask ventilation is being carried out, then a short period of time can be allocated to safe preparation. It is important to have two practitioners skilled in advanced airway management present where possible in case difficulties are encountered. The use of pre-intubation checklists is becoming more common to ensure that nothing is overlooked which may cause harm to the child during the procedure and to promote effective team working.

Oral intubation is the easier of the two methods and can usually be carried out rapidly with few complications. Disadvantages include the possibility of the child with teeth biting down on the tube, making ventilation and suctioning more difficult and excess oral secretions produced in response to the presence of the ETT make strapping and securing the tube more challenging.

Table 4.16 Clinical conditions in which intubation is indicated

Physiological problem	Possible cause
Upper airway obstruction	Croup
	Epiglottitis
	Bacterial tracheitis
	Foreign body aspiration
	Inhalation injury – house fire/ inhalation of chlorine gas
	Anaphylaxis (rare)
Respiratory failure	Pneumonia
	Bronchiolitis
	Asthma
	Acute respiratory distress syndrome (ARDS)
Respiratory depression	Seizures
	Neurological conditions, e.g. Guillain–Barré
	Poisoning
	Alcohol/drug intoxication
Systemic illness	Sepsis
	Multi-organ dysfunction
	Inborn errors of metabolism (often at initial presentation)
Trauma	Flail chest (rare)
	Penetrating lung injury (rare)
	Isolated head injury (common)
Cardiac	Severe cardiac failure
	Cardiogenic shock
	Cardioversion

Nasal intubation is advantageous as the tube tends to be more comfortable for the child and therefore better tolerated. Securing the tube is easier and the infant can also have a dummy or comforter as there is no risk of the tube being dislodged. However, nasal intubation is less straightforward and carries a greater risk of complications, such as traumatic haemorrhage due to the delicate nature of the tissue in the nasal passages, adenoidal trauma and, in long-term use, chronic sinusitis in the older child. Clinical contraindications for nasal intubation include:

- Basal skull fracture (confirmed or suspected).
- Presence of a cerebrospinal fluid (CSF) leak.

- Presence of clotting disorders, e.g. thrombocytopenia, disseminated intravascular coagulopathy (DIC).
- Nasal and/or mid-face deformities or trauma.

Rapid sequence induction (RSI)

Rapid sequence induction or intubation (both terms are used in the literature) is used when there is an unclear history from the patient or, more commonly in children, where there is a significant risk of gastric content aspiration due to a full stomach prior to intubation, e.g. when the child has been taking oral fluids or has received enteral nutrition prior to the need for intubation and there is insufficient time to ensure that gastric emptying has occurred. Aspiration of an NGT will facilitate gastric emptying but it is not a guarantee that the risk has been negated.

RSI involves pre-oxygenation of the child, the rapid administration of sedative and muscle relaxing agents, the application of cricoid pressure once the child is muscle-relaxed and oral intubation, without delivering positive pressure ventilation breaths before the ETT is inserted. The role of cricoid pressure in preventing regurgitation of gastric contents into the airway is crucial, therefore an experienced practitioner should be nominated for this task alone, and pressure should not be released until instructed to do so by the practitioner undertaking the intubation.

Fibreoptic bronchoscope intubation

The use of a flexible fibreoptic bronchoscope can assist with extremely difficult intubations where the bronchoscope is used to gain a view and then act as a guide over which the ETT can be passed. The bronchoscope is usually threaded through the ETT before the procedure begins and, once the scope has passed through the vocal cords, the ETT can be advanced into place. Accessibility to equipment (particularly out of hours) and the unpredictability of the need for such equipment matched to resource considerations mean that it is not an established routine or standard practice in the United Kingdom.

Intubation risks

The ease or difficulty with which a patient can be intubated can be graded according to the view of the larynx offered to the practitioner under direct laryngoscopy (Cormack and Lehane 1984):

- Grade 1: entire aperture visible (full view of cords).
- Grade 2: posterior arytenoids visible, some of glottic aperture (partial view of cords).
- Grade 3: epiglottis visible (minimal or no view of the cords).

Table 4.17 Clinical conditions predictive of difficult intubations

Condition	Characteristics
Pierre–Robin syndrome	Micrognathia (small lower jaw). Macroglossia (large tongue). Cleft defect of the soft palate.
Treacher–Collins syndrome	Auricular and ocular defects. Malar (zygomatic bone) and mandibular hypoplasia.
Down's syndrome	Poorly developed or absent bridge of the nose. Macroglossia.
Klippel–Feil syndrome	Congenital fusion of a variable number of cervical vertebrae, restriction of neck movement.

Source: Gupta et al. 2005.

- Grade 4: no visible structures (can see the soft palate only).

Grades 3 and 4 predict difficult intubations.

Certain congenital clinical conditions are predictors of potentially difficult intubations as a consequence of the anatomical/structural defects linked to the condition (Table 4.17).

Intubation medications

The aim of intubation medication is for the child to have no pain or awareness of the procedure and to be fully muscle-relaxed, thus reducing the risk of laryngospasm.

Three drug groups are usually required for intubation:

- Analgesics.
- Sedatives.
- Muscle relaxants.

The choice of drug and method of administration will depend on the clinical condition of the child and practitioner preference. Some of the commonly used intravenous intubation drugs are listed in Table 4.18; however it is the responsibility of the practitioner administering them to ensure that the dose is correct for the child. Practitioners should refer to the British National Formulary for Children (BNFc) for further information.

Depolarisation versus non-depolarising agents

Depolarising agents mimic the action of acetylcholine by binding to the post-synaptic membrane of the neuromuscu-

lar junction thus preventing acetylcholine from binding. This is a non-competitive binding. Unlike non-depolarising muscle relaxants they cannot be reversed and recovery is spontaneous (Rees 2005). Non-depolarising agents antagonise the neurotransmitter action of acetylcholine by binding competitively with cholinergic receptor sites on the motor end-plate. This antagonism is inhibited and neuromuscular block reversed by the administration of acetylcholinesterase inhibitors (e.g. neostigmine and pyridostigmine).

For children with *primary airway problems* such as croup, the use of inhalational anaesthetic agents is usually preferred as it is possible to maintain spontaneous breathing under its effects. Should intubation be unsuccessful, it is possible to lighten the child's level of anaesthetic, allowing them to maintain a degree of respiratory function and gas exchange.

Intubation procedure

The equipment required for intubation is discussed in (Table 4.19). A summary of essential checkpoints prior to beginning intubation is detailed in Table 4.20. Historically, non-cuffed ETTs have been used in children <8 years of age to account for the anatomical differences in the child's airway and the possibility of pressure-related mucosal trauma or post-extubation stridor. In recent years, low-pressure high-volume cuffed ETTs have become available for use in this age group. The evidence base for their use in the short term seems to suggest that the incidence of post-extubation stridor is comparable with children intubated with non-cuffed ETTs (Weiss et al. 2009), however there is little evidence relating to the incidence of long-term development of subglottic stenosis. It currently remains the choice of the medical team within the PICU whether to use cuffed ETTs in everyday practice or to reserve their use for selected cases where high airway pressures are anticipated during their intensive care stay, avoiding the need for reintubation because of air leak around the ETT.

Intubation attempts should take a maximum of 30 seconds and, if unsuccessful, the practitioner should withdraw the ETT and recommence bag–valve–mask ventilation and oxygenation. After successful intubation, hand ventilation should recommence while tube placement is confirmed through the following methods:

- Observe the chest for equal, bilateral movement.
- Attach $ETCO_2$ monitoring and assess waveform and reading.
- Auscultate for bilateral equal breath sounds.
- Chest X-ray.

Table 4.18 Commonly used intubation drugs in children

	Single dose	Considerations and notes
Analgesic agents		
Morphine sulphate	100–200 mcg/kg	May cause respiratory depression and hypotension. Causes histamine release and therefore potential bronchospasm.
Fentanyl	2–5 mcg/kg	May cause respiratory depression. Large doses given quickly may cause chest wall rigidity and bradycardia.
Sedatives/Anaesthetic agents		
Midazolam	100 mcg/kg	May cause respiratory depression and hypotension in large doses.
Ketamine	2 mg/kg	Causes increased HR and BP secondary to catecholamine release. May cause increased intracranial pressure as a consequence, so caution required in patients with suspected RICP.
Propofol	1 mg/kg	Excellent short-acting, general-purpose anaesthetic agent, not routinely used in children <3 years. May cause hypotension and bradycardia. Pain on administration.
Thiopentone	5 mg/kg	Causes decrease in cerebral metabolic rate, cerebral blood flow and reduces intracranial pressure. Causes apnoea. Suppresses myocardial performance, which can lead to hypotension.
Muscle relaxants (neuromuscular blockade)		
Suxamethonium	1–2 mg/kg	A depolarising drug with very rapid onset and short duration of action. Causes the release of acetylcholine, which produces vagal responses, the most notable of which is bradycardia. To prevent bradycardia administration of atropine may be considered alongside the first dose and should always be given with a second dose. Its effects cannot be reversed. Contraindicated in burns, crush injuries and renal failure as it promotes the release of potassium, which may cause profound hyperkalaemia and cardiac dysrhythmias/arrhythmias.
Vecuronium	100 mcg/kg	Non-depolarising agent. Longer duration of action; minimal cardiovascular effects. Metabolised by the liver.
Rocuronium	0.6–1.2 mg/kg	Non-depolarising agent. Minimal cardiovascular effects. Has a rapid onset of action and has been used in place of suxamethonium for RSI.
Pancuronium	100 mcg/kg	Non-depolarising agent. Increases HR as a consequence of vagolytic effects which may also increase BP. Metabolised by the liver and the kidneys, therefore should be used with caution in children with hepatic or renal dysfunction.
Atracurium	>2 years of age 0.4–0.5 mg/kg <2 years of age 0.3–0.4 mg/kg	Non-depolarising agent. Minimal cardiovascular effects. Not metabolised by the liver or kidneys.

Table 4.19 Equipment required for intubation

Equipment	Notes
Oxygen source	Ideally this will be from a main supply source. If using cylinder supply, nominate one member of the team to monitor it.
Bagging circuit and face mask (ambu-bag/ Ayres T piece)	Check face mask is appropriate size for the child. Choice of bagging circuit will depend on the individual practitioner however most PICU staff will use the Ayres T piece (open-ended anaesthetic-type circuit).
Laryngoscope	Check handle fit and the type of blade required:[*] • Neonate – small straight blade. • Infant/toddler – small curved blade. • Older child – large curved blade. Check the brightness of the bulb on each blade selected.
Introducer/ Stylette	Introducers may be inserted into the lumen of the ETT to assist with placement; however this must not protrude beyond the tip of the ETT as it will cause trauma to the airway.
Gum elastic bougie	A bougie is a straight, semi-rigid stylette-like device with a bent tip that can be used when intubation is known (or predicted) to be difficult. They are often helpful when the tracheal opening is anterior to the visual field. During laryngoscopy, the bougie is carefully advanced into the larynx and through the cords until the tip enters a main stem bronchus. The ETT can then be passed over the bougie and once in place, the bougie is removed.
Suction source Soft fine-bore suction catheters Yankauer	Ideally this will be from a main wall high pressure source. To calculate the required suction catheter size based on the size of the ETT required simply double the size of ETT, e.g. size 3.5 ETT = size 7Fr suction catheter. To clear secretions from the oropharynx.
Magill's forceps	For nasal intubation.
Guedel airway	Ensure correct size available for the child.
ETTs	When using a cuffed ETT, check that the cuff inflates successfully prior to insertion. ETTs are sized according to their internal diameter. To estimate the size of ETT required, the following formula can be used for infants over 1 year of age[**] *Size* Age (in years) $\div 4 + 4 =$ ETT size (Ensure that there is one size above and one size below the calculated size available) *Length* Oral – age (in years) $\div 2 + 12 =$ length in cm Nasal – age (in years) $\div 2 + 15 =$ length in cm
$ETCO_2$ monitoring	Positive $ETCO_2$ monitoring provides confirmation that the ETT has been correctly placed. Many units now use this method post-intubation and it is standard practice in theatres and emergency care situations.
Stethoscope	
Aqua gel	
Monitoring	The minimal standard of monitoring required is: • ECG. • Non-invasive blood pressure (NIBP). • Saturations (SpO_2). • $ETCO_2$.

Table 4.19 (*Continued*)

Equipment	Notes
Tape/ties	The chosen method of securing ETTs will depend on the individual unit's preference.
Skin protector	
Nasogastric tube (NGT)	Gastric decompression is usually necessary after intubation; the insertion of a nasogastric tube will allow this. Always check the NGT position on chest X-ray before using for enteral feeding.

*The choice of blade is ultimately that of the practitioner undertaking the procedure but is governed by the anatomy of the younger child. In infants < 1 year, the epiglottis is large and projects more posteriorly into the airway making the view more difficult. The straight blade is designed to pass over the whole of the epiglottis, moving it completely out of the way and therefore improving the view. Straight blades may be used up to the age of 5 years. As the child's airway matures, the epiglottis becomes smaller in comparison and assumes the same position as that found in adult anatomy. The curved blade used for these patients is designed to sit in the vallecula (just short of the epiglottis) and the upward lift of the blade moves the epiglottis out of view.

**Tube sizes in neonates are based on weight. Below 2 kg is not identified here; refer to local neonatal intensive care guidelines and protocols (Kattwinkel et al. 2010).

2 kg Size 3.0 ETT 7–8 cm at the lips

3 kg Size 3.5 ETT 8–9 cm at the lips

>3 kg Size 3.5–4.0 ETT 9–10 cm at the lips

Table 4.20 Key checkpoints prior to intubation.

- Oxygen on and working.
- Suction on and working.
- Stomach empty.
- Monitoring on and working.
- Laryngoscope light on and bright.
- Working access (IV or IO).
- All equipment readily at hand (including spares).
- Emergency drugs and volume to hand.
- All personnel aware of individual roles.
- Child and family prepared (where possible).

Once the position is confirmed, secure the ETT at the calculated desired length according to unit policy. Many units use Elastoplast™ or similar adhesive fabric tape to secure ETTs in infants and young children, while in the older child/adolescent white twill/cotton tape ties may be utilised. There are also a number of commercially available fixation devices, but again their use will be determined by local policy. Care should be taken to protect the skin to reduce the risk of epidermal stripping through contact with strong adhesives.

The complications associated with intubation may occur at any time during the intubation event and while many strategies have been put in place to minimise the risk to the child, there are occasions where adverse events will occur. These include blunt airway trauma, damage to dentition, hypoxia, oesophageal intubation, right/left main-stem bronchus intubation, vocal cord damage and exacerbation of cervical spine injury.

Tracheostomies

Some children require the formation of a tracheostomy to maintain a patent airway and help facilitate long-term ventilation. Most tracheostomies in children are elective surgical procedures involving an incision made below the cricoid cartilage through which a tube is inserted into the trachea through the 2nd and 4th tracheal rings. There is a variety of tracheostomy tubes available so it important to be aware of the differences between manufacturers' sizing, particularly in terms of tube length. Customised tracheostomy tubes can be ordered from manufacturers according to the individual child's needs. As with ETTs, tracheostomy tubes may be uncuffed or cuffed.

It is usual practice for the first tracheostomy tube to remain insitu for a week postoperatively, after which it is electively changed, normally by the ENT team responsible for the care of the child. The purpose of this delay is to allow time to promote healing of the surgical incision and for the stoma to form completely. 'Stay sutures' (stitches brought out from the sides of the wound and taped to the child's chest) are usually used to hold the edges of the stoma apart, maintaining stoma patency, and these are removed at the time of first tube change.

Consideration for practice

Securing the tracheostomy is usually done using either white twill cotton ties or Velcro™ fixation devices. Each unit will have its own policy and preferences for the type of material used. In the immediate postoperative period, cotton ties are used. With due care and attention these can be changed before the first tube change if they are blood-stained or soiled, however this should be done under medical or senior nursing staff supervision if possible. It is important that the tracheostomy tube is well secured to prevent accidental displacement, but the tapes should not be too tight as this has the potential to cause chafing and eventual breakdown of the skin.

Assessment of skin integrity should be undertaken at least twice a day, however this may need to be increased if there are any concerns about the skin surrounding the stoma or underneath the tapes/ties used to secure the tube.

The type of dressings used will depend on local unit policy or preference, for example, Lyofoam™ absorbent dressings designed to protect the skin underneath the tracheostomy tube phalanges from undue pressure and to keep the skin around the stoma dry. Dressings should be changed at least daily, and more often if wet or soiled.

When suctioning the child's tracheostomy tube, it is important to suction to a maximum of 0.5 cm beyond the length of the tube to avoid causing suction-related trauma to the airway beyond this.

Principles of ventilation

Children in PICU undergo multiple invasive interventions, such as line insertion, renal replacement therapy and placement of invasive monitoring lines, all of which are geared towards supporting the child until organ function or recovery occurs rather than curing the disease itself. Similarly, intubation and mechanical ventilation do not cure illness but facilitate the provision of intensive care and/or support the respiratory system while lung tissue and gas exchange recover. Mechanical ventilation is not without risk and the potential side-effects on the lungs include acute lung injury secondary to forces exerted by positive pressure ventilation, oxygen toxicity and the development of nosocomial infections (ventilator-associated or acquired pneumonia – VAP). In addition, adverse events (e.g. equipment malfunction) add to the potential harm a child may suffer secondary to this intervention.

Types of ventilation

Ventilation can be either positive or negative pressure, invasive or non-invasive. Determinants of ventilation will depend on the individual child and their underlying disease pathology or indication for ventilation. The practitioner is required to make a number of decisions when determining a ventilatory strategy for the child, based on the current clinical assessment and expected normal values for the age of the child. Ventilators vary in their methods of accessing the settings; the basic underlying settings of any ventilatory mode are highlighted in Table 4.21. It is important to achieve synchronicity or a smooth interaction between the ventilator and the child and wherever possible to maintain the child's own respiratory effort, if the child's clinical condition allows this.

Negative-pressure ventilation

This is not widely used in the paediatric critical care setting as its delivery can be problematic, although some units do have experience of its use. Historically, negative-pressure ventilation is associated with the 'iron lung', first used in the management of polio in children in 1928 in the United States at the Children's Hospital, Boston. During the worldwide epidemics of the 1950s these basic respiratory support devices were widely used in all age groups and continue to be used by some adults to this day. Smaller, more portable devices, such as the Hayek Cuirass™, have been available for a number of years and as a therapy it has been used successfully in patients with neuromuscular degenerative disorders (e.g. Duchenne's muscular dystrophy or spinal muscular atrophy – SMA) as well as in children post-cardiac surgery in whom the increased intrathoracic pressures seen with positive-pressure ventilation can significantly alter blood flow to the pulmonary circuit (e.g. post-Fontan procedure). Today this mode of ventilation has developed further and is known as biphasic cuirass ventilation rather than negative-pressure ventilation; however, it does mimic the action of normal respiration rather than exerting a positive pressure while assisting with respiratory effort.

Positive-pressure ventilation (PPV)

This can be delivered as a non-invasive support or as an invasive procedure following endotracheal intubation or formation of tracheostomy. Positive-pressure ventilation works on a simple basis – the ventilator causes alveolar ventilation by generating a positive pressure at the proximal airway which exceeds the alveolar pressure, thus creating a pressure gradient. This gradient forces gas to flow

Table 4.21 Basic ventilation parameters

Setting	Notes and considerations
Inspiratory time	Spontaneous inspiratory time is determined by lung compliance, airway resistance and flow rate. Settings for the inspiratory time on the ventilator mimic those anticipated in the well child – shortest in the neonate, gradually increasing with age: • Pre-term infants 0.3–0.5 seconds. • Full-term newborns – 0.5–0.7 seconds. • Infants/young children – 0.6–0.8 seconds. • Older children/adolescents – 1.0 second. Children with poor compliance ('stiff lungs') or those with narrowed airways may require long inspiratory times than may be anticipated for their age.
Peak inspiratory pressure (PIP)	The main factors that determine PIP are lung compliance, airway resistance, inspiratory time and tidal volume. Minimising PIP to avoid volutrauma is part of a lung protective strategy.
Positive end expiratory pressure (PEEP)	PEEP is applied at the end of expiration to maintain FRC and therefore maintain alveolar recruitment preventing areas of collapse developing in the lungs.
Tidal volume (V_t)	Tidal volumes should reflect expected tidal volumes for the spontaneously breathing child. As previously noted, tidal volume is constant at 6–8 ml/kg throughout life and the ventilator settings should aim to achieve this. In certain modes the V_t can be set, e.g. volume control (VC) or pressure-regulated volume control (PRVC). Increasing V_t over normal values will lead to hyperinflation and may cause a pneumothorax.
Inspiratory flow	In a spontaneously breathing child, flow rates and patterns are more variable than in the older child/adolescent in whom a more constant flow is typical. It is possible to adjust flow rate and pattern settings on most ventilators to optimise alveolar ventilation and improve patient comfort. Types of flow pattern include sinusoidal, decelerating and constant. Sinusoidal is the flow pattern seen in patients receiving CPAP. Decelerating flow patterns are seen in pressure-targeted ventilation – the majority of the flow is delivered on initiation of the breath with the remainder being delivered more slowly during the rest of the inspiratory phase which enhances oxygen distribution to alveoli.
Mean airway pressure (MAP)	MAP is the average airway pressure measured at the proximal airway from one inspiration to the beginning of the next. This value will vary according to the mode of ventilation used, e.g. in a pressure-controlled mode it will be an essentially static value, whereas in a pressure-regulated or volume-controlled mode it will be more variable. Factors that influence MAP include tidal volume, PIP, flow rate, respiratory rate and end expiratory pressure.

into the lungs. Expiration is essentially a passive process that occurs when the ventilator stops exerting the positive pressure (end of inspiration).

There is an increased risk of iatrogenic lung damage with positive-pressure mechanical ventilation because of children's developmental and anatomical differences:

• Increased chest wall compliance provides less protection against ventilator induced lung injury (VILI), especially if pressure-cycled ventilation leads to large tidal volumes.

• Concentrations of lung elastin (which correlates with the elastic recoil of the lung) are lower in children than in adults.

• Concentrations of lung collagen (which is associated with structural integrity of the lung) are lower in children compared to adults.

• An inverse relationship of chest wall compliance and the risk of microvascular damage with mechanical ventilation may lead to increased pulmonary oedema in the younger child/infant with higher chest wall compliance.

Each brand of ventilator has slightly different modes/terms used and it is the responsibility of the practitioner to become familiar with the ventilators used in their unit.

Non-invasive PPV (NIPPV)

As the name suggests, this is advantageous as it avoids the need for intubation with its associated risks. As a therapy it can be used in both the short and longer term and can be used to support children for whom intubation significantly increases their mortality and morbidity risk (Najaf-Zadeh and Leclerc 2011). In addition, NIPPV can be used very effectively as a weaning tool following a period of invasive ventilation, particularly in children with muscle weakness or those with acquired or congenital immune deficiency.

NIPPV provides two levels of support by delivering both inspiratory and expiratory positive pressure. The most commonly used mode of NIPPV in the acute setting is Bi-phasic Positive Airway Pressure (BiPAP) which is a form of CPAP that alternates between high and low positive airway pressures, permitting inspiration (and expiration) throughout. It reduces the work of breathing, improves alveolar ventilation and splints the alveoli open during the expiratory phase.

Characteristics of NIPPV ventilation

- Triggered or timed pressure-limited ventilation, combined with PEEP/CPAP.
- Permits spontaneous breathing during inspiration and expiration maintaining constant pressures.
- PIP, PEEP, rate, trigger sensitivity and inspiratory flow are set by operator.
- NIPPV ventilators can compensate for large leaks associated with the masks used for delivery of therapy.

One of the most important features of successful NIPPV is a well-fitting mask for effective delivery. Different types of mask are available, from small nasal masks, masks covering the nose and mouth, to full face masks and helmets, however finding a mask that fits well can be challenging in the infant/toddler age group. The consequences of a poorly fitting mask can be significant, causing pressure sores, especially on the bridge of the nose, and in long-term use this pressure can lead to mid-third facial deformities (Faroux et al. 2005).

Contraindications to NIPPV

- Severe hypoxaemia.
- Inadequate airway, e.g. croup/burns.
- Cardiovascular instability.

- Presence of a pneumothorax.
- Recent upper gastrointestinal surgery.

Considerations for practice – management of the child receiving NIPPV

The child's mask should be released every two hours to avoid the risk of pressure sores developing. Particular attention should be paid to the areas such as the bridge of the nose and the forehead as these are prone to pressure ulceration. In addition, the child's face should be washed and dried at the time of mask removal as constant contact with the mask can make the skin sweat.

Frequent eye care is required to reduce potential irritation from the leak around the mask and careful attention to oral hygiene is also necessary as the mucous membranes of the mouth can become dry and easily irritated.

The nature of NIPPV means that the child is at risk of increased of gastric distension therefore an oro-/nasogastric tube should be sited and aspirated every 2 hours along with mask care. Alternatively, if the child has a gastrostomy, this should be aspirated 2-hourly to minimise diaphragmatic splinting.

Invasive positive-pressure ventilation

Ventilation modes may be defined by the type of breath (mandatory or synchronised) based on patient effort and the amount of support delivered with any spontaneous breaths initiated (Table 4.22).

High frequency oscillatory (oscillation) ventilation (HFOV)

This ventilatory support is utilised when the child is unresponsive to conventional ventilation strategies. Historically, it was used as a treatment of last resort but it has in recent years gained a place in everyday practice. It is a useful alternative which may be used in combination with nitric oxide therapy for children who reach the referral criteria for extracorporeal membrane oxygenation (ECMO).

Indications for use in PIC include:

- Acute lung injury secondary to aspiration.
- Acute lung injury secondary to pulmonary infection.
- Severe sepsis.
- Smoke inhalation injury.
- Acute respiratory distress syndrome.
- Near-drowning.
- Prevention of barotrauma in children with severe restrictive lung disease.

Table 4.22 Ventilation modes in IPPV

Mode	Notes
Controlled or mandatory • Continuous mandatory ventilation (CMV) • Intermittent positive-pressure ventilation (IPPV) • Pressure control (PC) • Volume control (VC) • Pressure-regulated volume control (PRVC)	Suitable for the child who is apnoeic, e.g. use of muscle relaxants. All the breaths are ventilator breaths and the cycling is usually time-regulated. Can be pressure or volume-limited. All settings are controlled by the operator. Most suitable if deficiency in gas exchange is so severe that other modes are unable to achieve adequate ventilation and/or oxygenation.
Assist control	The ventilator delivers pre-set breaths in coordination with the respiratory effort of the patient. With each inspiratory effort, the ventilator delivers a full assisted tidal volume. Spontaneous breathing independent of the ventilator between the A/C breaths however is not enabled.
Synchronised • Synchronised intermittent mandatory ventilation (SIMV) • SIMV, PC and PS • SIMV, VC and PS • SIMV, PRVC and PS	The ventilator delivers a set number of breaths per minute but, unlike mandatory modes, these are synchronised breaths triggered by child's inspiratory effort. If the child makes no respiratory effort, the ventilator will continue to deliver the set breaths per minute. The size of breath (PIP or V_t), inspiration time, trigger sensitivity and rate are set by the operator. Inspiration is initiated when the child generates a small inspiratory gas flow or a small negative pressure in the ventilator tubing. This mode is often used in combination with pressure support which is a peak pressure above PEEP delivered to support breaths taken over the set breath rate. This level of support can be adjusted to increase or decrease the child's respiratory effort according to their clinical condition.
Pressure support • Pressure support (PS) • PS and CPAP	The ventilator supports every spontaneous breath with positive pressure during inspiration. The operator determines the level of support delivered with each breath. In the PS mode, there may be no back-up rate on the ventilator if the child tires, therefore it is often used in conjunction with SIMV. This mode decreases the work of breathing but allows the child to exercise inspiratory muscles. The combination of PS and CPAP ensures that the child receives end expiratory pressure in addition to inspiratory pressure support.

Improving oxygenation without increasing FiO_2
• Increase mean airway pressure (MAP).
• Increase PEEP.
• Increase PIP.
• Increase inspiration: expiration (I:E) ratio.
• Increase inspiratory flow rate (decrease rise time).

Decreasing $PaCO_2$
• Increase ventilator rate.
• Increase tidal volume either directly or by increasing PIP.

Principles of HFOV (Table 4.23)

The ventilator uses a diaphragm or piston to deliver oscillating pressure to the airway and drive a volume of gas into the lungs at a frequency of 60–3600/min (1–60 Hz). Exhalation is active as a consequence of the piston/diaphragm oscillations rather than passive and this has two benefits: first, it reduces the risk of air trapping, and second, it facilitates CO_2 clearance. The V_t delivered during each oscillation is ≤ anatomic dead-space and is approximately 1–3 ml.

Considerations for practice

In essence there are very few differences between the care of the child receiving conventional ventilation and the child receiving HFOV. A couple of points worthy of mention are:

- Suctioning – The use of a closed or in-line suction system is advocated to prevent alveolar derecruitment for patients with higher MAPs. Some units will use the in-line suction system with all their patients, while others reserve them for patients on HFOV. Some units routinely take the child off the oscillator once every 24 hours, hand ventilate and use that opportunity to provide deep suction using the open suction technique, however this practice is not supported by evidence and therefore cannot be advocated as regular practice. Effective humidification and the well-judged use of 0.9% sodium chloride through the instillation port on the suction system may have less of a detrimental effect on arterial oxygenation than the derecruitment associated with disconnection from the oscillator.

- Tubing management – The inflexible nature of the oscillator tubing makes repositioning the child receiving HFOV slightly more challenging than other children. It is prudent to have one practitioner allocated specifically to managing the child's tube to prevent accidental extubation during position changes. In addition, the child is at greater risk of pressure being exerted on the nares (if nasally intubated) or the corner of the mouth (if orally intubated) as it is more difficult to position the tubing of the oscillator to maintain a straight line between the machine and the child's ETT.

The best form of respiratory support, therefore, is one that gives the greatest chance of survival with the least risk

Table 4.23 HFOV parameter settings

Parameter	Notes
Mean airway pressure (MAP) Initial setting – 3–5 times higher than MAP on conventional ventilator, then reduce as able to avoid over-expansion	The MAP determines the degree of lung expansion and FRC. As such it is the principal mechanism for regulating oxygenation. It is important to avoid over-expansion, which will increase the resistance to gas flow, or under-expansion, which will cause areas of atelectasis. This must therefore be reviewed with a chest X-ray.
Power amplitude (ΔP) Initial setting – 35–45	This regulates the tidal volume by determining the amplitude (the amount of movement with each oscillation) of the piston. There is no magic formula that predicts the correct ΔP but initial settings are usually based on a clinical impression of the adequacy of chest 'wobble' or 'bounce' achieved with the set ΔP. Usual settings vary between 30 and 80 although higher settings may well be required based on blood gas analysis.
Frequency • Neonates 10 Hz • Older child 4–8 Hz	The frequency (in Hz) is similar to setting a rate on the conventional ventilator but it also directly influences V_t. Along with the ΔP, CO_2 clearance is determined by the frequency setting. Unlike conventional ventilation, to increase CO_2 clearance the frequency should be reduced or the ΔP increased.
Inspiratory time	As the oscillator can deliver up to 600 oscillations/min it is not possible to set an inspiratory time as used in conventional ventilation. An inspiratory time of 33% is most commonly used as setting higher than this (e.g. 50%) would not allow sufficient time for the expiration phase and air trapping would occur.

of long-term damage to other organs (Table 4.24). In order to facilitate this, targets for parameters, such as blood carbon dioxide levels, may be altered to prevent secondary lung damage (e.g. adopting a 'permissive hypercapnia' ventilation strategy). Examples of target parameters are detailed in Table 4.25.

Studies continue into the use of a permissive hypercapnia strategy, with discussion focusing on the possible detrimental effects, as well as its protective role in lung injury (Ijland et al. 2010; Laffey et al. 2009) and it is clear from the published literature, most of which is in the adult field, that it should not be used in isolation but should form part of a general lung protective strategy, including the use of reduced tidal volumes, effective lung recruitment and appropriate use of PEEP to prevent alveolar collapse at end expiration (Albuali et al. 2007; Matthay and Calfee 2005; Petrucci and Iacovelli 2007).

Acute lung injury or ventilator-induced lung injury (VILI) secondary to mechanical ventilation can occur in one of two phases of each mechanical breath delivered (Figure 4.8). The difficulty encountered when deciding on a ventilation strategy is finding the 'sweet spot', or the point at which all atelectatic alveoli are open and able to participate in ventilation without overextending the alveoli

Table 4.24   Clinical implications of positive pressure ventilation (PPV)

Body system	Effects
Cardiovascular	PPV causes a drop in cardiac output because: • Increased intrathoracic pressure decreases right atrial filling. • Pulmonary circulation is affected by changes in lung volume and this in turn affects right ventricular filling and afterload. • Left atrial filling is affected by increased pulmonary vascular resistance. • Left ventricular preload and afterload are affected by changes in intrathoracic pressure. • The increased pleural pressure generated by PPV decreases LV transmural pressure, which decreases cardiac output. Changes in lung volume and PVR are the major influences on variation in left ventricular output.
Neurological	PPV can exert significant effects on cerebral perfusion: • Decreased cardiac output can affect blood pressure and therefore cerebral perfusion pressure. • Increased intrathoracic pressure can impede systemic vascular return from the cerebral circulation and therefore and increase intracranial pressure. • Over-ventilation, which decreases CO_2, can cause cerebral vasoconstriction. The effects are normally overcome by cerebral autoregulation, but this is affected by neurological injury and compensation may not occur.
Renal	The effects of PPV on the renal system are complicated and linked to the effects exerted on the cardiovascular system: • Reduced glomerular filtration can occur as a consequence of lower blood pressure and reduced renal perfusion. • Reduced right atrial filling stimulates release of atrial natriuretic peptide, which increases water retention. • Increased ADH secretion (through sympathetic activity) increases water retention. • Increased aldosterone secretion increases reabsorption of sodium and water.
Gastrointestinal	• Abdominal and intestinal distension can occur due to ventilation and air swallowing. • Reduced cardiac output can effect splanchnic/mesenteric (gut) perfusion. • High PEEP may directly increase intra-abdominal pressure, which will reduce perfusion to the gastrointestinal tract. • Hepatic perfusion is affected by reduced cardiac output and increased hepatic venous pressure secondary to the increased intrathoracic pressures generated by PPV.

Table 4.25 Parameter targets for lung protective ventilation

	Normal	Targets to minimise lung damage
pH	7.35–7.45	>7.25
$PaCO_2$	35–45 mmHg	<80 mmHg
	4.5–5.5 kPa	<10.5 kPa
PaO_2	>80 mmHg	$FiO_2 < 50\%$
	10.5 kPa	
PIP		<35 cmH$_2$O
PEEP		5–15 cmH$_2$O

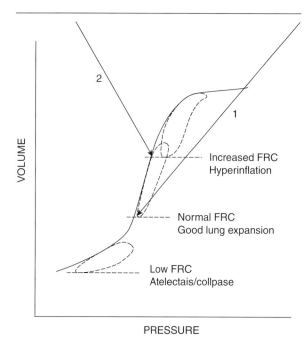

Figure 4.8 Ventilation curve with lower and upper inflection points.

to the point at which compliance decreases and gas exchange is compromised (Froese 1997; Matthews and Noviski 2001). These two points are referred to in the literature as the lower inflection point (LIP) and the upper inflection point (UIP).

On the ventilation curve of each breath the area below the LIP (Figure 4.8, no.1) is the zone of derecruitment and alveolar atelectasis, while the area above the UIP (Figure 4.8, no.2) is the zone of over-distension and potential

alveolar rupture. Pressure and volume both contribute to achieving the 'safe window zone'; therefore each can contribute to over-distension or derecruitment, both of which can have adverse effects.

There are a number of different processes through which damage to the lung tissues can occur during mechanical ventilation and practitioners should be mindful of these when considering ventilation strategies.

Barotrauma usually occurs as a consequence of alternating high pressures being exerted inside the alveolar sacs, which leads to over-distension of the walls and eventual rupture of the sacs. Consequences include:

- Air leaking into the pleural space.
- Air leaking into interstitial space (pulmonary interstitial emphysema).
- Tearing at the broncho-alveolar junction as lung is recruited and then allowed to collapse as the pressure drops at the beginning of expiration.

Volutrauma is caused by 'cycling' of the lung (change in surface area associated with altering volumes of gas within the alveolar sacs), independent of the pressures required to move air into the lungs. The forces exerted on the individual cells within the wall of the alveolus have some significant effects during this phase:

- Altered surfactant function which contributes to the promotion of atelectasis.
- Increase in the capillary leak of proteinaceous material which contributes to areas of consolidation and or atelectasis.

Stretch injury occurs as a consequence of both the pressure and volumes being used in mechanical ventilation. Alteration in the capillary transmural pressures causes structural defects in the capillary walls, which in turn eventually cause a breakdown in the capillary endothelium and epithelium. Widening gaps in the walls of the capillaries allow proteinaceous material to leak across, promoting atelectasis.

Biotrauma occurs as a result of damage to the lung parenchyma and as a consequence of the localised inflammatory responses seen in these areas of damage. The release of certain inflammatory mediators causes ongoing damage to the cells of the capillaries and the alveolar sacs themselves. Some of the inflammatory mediators implicated include:

- Interleukins.
- Tumour necrosis factor (TNF).

- Endothelin.
- Bradykinin.
- Histamine.
- Thromboxane A_2.
- Complement system.
- Oxygen-free radicals.

It is important to note that while VILI is usually associated with invasive mechanical ventilation, it can also manifest in children receiving non-invasive mechanical ventilation and careful consideration should be given to the strategies employed when managing this group of children.

Ventilator-associated pneumonia

Ventilator-associated (acquired) pneumonia (VAP) is widely acknowledged as a contributor to morbidity and mortality in intensive care as well as increasing length of stay with the associated costs this generates (Melsen et al. 2009; Richardson et al. 2010; Sevketoglu and Karabocuoglu 2007). VAP is well documented in the adult population in terms of both mortality and morbidity, and prevention of VAP is one of the key high-impact intervention priorities of the 'Saving Lives' initiative instituted by the Department of Health in general ICUs in 2005. In PIC, this is an area that is only recently receiving the attention it merits and many centres have introduced care bundles (extrapolated from the adult care bundle) aimed at reducing the incidence of VAP. Venkatachalam et al. (2011) note the challenges of producing data are due in the main to the problematic diagnosis. They note that clinical, radiological and microbiological criteria lack the sensitivity and specificity relative to autopsy, histopathology and culture, and there is a lack of consistency in the application of diagnostic criteria within the published studies. Although the evidence base seems limited in paediatrics, the principles of care outlined in the care bundle are inherently good practice standards. As they are not costly to implement they should be used in daily clinical practice.

Clinical indicators of VAP

There is no generally accepted definition of VAP in mechanically ventilated patients, but it is often defined as pneumonia that develops 48 hours or more after intubation with either an ETT or a tracheostomy tube and that was not present before intubation. Definite diagnosis, as noted above, may not be straightforward because there are no firm diagnostic criteria for VAP; it is generally diagnosed therefore on the basis of clinical signs: fever not attribut- able to other causes, chest X-ray changes consistent with infective processes and microbiological confirmation.

Interventions to minimise the incidence of VAP

There are four key interventions identified within the adult population which include deep vein thrombosis (DVT) prophylaxis. This needs to be a consideration for the older child/adolescent in PIC, however each unit will have its own policy and guidelines and practice will be determined by these. The evidence base for DVT prophylaxis in young children is not established. The most frequently identified interventions and general management of the ventilated child are detailed in Table 4.26.

Extracorporeal membrane oxygenation

Extracorporeal membrane oxygenation (ECMO) has been one of the most exciting developments to have taken place in critical care. It is a relatively simple circuit which is primed with a compatible group of blood to the child. When the child is cannulated and attached to the circuit oxygen-deficient blood is conveyed to perfuse through an oxygenator before being returned to the child. Although ECMO has been refined since it was first introduced into the United Kingdom in the late 1980s, the general principles today are the same as those first used.

ECMO is needed because there are a small but significant number of critically ill infants and children who fail to respond to maximum ventilator therapy and pharmacological support. Typically, this group become more and more hypoxic and either die or survive with damaged lungs and neurological deficit. ECMO support buys time and allows the lungs to rest and recover (Harvey and Crawford, in press). ECMO is not a therapy to delay the dying process in any of the age ranges or avert an outcome of death regardless of quality of life. ECMO will not be considered if there has been major neurological insult; the child has a lethal malformation, uncontrollable coagulopathy or has been on ventilation for so long that the probability of lung recovery is unlikely. (See also Chapter 5.)

Examples of ECMO indications

In neonates

ECMO is suitable for use in the newborn of 35 or more weeks' gestation for conditions such as persistent pulmonary hypertension either primary or secondary to other treatable pathology. These range from respiratory distress syndrome (RDS) to overwhelming sepsis, pneumonia and massive barotrauma rendering management on conventional ventilation impossible. It is also used for meconium aspiration syndrome (MAS) which has remained

Table 4.26 Care of the ventilated child to minimise VAP

Intervention	Notes and considerations
Elevation of the head of the bed	All children should be nursed at an angle of 30–45° unless there is a clinical reason not to (e.g. spinal injuries). Studies in the adult population indicate a lower incidence of VAP in those nursed in the semi-recumbent position versus those nursed supine. In practice it is extremely difficult to achieve a 45° angle, therefore the range of 30–45° is noted (NICE and the National Patient Safety Agency 2008). It is thought that this helps to prevent the aspiration of secretions from the oropharynx which are implicated in the VAP process (Peace 2007).
Daily muscle relaxant holds	In those patients who are on infusions of muscle-relaxing agents, these should be stopped daily until there is evidence that it has worn off. In addition, sedation should be reviewed every morning to ensure accumulation is not occurring and adding to an increased number of ventilator days.
Appropriate humidification of inspired gases	Adequate humidification of inspired gases ensures that secretions are easier to clear from the ETT, particularly in the infant/child with a weak cough.
Appropriate ventilator tubing management	Prevents the condensate from the ventilator tubing entering the lower respiratory tract. Changing tubing sets according to the manufacturer's guidelines (or more frequently if soiled) reduces the risk of lower respiratory tract colonisation with pathogens likely to cause VAP.
Suctioning of respiratory secretions with good technique	Regular effective suctioning of the ETT/tracheostomy using a clean technique may help to prevent the accumulation of pathogens thought to contribute to the development of VAP.
Oral hygiene practice	Good oral hygiene practices have been identified as one of the key factors in the prevention of VAP. Deep oropharyngeal suction prior to ETT suctioning is advocated alongside robust oral hygiene practices, including the use of oral assessment tools and frequent mouth care. Some authors advocate the use of chlorhexidine solution and many of the pre-prepared oral hygiene packs now contain this. However, caution should be taken with the use of chlorhexidine solution in the neonatal/infant population due to its strength and most neonatal units continue to use sterile water instead. When carrying out oral hygiene consideration must be given to children with clotting disorders or those with mucositis.
Gastric ulcer prophylaxis	There is no evidence base for the prevention of gastric ulcers in children. Many units use non-nutritive feeds (e.g. 5 ml milk via oro-/nasogastric tube 3-hourly) to minimise potential gastric mucosal irritation. The use of ranitidine is advocated in some literature, however local policy will determine the individual practitioner's approach.

the greatest indication for non-adult ECMO in the United Kingdom with 50.6% of ECMO applications (Brown et al. 2010).

- Selectively with congenital diaphragmatic hernia.
- Selectively with congenital cardiac abnormalities.
- Selectively with cardiomyopathy.

Children and young people

Indicators for paediatric use include pneumonia, near-drowning, sepsis and other reversible conditions which have made the child non-responsive to maximum ventilator therapy including HFOV and nitric oxide. For the adolescent, young person and adult use, the reasons for need are more varied. ECMO can be considered for any reversible pulmonary disease, trauma or insult. Its usefulness was demonstrated during the 2009–10 H1N1 epidemic (Harvey and Crawford, in press).

- Reversible pulmonary disease, trauma or insult.
- Selectively following inhaled smoke inhalation (house fires).

- Selectively following inhaled foreign bodies.
- Selectively as part of the management of cardiac conditions.

Clinical indicators

- Clinical picture and assessment of the balance of risk between conventional management and the need for the rescue therapy.
- Oxygen index (OI) >40 on two or more arterial blood gas measurements.
- PaO_2 < 40 mmHg or 5.3 kPa for 4 hours in 100% O_2.
- Intractable metabolic acidosis.
- Intractable shock.
- Progressive, intractable pulmonary or cardiac failure.
- Inability to come off cardiopulmonary bypass at operation.

Clinical application

Clinical application is most commonly by way of veno-arterial (VA) cannulation or veno-veno (VV) cannulation. In VA cannulation deoxygenated blood is taken out of the venous system by way of a line in the right atrium via the right internal jugular vein. The return of oxygenated blood is via the right common carotid artery into the aortic arch. This method has the ability to support cardiac function as well as oxygenation, so in the very sickest of neonates and young children this is the method of choice. However, it is not without complications; for example, the repair of such small vessels can be difficult so the vessel may be tied off and this leads to changes in the way the brain is perfused. In VV cannulation a venous exit route, such as the vena cava, is used and the blood is either returned to the child via the same blood vessel using a dual lumen cannula or blood is removed via the inferior vena cava and returned using a second insert point, such as the femoral vein. Significant improvements may be seen in VV ECMO because of the benefits of good oxygenation and CO_2 removal and improvements in the blood gas results.

While on ECMO the child has serial chest X-rays to monitor their progress. Pulmonary ventilation continues at rest settings appropriate for the size of the child. This acts as physiotherapy for the lungs and helps to remove CO_2. The physiotherapy team see the child several times a day and provide therapy which conditions the lungs in preparation for when the ECMO support is weaned and a trial off the circuit takes place after which, if successful, the child is decannulated.

Suctioning the artificial airway

Suctioning is the technique used to clear the airways of a child who is unable to do this for themselves (Knox 2011). It is not a routine procedure and indications that a child requires this include audible secretions, visual secretions and a distressed and uncomfortable child struggling to cough and diminished breath sounds (Ireton 2007). When an arterial line is in situ a change in the blood gas results which indicate that CO_2 is being trapped. Whenever possible it is preferable not to break the ventilator circuit and make use of an inline suctioning port. There are clear benefits in keeping an intubated child's airway clear, particularly where small diameter endotracheal tubes are used. The procedure should be performed with care using a catheter no more than half the diameter of the ETT (Biarent et al. 2010) and the minimal amount of negative pressure which is effective in aspirating the secretions employed. Catheters should be measured so that they go only to the end of the ETT to avoid possible trauma to the bifurcation of the trachea. The process should be performed smoothly and swiftly with an aim to avoid any corkscrewing and jabbing actions. Suctioning is not without risks and potential complications.

Risks of poor suction technique

- Sudden collapse.
- Bradycardia.
- Desaturation.
- Hypoxia.
- Hypo- or hypertensive incident.
- Arrhythmia.
- Bronchospasm.
- Airways stimulated to make more secretions.
- VAP.
- Trauma.

One of the longer-running controversies in PIC is the use of 0.9% sodium chloride in ETT management. Historically, 0.9% sodium chloride has been used to assist with maintaining ETT patency and secretion removal. It is, however, a controversial practice, with evidence from as far back as 1999 (Blackwood 1999) suggesting that it may well be detrimental to the patient in terms of gas exchange, in particular arterial oxygenation levels, after its use. The majority of studies have been carried out in the adult population, but Riding et al. (2003) suggest that this detrimental effect is also seen in children. Included in these effects are increased intracranial pressure, nosocomial infections and cardiovascular instability (Celik and Kanan 2006) and current recommendations advocate use only after careful assessment and evaluation of the child's response.

More recent studies have explored the use of 0.9% sodium chloride in the prevention of VAP and in one small study it was found to be significant in the reduction of VAP in an adult population (Caruso et al. 2009). Additional factors to be considered include the level of sedation utilised and the effects this may have on the child's ability to cough as well as the infant/child's physiological response to decreased oxygen levels. What is clear from the evidence base is that there is a dearth of evidence from the PIC population and further studies are needed to continue advocating the routine use of 0.9% sodium chloride in the management of tube patency in intubated children.

Weaning and extubation

There is no easy way to predict how long a child's course of ventilation will be and weaning of mechanical ventilation will be determined by resolution of the underlying disease process, improvement in gas exchange and the child's general clinical condition. Prolonged critical illness and its increased calorific demands can leave the child with inadequate energy stores, which may contribute to muscle weakness and fatigue. This may well delay the weaning process beyond the anticipated timeframe. It is important that parents/carers are aware of these factors as perceived 'failures' of either weaning or extubation can lead to significant stress.

General indicators for readiness to wean or extubate

- Cardiovascular stability – reduced or stable levels of inotropic support without ongoing volume requirements.
- FiO_2 requirements of 0.40 or less with $SpO_2 > 94\%$ (or appropriate determined level for the child).
- PEEP level of 5 cm H_2O or less.
- Adequacy of respiratory muscles to maintain spontaneous ventilation.
- Adequate level of consciousness with good respiratory effort present.
- Good cough and gag reflex present.
- Pain well controlled without excessive sedative agents.
- $PaCO_2$ within a range acceptable for the child.

If the child has been ventilated for a very short period, then a rapid wean of ventilator settings and early extubation may be possible if the above indicators are achieved. In these children, a readiness to extubate test may be carried out by providing CPAP via an Ayre's T-piece circuit rather than the ventilator which allows for assessment of respiratory effort in a controlled fashion.

For the child whose ventilation has been prolonged, a more planned, step-by-step reduction in the level of support is necessary. The use of pressure support (PS)/CPAP modes on the ventilator can be useful in facilitating readiness for extubation or as a method of cycling a child with a tracheostomy off ventilatory support. When using a ventilatory mode with PS (e.g. SIMV PC or VC with PS) weaning of the PS is equally important or the child may end up with their own breaths receiving more support than the set machine breaths.

Preparation for extubation

Just as with intubation, wherever possible extubation should be undertaken in a controlled manner and it is important, where possible, to have two practitioners skilled in advanced airway management present in case difficulties are encountered once the tube has been removed. Essentially, the same preparations should be made as when preparing for intubation with the additional consideration of what method of supplementary oxygen therapy will be needed. For some infants/children, a decision may have been made to have NIV or CPAP instituted immediately after extubation, while others may require this additional support when it has not been anticipated. For children who have been intubated for prolonged periods or those with known upper airway concerns the use of a pre-extubation course of a corticosteroid (e.g. dexamethasone) may be beneficial in reducing post-extubation stridor or extubation failure. Although the evidence base for this in children is not established, empirical practice is suggestive of benefits in these particular children (Khemani et al 2009). A small number of children without pre-existing upper airway pathology may experience post-extubation stridor and the administration of nebulised adrenaline can successfully manage this.

After successful extubation close nursing observation and assessment are necessary for at least an hour and a blood gas should be taken during this time. Practitioners need to be aware that respiratory muscle fatigue may take a few hours to manifest and therefore continued monitoring is important, the duration of which will be based on clinical assessment of the child.

Upper airway conditions

Croup

Croup (acute laryngo-tracheitis/laryngo-tracheobronchitis) is an acute clinical syndrome in which the child presents with respiratory stridor, a barking cough, hoarseness of voice and variable degrees of respiratory distress (Figure 4.9). It can be associated with atopic disease. The peak incidence of viral croup is around the second year of life but the condition may be seen in infants as young as 3 months and in school-aged and older children. Fewer than 2% of children admitted to hospital will require intubation for airway protection.

Almost all (95%) croup is caused by viral pathogens, with the most common types being parainfluenza types I, II, III and IV, adenovirus or respiratory syncytial virus (RSV).

Less than 5% of cases can be attributed to a bacterial infection. Bacterial tracheitis or pseudomembranous croup is uncommon but can be distinguished by the presence of copious secretions and mucosal necrosis.

Clinical features

Acute presentation is usually preceded by a 1–3 day history of coryzal symptoms with symptoms worsening at night:

- Barking cough.
- Stridor.
- Hoarseness.
- Mild fever (usually < 38.5°C).
- Tachypnoea.

- Tachycardia.
- Respiratory distress (usually mild to moderate).
- Hypoxaemia (usually mild).
- Presence of a wheeze if the infection had spread to lower respiratory tract.

Differential diagnosis

The child with croup does not usually look systemically unwell and croup is not usually associated with dysphagia. In addition, croup has a relatively slow onset, therefore if symptoms occur acutely, consideration should be given to an alternative diagnosis including:

- Bacterial tracheitis.
- Epiglottitis.
- Peritonsillar abscess.
- Retropharyngeal abscess.
- Foreign body aspiration.

Croup scores

A number of croup scores are used in clinical practice, most of which are adaptations of the Westley Clinical Scoring System for Croup (Westley et al 1978). The use of a croup scoring tool probably has limited use in the urgent care of a child with croup, although it may be used to assess response to interventions and as a tool to consider

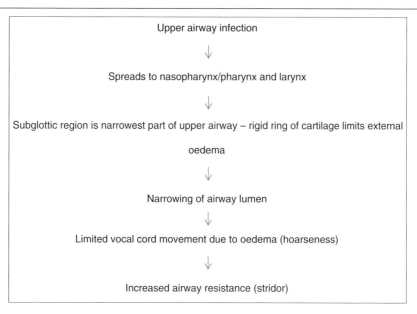

Figure 4.9 Pathophysiology of croup.

admission to hospital care or discharge home from an Emergency Department.

No scoring tool replaces astute clinical assessment based on the individual child and the presence of certain 'red flags' which indicate the need for urgent intervention, such as intercostal recession which disappears despite increasing respiratory distress, drowsiness, lethargy and cyanosis.

Management of the child with moderate to severe croup

- Keep the child comfortable and avoid wherever possible painful interventions that will cause or increase the child's distress. The presence of a parent, if possible, is beneficial.
- Administration of humidified O_2 to relieve hypoxaemia. This may not be possible via a close-fitting face mask if this further distresses the child – in these instances 'wafting' oxygen therapy which is positioned as close to the child as possible (often held in place by the parent) to maintain oxygen saturations > 93% is used.
- Nebulised adrenaline is used to provide short-term symptomatic relief. The usual dose is 0.5 ml/kg of 1:1000 solution up to a maximum of 5 ml per dose. This can be repeated after 30 minutes (Barry et al 2010). The effects of nebulised adrenaline can be maintained for between 2 and 3 hours, therefore continued close observation is essential.
- ECG and SpO_2 monitoring are required to assess effectiveness of interventions such as nebulised adrenaline and supplementary oxygen therapy and to detect signs of deterioration in the child's condition.
- Steroids – the use of glucocorticoids such as dexamethasone has been shown to be effective in the management of mild to moderate croup (Amir et al. 2006; Barry et al 2010). In the published studies no difference has been shown in the effects based on route of administration therefore a dose of 150 mcg/kg of dexamethasone (oral or IV) or budesonide 2 mg (by nebuliser) are advocated. The dose may be repeated after 12 hours if necessary (BNFC 2012).
- Anti-pyretics can be administered to reduce the effects of the child's fever and ease any discomfort. Current guidelines note that anti-pyretics should only be administered to the child if they are unwell or distressed with their illness and should not be administered with the sole intention of reducing the fever (NICE 2007).
- Intravenous fluids should be delivered to maintain hydration status and serum blood glucose levels within normal limits. Oral fluids should not be offered until there is clear clinical evidence that the child's condition has

improved. There should be no attempt at nasogastric tube insertion as this is highly likely to compound the child's distress and degree of airway obstruction.

The decision to intubate a child with croup is based on clinical assessment – there is no place for blood gas analysis prior to the decision being made. In these cases the child will require a gas induction prior to intubation and the procedure should be undertaken by an experienced practitioner with advanced airway skills. It is prudent to ensure that there is ENT support available in the locality before the procedure is carried out.

Once the child is intubated with a secure airway, it is possible for them to be maintained breathing spontaneously without the need for mechanical ventilation and the associated use of sedative agents. The length of time required before extubation can be considered varies from 2 to 10 days and the ease with which the child moves towards extubation will depend in part on the size of ETT used at initial intubation. Some units will upsize a child's ETT (e.g. from size 3.0 to size 3.5/4.0) once before attempting extubation, particularly if the original tube was significantly smaller than the anticipated tube size for the child. The development of a measurable or audible leak around the child's ETT is indicative of a reduction in the degree of oedema present. A course of steroids is usually prescribed prior to extubation being attempted.

Parental support with full explanations of their child's planned care and the responses to prescribed interventions

A daily meeting with the intensivist responsible for the child (or their nominated doctor) should take place to maintain a therapeutic relationship with the child's family. Where possible and if appropriate to the child's age, cognitive ability and clinical condition, the child's involvement in update discussions should be considered.

Considerations for practice

Humidification and supplementary oxygen therapy can be administered via a heat–moisture exchanger (HME) or a 'swedish nose'. Play and distraction therapy plus presence of a parent is important in this group of children as accidental self-extubation is to be avoided at all costs. Some children cannot tolerate the presence of the ETT without the use of sedative agents and this group may need to be ventilated for the duration of their illness. Arm splints to prevent the child from reaching their ETT but otherwise allowing movement are used in many units. It is pertinent to review the individual Trust's holding/restraining policies as well as national guidance such as that issued by the Royal College of Nursing before advocating this practice. There are many concerns relating to the use of physical restraints, particularly in children, but these should be matched to the side-effects of sedation use and a balanced judgement made in partnership with the child's parents.

Bacterial tracheitis

Bacterial tracheitis is a rare clinical presentation (Tebruegge et al. 2009) and is a diffuse inflammatory process involving the larynx, trachea and bronchi characterised by the formation of adherent or semi-adherent muco-purulent membranes within the trachea. The main focus of the disease is around the cricoid cartilage level and in children around the subglottis, which is the narrowest part of the airway.

Acute airway obstruction may develop secondary to both subglottic oedema and sloughing of epithelial lining or accumulation of a muco-purulent membrane within the trachea. Clinical signs of bacterial tracheitis often mimic those of croup but the child does not respond to croup treatment strategies (e.g. nebulised adrenaline) and may also present with some clinical features similar to a child with epiglottitis.

It can affect any age group and in the paediatric population most commonly occurs between the ages of 4 and 8 years. The common causative pathogens include:

- *Staphylococcus aureus.*
- *Streptococcus pyogenes.*
- *Streptococcus pneumoniae*
- *Haemophilus influenzae.*
- *Moraxella catarrhalis.*

Viral co-infection may also be identified in children presenting with bacterial tracheitis including influenza A, parainfluenza I and III and adenovirus.

Clinical features of bacterial tracheitis

A mixed presentation is possible with some features of a croup-type illness and others similar to epiglottitis. In addition, clinical presentation will depend on whether it is a primary bacterial tracheitis or a secondary bacterial infection to an existing viral infection (Barry et al. 2010). The prodrome is usually an upper respiratory infection, followed by progression to higher fever, cough, inspiratory stridor and a variable degree of respiratory distress. In the classic presentation children present acutely with:

- High fever (>39.0°C).
- Toxic (systemically unwell) appearance.

- Stridor.
- Tachypnoea.
- Elevated white blood cell count.
- Presence of a frequent but not painful cough.

Children may acutely decompensate with worsening respiratory distress due to airway obstruction from a purulent membrane that has loosened. There may also be signs of lower airway infection indicated by the presence of wheeze on auscultation, but a significant consideration in terms of a differential diagnosis is that the child's airway is not affected by positioning as would be found in the child with epiglottitis.

Management of the child with bacterial tracheitis

The management of the child with bacterial tracheitis is essentially the same as that of a child with croup or epiglottitis requiring airway protection. At intubation it is possible to make a definitive diagnosis based on the appearance of supraglottic structures and the presence of thick purulent secretions in the airway. Once the child is intubated frequent ETT suctioning is usually necessary due to the volume of secretions produced by the sloughing of the epithelial lining of the main airways. Children with bacterial tracheitis require antibiotics for up to 2 weeks, although the duration of intubation and ventilation is between 5 and 7 days.

Parental support with full explanations of their child's planned care and the responses to prescribed interventions

A daily meeting with the intensivist responsible for the child (or their nominated doctor) should take place to maintain a therapeutic relationship with the child's family. Where possible and if appropriate to the child's age, cognitive ability and clinical condition, the child's involvement in update discussions should also be considered.

Retropharyngeal abscess

A retropharyngeal abscess forms in the deep space of the neck tissues involving the surrounding connective tissues and the lymph nodes. These abscesses form either as a consequence of penetrating trauma to the area (e.g. from accidental lacerations caused when the child places a sharp object in their mouth and then falls) or as a consequence of an upper respiratory tract infection spreading to the retropharyngeal lymph nodes. Sources of the infection may be pharyngitis, tonsillitis or sinusitis (Grisaru-Soen et al. 2010). Retropharyngeal abscesses are almost exclusively a paediatric diagnosis. Most incidents occur in children aged between 6 months and 6 years, with a mean age of 3–5 years. Other deep neck abscesses (e.g. parapharyngeal or peritonsillar) are observed more frequently in older children or adults.

The child is at risk of airway obstruction as the size of the abscess enlarges and starts to encroach on the surrounding structures. In addition, the infection can spread, resulting in inflammation and destruction of adjacent tissues. Spread of the infection to the mediastinum can result in mediastinitis, a purulent pericarditis with possible tamponade, empyema or bronchial erosion. If the infection spreads posteriorly to the retropharyngeal space, there is a risk of the child developing osteomyelitis of the vertebrae.

If the child presents with respiratory compromise, then intubation (for airway protection) is indicated followed by surgical incision and drainage of the abscess. Antibiotics should be prescribed for 1 or 2 weeks depending on the sensitivity of cultures.

Parental support with full explanations of their child's planned care and the responses to prescribed interventions

A daily meeting with the intensivist responsible for the child (or their nominated doctor) should take place to maintain a therapeutic relationship with the child's family. Where possible and if appropriate to the child's age, cognitive ability and clinical condition, the child's involvement in update discussions should also be considered.

Epiglottitis

Epiglottitis is a severe bacterial infection most commonly caused by *Haemophilus influenzae B* (HIB) which causes inflammation and swelling of the epiglottis and surrounding tissues leading to severe airway obstruction. It affects any age group, although it is most common between the ages of 1 and 8 years. It is characterised by a rapid onset without a preceding history of coryzal symptoms associated with the presentation of croup. Incidence of the disease decreased dramatically after the introduction of the conjugate HIB vaccine during the 1990s which is considered to be very effective in affording the required protection. The successful uptake of the vaccination programme has also conferred herd immunity to unvaccinated children by reducing nasopharyngeal carriage in asymptomatic carriers (Swingler et al 2007). HIB remains a key pathogen in the development of meningitis and pneumonia worldwide. Children presenting with recent arrival from developing countries may not have received the HIB vaccine

and therefore may be at greater risk for developing systemic disease.

Clinical features of epiglottitis

This will be an acute presentation in a child who looks systemically unwell:

- Absent or weak cough.
- Unable to swallow – drooling saliva.
- Septic appearance.
- Fever > 38.5°C
- Soft inspiratory stridor.
- Sternal recession.
- Tachypnoea.
- Tachycardia.
- Need to sit up.
- Late signs – listlessness, cyanosis, bradycardia, hypoxia.

Management of the child with epiglottitis

This must be managed as a medical emergency and no intervention should be attempted before all preparations have been made and the necessary personnel are available in the area where the child is being cared for.

Keep the child under constant observation but do not attempt to attach monitoring at this point. Avoid any interventions as this will increase the degree of airway obstruction and cause complete airway occlusion. The child will usually adopt a position of comfort themselves and this should be maintained, with the presence of a parent being essential. Keep the number of people in the area immediate to the child to a minimum and offer quiet explanations to the child (where appropriate) and their parents.

Prepare for a gas induction and intubation and ensure that there is the appropriate equipment and experienced personnel present to carry out a surgical airway/emergency tracheostomy if necessary.

Consider the administration of humidified O_2 if possible to relieve hypoxaemia without causing any distress to the child – in these instances the use of 'wafting' oxygen therapy which is positioned as close to the child as is possible (often held in place by the parent) is advocated to maintain oxygen saturations > 93%.

Once the child's airway is secure it is possible to gain IV access, take and send bloods for a full blood count (FBC) and cultures (MC&S). Antibiotics are indicated and cefotaxime or ceftriaxone are the most commonly used, however check the prescription against the unit's antibiotic prescribing policies prior to administration. Corticosteroids are not routinely indicated in the management of epiglottitis as there is no established evidence base for the efficacy of their use (Barry et al. 2010).

Parental support with full explanations of their child's planned care and the responses to prescribed interventions

A daily meeting with the intensivist responsible for the child (or their nominated doctor) should take place to maintain a therapeutic relationship with the child's family.

The majority of children are extubated within 48–72 hours of initial intubation, in the presence of a measurable or audible leak around the ETT and when afebrile. Local variations in practice between units means that some children may be managed in the same way as a child with croup and allowed to maintain spontaneous ventilation via the ETT with added humidification and supplementary oxygen therapy while other units will leave the child mechanically ventilated until ready for extubation.

Subglottic stenosis

Subglottic stenosis is a narrowing of the subglottic airway, which is housed in the cricoid cartilage. The subglottic airway is the narrowest area of the airway because it is a complete, non-expandable, non-pliable ring, unlike the trachea, and stenosis may be congenital or acquired. The cause of congenital subglottic stenosis is in utero malformation of the cricoid cartilage, while the causes of acquired subglottic stenosis are usually related to trauma to or injury of the subglottic mucosa. Injury can be caused by infection or mechanical trauma, usually from endotracheal intubation, and this is the commonest cause of acquired subglottic stenosis in children. Factors implicated in the development of acquired subglottic stenosis include:

- The size of the endotracheal tube relative to the child's larynx – the larger the ETT the greater the risk of the infant/child developing subglottic stenosis.
- The length of time the child is intubated.
- The repetitive movement of the tube in the trachea.
- Repeated intubations.

Infants and children with subglottic stenosis will often present with stridor, which may be exacerbated by upper respiratory tract infections. Investigations through a micro laryngoscopy and bronchoscopy (MLB) will confirm the diagnosis and treatment options may include formation of a tracheostomy followed by surgical repair known as a laryngotracheal reconstruction (LTR). Children require a period of mechanical ventilation of 4–6 days following surgery and are usually nursed in the midline position to avoid placing excessive tension on the area of reconstruction. They may require muscle relaxants in addition to sedative and analgesic agents to facilitate this.

Parental support with full explanations of their child's planned care and the responses to prescribed interventions

A daily meeting with the intensivist responsible for the child (or their nominated doctor) should take place to maintain a therapeutic relationship with the child's family.

Other causes of stridor

Vascular rings

Vascular rings are congenital vascular abnormalities of the aortic arch complex which result in extrinsic compression of the trachea and/or the oesophagus. The incidence of vascular rings is rare, accounting for around 1% of all reported congenital cardiovascular conditions (Park 2010). Vascular rings can be classified as true rings (which are anatomically complete) or partial rings (which are not complete), though both can have similar clinical presentations. The complete vascular rings include double aortic arch and right aortic arch with aberrant left subclavian artery and left ligamentum. The incomplete vascular rings include innominate artery compression and pulmonary artery sling. Infants with a double aortic arch present with predominant airway symptoms (stridor, respiratory distress and cough). The pulmonary artery sling is a rare defect in which the left pulmonary artery arises from the right pulmonary artery and encircles the right main stem bronchus and trachea as it passes between the trachea and oesophagus prior to entering the left lung. This causes oesophageal compression anteriorly. Due to the degree of compression present, infants usually present early in life with respiratory symptoms (Shah et al. 2007).

Management is dependent on the type of vascular ring. Surgery is always required to repair the double aortic arch and pulmonary artery sling, but the anomalous innominate artery defect or the aberrant right subclavian artery can be managed conservatively (Park 2010).

Inhaled or aspiration of a foreign body

Inhalation or aspiration of a foreign body is a relatively common presentation in the paediatric Emergency Department (Glynn et al 2008). Foreign body aspiration can result in a spectrum of clinical presentations from minimal, often unobserved symptoms, to respiratory compromise or failure, and even death. In young children, who present with acute stridor and a cough/wheeze but with no underlying symptoms or history of upper respiratory tract infection, as would be seen in croup for example, foreign body aspiration should be considered as a matter of course. Often the presenting history includes a short period of unsupervised activity and it is on the return of the parent/carer that the change in the child is apparent. Examples of common foreign bodies inhaled include small beads, food particles and micro-toys or bits of a toy. Children aged 1–3 years are particularly at risk and are the group unable to provide a history on presentation.

The foreign body can lodge at any site from supraglottic region to the terminal bronchioles and may or may not be evident on chest X-ray. The removal of a foreign body in the upper airways of young children, particularly those lodged posteriorly, should always be attempted under general anaesthesia as it can be dislodged further down into the lower airways leading to potentially fatal complications, with the use of flexible bronchoscopy to retrieve foreign bodies from the lower airways.

Lower respiratory tract conditions

Bronchiolitis

Bronchiolitis is an acute seasonal viral illness of the lower respiratory tract which affects mainly infants and children <2 years. It can also be seen in older children with immune insufficiency, for example following bone marrow transplant.

Bronchiolitis is primarily a disorder of oxygenation which, if unresolved, will lead to respiratory failure indicated by hypercapnia/acidosis in addition to the hypoxaemia present.

The causative pathogen in 75% of bronchiolitis episodes in the under 1 year old is the respiratory syncytial virus (RSV). Other pathogens include parainfluenza types 1, 2 and 3, influenza B, adenovirus types 1, 2 and 5 (approximately 11%) and mycoplasma in older children.

RSV infection

In temperate climates the RSV season occurs in the winter through to the spring, while parainfluenza season occurs in autumn. There are two RSV subgroups (A and B) and one subtype predominates during a given season. Nearly 100% of children will experience an RSV infection within two RSV seasons and of these approximately 1% will be hospitalised – this equates to around 7 200 infants hospitalised each year with 1% of these requiring admission to PICU. Fifty per cent of the infants hospitalised are between 1 and 3 months of age. Infection with RSV provides temporary immunity only, therefore infants can develop symptomatic illness during the following season.

RSV is also a major cause of upper respiratory tract infections in small children. It is responsible for:

- 25% of URTIs in children < 1 year of age.
- 13% of URTIs in children aged 1–2 years.

There are a number of identified risk factors for symptomatic RSV infection:

- Low birth weight.
- Prematurity.
- Lower socioeconomic group.
- Crowded living conditions.
- Parental smoking.
- Day care.
- Absence of breast feeding (colostrum appears to be protective).

Clinical presentation of bronchiolitis (Figure 4.10)

Regardless of the causative pathogen the clinical presentation of bronchiolitis follows a predictable pattern. There is a history of coryzal symptoms, low-grade fever and upper airway congestion. This may affect the infant's ability to feed, but hydration is usually adequately maintained at this point. Within 2–5 days of the onset of symptoms, 40% of infants affected will progress to lower respiratory tract symptoms including:

- Cough and wheezing.
- Dyspnoea.
- Feeding difficulties.
- Apnoeas.

In severe infections clinical signs will also include nasal flaring, recession and cyanosis at presentation.

Apnoeas and bronchiolitis

Apnoeas occur in 18–20% of hospitalised infants with bronchiolitis, especially if they were born at <32 weeks of gestation (pre-term infants) or are aged <28 days of age at presentation in the term infant.

Apnoeas may occur early in the illness course and can often be the presenting symptom into the Emergency Department. These apnoeas are usually non-obstructive, centrally mediated and often occur when the infant is asleep. Apnoeas may last for a few days and usually require minimal intervention, however approximately 10% of these infants need respiratory support in the form of nasal CPAP or intubation and ventilation. Caffeine citrate (either intravenous or oral) is often used to manage the apnoeic episodes. The efficacy of caffeine use in preterm infants is well described in the literature and it is now used in prefer-

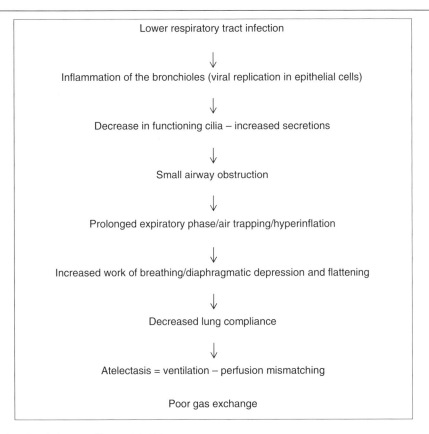

Lower respiratory tract infection

↓

Inflammation of the bronchioles (viral replication in epithelial cells)

↓

Decrease in functioning cilia – increased secretions

↓

Small airway obstruction

↓

Prolonged expiratory phase/air trapping/hyperinflation

↓

Increased work of breathing/diaphragmatic depression and flattening

↓

Decreased lung compliance

↓

Atelectasis = ventilation – perfusion mismatching

Poor gas exchange

Figure 4.10 Pathophysiology of bronchiolitis.

ence to other agents such as theophylline due to its dosing regime and lower risk of toxicity (Buck et al. 2008).

Clinical assessment findings

Physical examination

- Tachypnoea, often at rates > 60–70 breaths/min (most common physical sign).
- Tachycardia.
- Fever, usually in the range of 38–38.5°C.
- Presence of mild conjunctivitis or pharyngitis.
- Nasal flaring.
- Intercostal recession/tracheal tug.
- Cyanosis.
- Otitis media.
- Palpable liver and spleen from hyperinflation of the lungs and consequent depression of the diaphragm.

CXR findings

- Hyperinflation (indicated by rib count).
- Flattened diaphragm.

- Peribronchial thickening (heart borders).
- Lobar infiltrates present in 20–30% of infants.

Auscultation

- Diffuse, fine wheezing.
- Prolonged expiratory phase.
- Fine crackles.

Management of the infant with bronchiolitis

After assessment in the Emergency Department, admission to hospital is likely to be required when any of the following criteria are met:

- Sustained SpO_2 < 92% in room air.
- <6 months of age.
- Inability to maintain oral hydration.
- Markedly elevated respiratory rate.

Infants with established chronic lung disease and home O_2 dependency, as well as those with congenital heart disease

Table 4.27 Summary of outcomes in bronchiolitis

Healthy infants presenting with bronchiolitis	Infants with chronic lung/congenital heart disease presenting with bronchiolitis
Of those requiring hospitalisation:	Of those requiring hospitalisation:
Median length of stay = 4 days	69% are hospitalised for > 7 days
12% require PIC admission	35% require PIC admission
10% receive mechanical ventilatory support	19% receive mechanical ventilatory support
Of those who do require ventilation:	Of those who do require ventilation:
• mean length of ventilation = 5 days	• mean length of ventilation = 10 days
• mean oxygen therapy = 7 days	• mean oxygen therapy = 18 days
• mean discharge by 9 days	• mean discharge by 21 days

and pulmonary hypertension, should be admitted even if their presenting symptoms are relatively mild as they have the potential to become severely compromised by the illness and are more likely to require intensive care admission than the infant with no underlying comorbidity (Table 4.27).

In 2010, the use of palivizumab (Synagis®), a monoclonal antibody drug that provides passive immunity against RSV, was approved by the Joint Committee on Vaccination and Immunisation (JCVI) and the Department of Health in the UK for use in certain clinical conditions and added to the immunisation programme. The vaccine has a half-life of 18–21 days per dose and the schedule involves monthly injections through the RSV season (up to five doses required per season). The vulnerable populations include infants with chronic lung disease and oxygen dependency or congenital heart disease. In addition, it is recommended that its use should be considered in children with severe combined immunodeficiency syndrome (SCIDS) and those receiving long-term ventilation (DH 2010).

Management of the infant with bronchiolitis is essentially supportive and matched to the symptoms. Key priorities include:

- Strict hand washing and standard isolation practice.
- Monitoring – ECG, SpO_2 and NIBP/CBGs as clinically indicated; routine bloods.
- Supplementary oxygen therapy which is warmed and humidified.
- IV fluids; orogastric tube; small-volume feeds.
- Bronchodilators and/or steroids are not routinely indicated in the management of bronchiolitis but may provide symptomatic relief. Opinion remains divided about their use. In a recent systematic review of studies of bronchodilator/steroid administration (Hartling et al. 2011) none of the interventions examined showed clear benefits for length of stay for inpatients, however some limited evidence suggested benefits on clinical score for adrenaline use as well as for steroids and salbutamol compared with placebo.
- Comfort measures – administration of paracetamol; careful positioning; parental advice and support.

Parental support with full explanations of their child's planned care and the responses to prescribed interventions

A daily meeting with the intensivist responsible for the child (or their nominated doctor) should take place to maintain a therapeutic relationship with the child's family.

Bronchiolitis is a relatively short illness in the acute phase, however a cough and/or wheeze may persist for up to 2 months after acute symptoms resolve. There is a possibility of the infant developing asthma in later life and infants with a persistent wheeze that lasts longer than expected after a bronchiolitic illness merit follow-up.

Asthma and status asthmaticus

Asthma is defined as a disease which results from the interaction of genetic and/or environmental influences on the tone or reactivity of the airways causing symptoms of breathlessness, cough and wheezing. There are currently 5.4 million people in the UK receiving treatment for asthma: 1.1 million children (1 in 11) and 4.3 million adults (1 in 12). Additional epidemiological facts relating to asthma include:

- It is the most common long-term medical condition requiring management.
- On average there are two children with asthma in every UK classroom.
- The UK has the highest prevalence of severe wheeze in children aged 13–14 years worldwide.

- If one parent has asthma, the chance of their child developing asthma is approximately double that of children whose parents do not have asthma.
- Smoking during pregnancy brings a 35% increased risk of the infant being wheezy or having breathing difficulties.
- Children whose parents smoke are 1.5 times more likely to develop asthma.

(Asthma UK 2011).

Development of asthma

Genetics: There is a strong genetic component to development of asthma. Identical twins have a greater chance of both developing asthma than non-identical twins.

There is an increased risk of developing asthma as a child if both parents suffer from the disease.

Bronchial muscle: Evidence suggests that the smooth muscle in asthmatic airways has altered mechanical properties, which predisposes them to hyper-reactivity. Asthmatic airways also have increased sensitivity to histamine.

Atopia: It is estimated that 90% of asthmatics are atopic – they have the inherited ability to produce immunoglobulin E (IgE) in response to allergenic stimulation. IgE is known to bind to mast cells causing the release of mediators such as histamine. Other causes are identified in Table 4.28.

Status asthmaticus is defined as severe asthma which fails to respond to inhaled β_2 agonists, oral or IV steroids and oxygen therapy, necessitating hospital admission. Less than 1% of children with asthma require admission to PICU. There are a number of identified risk factors which are linked to an increased risk of a fatal asthma episode (Table 4.29).

The pathophysiology of asthma can be divided into four interdependent pathways, the physiological effects of each having an impact on the other:

- Inflammatory cytokine responses.
- Airway/pulmonary effects.
- Cardiovascular effects.
- Metabolic effects.

Inflammatory cytokine responses

Airway inflammation is characterised by the submucosal cellular infiltrate of eosinophils, mast cells and CD4 lymphocytes. The presence of these cells correlates with the disease severity. The cascade of inflammation begins with degranulation of mast cells, usually in response to allergen

Table 4.28   Causes of acute asthma

1. Food and or drink – almost 10% of all asthmatics are affected by certain types of food and/or drink. Common causes include:
    - Milk.
    - Eggs.
    - Fish.
    - Cereals.
    - Nuts.
    - Chocolate.
    - Flavourings/preservatives in soft drinks (e.g. tartrazine).
2. Air pollution/tobacco smoke.
3. Viral infections in early years.
4. Gastro-oesophageal reflux disease (GORD).
5. Exercise.
6. Animals – up to 25% of asthmatics are sensitive to animal dander.
7. Pollen – the most common pollen in Europe is grass pollen.
8. Psychological factors – stress, shock, excitement or laughter can all provoke asthmatic responses.
9. House dust/house dust mites – most asthmatics (approximately 80%) report symptoms following exposure to house dust.

Table 4.29   Risk factors for increased morbidity associated with status asthmaticus

- Poorly controlled disease.
- Previous life-threatening exacerbations with ICU admission requiring ventilation.
- History of sudden and rapid deterioration.
- Failure to respond to treatment; deterioration on steroids.
- Lack of perception of severity of attacks, especially the degree of hypoxaemia present.
- Lack of compliance; risk-taking behaviours in adolescents.
- Lack of adequate social support.
- Psychosocial disease, including overt depression and manipulative use of asthma.

exposure. Activated mast cells and lymphocytes produce pro-inflammatory cytokines (e.g. histamine, leukotrienes, platelet activating factor – PAF), which are increased in asthmatics. Inflammatory cytokine responses may be triggered early or late in the acute episode (Figure 4.11). The

Early phase	Late phase
Activated mast cells release histamine and leukotrienes, both activators of early airway smooth muscle spasm	Submucosal infiltration by eosinophils, neutrophils and activated lymphocytes is responsible for delayed bronchospasm
↓	↓
The activated mast cells further activate T lymphocytes, which produce more inflammatory cytokines (TH2) and IL-4, -5 and -13	Early bronchospasm may be more sensitive to bronchodilating agents, while late bronchospasm is refractory to bronchodilators and more sensitive to anti-inflammatory therapy
↓	↓
In addition, chemokines (leukotriene B4) are released which attract neutrophils and promote further activation of the pro-inflammatory cascade	This inflammatory environment results in overproduction of mucous; injury to airway epithelium that exposes nerve endings, which augments airway irritability, hyper-responsiveness and mucosal oedema

Figure 4.11   Inflammatory cytokine responses in asthma.

final common pathway for the inflammatory cascade is bronchoconstriction and mechanical airway obstruction by oedema and mucous.

Airway and pulmonary effects

The characteristics of the disease process within the airways starts with the hyper-responsiveness of the bronchial muscle, leading to the release of increased numbers of inflammatory cells (mast cells, neutrophils, T-lymphocytes, eosinophils) in the bronchi. These processes lead to:

- Narrowing of the airways.
- Hypersecretion of mucous.
- Associated oedema and vascular leak.
- Epithelial shedding, reflected by presence of Curschmann's spirals in the mucous.

As a consequence there is an increase in intrapulmonary shunting. There is an increased V/Q mismatch from increased dead space (airway over-distension), which results from small airway obstruction due to mucous plugging, oedema and bronchoconstriction. Small-airway obstruction causes areas of decreased ventilation but adequate pulmonary blood flow – the resultant shunt leads to arterial hypoxaemia. As disease severity worsens, greater distal airway obstruction causes alveolar distension and increased pulmonary dead space, worsening the shunt/hypoxaemia (Figure 4.12).

To compensate for this V/Q mismatch, tachypnoea occurs. Despite increasing dead space to tidal volume ratio (Vd/Vt), hypocarbia persists because minute ventilation increases. Finally, intercostal and diaphragmatic muscles fatigue. Increased minute ventilation is unable to compensate for the greatly increased Vd/Vt ratio and hypercarbia

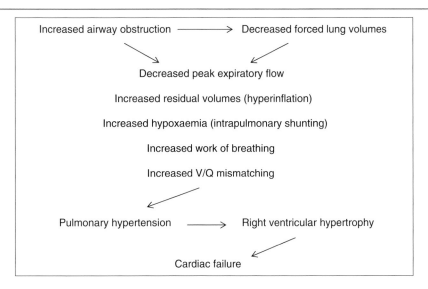

Figure 4.12   Airway and pulmonary effects of acute asthma.

results. As fatigue worsens, progressive hypoxaemia and hypercarbia ensue and result in respiratory failure.

Cardiovascular effects

Right ventricular function

Increased residual lung volumes stretch the pulmonary vasculature, increasing pulmonary vascular resistance and right ventricular afterload, which may compromise right ventricular function. In addition, fluctuations in pleural pressures produce significant effects on the intrathoracic vessels and right atrial venous return.

Left ventricular function

During the large negative intrathoracic pressure created during inspiration, left ventricular afterload is increased and systolic blood pressure is decreased. Exaggerated variation in systolic blood pressure associated with intrathoracic pressure variation during inspiration is termed pulsus paradoxus.

Metabolic effects

There are significant metabolic changes that occur during an acute episode of asthma; these are detailed in Figure 4.13. The metabolic changes and effects are often underestimated as respiratory symptoms require more urgent evaluation and intervention.

Clinical assessment findings

Wherever possible it is important to gain a history of the episode from the child's parents/carers. The key points to elicit are the duration of symptoms, the treatments already given with the child's response and finally, the course of any previous attacks.

Physical examination

Physical examination is based on assessment of:

• Work of breathing.
• Effectiveness of effort.
• Auscultation.

Key points:

• Respiratory rate and sound of a wheeze are poor indicators of the severity of illness in children.
• Cyanosis is a late sign of life-threatening asthma.
• A silent chest is a sign of life-threatening asthma.

Peak expiratory flow readings (PEFR) are helpful indicators of the severity of the episode but are not reliable in the under-5 year olds or in children presenting with severe dyspnoea (Table 4.30).

Chest X-rays are not normally indicated in the assessment of acute asthma unless there are signs and/or a presenting history of severe infection, asymmetry of chest

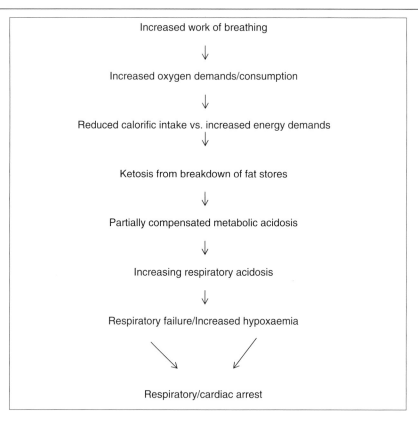

Increased work of breathing

↓

Increased oxygen demands/consumption

↓

Reduced calorific intake vs. increased energy demands

↓

Ketosis from breakdown of fat stores

↓

Partially compensated metabolic acidosis

↓

Increasing respiratory acidosis

↓

Respiratory failure/Increased hypoxaemia

Respiratory/cardiac arrest

Figure 4.13   Metabolic effects of acute asthma.

Table 4.30   Expected peak flow readings

Height (cm)	Peak flow (l/min)
110	150
120	200
130	250
140	300
150	350
160	400
170	450

Source: ALSG 2005.

signs or uncertainty regarding the diagnosis. Only 1–5% of chest X-rays will show abnormalities in status asthmaticus.

Arterial blood gases (ABGs) are not usually helpful and as such are not routinely indicated unless the child is already intubated and ventilated. Obtaining ABGs from a child without indwelling IA access can be difficult for the practitioner and traumatic for the child. The decision to intubate, therefore, should depend on frequent clinical assessment not blood gas results.

Progression of altered acid base environment in status asthmaticus

EARLY PHASE:
• Non-hypoxaemic but hyperventilating.
• Low $PaCO_2$ and normal PaO_2.

PROGRESSIVE PHASE:
• Hyperventilating and hypoxaemic.
• Low $PaCO_2$ and low PaO_2.

LATE PHASE:
• Worsening hypoxaemia.
• Work of breathing increasing but respiratory effort slowing.

- Normal $PaCO_2$ (due to respiratory muscle fatigue) and low PaO_2 ($PaCO_2$ is false normal which is a sign of impending failure).

Respiratory failure

$PaCO_2$ is high; PaO_2 is low – significant hypercarbia and hypoxaemia present. At this point intubation and ventilation are indicated.

Clinical assessment features of severe asthma

- The child cannot complete sentences in one breath or is too breathless to talk or feed.
- Recession/use of accessory muscles.
- Respiratory rate > 30 breaths/min (>5 years) or > 40 (2–5 years).
- SpO_2 < 92% in room air.
- Tachycardia > 140 bpm (2–5 years) or > 125 bpm (>5 years).
- Widespread audible expiratory wheeze.
- PEFR 33–50% of expected/known best.

(British Thoracic Society 2011).

Clinical assessment features of life-threatening asthma

- Depressed level of consciousness.
- Exhaustion.
- Hypotension.
- Poor respiratory effort.
- SpO_2 < 85% in room air.
- Central cyanosis.
- Silent chest.
- Peak flow < 33% of expected/known best.

(British Thoracic Society 2011).

Management of the child with asthma

Management priorities are structured around the guidelines issued by the British Thoracic Society and the Scottish Intercollegiate Guidelines Network. These guidelines are subject to review and revision on an annual basis as the evidence base develops. These guidelines are accessible in their electronic format:

www.brit-thoracic.org.uk/guidelines/asthma-guidelines. aspx and www.sign.ac.uk.

Treatment is directed towards improving or maintaining oxygenation, ensuring adequate CO_2 clearance and reversing the characteristic bronchoconstriction (Table 4.31). Initially high flow oxygen (15 litres via non-rebreathe mask) should be administered to maintain oxygen saturations (SpO_2) above 95%. Once the child is clinically stable, warmed and humidified oxygen to maintain saturations above 95% should be administered. As chronic hypoxaemia is not a clinical finding in asthmatics between acute exacerbations, treatment should be directed towards maintaining normal saturations during the child's hospitalisation.

Antibiotics are not routinely indicated in the management of the child in status asthmaticus unless there is clear evidence of underlying bacterial infection, for example, infiltrates on a CXR, fever and elevation of septic markers.

Careful fluid management is also required. Although most children will present partially dehydrated, restoration of euvolaemia (normal fluid status) is essential as there is the potential for pulmonary oedema with over-hydration secondary to inappropriate anti-diuretic hormone (ADH) secretion. Altered atrial pressures, both left and right, induce a false hypovolaemia status. ADH is secreted by the posterior pituitary gland and acts on the kidneys to induce water retention, primarily at the level of the collecting ducts. This leads to relative fluid overload (normal sodium management within the body). The child is at risk of pulmonary oedema due to increased microvascular permeability and alveolar fluid migration associated with the inflammatory processes in the lung.

Intubation and ventilation in the asthmatic child

The need for intubation and ventilation is made based on clinical assessment in the presence of decreased respiratory effort with fatigue or shallow tachypnoea, an inability to speak single words, absence of wheeze on auscultation or increasing hypercapnia with refractory hypoxaemia.

Considerations for practice

Intubation drugs used in this scenario should avoid those known to trigger significant histamine release, such as morphine and atracurium. Useful medications to consider are ketamine and midazolam or propofol for the older child, alongside a muscle relaxant such as Rocuronium™, Pancuronium™ or Vecuronium™.

While spontaneously breathing, asthmatics generate significant negative intrathoracic pressures which can augment venous return and cardiac output. Once intubation drugs have been administered and there is a loss of intrinsic respiratory effort, a significant decrease in venous return may occur, the effects of which may be worsened by the instigation of positive-pressure ventilation. This in turn may lead to cardiovascular instability during intubation, therefore it is advantageous to have prepared either crystalloid or

Table 4.31 Drugs targeting bronchoconstriction in acute asthma

Drug therapies	Notes and considerations
Inhaled bronchodilators	
Salbutamol (Ventolin™) (sympathomimetic)	Short acting β2 agonists
Ipratropium bromide (Atrovent™) (anticholinergic)	Works by stimulating the β2 receptors on bronchial smooth muscle and mediates muscle relaxation as a consequence. Their method of action is through activation of adenylate cyclase with increases in the level of cyclic adenosine monophosphate (cAMP) and functional antagonism of the bronchoconstriction. *Side-effects* • Tachycardia, agitation, tremors. • Hypokalaemia. Works by blocking parasympathetic (vagal) receptors found in the pulmonary tissue, promoting bronchodilation. Less than 10% of nebulised drug reaches the lung under ideal conditions. Drug delivery depends on breathing pattern, tidal volumes, gas flow and nebuliser type. In patients with severe air flow limitation or those who show no clinical signs of improvement with continuous nebulised therapy a switch to intravenous therapy should be made.
Intravenous bronchodilators	
Salbutamol (Ventolin™)	The current recommendations prompt consideration of the early addition of a single bolus dose of IV salbutamol (15 mcg/kg over 10 minutes) in severe cases where the patient has not responded to initial inhaled therapy (British Thoracic Society 2011). *Side-effects* • Tachycardia, agitation, tremors. • Hypokalaemia.
Aminophylline	Conflicting reports in the published literature on the efficacy of aminophylline therapy have made its use controversial. The current consensus in the published guidelines is that its use should be considered in the HDU or PIC setting for children with severe or life-threatening bronchospasm unresponsive to their maximum doses of both bronchodilators and steroids. Data suggest that aminophylline may have an anti-inflammatory effect in addition to its bronchodilator properties. The loading dose is usually 5 mg/kg, followed by a continuous infusion of 0.5–0.9 mg/kg/h. Aminophylline is not currently recommended in children with mild to moderate acute asthma.
Steroids	
Prednisolone (oral) Hydrocortisone (IV)	Works by dampening the host response to the trigger/stimulus thereby suppressing the innate immune response, the release of mediators such as histamine and decreasing the production of cytokines. Steroids have also been shown to reduce the number of eosinophils in the airway which are significant in the pathophysiology of asthma. *Side-effects* • Hyperglycaemia. • Hypertension. • Unusual or unusually severe infections. Steroid therapy should be weaned over a number of days after an acute episode.

Table 4.31 (*Continued*)

Drug therapies	Notes and considerations
Other agents	
Magnesium sulphate	Magnesium's primary pharmacological action in asthma is based on its ability to inhibit the release of calcium from vesicles in the sarcoplasmic reticulum, resulting in bronchial smooth muscle relaxation (Cheuk et al. 2005). In addition, it has been shown to decrease histamine release from mast cells.
Leukotriene receptor antagonists, e.g. montelukast	Work by blocking the action or synthesis of cysteinyl leukotrienes responsible for causing bronchoconstriction, mucous secretion, altered vascular permeability and eosinophil migration to the airways (Bisgaard and Nielsen 2000). These drugs are not first-line agents in the treatment of status asthmaticus, however if the child has been taking them prior to admission, they are usually continued during their hospitalisation.

colloid (depending on unit preference) for volume resuscitation prior to beginning the intubation.

Once intubated, it can be difficult to achieve satisfactory ventilatory support for asthmatic patients in the light of the degree of bronchoconstriction present, the presence of thick secretions and mucosal oedema, all of which may contribute to increased airway resistance.

Practitioners also need to be aware of the risk of hyperinflation and air trapping when determining ventilation strategies. The use of a pressure-regulated volume control ventilation (PRVC) mode, which allows control of both pressure and volume indices, offers more targeted parameters matched to the individual child's clinical picture. Reducing the set ventilation rate even to a rate lower than would be anticipated for the child's age allows a longer expiratory time to be used, minimising the effects of air trapping and hyperinflation. The judicious use of PEEP is essential, balancing the need to avoid increasing the FRC which is already elevated in the asthmatic, while managing refractory hypoxaemia, where the use of PEEP to recruit atelectic alveoli would be beneficial.

It may be necessary to keep the child well sedated and muscle relaxed for the first 24–48 hours after intubation according to the clinical stability of the child.

Indications for weaning are improvement in oxygenation and reducing peak inspiratory pressures, which can take as little as 48 hours after intubation in some children. The aim should be to extubate the child as soon as possible as the presence of the ETT in a hypersensitive airway itself can exacerbate the underlying process.

As previously noted, PICU admission and intubation/mechanical ventilation are among the risk factors for increased mortality, and parental advice and support are important considerations as part of family care within the

Table 4.32 Complications of status asthmaticus

- Respiratory failure despite maximal therapy.
- Atelectasis.
- Pneumothorax.
- Pneumomediastinum.
- Superimposed infections.
- Inappropriate ADH secretion.
- Hyponatraemia.
- Hypokalaemia.
- Cardio-respiratory arrest.
- Hypoxic brain damage.
- Death.

PICU alongside liaison with an asthma or respiratory nurse specialist.

The immediate complications of status asthmaticus are detailed in Table 4.32.

Parental support with full explanations of their child's planned care and the responses to prescribed interventions

A daily meeting with the intensivist responsible for the child (or their nominated doctor) should take place to maintain a therapeutic relationship with the child's family. Where possible and if appropriate to the child's age, cognitive ability and clinical condition, the child's involvement in update discussion should also be considered.

Pneumonia

Pneumonia can be generally defined as inflammation of the lung parenchyma, in which there is consolidation of the affected part and a filling of the alveolar air spaces with exudate and inflammatory cells. Pneumonia is one of the commonest clinical presentations in the critically ill child and may be bacterial, viral or fungal in origin (Table 4.33). It is also possible for the child to present with both bacterial and viral pneumonia. The exact mechanism for this is not clearly understood. Initially, it was proposed that the explanation for the viral–bacterial relationship focused on the disruption of the respiratory epithelium by the virus, which cleared the way for bacterial pathogens to invade. However, it is thought that there are far more complex and possibly synergistic interactions between viruses and bacteria, which include the alteration of pulmonary physiology, down-regulation of the host immune defence, changes in expression of receptors to which bacteria adhere and enhancement of the inflammatory process (McCullers 2006).

The child may be admitted with a primary pneumonia or may develop a secondary pneumonia as a consequence of intubation and ventilation (ventilator-acquired pneumonia). Treatment strategies and prognosis are dependent on the causative organism, the severity of the illness and any underlying or pre-existing comorbidity factors such as children with immunocompromise/immunoinsufficiency. Community-acquired pneumonia (CAP) has a significant mortality risk (Barry et al. 2010) and some of the presenting pathogens are particularly virulent, such as the strain of *Staphylococcus aureus* identified as PVL (Panton-Valentine Leukocidin)-MRSA, which is also known as community-associated MRSA (CA-MRSA) (Health Protection Agency 2011) (Table 4.33).

Table 4.33 Common pathogenic causes of pneumonia

Type of pneumonia	Common pathogens
Bacterial	*Streptococcus pneumoniae*
	Haemophilus influenzae B
	Group A or Group B streptococci
	Staphylococcus aureus
	Pseudomonas aeruginosa
Viral	Respiratory syncytial virus (RSV)
	Adenovirus
	Influenza A and B
	HIN1 influenza
	Measles
	Mycoplasma
Fungal	Aspergillus
	Candida albicans

Pneumonia may be classified according to the area of the lung(s) affected:

- Lobar.
- Multifocal/lobular (bronchopneumonia).
- Interstitial (focal diffuse).

Clinical features of pneumonia

- Fever (may be a single presenting sign or in combination with other signs).
- Cough.
- Abdominal, chest and or neck pain.
- Tachypnoea.
- Tachycardia.
- Increased work of breathing – use of accessory muscles, head bobbing and grunting in infants.
- Presence of hypoxaemia (SpO$_2$ < 92%).
- Adventitious breath sounds on auscultation (presence of coarse crackles, bronchial breathing).
- Pale and mottled skin.

Clinical investigations

- Blood cultures.
- Respiratory secretions for MC&S and virology.
- Chest X-ray which will show areas of consolidation and or collapse. There may also be evidence of hyperinflation and localised or general infiltrates.

Management of the child with pneumonia

This is targeted towards organ support and treatment of the underlying causes until function recovers. Key priorities include:

- Strict handwashing and standard isolation practice dependent on the identified organism(s) responsible for the illness.
- Monitoring – ECG, SpO$_2$ and NIBP with capillary blood gases as a minimum in the non-ventilated child. If the child requires intubation and ventilation, then arterial line siting is beneficial to facilitate close monitoring of the child's respiratory status and responses to change in ventilatory support.
- If the child is self-ventilating, supplementary oxygen therapy which is warmed and humidified should be administered in the method most appropriate for the child's age.
- The use of NIPPV may avoid the need for intubation and ventilation. However, the decision to intubate should be made based on the presence of respiratory failure (indicated by increased PaCO$_2$ and low pH), the presence of

persistent hypoxaemia refractory to supplementary oxygen therapy or in the face of a clinical picture of a child who is exhausted (decreased respiratory effort and slowing respiratory rate) on initial presentation.

- It is usual to fluid-restrict children presenting with significant respiratory illness to 75 or 80% of their calculated daily requirements as there is a risk of them developing inappropriate anti-diuretic hormone secretion which causes fluid retention. These children may also require diuretic therapy such as furosemide to promote effective fluid removal.

- Careful positioning is an essential part of treatment alongside physiotherapy in clearing secretions from the lower airways and re-inflating areas of alveolar collapse. Not all children will tolerate aggressive physiotherapy in the initial phase of their illness. Lateral lying is beneficial in treating a child with pneumonia. Whereas adults with unilateral lung disease tolerate lying with their normal lung in the dependent position, the reverse is applicable in infants and young children and they often need to be positioned with their good lung uppermost. Although this is a good rule of thumb when considering the best position for the child, some children will not tolerate side-lying at all in the initial phase of their illness. For these children, or those for whom oxygenation is a significant issue, the use of the prone position may be considered.

- Administration of appropriate antimicrobial agents according to local prescribing guidelines and identified sensitivities from cultures.

- General comfort cares, including meeting the child's basic hygiene needs, regular eye care and oral hygiene as well as regular skin assessment to minimise the potential for the child to develop sore skin secondary to monitoring lines/wires.

Parental support with full explanations of their child's planned care and the responses to prescribed interventions

A daily meeting with the intensivist responsible for the child (or their nominated doctor) should take place to maintain a therapeutic relationship with the child's family. Where possible and if appropriate to the child's age, cognitive ability and clinical condition, the child's involvement in update discussion should also be considered.

Aspiration pneumonia

Aspiration pneumonia is a clinical condition seen as a consequence of the inhalation of gastric or oropharyngeal contents into the lower airways where it causes inflamma-

tory changes and initiates a pneumonitis. Chronic aspiration secondary to gastro-oesophageal reflux disease can manifest in frequent presentations with lower respiratory tract symptoms or pneumonia. Acute aspiration events may often be attributable to episodes of vomiting in children with either a decreased level of consciousness or children with underlying neuromuscular weaknesses, however any condition that impairs the child's ability to swallow can lead to an aspiration episode. Aspiration events secondary to the misplacement of an oro-or nasogastric tube were identified as 'never events' by the Department of Health in 2010. Never events are deemed to be serious adverse patient events that are largely preventable with the correct preventative measures in place (DH 2011).

The management of an aspiration episode is to follow the ABC approach – clear the child's airway using suction, provide bag–valve–mask ventilation and/or supplementary oxygen therapy based on the child's clinical condition and institute cardiovascular monitoring. If the child continues to require oxygen therapy or shows signs of increasing respiratory distress, the child should be transferred to the PICU (if not already there) and either NIPPV or intubation and mechanical ventilation should be considered. Clinically, aspirated gastric or oropharyngeal contents will usually end up in the right middle and lower lobes due to the position of the right mainstem bronchus, however CXR changes in these areas may not manifest in the immediate period following the event. The lack of changes on initial CXR is not predictive of the child not subsequently developing a pneumonitis. The management of a child who is intubated and ventilated following an aspiration event is no different from that of the child with pneumonia of any other cause. Consideration should be given to the potential management of severe gastro-oesophageal reflux disease or further investigations of underlying neuromuscular weaknesses if these have not already been instigated.

Acute respiratory distress syndrome

First described by Ashbaugh et al. in 1967, acute respiratory distress syndrome (ARDS) is a clinically defined entity describing the severity of diffuse alveolar injury caused by direct (pulmonary) or indirect (systemic) injury to the lung parenchyma (Table 4.34) and occurs as a consequence of critical illness.

Acute lung injury or ARDS?

In 1994 a consensus statement from the North American–European Consensus Conference defined the spectrum of respiratory failure in the adult population into two categories: Acute Lung Injury – PaO_2/FiO_2 ratio ≤ 300; and

Table 4.34   Causes of ARDS

Direct (pulmonary) causes	Indirect (systemic) causes
Pneumonia	Common causes
Aspiration events	• Sepsis
Pulmonary contusion	• Trauma
Smoke inhalation	• Shock
Near-drowning	• DIC
Drugs	Rarer causes
Radiation	• Multiple transfusions
Pulmonary embolism	• Re-perfusion injury
	• Anaphylaxis

ARDS – PaO_2/FiO_2 ratio ≤ 200 (Table 4.34). Rodriguez Martinez and colleagues (2006) concluded that these figures lack the validity to apply within the PIC population making definition more difficult in the paediatric population, although other authors have accepted their validity (Cheifetz 2011; Zimmerman et al. 2009). Similar divergent opinions are to be found in published literature advocating different treatment approaches. What is clear is that, historically, the majority of studies have been conducted in the adult population with results being extrapolated to the paediatric population. Children will present with ARDS-type illnesses, however the complex nature of the disease process and the immaturity and resilience of paediatric organ systems make it more difficult to quantify. It is therefore a relatively rare disease within PIC compared to general intensive care and one that has a variable mortality association. Mortality remains relatively high at approximately 50% in the adult population, although this can be divided into those who die as a consequence of the triggering event (death within 7 days) and those who die as a consequence of respiratory failure (death after 7 days). Mortality in the paediatric population is reported as between 8 and 70% and there is a correlation between severity of presenting hypoxia and mortality in children (Randolph 2009).

ARDS is a complex clinical syndrome characterised by non-cardiogenic pulmonary oedema, damage to the alveolar capillary membrane and increased microvascular permeability. These physiological abnormalities result in refractory hypoxaemia, decreased lung compliance and altered gas exchange.

The characteristics of the disease are summarised as:

• Acute onset, which may follow a catastrophic event.
• Widespread bilateral infiltrates on CXR (diffuse pulmonary inflammation).

• Severe hypoxaemia resistant to supplementary oxygen therapy.
• No clinical evidence of left atrial hypertension.

Pathophysiology of ARDS

The ARDS process can be delineated into four clinical phases: acute exudative phase, sub-acute proliferative phase, chronic phase and recovery phase.

Acute exudative (alveolar injury) phase: This phase occurs within hours of the triggering event. Although the mechanism is not fully understood, tissue injury may be related to the production of endogenously released products from macrophages and neutrophils. Neutrophil activation is thought to be one of the key factors of the ARDS process, however neutropenic patients also develop ARDS, therefore other vasoactive mediators and bioactive compounds are just as important in the pathophysiology. An example of the process in sepsis is detailed in Figure 4.14.

The damage to the endothelium causes the further release of bioactive compounds.

Within the lungs the following picture emerges:

• Leak of proteinaceous material containing fibrin results in the inhibition of surfactant activity and the formation of hyaline membranes around the alveolar lining.
• Damage to the pneumocytes (Type 2 cells) reduces the availability of surfactant.

The combination of these two events causes a loss of lung elasticity.

A further chain of events takes place at the same time involving plugging of the pulmonary microcirculation with platelet thrombi and the release of thromboxane A2. This leads to an increase in the pulmonary vascular resistance and the development of pulmonary hypertension which contribute to the increasing refractory hypoxaemia present. There are cardiovascular implications of ARDS which should be considered. The development of pulmonary hypertension results in increased right ventricular afterload, while the application of high PEEP levels necessary to improve oxygenation results in decreased preload. The combination of these two factors results in decreased cardiac output.

Sub-acute proliferative phase: It is thought that the high level of ventilation and oxygen required at this time continues to trigger the release of bioactive compounds from the pulmonary macrophages, which in turn increases the damage to the structure of the alveoli and the lungs. At a cellular level this phase is characterised by an energy crisis

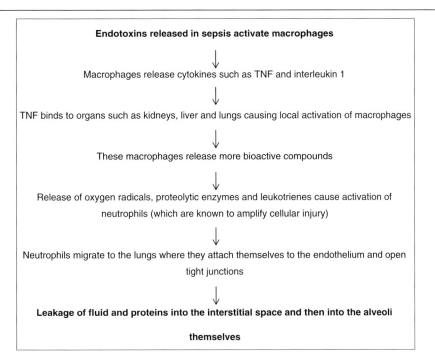

Figure 4.14   Basic pathophysiology of ARDS in sepsis.

in the cells, while clinically there is an increasing V/Q mismatch, the development of hypercarbia and ongoing pulmonary hypertension. The energy crisis in the cell is described in Figure 4.15.

The increased V/Q mismatch occurs as a consequence of alveolar oedema and the formation of a fibrous membrane over the surface of the alveoli, which inhibits the diffusion of oxygen across the alveolar–capillary membrane. Changes in the cells lining the alveolus further reduce the gas exchange abilities of the lungs. The type 1 pneumocytes swell and become ineffective in terms of their primary function (gas exchange) while the type 2 pneumocytes proliferate and eventually replace type 1 pneumocytes. These are non-functioning and therefore produce no surfactant. In addition, pulmonary interstitial oedema develops as the lymphatics are overwhelmed by the fluid changes within the lung parenchyma.

Structurally, there is small airway and alveolar compression which leads to increased airway resistance. The presence of atelectasis decreases FRC and further decreases compliance, making ventilation management more challenging.

Chronic phase: This is characterised by a period of relative stability but little progress clinically in terms of ventilation requirements.

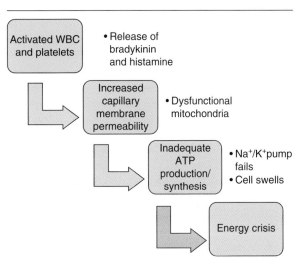

Figure 4.15   Sub-acute proliferative phase – energy crisis in the cell.

Recovery phase: As the child moves into the recovery phase there is a gradual improvement in respiratory function which allows for the weaning of ventilatory support and a move towards extubation. This final phase is characterised by a resolution of hypoxaemia, resolution in the radiological abnormalities and improved lung compliance.

Management of the child with ARDS

The primary aim of management is to optimise oxygen transport/delivery to the cells (DO_2), while supporting other body systems to prevent deterioration in function (Table 4.35 and Table 4.36). Factors affecting DO_2 include haemoglobin (oxygen-carrying capacity), cardiac output (preload, afterload and contractility) and arterial oxygen content. Manipulation of these factors can increase oxygen delivery to the cells and prevent the switch from aerobic to anaerobic metabolism with associated acidosis.

Drugs available for use in the management of ARDS are few and the evidence base for their use is limited, although empirical practice has shown clinical improvement in some children.

Nitric oxide therapy– does it work?

Empirical evidence suggests that if it is going to be effective, there will be a relatively rapid improvement in oxygenation after commencing therapy and early use may prolong and maximise its effectiveness (Fioretto et al. 2004). This early view is supported by many of the published studies reviewed by Adhikari et al. (2007) in their systematic review and meta-analysis, however only two of these trials involved children. The summary of the trials found that there was no demonstrable improvement in:

- Mortality.
- Duration of ventilation.
- Ventilator-free days.

In addition, there is the potential that nitric oxide therapy may cause harm and careful monitoring of methaemoglobin levels is required while the child is receiving inhaled nitric oxide therapy. Methaemoglobin is formed when the iron within haemoglobin is oxidised from the ferrous (Fe^{2+}) state to the ferric (Fe^{3+}) state. Because iron needs to be in the ferrous state to allow haemoglobin-to-oxygen binding, methaemoglobinaemia results in variable degrees of deficiencies of oxygen transport. This effect is usually associated with the delivery of 20 ppm (or greater) of nitric oxide and it is rare for that concentration of nitric oxide to be maintained for a prolonged period of time.

Parental support with full explanations of their child's planned care and the responses to prescribed interventions

A daily meeting with the intensivist responsible for the child (or their nominated doctor) should take place

to maintain a therapeutic relationship with the child's family.

Near-drowning

Although there is no universally accepted classification for submersion injuries, drowning is usually defined as death resulting from asphyxia within 24 hours of submersion in a liquid medium. Near-drowning therefore refers to survival (even if temporary) beyond 24 hours after a submersion episode (Papa et al. 2005), although conflicting terms are used in the literature. Further delineation relating to the type of water (fresh or saltwater), the place containing the water (natural or man-made) and the temperature of the water (warm or cold) can be made and maybe significant in the management of the child, but are considered as unimportant in the actual submersion event (Suominen et al. 2002). The number of water-related fatalities in the UK in 2009 in the under 18s is reported as 59 (National Water Safety Forum 2011).

Pathophysiology of drowning

Aspiration of large volumes of water is uncommon in submersion episodes. The most important contributory factors to morbidity and mortality from submersion events are hypoxaemia with inadequate oxygen delivery to vital tissues. The pathophysiology of near-drowning is clearly related to the multi-organ effects of hypoxaemia (Ibsen and Koch 2002; Ross 2005).

Pulmonary effects

Increased airway resistance secondary to plugging of the patient's airway with debris, as well as the release of inflammatory mediators that result in vasoconstriction, may impair gas exchange post-injury. Fluid aspiration of as little as 1–3 ml/kg can result in significantly impaired gas exchange secondary to impaired surfactant function. Altered surfactant volume and/or function result in atelectasis and significant injury to the alveolar–capillary unit, resulting in lower functional residual capacity and the development of pulmonary oedema. Acute respiratory distress syndrome (ARDS) from altered surfactant function and neurogenic pulmonary oedema is a common complication in children following submersion injury.

Pneumonia is a relatively rare consequence of submersion injury and is more common with submersion in stagnant, warm, fresh water.

Cardiovascular effects

Although initial cardiovascular effects may be significant, they are usually transient compared to the severity of brain injury suffered. Myocardial dysfunction may occur as a

Table 4.35 Management strategies in ARDS

Management strategies	Notes and considerations
Permissive hypercapnia	A strategy where the targets for $PaCO_2$ and therefore pH are widened in an attempt to reduce the detrimental effects of mechanical ventilation on the lung parenchyma. An elevated $PaCO_2$ will cause a respiratory acidosis with a pH of less than 7.35. While acknowledging the effects on the body systems of a persistent acidosis, it is generally accepted that as long as the pH remains above 7.25, $PaCO_2$ levels should be allowed to rise to around 80mmHg or 10.6 kPa without adjustment or increases in ventilation to achieve more normal values.
Use of PEEP and appropriate tidal volumes ($V_t = 6$ ml/kg)	The use of PEEP (8–10 cmH$_2$O) is advocated for its positive effects in terms of increasing the transpulmonary distending pressure, which: • Displaces oedema from the alveolar space. • Decreases atelectasis. • Decreases right-to-left shunts. • Increases compliance. • Improves oxygenation. These positive effects have to be balanced against the negative effects of PEEP on cardiovascular performance. In addition, a leak of >20% around the ETT will reduce the effectiveness of the application of PEEP. Tidal volumes of 4–6 ml/kg are advocated as the appropriate volumes in the adult field and while there is no clear evidence in the paediatric field, this strategy is widely used.
High frequency oscillatory ventilation (HFOV)	Lung-protective ventilation using high frequency very low tidal volumes generated by the oscillator is commonly used in PIC for the management of ARDS. The evidence base for its use remains limited, with only one published RCT (Arnold et al.1994), which suggested improvement in oxygenation and a reduction in the need for supplementary oxygen therapy at 30 days. Empirical reports confirm these findings. Positive effects of oscillation include: • Rises in the mean airway pressure and therefore improvement in oxygenation. • Re-recruitment of collapsed lung volume. • Uniform alveolar inflation – reduces possibility of barotrauma and associated release of vasoactive mediators from damaged cells. HFOV can impede venous return, necessitating intravascular volume expansion and/or inotropes.
Prone positioning	The use of the prone position is advocated as an intervention for improving oxygenation and there is a wealth of evidence in the adult and neonatal populations. The positive attributes of prone positioning in respiratory distress include: • More uniform alveolar ventilation. • Recruitment of atelectasis in dorsal regions. • Improved postural drainage. • Redistribution of perfusion away from oedematous-dependent regions. In children there is limited evidence of its efficacy, but one RCT (Curley et al. 2005) showed improvement in oxygenation in the short term but no significant benefit of prone positioning (20 hours a day for 7 days) in terms of clinically important outcome measures of ventilator-free days, mortality and morbidity.
ECMO	ECMO is indicated in children who continue to deteriorate despite maximal therapy or in children who are continuing to receive high ventilatory settings and are therefore at risk of significant barotrauma. Rescue ECMO has shown positive outcomes in the adult and neonatal population and retrospective studies support its use in children. Prior to referral for ECMO, the child will need to meet certain criteria, such as a reversible underlying pathology and a limited number of days (usually <10) of mechanical ventilation. ECMO is only provided in a small number of UK centres, therefore the need for transfer should be considered early in the child's illness course if they appear to be refractory to maximal treatment. There is currently only one specialised paediatric team who transfer children already established on ECMO.

Table 4.36 Drugs used in the management of ARDS

Drug therapy	Notes
Surfactant	Surfactant production in ARDS is impaired, with the changes identified in the cells of the alveolar wall. In neonatal patients treated for infant ARDS, the use of surfactant has been clinically shown to improve outcome. In adult patients, trials have not produced similar significant benefits. Evidence suggests that surfactant use may be beneficial in children with ARDS by reducing mortality and ventilator-dependent days (Randolph 2009). Young children with ARDS due to a primary pulmonary insult may be the most likely to benefit from exogenous surfactant. There are a number of different types of surfactant available, derived from animal or synthetic sources. In the United Kingdom there are currently two versions available (Survanta® and Curosurf®) and doses are product-dependent. Practitioners should refer to their local guidelines or the BNFC for further information. The administration of surfactant can be difficult and may cause haemodynamic instability and profound hypoxia in the child (Been and Zimmermann 2007).
Steroids	Corticosteroids have anti-inflammatory and immunosuppressive properties and modify the body's immune response to a diverse range of stimuli. They have been used to manage refractory ARDS unresponsive to maximal therapies. Some published data in the adult field suggest that the use of corticosteroids may be beneficial in patients with severe ARDS. No trials have been conducted with published results to evaluate their use in children with ARDS in either the early (<7 days) or late (>7 days) phases of the disease process (Randolph 2009; Foster 2010). The timing of the use of corticosteroids continues to be based on empirical evidence.
Nitric oxide	Pulmonary vasodilator • Selectively improves perfusion of ventilated areas. • Reduces intrapulmonary shunting. • Improves arterial oxygenation. • No systemic haemodynamic effects. Hypoxia associated with ARDS increases endothelin-1 production, the presence of which decreases endogenous nitric oxide synthesis. Inhaled nitric oxide activates pathways in the smooth muscle which end in the relaxation of alveolar vascular smooth muscle tone and therefore improvement in ventilation–perfusion matching.

consequence of hypoxaemia and acidosis or less commonly electrolyte abnormalities which will decrease cardiac output. This dysfunction may manifest in cardiac dysrhythmias, such as pulseless electrical activity (PEA) or ventricular fibrillation (VF). Pulmonary hypertension may result from the release of pulmonary inflammatory mediators which will increase right ventricular afterload and consequently decrease both pulmonary perfusion and left ventricular preload.

Central nervous system (CNS) effects

CNS injury is the major determinant of subsequent survival and long-term morbidity in cases of near-drowning. Primary CNS injury is initially associated with tissue hypoxia and ischaemia. If the period of hypoxia and ischaemia is brief or in the very young child who rapidly develops core hypothermia, primary injury may be limited and the child may recover with minimal neurological sequelae. In contrast, submersion injuries associated with prolonged hypoxia and or ischaemia are likely to lead to significant primary injury and secondary injury from reperfusion, sustained acidosis, cerebral oedema, hyperglycaemia, release of excitatory neurotransmitters, seizures, hypotension and impaired cerebral auto regulation, especially in older patients who cannot rapidly achieve core hypothermia.

Autonomic instability (diencephalon/hypothalamic storming) may occur following severe traumatic, hypoxic or ischaemic brain injury. Clinical features are symptoms of hyperstimulation of the sympathetic nervous system, including tachycardia, hypertension, tachypnoea, diaphoresis, agitation and muscle rigidity.

Other effects

The child's clinical course may be complicated by multi-organ system failure as a consequence of prolonged hypoxia and/or acidosis. Additional critical care problems, including disseminated intravascular coagulation (DIC) and hepatic and renal dysfunction, should be anticipated and managed appropriately if they arise.

Smoke inhalation

Smoke inhalation injury is the commonest cause of mortality in fire-associated deaths in children, although many but not all of these children will also suffer significant skin thermal injury. In the UK in 2010–11, 23 children under the age of 16 died in house fires while a further 1276 suffered non-fatal injuries (Department of Communities and Local Government 2011). The clinical signs of smoke inhalation injury may not manifest until 24–48 hours after the event and therefore early CXRs may have a normal appearance. The mortality rate for smoke inhalation alone is around 7% and this increases to around 22% in the presence of simultaneous carbon monoxide (CO) poisoning (Barry et al. 2010).

Pathophysiology of smoke inhalation injury

The mechanism of injury in smoke inhalation is complex and multifactorial and when smoke inhalation injury is combined with burn injury or pneumonia, the physiological responses are different and more severe than those of smoke inhalation injury alone (Murakami and Traber 2003). A number of factors have been identified in the literature and include changes in bronchial blood flow which contributes to increased fluid and protein shifts into the alveoli alongside complex interactions between endogenous nitric oxide and other mediators of the inflammatory response such as interleukin-1, culminating in an up-regulation of nitric oxide in the lungs, which contributes to an increased ventilation perfusion mismatch (Enkhbaatar and Traber 2004). The very specific interactions and detailed physiology of smoke inhalation injury (and burn injury) are beyond the scope of this chapter, however they can be summarised as:

- Direct damage to the lung parenchyma as a consequence of the inhalation of both hot gases and soot particles, which are both profound irritants. The presence of these triggers the inflammatory response seen in the ARDS process, leading to increased permeability across the alveolar–capillary membrane, the leak of proteinaceous fluid into the alveoli and subsequent changes in the function of the pneumocytes. This leads to a clinical picture of increasing pulmonary oedema, decreased lung compliance and refractory hypoxaemia.
- Asphyxiation resulting in hypoxia secondary to the presence of carbon monoxide (CO) in the inhaled gases. CO is very rapidly absorbed into the blood stream and once there, preferentially binds with haemoglobin (in place of O_2) forming carboxyhaemoglobin. CO binding prevents O_2 binding with haemoglobin. There is a left shift in the oxygen dissociation curve, which reduces the release of O_2 to the tissues causing tissue hypoxia and abnormal tissue metabolism. In addition, CO affects the ability of the cells effectively to metabolise energy sources and release adenosine triphosphate (ATP). As a consequence, CO increases free oxygen radicals production, which are known to be harmful to tissue cells.
- Cyanide poisoning – cyanide is a toxic substance given off when certain materials burn, which is rapidly absorbed into the blood stream. Cyanide affects both the myocardium and the central nervous system causing tissue damage.

Clinical features of smoke inhalation and airway burns

- Presenting history – type and location of fire, length of time the child remained in a smoke-filled space as these will influence the possibility of the child developing a significant lung injury.
- Initial examination:
  - Burn injury: site, assessment of percentage of injury, degree of thickness of burn and potential concerns if there are circumferential burns to the chest wall which may impact on respiratory performance.
  - Respiratory: presence of soot around the nares, sputum containing soot particles, audible stridor and/or presence of wheeze on auscultation are indicative of significant airway involvement, however the presence of soot around the nares alone is a clinical sign that the child has the potential to develop pulmonary sequelae.
  - Cardiovascular: assessment of cardiac function (heart rate, blood pressure and capillary refill time) although this may prove difficult in the child with significant external burn injuries. Initial management should follow approved resuscitation algorithms if the child presents in cardiac arrest. As CO binds to virtually all the haem molecules, myocardial myoglobin is affected and consequently myocardial contractility is decreased.
  - Other injuries: depending on the history and location of the child, there may well be additional trauma such

as bone fractures which need to be assessed and managed.

Considerations for practice

Although detailed respiratory assessment is essential in the management of the child with inhalation injury, pulse oximetry and PaO_2 measurements are unreliable in children with carbon monoxide poisoning. It is important to have a detailed breakdown of the levels of different types of haemoglobin present in the child's blood provided by the co-oximetry measurements on blood gas analysers. The delivery of high-flow oxygen therapy should be instigated in the self-ventilating child while the intubated child should receive a set FiO_2 of 1.0 via the ventilator until there is clear evidence of the level of carboxyhaemoglobin present. If there is, then this treatment should be continued.

The half-life of CO is 320 minutes in room air, 90 minutes in 100% oxygen and 23 minutes in a hyperbaric chamber at 3 atmospheres absolute (ATA). Elimination of CO depends primarily on the law of mass action, so alveolar PO_2, rather than alveolar ventilation, is the critical factor in its removal (Kao and Nanagas 2006)

Renal function and CK levels should be monitored closely as the child with significant burns is at risk of developing rhabdomyolysis (see Chapter 6).

Respiratory management of the child with smoke inhalation injury

- Early intubation and ventilation if there is strong suspicion or evidence of airway involvement.
- Delivery of high levels of supplementary oxygen.
- Ventilation strategy should be lung-protective and may require the use of HFOV as in the management of ARDS.
- Bronchoscopy and bronchoalveolar lavage are advocated in adult practice and published results suggest that it may be a benefit in terms of measurable outcomes such as ventilator-free days and overall mortality (Carr et al. 2009).

Further management of the child with thermal injury is detailed in Chapter 10.

Persistent pulmonary hypertension of the newborn (PPHN)

Persistent pulmonary hypertension of the newborn (PPHN) with right to left shunting occurs in a variety of clinical situations in the newborn infant including:

- Meconium aspiration syndrome (MAS).
- Hypoplastic lungs.
- Transient tachypnoea of the newborn (TTN).

Normal transition of circulation	In a baby with PPHN
Rapid dilation of pulmonary vascular beds (as lungs receive 100% of cardiac output)	Delayed relaxation of the pulmonary vascular beds
↓	↓
Decreases in pulmonary vascular resistance (PVR) aided by: • Presence of spontaneous respiration • Increased PaO_2 • Altered production of vasoactive agents such as endothelin-1/prostacyclin and nitric oxide	Pulmonary vascular resistance (PVR) does not drop therefore right-sided pressures do not fall Increased right-sided pressures which exceed left-sided pressures result in the foramen ovale (and the ductus arteriosus) remaining open
↓	↓
Closure of foramen ovale and the ductus arteriosus as left-sided pressures increase and right-sided pressures decrease	PERSISTENT FOETAL CIRCULATION

Figure 4.16 Pathophysiology of PPHN.

- Congenital pneumonia.
- Respiratory distress syndrome.

Secondary disturbances, such as hypoglycaemia, cold stress, sepsis and myocardial failure are also contributory factors. There may be a history of chronic in utero hypoxia, but some cases remain idiopathic. The pathophysiology of PPHN is detailed in Figure 4.16.

Clinical features of PPHN
- Systemic/suprasystemic pulmonary artery pressures.
- Right to left shunting through the foramen ovale.
- Myocardial dysfunction – varies from mild RV dysfunction to biventricular failure leading to congestive cardiac failure.
- Hypoxia.
- Acidosis.

Management priorities for PPHN (Table 4.37)
- Lower PVR/SVR ratio – improve pulmonary blood flow and improve oxygenation without inducing systemic hypotension.
- Reduce intracardiac shunting.
- Reduce RV afterload – manage myocardial dysfunction.
- Correct underlying cause of PPHN (if possible).

Congenital diaphragmatic hernia

Congenital diaphragmatic hernia occurs in 1/2000–3000 live births and accounts for 8% of all major congenital anomalies. The risk of recurrence of isolated (non-syndromic) congenital diaphragmatic hernia in future siblings is approximately 2%. Familial congenital diaphragmatic hernia is rare (<2% of cases), and both

Table 4.37 Management priorities in PPHN

Intervention	Notes and considerations
Mechanical ventilation	The aim is to achieve lung volumes greater than FRC to improve and reverse hypoxia and increased PVR.
HFOV	Short inspiration times to avoid alveolar over distension (0.15–0.3 seconds) • Improves gas exchange. • Promotes uniform alveolar inflation. • Decreases V–Q mismatch. • Decreases air leaks. • Reduces release of inflammatory mediators associated with barotrauma from conventional ventilation. • Has been shown to decrease need for ECMO.
Nitric oxide therapy (iNO)	Hypoxia associated with PPHN increases endothelin-1 production, the presence of which decreases endogenous nitric oxide synthesis. Inhaled nitric oxide activates pathways in the smooth muscle which end in the relaxation of alveolar vascular smooth muscle tone and improvement in ventilation–perfusion matching.
Sildenafil	Works by increasing the levels of GMP* which results in pulmonary vascular relaxation. • Augments the effects of iNO. • Prevents the pulmonary vasoconstriction and rebound PHT associated with weaning of iNO. • Has been shown to increase cardiac output by as much as 30%. *Cyclic guanosine monophosphate which acts at the cellular level as a regulator of various metabolic processes.*
General cares	• Use of alkalising agents ($NaHCO_3$) to treat metabolic acidosis. • Cardiovascular support – improve cardiac output and systemic oxygen transport through use of inotropes/inodilators. • Sedation/minimal handling to reduce oxygen demands (+/– muscle relaxants). • Effective thermoregulation to avoid cold stress. • Maintain serum glucose levels within normal parameters to promote effective cellular metabolism.

autosomal recessive and autosomal dominant patterns of inheritance have been reported.

Congenital diaphragmatic hernia is a recognised finding in Cornelia de Lange syndrome and also occurs as a prominent feature of Fryns syndrome. It occurs as a consequence of the failure of the pleuro-peritoneal canal division due to inadequate development of the muscular components (weeks 8–10). The majority are diagnosed antenatally at the 18-week scan or after investigation of polyhydramnios. Postnatal diagnosis can be described as early (<24 hours of age) or late (>24 hours of age).

Types of congenital diaphragmatic hernia
• Morgagni hernia: This is rare (2% of cases) and involves an opening in the front (anteromedial) of the diaphragm, just behind the sternum. The intestines may move up into the thoracic cavity.
• Bochdalek hernia: This involves an opening on the back (posterolateral) of the diaphragm. The stomach, intestines and liver or spleen usually move up into the thoracic cavity. These account for over 80% of cases with left-sided defects outnumbering right.

The remaining classification of diaphragmatic hernia is the para-oesophageal or hiatus hernia. Bilateral defects are extremely rare and are usually fatal.

The prognosis for infants with single defects is related to the degree of pulmonary hypoplasia and age at presentation (Levene et al. 2008).

• Infants presenting with respiratory distress by <6 hours of age have a mortality of around 70%.
• Infants presenting between 6 and 24 hours have a mortality of between 10 and 15%.
• Later presentations tend not to be associated with pulmonary hypoplasia and therefore have a very good prognosis.
• Poor prognostic indicators:
  – Presence of polyhydramnios.
  – Persistently elevated $PaCO_2$ levels with mean airway pressures of >20 cmH$_2$O.
  – Hypoxia requiring management with pulmonary vasodilators.

Pathophysiology of congenital diaphragmatic hernia
Congenital diaphragmatic hernia is characterised by a variable degree of pulmonary hypoplasia associated with a decrease in the cross-sectional area of the pulmonary vasculature and alterations of the surfactant system. The lungs have a small alveolar capillary membrane for gas exchange, which may be further decreased by surfactant dysfunction. In addition to parenchymal disease, increased muscularisation of the intra-acinar pulmonary arteries appears to occur. In very severe cases, left ventricular hypoplasia is observed. Pulmonary capillary blood flow is decreased because of the small cross-sectional area of the pulmonary vascular bed, and flow may be further decreased by abnormal pulmonary vasoconstriction.

Clinical features of congenital diaphragmatic hernia
• Scaphoid abdomen and barrel-shaped chest.
• Signs of respiratory distress:
  – Recession.
  – Cyanosis.
  – Grunting respirations.
• In left-sided posterolateral hernia, auscultation of the lungs reveals poor air entry on the left, with a shift of cardiac sounds over towards the right chest.
• In infants with severe defects, signs of pneumothorax (poor air entry, poor perfusion) may be found.

Management of congenital diaphragmatic hernia is detailed in Table 4.38.

Tracheomalacia/Bronchomalacia

Malacia is defined as softness in either cartilage or bone and in relation to the airway refers to a softness of tracheal cartilage in tracheomalacia or the bronchial cartilage in bronchomalacia (Austin and Ali 2003). Malacia disorders are essentially disorders of airway resistance. In a dynamic sense, the expiratory phase is usually worse, but the variable nature of the lesions in paediatrics means that the partial airway closure may affect inspiration as well.

Tracheomalacia refers to narrowing of the trachea during expiration with no involvement of the lower airways (bronchi). It may occur as an isolated lesion or can be found in combination with other lesions that cause compression or damage of the airway. Tracheomalacia is usually benign, with symptoms due to airway obstruction.

Bronchomalacia refers to either unilateral or bilateral narrowing of the mainstem bronchi without any tracheal involvement.

Tracheobronchomalacia refers to conditions in which both the trachea and mainstem bronchi narrow during expiration.

The causes may be divided into primary which may arise in isolation as a structural defect or in association

Table 4.38 Management of the infant with congenital diaphragmatic hernia

Pre-operative management priorities	Postoperative management priorities
Orogastric tube placement for gastric decompression	Management of pulmonary hypertension
No bag–valve–mask ventilation	Strategies to minimise right–left shunting (inotropes/volume)
Intubation/ventilation to support respiratory function	Muscle relaxants/sedation
	Nutrition
HFOV (evidence base not established)	There is often a 'honeymoon period' in the immediate postoperative phase followed by deterioration in the infant's clinical condition associated with:
Use of nitric oxide/prostacyclin for pulmonary vasodilation to improve hypoxia associated with increased ventilation/perfusion mismatch	• Increased abdominal pressure • Impaired peripheral and visceral perfusion • Limited diaphragmatic excursion • Worsening of pulmonary compliance
Referral for ECMO (52% survival rate – ELSO registry)	

with another congenital presentation, and secondary where they are acquired as a consequence of a disease process.

Examples of primary causes
- Isolated defect in an otherwise healthy infant.
- Congenital abnormalities of cartilage structure.
- Tracheo-oesophageal fistula.
- VATER anomaly.
- Pierre–Robin syndrome.
- Trisomy 21.

Examples of secondary causes
- Prolonged intubation.
- Presence of tumours or cysts.
- Traumatic injury.
- Secondary to vascular compression, e.g. double aortic arch.

Clinical features

The clinical features will depend on the area of the airway involved and the severity of the narrowing experienced. Each of these three conditions has a significant associated morbidity and mortality risks depending on the extent and severity of the narrowing. Investigations such as bronchoscopy with the child spontaneously ventilating are required for confirmation of the diagnosis. Common presenting features include:

- Difficulty in feeding and faltering growth.
- Recurrent episodes of respiratory distress or frequent presentation with symptoms of respiratory illness but no identified underlying pathology.
- Stridor (may be present on inspiration and expiration).
- Selective positioning by the infant to improve patency of airway.
- In severe cases, recurrent, acute life-threatening episodes (ALTEs), such as prolonged apnoeas with bradycardia leading to collapse.

Management of tracheomalacia/bronchomalacia will be governed by the severity and extent of the narrowing. Treatment can vary from conservative management in infants who have mild symptoms only involving maximising the infant's nutritional status, and parental support/advice relating to positioning, through to the formation of a tracheostomy and long-term ventilation provision. Children with severe disease or those in whom there is a significant risk of death secondary to ALTEs may require surgical intervention, such as aortopexy, which is a procedure in which the aortic arch is surgically fixed to the sternum, resulting in the tracheal lumen being pulled open and which can be used to treat severe localised tracheomalacia; or stenting of the segment of the airway that is affected.

Intercostal drain insertion

There are a number of clinical conditions in which intercostal drain insertion may be necessary as part of the child's treatment. These are detailed in Table 4.39.

Conclusion

This chapter has reviewed the growth and development of the respiratory system, considered applied physiology and provided an overview of current airway management and ventilation strategies designed to provide support to the child who requires these for a primary respiratory reason or needs to be ventilated for another reason.

Table 4.39   Clinical conditions requiring intercostal drain insertion

Condition	Notes and considerations
Pneumothorax	May be either a simple pneumothorax or a tension pneumothorax. Simple – the presence of air/free gas between the pleural and visceral layers of the pleural cavity. The underlying degree of lung collapse is related to the volume of air present. A small pneumothorax may resolve with the administration of a high concentration of supplementary oxygen, if this is not contraindicated by any coexisting disease process. Tension – the presence of air between the pleural and visceral layers of the pleural cavity which increases in volume with each breath, resulting in mediastinal shift and potential cardiac tamponade. This is a life-threatening emergency which requires immediate needle decompression followed by formal chest drain insertion.
Haemothorax	An accumulation of blood within the chest which most often results from injury to intrathoracic structures or the chest wall. It may be seen post-cardiac or thoracic surgery. Consideration should be given to the volume of blood drained after insertion of a chest drain. There are two long-term complications: an empyema and a fibrothorax. An empyema results from bacterial contamination of the retained haemothorax. If undetected this can lead to bacteraemia and septic shock. A fibrothorax occurs when fibrin deposits develop within a haemothorax and coat the parietal and visceral pleural surfaces, trapping the lung. The lung is fixed in position by this adhesive process and is unable to fully expand. Persistent atelectasis of portions of the lung and reduced pulmonary function result from this process.
Pleural effusions	A pleural effusion is the abnormal collection of fluid in the pleural space. There are a number of types of pleural effusions, the classification of which are dependent on the underlying processes leading to their development. • Effusions that develop as a consequence of a lower respiratory tract infection are known as para-pneumonic effusions and are commonly associated with bacterial infections such as *Pneumococcus pneumoniae* although they may develop secondary to viral and atypical infections as well. These effusions can develop into an empyema if they are not managed in the initial stages. A relatively common presentation into the ED from the community is that of a child 2–3 weeks after a LRTI who has increased symptoms of respiratory distress and is generally unwell. • Other effusions may develop as a consequence of non-infective processes such as those seen in postoperative cardiac patients, particularly those with high right-sided pressures, or as a consequence of renal failure. • Pleural effusions may also occur as a consequence of malignancies and unless the child presents as acutely compromised from a respiratory/cardiac perspective, these are often managed through the use of diuretics, fluid restriction and therapies targeting the underlying disease process rather than through the use of a chest drain. Management of the child with a pleural effusion will depend on the underlying cause, the size of the effusion and the clinical stability of the child.
Empyema	An empyema develops secondary to the presence of a pleural effusion and is a mixture of viscous fluid and cells which form pus. The characteristics of empyema development mean that small, isolated pockets of pus form as a consequence of fibrin membranes developing around the collection. This in known as loculation or a loculated collection. The fluid at this stage is extremely thick. Children who present with empyema usually require a 3-week course of high-dose IV antibiotics and fibrinolysis therapy targeting the fibrin membrane which dissolves it and enables the collection to drain.

Table 4.39   (*Continued*)

Condition	Notes and considerations
Chylothorax	A chylothorax is a pleural effusion which occurs as a consequence of lymph fluid collecting in the pleural space secondary to a leak from the thoracic lymph duct or one of its main branches. It occurs as a consequence of either cardiac or thoracic surgery in which there is damage to the lymph ducts or in children with high-sided right pressures where this leads to mechanical obstruction of the lymph ducts.
	The management of the child with a chylothorax depends on the effects of the effusion. The majority of children will already have a chest drain in situ, therefore monitoring of the amount of drainage is easy to achieve. The child should receive modified enteral feeds with medium chain triglycerides (MCT) providing their fatty acids. In children in whom the change in enteral nutrition does not resolve the chylothorax, total parental nutrition may be instituted for a short period followed by the re-introduction of modified enteral feeds.

References

Adhikari NK, Burns KE et al. 2007. Effect of nitric oxide on oxygenation and mortality in acute lung injury: systematic review and meta-analysis. British Medical Journal, 334:779–86.

Advanced Paediatric Life Support (ALSG). 2005. Advanced Paediatric Life Support: The practical approach (4th edition). Oxford: Wiley-Blackwell.

Albuali WH, Singh RH et al. 2007. Have changes in ventilation practice improved outcome in children with acute lung injury? Pediatric Critical Care Medicine, 8(4):324–30.

Amir L, Hubermann H et al. 2006. Oral betamethasone versus intramuscular dexamethasone for the treatment of mild to moderate croup. Pediatric Emergency Care, 22(8):541–4.

Arnold JH, Hanson JH et al. 1994. Prospective randomized comparison of high-frequency oscillatory ventilation and conventional mechanical ventilation in pediatric respiratory failure. Critical Care Medicine, 22(10):1530–9.

Ashbaugh D, Bigelow D et al. 1967. Acute respiratory distress in adults. Lancet, 2(7511):319–23.

Asthma UK. 2011. Asthma Basics. www.asthma.org.uk/about-asthma/asthma-basics.

Austin J, Ali T. 2003. Tracheomalacia and bronchomalacia in children: pathophysiology, assessment, treatment and anaesthesia management. Paediatric Anaesthesia, 13:3–11.

Barry P, Morris K, Ali T. (Eds). 2010. Paediatric Intensive Care. Oxford: Oxford University Press.

Been JV, Zimmermann LJI. 2007. What's new in surfactant? A clinical view on recent developments in neonatology and paediatrics. European Journal of Pediatrics, 166(9): 889–99.

Biarent D, Bingham R, Eich C, et al. 2010. European Resuscitation Council Guidelines 2010. Section 6: Paediatric life support. Resuscitation, 81(10):1364–88.

Bisgaard H, Nielsen KG. 2000. Bronchoprotection with a leukotriene receptor antagonist in asthmatic preschool chil-dren. American Journal of Respiratory Critical Care Medicine, 161:1–4.

Blackwood B. 1999. Normal saline instillation with endotracheal suctioning: primum non nocere (first do no harm). Journal of Advanced Nursing, 29:928–34.

British National Formulary for Children (BNFC). 2012. British Medical Association, Royal Pharmaceutical Society, Royal College of Paediatrics and Child Health, Neonatal and Paediatric Pharmacists Group. www.medicinescomplete.com/mc/bnfc/tinyurl.com/c7tlbcc.

British Thoracic Society. 2011. Managing Asthma in Children. www.brit-thoracic.org.uk/Portals/0/Guidelines/AsthmaGuidelines/pat101_children.pdf.

Brown K, Sriram S, et al. 2010. Extracorporeal membrane oxygenation and term neonatal respiratory failure deaths in the United Kingdom compared with the United States 1999 to 2005. Pediatric Critical Care Medicine, 11(1):60–5.

Buck ML. 2005. The use of chloral hydrate in infants and children. Pediatric Pharmacotherapy, 11(9).

Buck ML, Hofer KN, McCarthy MW. 2008. Caffeine citrate for the treatment of apnea of prematurity. Pediatric Pharmacotherapy, 14(6).

Cambonie G, Milesi C et al. 2008. Nasal continuous positive airway pressure decreases respiratory muscles overload in young infants with severe acute viral bronchiolitis. Intensive Care Medicine, 34:1865–72.

Carr JA, Phillips BD, Bowling WM. 2009. The utility of bronchoscopy after inhalation injury complicated by pneumonia in burn patients: results from the National Burn Repository. Journal of Burn Care and Research, 30(6): 967–74.

Caruso P, Denari S et al. 2009. Saline instillation before tracheal suctioning decreases the incidence of ventilator-associated pneumonia. Critical Care Medicine, 37(1):32–8.

Celik SA, Kanan N. 2006. A current conflict: use of isotonic sodium chloride solution on endotracheal suctioning in critically ill patients. Dimensions of Critical Care Nursing, 25(1):11–14.

Cheifetz IM. 2011. Paediatric acute respiratory distress syndrome. Respiratory Care, 56(10):1589–99.

Cheuk DKL, Chau TCH, Lee SL. 2005. A meta-analysis on intravenous magnesium sulphate for treating acute asthma. Archives of Disease in Childhood, 90:74–7.

Cormack RS, Lehane J. 1984. Difficult tracheal intubation in obstetrics. Anaesthesia, 3:1105–11.

Curley MAQ, Hibberd PL et al. 2005. Effect of prone positioning on clinical outcomes in children with acute lung injury. JAMA, 294(2):229–38.

Department of Communities and Local Government. 2011. Fire Statistics: Great Britain 2010–2011. http://www.communities.gov.uk/publications/corporate/statistics/firestatsgb201011

Department of Health. 2010. Immunisation against Infectious Diseases – The Green Book. www.dh.gov.uk/en/Publicationsandstatistics/Publications.

Department of Health. 2011. The Never Events List for 2011–2012. www.dh.gov.uk/en/Publications.

Enkhbaatar P, Traber DL. 2004. Pathophysiology of acute lung injury in combined burn and smoke inhalation injury. Clinical Science, 107:137–43.

Faroux B, Lavis J-F et al. 2005. Facial side effects during non-invasive positive pressure ventilation in children. Intensive Care Medicine, 31(7):965–9.

Fassassi M, Michel F et al. 2007. Airway humidification with a heat and moisture exchanger in mechanically ventilated neonates. Intensive Care Medicine, 33:336–43.

Fioretto JR, de Moraes MA et al. 2004. Acute and sustained effects of early administration of inhaled nitric oxide to children with acute respiratory distress syndrome. Pediatric Critical Care Medicine, 5(5):469–74.

Fontanari P, Burnet H et al. 1996. Changes in airway resistance induced by nasal inhalation of cold dry, dry, or moist air in normal individuals. Journal of Applied Physiology, 81(4):1739–43.

Foster JR. 2010. Steroids for early acute respiratory distress syndrome: critical appraisal of Meduri GU, Golden E et al: Methylprednisolone infusion in early severe ARDS: results of a randomized controlled trial. Chest, 2007, 131:954–963. Pediatric Critical Care Medicine, 11(3):404–7.

Froese AB. 1997. High-frequency oscillatory ventilation for adult respiratory distress syndrome: let's get it right this time. Critical Care Medicine, 25(6):906–8.

Glynn F, Amin M, Kinsella J. 2008. Nasal foreign body in children: should they have a plain radiograph in the accident and emergency? Pediatric Emergency Care, 24:217–20.

Grisaru-Soen G, Komisar O et al. (2010. Retropharyngeal and parapharyngeal abscess in children–epidemiology, clinical features and treatment. International Journal of Pediatric Otorhinolaryngology, 74(9):1016–20.

Gupta S, Sharma R, Jain D. 2005. Airway assessment: predictors of difficult airway. Indian Journal of Anaesthesia, 49(4):257–62.

Haines C. 2009. Respiratory. In M Dixon, D Crawford et al. (Eds). Nursing the Highly Dependent Child or Infant: A Manual of Care (chapter 3). Oxford: Wiley–Blackwell.

Hartling L, Fernandes RM et al. 2011. Steroids and bronchodilators for acute bronchiolitis in the first two years of life: systematic review and meta-analysis. British Medical Journal, 342.ncbi.nlm.nih.gov.

Harvey B, Crawford D. In press. A review of ECMO use in the UK. Nursing Children and Young People.

Health Protection Agency. 2011. Latest Results for MRSA, MSSA, E. coli, CDI and GRE. www.hpa.org.uk/Topics/InfectiousDiseases/InfectionsAZ/HCAI/LatestPublicationsFromMandatorySurveillanceMRSACDIAndGRE.

Ibsen LM, Koch T. 2002. Submersion and asphyxial injury. Critical Care Medicine, 30(11) (Suppl.):S402–S408.

Ijland MM, Heunks LM, van der Hoeven JG. 2010, Bench-to-bedside review: hypercapnic acidosis in lung injury –from 'permissive' to 'therapeutic'. Critical Care, 14(6):1–10.

Ireton J. (2007) Tracheostomy suction: a protocol for practice. Paediatric Nursing, 19(10):14–18.

Kao LW, Nanagas KA. 2006. Toxicity associated with carbon monoxide. Clinics in Laboratory Medicine, 26(1):99–125.

Kattwinkel J, Perlman J et al. 2010. Neonatal Resuscitation: American Heart Association Guidelines for Cardiopulmonary Resuscitation and Emergency Cardiovascular Care. Pediatrics, 126(5):1400–13.

Khemani RG, Randolph A, Markovitz B. 2009. Corticosteroids for the prevention and treatment of post-extubation stridor in neonates, children and adults. Cochrane Database of Systematic Reviews 3: Art. CD001000.

Knox T. (2011) Practical aspects of suctioning in children. Nursing Children and Young People, 23(7):14–17.

Laffey JG, O'Croinin D et al. 2009. Permissive hypercapnia – role in protective lung ventilatory strategies. (pp. 241–50). In G Hedenstierna, J Mancebo et al. (Eds). Applied Physiology in Intensive Care Medicine. Berlin: Springer.

Levene MI, Tudehope DI, Sinha S. 2008. Essential Neonatal Medicine (4th edition). Oxford: Blackwell.

Matthay MA, Calfee CS. 2005. Therapeutic value of a lung protective ventilation strategy in acute lung injury. Chest, 128(5):3089–91.

Matthews BD, Noviski N. 2001. Management of oxygenation in pediatric acute hypoxemic respiratory failure. Pediatric Pulmonology, 32(6):459–70.

McCoskey L. 2008. Nursing care guidelines for the prevention of nasal breakdown in neonates receiving nasal CPAP. Advances in Neonatal Care, 8(2):116–24.

McCullers JA. 2006. Insights into the interaction between influenza virus and pneumococcus. Clinical Microbiological Reviews, 19(3):571–82.

Melsen WG, Rovers MM, Bonten MJ. 2009. Ventilator-associated pneumonia and mortality: a systematic review of observational studies. Critical Care Medicine, 37(10): 2709–18.

Murakami K, Traber DL. 2003. Pathophysiological basis of smoke inhalation injury. Physiology, 18(3):125–9.

Najaf-Zadeh A, Leclerc F. 2011. Non-invasive positive pressure ventilation for acute respiratory failure in children: a concise review. Annals of Intensive Care, 1(15).

National Institute for Health and Clinical Excellence. 2007. Feverish Illness in Children. guidance.nice.org.uk/CG47.

National Institute for Health and Clinical Excellence and the National Patient Safety Agency. 2008. Technical Patient Safety Solutions for Ventilator-Associated Pneumonia in Adults. www.nice.org.uk/PSG002.

National Water Safety Forum. 2011. UK Water-related Fatalities 2009.WAID database report. www.nationalwatersafety. org.uk/waid/reports.asp.

Papa L, Hoelle R, Idris A. 2005. Systematic review of definitions for drowning incidents. Resuscitation, 65(3):255–64.

Park MK. 2010. The Pediatric Cardiology Handbook, 4th edition. Philadelphia: Mosby Elsevier.

Peace D. 2007. Oral care during mechanical ventilation significantly reduces the incidence of ventilator-associated pneumonia. American Journal of Infection Control, 35(5): E67.

Petrucci N, Iacovelli W. 2007. Lung protective ventilation strategy for the acute respiratory distress syndrome. Cochrane Database of Systematic Reviews 3: Art. CD003844.

Pryor J, Prasad S. 2002. Physiotherapy for Cardiac and Respiratory Problems: Adults and children. Edinburgh: Churchill Livingstone.

Randolph AG. 2009. Management of acute lung injury and acute respiratory distress syndrome in children. Critical Care Medicine, 37(8):2448–54.

Rees JE. 2005. Suxamethonium apnoea. Anaesthesia, 19 (16): 1.

Richardson M, Hines S et al. 2010. Establishing nurse-led ventilator-associated pneumonia surveillance in paediatric intensive care. Journal of Hospital Infection, 75(3):220–4.

Riding DA, Martin LD, Bratton SL. 2003. Endotracheal suctioning with or without instillation of isotonic sodium chloride solution in critically ill children. American Journal of Critical Care, 12(3):212–19.

Rodriguez Martinez CE, Guzman MC et al. 2006. Evaluation of clinical criteria for the acute respiratory distress syndrome in pediatric patients. Pediatric Critical Care Medicine, 7(4):335–9.

Ross J. 2005. Summer Injuries Series. Near drowning]. RN68 (7) CINAHL with full text. EBSCOhost.

Sevketoglu E, Karabocuoglu M. 2007. Ventilator-associated pneumonia in children. Journal of Pediatric Infectious Diseases, 2(3):127–34.

Shah RK, Mora BM et al. 2007. The presentation and management of vascular rings: an otolaryngology perspective. International Journal of Pediatric Otorhinolaryngology, 71:57–62.

Suominen P, Baillie C et al. 2002. Impact of age, submersion time and water temperature on outcome in near-drowning. Resuscitation, 52(3):247–54.

Swingler G, Fransman D, Hussey G. 2007. Conjugate vaccines for preventing Haemophilus influenzae type B infections. Cochrane Database of Systematic Reviews 4: CD001729.

Tebruegge M, Pantazidou A et al. 2009. Bacterial tracheitis: A multi-centre perspective. Scandinavian Journal of Infectious Diseases, 41(8):548–57.

Venkatachalam V, Hendley JO, Willson DF. 2011. The diagnostic dilemma of ventilator-associated pneumonia in critically ill children. Pediatric Critical Care Medicine, 12(3):286–96.

Weiss M, Dullenkopf A et al. 2009. Prospective randomized controlled multi-centre trial of cuffed or uncuffed endotracheal tubes in small children. British Journal of Anaesthesia, 103:867.

Westley C, Cotton EK, Brooks JG. 1978. Nebulized racemic epinephrine by IPPB for the treatment of croup: a double-blind study. American Journal of Diseases in Children, 132(5):484–7.

Zimmerman JJ, Akhtar SR et al. 2009. Incidence and outcomes of pediatric acute lung injury. Pediatrics, 124(1): 87–95.

Chapter 5
CARE OF AN INFANT OR CHILD WITH A CARDIAC CONDITION OR DISEASE

Sandra Batcheler and Michaela Dixon

Paediatric Intensive Care Unit, Bristol Royal Hospital for Children,
University Hospitals Bristol NHS Foundation Trust, Bristol, UK

Introduction

Cardiovascular performance in the critically ill child is often impaired or decreased secondary to hypoxia, acidosis or the presence of both. Causes of myocardial dysfunction may be primary, relating to structural defects (Congenital Heart Disease), rhythm disturbances or disease processes directly affecting the myocardium or secondary, relating to systemic illness such as sepsis, or ARDS. Effective cardiovascular assessment, recognition of the factors affecting cardiovascular performance and timely management are all essential in preventing further deterioration in the child's condition. This chapter will consider the developmental anatomy and physiology of the child and consider the deviations from normal. Medical and nursing care will be considered in the management of these conditions and an overview of some of the pharmaceutical management will be provided. The care of these children and their families is complex and the progress in what can be offered is at times startling. Infants and children for whom surgical and medical intervention would not have been possible only a few years ago can now be managed and the future continues to look promising.

Cardiac embryology

The heart is one of the first structures to form in the developing foetus and by 8 weeks' gestation the four chambers, the valves and the vessels are clearly identifiable. Any malfunction of this complex process will lead to the presence of a congenital heart lesion, although the reason for the cause of the abnormality is not always clearly understood.

Key stages in the development of the foetal heart (Figure 5.1)

- The origin of cardiac tissue is the mesoderm of the embryo.
- Around day 18, bilateral cardiogenic cords are formed from the mesoderm which in turn form the paired endocardial heart tubes.
- The endothelial tubes fuse and grow, establishing a single straight primitive heart tube at around day 21.
- A rhythmic ebb and flow of blood (which precedes heart beats) is a chief characteristic of the primitive heart.

Between days 21 and 28 the primitive heart tube elongates, thickens and twists to the right. This is referred to as dextral or D looping and results in the correct anatomical positioning of the two ventricles. If the heart loops to the left at this stage (levo or L looping) then ventricular inversion occurs. By day 28 there is blood flow through the four identifiable heart chambers.

Atrial septation begins at day 28. The septum primum grows from a fold in the upper portion of the atria down

Paediatric Intensive Care Nursing, First Edition. Edited by Michaela Dixon and Doreen Crawford.

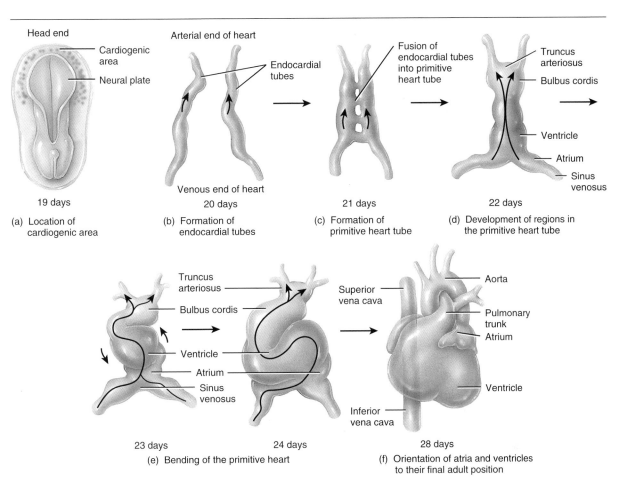

Figure 5.1 Development of the heart. From Tortora, G.J. and Derrickson, B.H. (2009) *Principles of Anatomy and Physiology*, 12th edn. Reproduced with permission from John Wiley and Sons, Inc.

towards the endocardial cushion, closing the opening known as the ostium primum. Fenestrations then appear in the upper section of the septum primum and these become the ostium secundum.

Next the septum secundum grows from the upper portion of the atria and this, in conjunction with the septum primum, forms the flap-like structure of the foramen ovale which permits blood to flow from the right to the left atrium when right atrial pressures are high, as they are in utero.

Ventricular septation occurs between weeks 4 and 8. A muscular fold appears at about day 30 and grows from the anterior wall and floor of the developing ventricles towards the endocardial cushion. The ventricles continue to grow downwards on either side of the evolving septum and septation is completed by growth of the bulbar ridges and the endocardial cushion at the end of week 7.

The developing ventricles initially share a single outflow tract, known as the truncus arteriosus. By day 40 the base begins to rotate clockwise, placing the evolving aorta anteriorly and the pulmonary artery posteriorly. Truncoconal swellings form from the truncal endocardium and these grow and rotate inwards before joining and separating the aorta and pulmonary artery.

Fusion of the endocardial cushions at week 6 divides the atrioventricular canal into two channels. The septal leaflets of the mitral and tricuspid valves develop from the endocardial cushion tissue while the mural leaflets develop from the myocardial wall (Kirby 2007).

Foetal circulation

The foetal circuit (Figure 5.2) consists of two arteries and one vein and three key openings or passages, the ductus

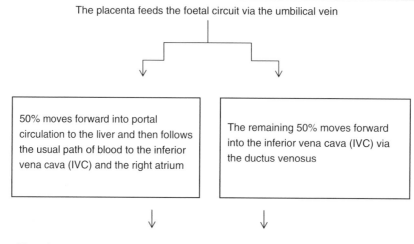

The placenta feeds the foetal circuit via the umbilical vein

| 50% moves forward into portal circulation to the liver and then follows the usual path of blood to the inferior vena cava (IVC) and the right atrium | The remaining 50% moves forward into the inferior vena cava (IVC) via the ductus venosus |

Blood from the IVC passes into the right atrium and the majority then moves across to the left atrium via the foramen ovale

Left ventricle to ascending aorta (supplies brain, coronaries and arms)
Blood from these areas returns to heart via SVC as normal

Blood not directed towards the left atrium passes into the right ventricle and moves into the pulmonary artery to supply the lower body: 90% will enter the descending aorta via the ductus arteriosus to supply the lower body and the remaining10% will move forward into the pulmonary vasculature to supply the cells of the lungs. Blood returns to the placenta via the umbilical arteries.

Figure 5.2   Schematic representation of the foetal circulation pulmonary artery.

venosus, foramen ovale and ductus arteriosus, which move blood around the foetus, bypassing the pulmonary circulation.

The foetal circuit is relatively hypoxic as it is passively fed from the maternal circulation and the pulmonary vascular resistance is high due to hypoxia-induced vasoconstriction and fluid rather than air-filled alveoli.

Changes in pulmonary vascular resistance (PVR) secondary to the reversal of hypoxia-induced vasoconstriction in the lungs at birth cause pressures in the right side of the heart to fall. Cord clamping and removal of low-resistance placental circulation cause closure of the ductus venosus and produces an increase in systemic vascular resistance (SVR) and increased pressure in the left ventricle. The combination of the fall in RA pressure and rise in LA pressure produces functional closure of the foramen ovale, however obstructive lesions on the right side of the heart may lead to delayed closure. Constriction of ductal smooth muscle leads to gradual closure of the ductus arteriosus over the first 7–10 days of life. During the first 2–9 weeks

of life, in a structurally normal heart, there is a gradual thinning of the medial smooth muscle layer of the pulmonary arteries, which leads to further reduction in PVR. At 3 months, therefore, in a normal healthy term infant PVR is equal to that found in adults.

Brief overview of cardiac anatomy and physiology (Figure 5.3)

External structure of the heart

The heart is surrounded by the pericardium, a loose-fitting, inextensible sac, which consists of two layers:

- Fibrous pericardium – a tough, loose-fitting and inelastic sac around the heart.
- Serous pericardium– consists of two layers:
  - The parietal layer is the lining of the fibrous pericardium.
  - The visceral layer adheres to the outside of the heart.

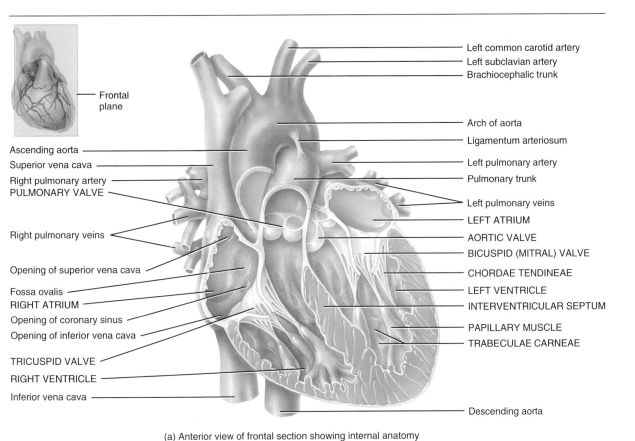

Left common carotid artery
Left subclavian artery
Brachiocephalic trunk

Frontal plane

Arch of aorta
Ligamentum arteriosum

Ascending aorta
Superior vena cava
Right pulmonary artery
PULMONARY VALVE

Left pulmonary artery
Pulmonary trunk

Left pulmonary veins
LEFT ATRIUM
AORTIC VALVE
BICUSPID (MITRAL) VALVE

Right pulmonary veins

CHORDAE TENDINEAE
LEFT VENTRICLE
INTERVENTRICULAR SEPTUM

Opening of superior vena cava

Fossa ovalis
RIGHT ATRIUM
Opening of coronary sinus
Opening of inferior vena cava

PAPILLARY MUSCLE
TRABECULAE CARNEAE

TRICUSPID VALVE
RIGHT VENTRICLE
Inferior vena cava

Descending aorta

(a) Anterior view of frontal section showing internal anatomy

Figure 5.3   Gross anatomy of the heart. From Tortora, G.J. and Derrickson, B.H. (2009) *Principles of Anatomy and Physiology*, 12th edn. Reproduced with permission from John Wiley and Sons, Inc.

The gap between these layers is known as the pericardial space and contains a small amount of pericardial fluid whose purpose is to reduce surface friction between the two layers of the serous pericardium. Any condition that leads to fluid accumulating in this sac will cause restriction of cardiac output and cardiac tamponade if it is not recognised and managed. The heart wall is made up of three layers of tissue: epicardium, myocardium and endocardium.

Epicardium

This is the outer layer of the heart wall and is the visceral layer of the serous pericardium; therefore, these two layers are one and the same.

Myocardium

This is the middle layer of the heart wall and is a thick, contractile layer of specially constructed and arranged cardiac muscle cells.

Endocardium

This is the lining of the interior of the myocardial wall and is a delicate layer of endothelial tissue. The endocardium covers projections of myocardial tissue from the ventricular walls known as trabeculae. Specialised folds or pockets formed by the endocardium make up the functional components of the intra-cardiac valves.

Intracardiac valves

There are four sets of valves in the heart which ensure that blood flows in one direction only, preventing an increase in the pressures within the atria and or ventricles which may cause damage to the structure or function of the myocardium.

- Atrioventricular valves (also called cuspid valves).
  - Tricuspid valve (RA–RV) is a three-leaflet valve.
  - Bicuspid valve (LA–LV) is a two-leaflet valve (the mitral valve).

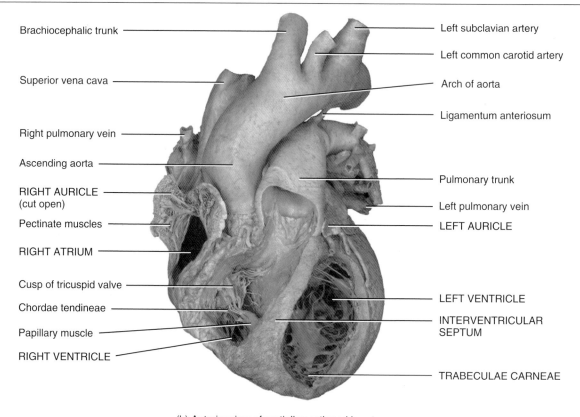

(b) Anterior view of partially sectioned heart

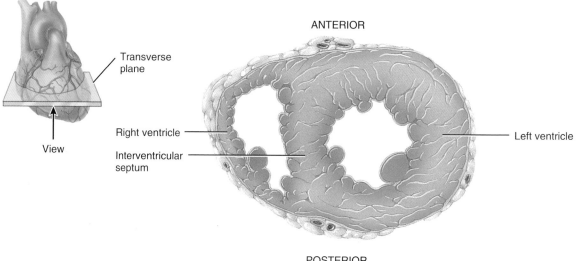

(c) Inferior view of transverse section showing differences
in thickness of ventricular walls

Figure 5.3   (*Continued*)

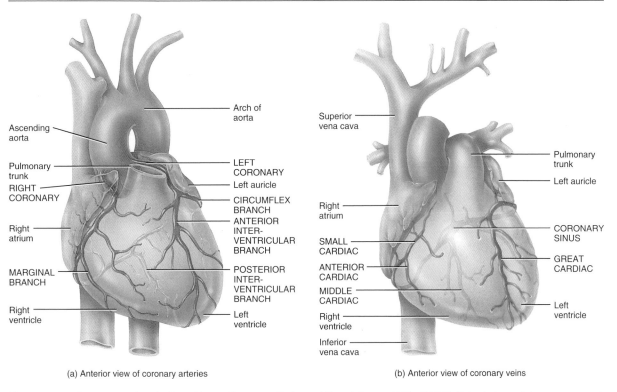

(a) Anterior view of coronary arteries

(b) Anterior view of coronary veins

Figure 5.4 Coronary circulation. From Tortora, G.J. and Derrickson, B.H. (2009) Principles of Anatomy and Physiology, 12th edn. Reproduced with permission from John Wiley and Sons, Inc.

These valves are held in place by the papillary muscle and additionally in the right ventricle by structures known as the chordae tendineae.

- Semilunar valves – consist of half-moon-shaped flaps growing out of the lining of the pulmonary artery and the aorta. The purpose of these valves is to prevent blood flowing back into the right or left ventricle from the pulmonary artery or aorta respectively at the end of ventricular systole.

Myocardial blood supply (Figure 5.4)

Myocardial cells receive blood to meet their metabolic demands from two small vessels known as the coronary arteries. The coronary arteries are found in the aorta behind the flaps of the aortic semilunar valves. The location of the coronary arteries has significance in terms of myocardial performance in the presence of a sustained tachycardia or low diastolic blood pressure.

Both coronary arteries have two main branches, but while the ventricles receive their blood supply from branches of both of the coronary arteries, the atria by con- trast receive blood from a small branch of the correspond- ing coronary artery.

Venous return

Once blood has passed through the capillary beds in the myocardium it enters a series of cardiac veins before drain- ing into the right atrium through a common venous channel known as the coronary sinus. (Several veins which collect blood from a small area of the right ventricle do not end in the coronary sinus but drain directly into the right atrium.)

The cardiac cycle

Innervation of the heart

Both divisions of the autonomic nervous system send fibres to the heart:

- Sympathetic fibres are contained in the middle, superior and inferior cardiac nerves.
- Parasympathetic fibres are contained in branches of the vagus nerve.

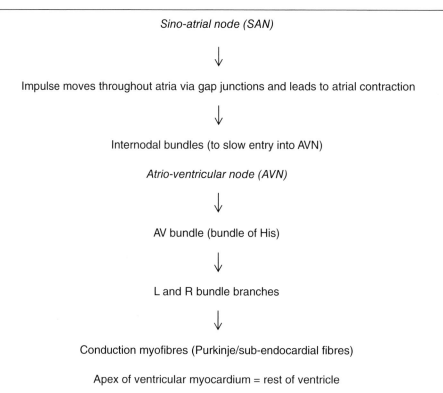

Sino-atrial node (SAN)

↓

Impulse moves throughout atria via gap junctions and leads to atrial contraction

↓

Internodal bundles (to slow entry into AVN)

Atrio-ventricular node (AVN)

↓

AV bundle (bundle of His)

↓

L and R bundle branches

↓

Conduction myofibres (Purkinje/sub-endocardial fibres)

Apex of ventricular myocardium = rest of ventricle

Figure 5.5   Impulse pathway.

These fibres combine to form the cardiac plexuses located close to the arch of the aorta. From the cardiac plexuses fibres accompany the coronary arteries to enter the heart, where most will terminate in the sino-atrial node (SAN), some in the atrio-ventricular node (AVN) and some in the atrial myocardium. From the SAN the impulse is transmitted through the conduction pathways of the atria and ventricles to generate contraction of both sets of chambers (Figure 5.5).

Structure and function of cardiac muscle fibres

The structure and properties of cardiac muscle are essentially a cross between that of the smooth muscle layers of the lungs, blood vessels and the gut and that of the striated muscle in the musculoskeletal system. While the basic contractile machinery is similar there are several important morphological and functional differences between cardiac muscle and skeletal muscle:

• Smooth (cardiac) muscle contracts and relaxes slowly, can initiate contraction and does not tire, whereas stri-ated (skeletal) muscle can contract and relax more rapidly but cannot initiate contraction and tires quickly.
• Cardiac muscle fibres are shorter than skeletal muscle fibres, but they have a larger diameter.
• Cardiac muscle has limited intracellular reserves of Ca^{++} compared to skeletal muscle.

The cells in the heart are known as myocytes (myocardial cells). The ends of individual myocytes connect to neighbouring cells through irregular transverse thickenings of the cell membrane, known as intercalated discs. These discs contain desmosomes, which hold the fibres together, and gap junctions, which allow action potentials to spread from one muscle fibre to another; consequently the walls/septum of the atria and the walls/septum of the ventricles form functional networks. This ensures that the impulse moves smoothly from the top of the atria downwards and from the apex of the ventricle upwards. Myocytes contain a large number of mitochondria and are surrounded by a strong capillary network to ensure that the oxygen demands of the cells are constantly addressed.

Each myocyte is made up of myofibrils, which in turn are made up of structures known as sarcomeres, which are the basic contractile units. The myofibrils are surrounded by the sarcoplasmic reticulum, the function of which is to act as a reservoir for calcium stores within the cell. Coordinated shortening of all the sarcomeres within each cell is the process through which contraction occurs.

The sarcomere is made up of filaments which interlace with each other. Some of the filaments are thick and contain the protein myosin while the remainder are thin and contain the protein actin. Heads on the myosin filaments stick out and are attracted to binding sites on the actin filaments. When activated, the myosin head attaches to the binding site (called a cross-bridge) on the actin filament. Each myosin head has two actin binding sites and two enzymatic sites which can change ATP to ADP and inorganic phosphate (involved in chemomechanical transduction, which is the molecular basis of energy transformation in all muscles). The interactions between the individual cross-bridges and the actin filaments is dependent on the presence of ATP, but is inadequate to generate enough force to affect muscle contraction. However, millions of cross-bridges cycling asynchronously can combine to generate considerable force, which contributes to the overall muscle cell shortening and contraction.

At rest actin and myosin are prevented from contacting each other by two other proteins: tropomyosin and the Ca^{++} binding protein troponin. Troponin is a complex protein which has three parts: troponin C, which binds calcium, troponin I; which prevents the interaction between actin and myosin; and troponin T, which binds the troponin molecule to tropomyosin. Upon stimulation, Ca^{++} is released from internal stores and binds to troponin C which induces a conformational change of tropomyosin and allows actin–myosin interaction. This process is outlined in Figure 5.6.

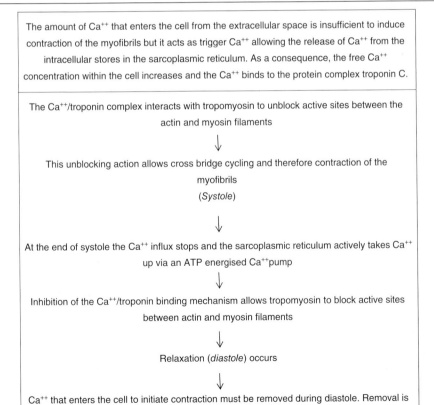

Figure 5.6   Mediation of cell contractility by calcium.

Considerations for practice

- Removal of Ca^{++} from the extracellular fluid decreases contractile force and will eventually cause arrest in diastole.
- Increases in the concentration of extracellular Ca^{++} enhance contractile force but very high Ca^{++} concentrations will eventually induce cardiac arrest in systole (rigor).

Cardiac action potentials

There are two general types of cardiac action potentials:

- Non-pacemaker action potentials (also called fast response action potentials because of their rapid depolarisation) are found throughout the heart, except for the pacemaker cells.
- The pacemaker cells generate spontaneous action potentials (also termed slow response action potentials because of their slower rate of depolarisation). These are found in the SA and AV nodes.

The action potential generated in the cardiac cells is different from that generated in the other types of cell as it contains a plateau phase which is essential to prevent myocardial tetany. The phases of a cardiac cell action potential are detailed in Figure 5.7.

Phase 4 – Resting membrane potential *(RMP)*
- *Cell is ready to generate an action potential*

Phase 0 – Depolarisation
- *Sodium moves into cell via the fast channels*
- *Cell becomes $^+$ve charged*
- *Slow channels open allowing movement of calcium into the cell*

Phase 1 – Short phase partial re-polarisation
- *Results from closure of fast channels*

Phase 2 – Plateau
- *Plateau in AP caused by continued diffusion of calcium into the cell and delays repolarisation*

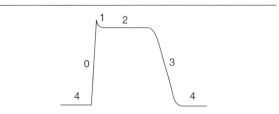

Figure 5.7   Phases of a cardiac action potential.

Phase 3 – Repolarisation
- *Slow calcium channels close and potassium channels open*
- *Membrane permeability to potassium is restored*
- *Significant potassium efflux to the outside of the cell*

Phase 4 – Restoration of RMP
- *Cell is ready to generate another action potential*

Regulation of cardiac action potentials

To maintain a normal rhythm it is vital that the cardiac muscle cells cannot generate a second action potential until completion of the previous cycle. The regulation of action potentials within the heart is achieved through the division of the action potential into four periods which control whether the cell can generate an action potential:

- Actual refractory period (ARP) –no matter how large a stimulus (i.e. inward current), the cell is unable to generate a second action potential during the absolute refractory period (ARP), because most of the Na$^+$ channels are closed. The absolute refractory period includes the upstroke, the entire plateau and a portion of the repolarisation. This period concludes when the cell has repolarised to approximately −50 mV.
- Effective refractory period (ERP) –includes and is slightly longer than the absolute refractory period. At the end of the effective refractory period, the Na$^+$ channels start to recover (i.e. become available to carry inward current).

  (The distinction between the absolute and effective refractory periods is that absolute means absolutely no stimulus is large enough to generate another action potential; effective means that a while an action potential may be generated it will not be a conducted action potential as there is not enough inward current to conduct it forward to the next site.)

- Relative refractory period (RRP) –begins at the end of the effective refractory period and continues until the cell membrane has repolarised to about −70 mV. During the relative refractory period even more Na$^+$ channels have recovered and it is possible to generate a second action potential, although a greater than normal stimulus is required. If a second action potential is generated during the relative refractory period, it will have an abnormal configuration and a shortened plateau phase.
- Supranormal period (SNP) –follows the relative refractory period. It begins when the membrane potential is −70 mV and continues until the membrane is fully repolarised to −85 mV. As the name suggests, the cell is more excitable than normal during this period and therefore

Table 5.1   Clinical implications of electrolyte imbalance, hypoxia and acidosis

Clinical state	Effects
Hypokalaemia (decreased extracellular potassium)	Affects the resting membrane potential and causes cardiac cells to become irritable; delays the repolarisation which leads to tachycardias and irregular beats (ectopics).
Hyperkalaemia (increased extracellular potassium)	Hypopolarises cardiac myocytes and causes a decrease and lengthening of depolarisation and repolarisation; heart block/arrhythmias common with fibrillation at higher serum K levels.
Hypocalcaemia (decreased extracellular calcium)	Reduces the strength of cardiac contraction by affecting the intracellular release of calcium necessary for actin–myosin binding, which reduces cardiac output and may also produce ectopic foci.
Hypercalcaemia (increased extracellular calcium)	Causes premature repolarisation and may produce spasmodic contractions of the cardiac muscle.
Hypoxia	Affects the function of the sodium–potassium pump which is ATP-dependent. This reduces the ability of the cells to maintain ionic balance and may lead to cell death.
Acidosis	Alters the function of the sodium and calcium channels reducing their specific conductance. This will lead to reduced cardiac contractility and cardiac output.

less inward current is required to depolarise the cell to the threshold potential. The physiological explanation for this increased excitability is that the Na^+ channels are recovered (i.e. the inactivation gates are open again), and because the membrane potential is closer to threshold than it is at rest, it is easier to fire an action potential than when the cell membrane is at the resting membrane potential.

Disorders of electrolyte balance, particularly potassium and calcium, as well as hypoxia and acidosis all have significant implications for cardiac rhythm (Table 5.1).

Each part of the cardiac cycle is associated with the movement of blood through the heart (Figure 5.8).

Atrial systole (ventricular diastole)

Onset of atrial systole occurs soon after the beginning of the P-wave on the ECG (curve of atrial depolarisation). Transfer of blood from the atrium to the ventricle is accomplished by a peristaltic-like wave of atrial contraction. The atrial pressure barely exceeds the ventricular pressure and the resistance of the pathway via the AV valves is normally very low.

Isovolumetric contraction (first heart sound)

The onset of ventricular contraction coincides with the peak of R-wave on the ECG and is the earliest rise in ventricular pressure after atrial contraction. The interval between the start of ventricular systole and the opening of the semilunar valves (when ventricular pressures rises sharply) is known as isovolumetric contraction because ventricular volume is constant during this period.

Ejection (R–S–T)

The opening of semilunar valves marks onset of the ejection phase which can be divided into two phases – rapid and reduced:

Rapid:

- Sharp rise in ventricular and aortic/pulmonary pressure.
- Decrease in ventricular volume.
- Large forward aortic/pulmonary blood flow.

Reduced:

- Decline in ventricular and aortic/pulmonary pressure.
- Reduced forward blood flow to the aorta/pulmonary artery.
- Stored energy in the arterial walls continues to move blood forward.

At the end of ejection a volume of blood which equals the volume of blood ejected in systole remains in the ventricle and is known as the residual volume. Closure of semilunar valves gives rises to the second heart sound.

- If outflow resistance decreases = reduced residual volume
- If outflow resistance increases = increased residual volume

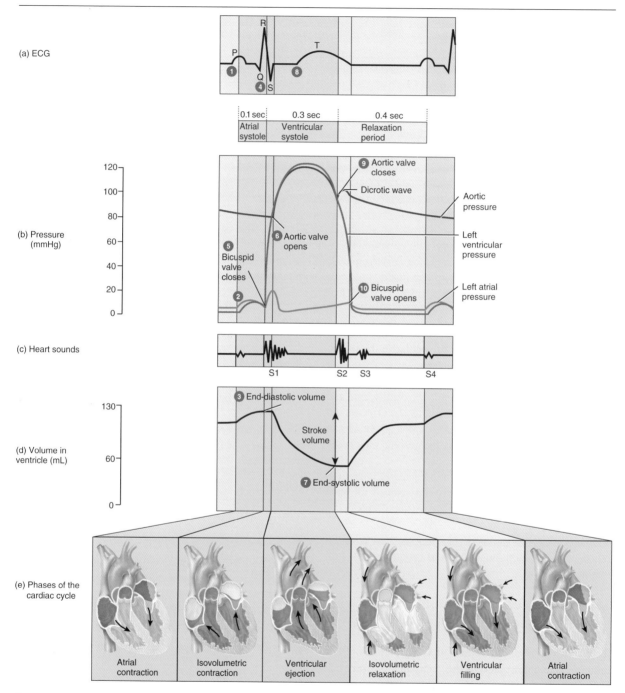

Figure 5.8   The cardiac cycle. From Tortora, G.J. and Derrickson, B.H. (2009) *Principles of Anatomy and Physiology*, 12th edn. Reproduced with permission from John Wiley and Sons, Inc.

Isovolumetric relaxation (end of T-wave to beginning of P-wave)

The gap between the closure of the semilunar valves and the opening of the AV valves is called isovolumetric relaxation. There is a large drop in ventricular pressure without a corresponding change in the ventricular volume.

Rapid filling phase (end of T-wave to beginning of P-wave)

Most ventricular filling occurs immediately after the AV valves open when blood which has returned to the atria during ventricular systole is released into the relaxing ventricles. The atrial and ventricular pressures both drop despite increases in ventricular volume because the relaxing ventricles exert less force on the blood.

Diastasis (slow filling phase)

Blood returning from the peripheries flows into the right ventricle from the right atria and blood from the pulmonary circulation into the left ventricle. Small slow additions to ventricular filling are indicated by gradual increases in atrial, ventricular and venous pressures.

Cardiac output

Cardiac output is defined as the volume of blood ejected from the heart in one minute and is determined by heart rate and stroke volume (amount of blood ejected from the ventricle per beat/cardiac cycle).

Heart Rate

When the heart rate is normal for the individual's age the following applies:

- Systolic component = 30% of each cardiac cycle.
- Diastolic component = 70% of each cardiac cycle.

If the heart rate increases, the systolic component remains relatively static but the diastolic component is reduced. This has two significant consequences. First, the period for ventricular filling is reduced, and second, myocardial oxygen supply decreases because the coronary arteries are filled and the myocardium is perfused during diastole. A persistent tachycardia may result in reduced cardiac output because of suboptimal myocardial performance, while in infants and children in particular bradycardia will reduce cardiac output because the stroke volume is relatively limited by the size of the heart and the fewer contractile elements in the immature heart. To maintain cardiac output, therefore, infants and young children need to increase their heart rate.

Factors affecting heart rate include:

- Chemicals such as adrenaline and noradrenaline.
- Electrolytes – mainly K^+, Na^+, Ca^{++} and magnesium.
- Age and gender.
- Body temperature – hyperthermia gives rise to tachycardia, hypothermia to bradycardia.
- Emotions.

In addition, there are a number of baroreceptors located in the carotid sinus, the aortic arch and the right atrium which work with the autonomic nervous system (ANS) to regulate the heart rate. Structures of the ANS include the cardioacceleratory and cardioinhibitory centres in the medulla, the vagal nerve and the SA and AV nodes.

Stroke Volume

This is determined by preload, afterload, contractility and compliance.

Preload – key points

This is the distending force or stretch exerted on the myocardial muscle fibre just prior to electrical stimulation and ventricular contraction. The force of myocardial muscle contraction is directly related to the initial length of the muscle fibres.

Preload determines the force and efficiency of ventricular contraction because it:

- Regulates the resting sarcomeres' length.
- Determines the number of actin–myosin cross bridges formed during systole.

Preload is dependent on venous return. A decrease in venous return will cause a decrease in cardiac output. The relationship between preload and its effects on stroke volume is described by Starling's law of the heart. The greater the diastolic volume or fibre stretch at end diastole, the greater the force of the next contraction during systole. However, once maximum stretch is achieved any further volume loading will reduce rather than increase stroke volume.

Afterload – key points

The amount of resistance to ventricular ejection and stroke volume is inversely proportional to afterload, therefore the greater the afterload the smaller the stroke volume. Influences on afterload include:

- Ventricular size.
- Ventricular shape.

- Aortic/pulmonary artery impedance.
- Systemic and/or pulmonary vascular resistance.

Compliance – key points

This is defined in terms of the relationship between end diastolic pressure (EDP) and end diastolic volume (EDV) and is the ability of the ventricle to relax and fill during diastole. In a normal mature heart compliance is high, allowing it to accept large increases in EDV without a significant increase in ventricular pressure. At birth infants have a greater proportion of non-contractile myocardial fibres, consequently their ventricular compliance is less. Postoperative myocardial wall oedema or either unilateral or bilateral ventricular hypertrophy will reduce compliance and will manifest as reduced diastolic function.

Considerations for practice

- Volume loading an infant who is not hypovolaemic will reduce cardiac performance because the immature ventricle cannot tolerate increased EDV without significantly increasing EDP.
- Right ventricular volume overload will displace the ventricular septum towards the left ventricle. This will inhibit the filling ability of the left ventricle, leading to obstruction of the left ventricular outflow tract and therefore reduce cardiac output.

Contractility – key points

This is the ability of the heart to modify its contractile performance independently of fibre length and therefore independent of volume loading. Sympathetic stimulation increases contractility as a result of the direct release of noradrenaline into the cardiac tissues (from intra-cardiac stores).

Other influences on contractility independent of fibre length are K^+, Na^+, Ca^{++}, hypoxia and acidosis.

Neonatal hearts function at near-capacity with minimal reserves as a consequence of both structural and functional immaturity, the key points of which are:

- Myocardial cells in infants are smaller and have more non-contractile elements.
- The degree and velocity of fibre shortening are less in the newborn heart, therefore less force is generated.
- Increased afterload decreases functional capacity far quicker in neonates than in the mature heart.
- Newborn myocardium lacks complete development of sympathetic innervation but parasympathetic innervation is complete at birth.

- Cardiac stores of noradrenaline in the ventricular myocardium are low, therefore there is a limited response in the neonate to alter contractility.

Cardiac assessment

A thorough cardiovascular assessment is essential to ensure the child's condition and any changes to that condition are quickly identified. It is therefore vital to have a good knowledge of normal cardiovascular parameters and the ability to link any variants with underlying cardiac pathophysiology.

- At birth the heart is classed as transverse and is large in proportion to the diameter of the thoracic cavity.
- In the infant, the heart is 1/130 of the total body weight, whereas in the adult it is 1/300.
- While myocardial performance reaches maturity around the age of 8 years, the heart continues to develop in terms of size and shape up to the age of 25.
- The size of the heart is normally roughly that of the individual's closed fist.
- In adulthood the heart's shape tends to resemble the shape of the chest – in tall thin individuals it is often elongated, in short stocky individuals it is transverse.

Practitioners also need to be aware of the maturational changes in cardiovascular performance.

Some key points to consider:

- Ventricular size – at birth both the right and left ventricle are similar in size. Over the next few months, as pulmonary vascular resistance decreases and systemic vascular resistance increases, the left ventricular (LV) wall thickens while the right ventricular (RV) wall remains the same size (Blackburn 2007). This change in size and power of the ventricles is reflected on a 12-lead ECG which demonstrates RV dominance up to around 4 months and then subsequently LV dominance. ECGs that demonstrate RV dominance in older infants and children merit further investigation. While the changes in PVR are usually complete by the age of 3–4 months the reciprocal changes in SVR occur throughout childhood. SVR is low in utero and rises immediately after birth, continuing to increase until adulthood is reached.
- Stroke volume – infants have a small stroke volume of about 1.5ml/kg at birth and this will increase as the ventricular size develops. In infants the stroke volume is also relatively fixed; to increase cardiac output their heart rate will need to increase and tachycardia in infants always reflects some degree of cardiovascular compro-

mise. By the age of 2 years myocardial function is similar to that of an adult, although their reserves remain limited in comparison.

- Circulating volume – an infant's circulating blood volume is approximately 80–90ml/kg which is higher per kg body weight than that of an adult. However, the much smaller actual volumes make the infant more vulnerable to the changes in fluid distribution associated with blood loss from trauma or surgery or the increased capillary permeability associated with sepsis, for example.

Physical inspection

As time allows, a detailed history should be taken of pre-natal, perinatal and family health, feeding patterns, fatigue and psychosocial history. Where appropriate, in an awake child the physical assessment should employ developmentally appropriate techniques to engage or distract the child as distress will affect the values gained from the examination. In the PICU the effects of critical illness such as the response to fever or the hormonal/neural compensatory mechanisms in the shock process need to be taken into account. During the physical examination, although focusing on cardiovascular assessment, other systems should not be ignored and any scars from previous surgery, respiratory distress or hepatomegaly in particular should be noted.

Physical assessment should begin with general observation of the child, paying attention to any dysmorphic or unusual features which may suggest a chromosomal abnormality. A number of chromosomal abnormalities such as Trisomy 21 (Down's syndrome), DiGeorge syndrome (micro-deletion of 22q11.2) or Marfan syndrome are associated with a higher incidence of cardiac defects (Park 2010).

Assessment of the child's state of growth and nutrition is a key part of cardiovascular assessment. Infants with a cardiac problem often present with or have clinical signs of tachypnoea and reduced cardiac output, indicated by increased respiratory effort and tachycardia, which mean they will tire easily during feeding and have difficulty coordinating their breathing with feeding and swallowing. This inability to maintain adequate calorific intake can result in faltering growth (Nydegger and Bines 2006; Steltzer et al. 2005).

Signs of pallor, mottling, diaphoresis (excessive sweats where the skin is cool to touch, thought to be triggered by continued stimulation of the sympathetic nervous system) or cyanosis should be noted. The presence and severity of clubbing of the fingers and toes, which is indicative of chronic hypoxaemia, may be observed in any child with a long-standing arterial desaturation (usually of more than 6 months). Clubbing is bulbous enlargement of soft parts of the terminal phalanges with both transverse and longitudinal curving of the nails. This occurs due to interstitial oedema and dilation of the arterioles and capillaries. The exact mechanism for the development of clubbing is uncertain but it does appear to be a consequence of hypoxia.

Palpation should be undertaken by an experienced practitioner or under the direct supervision of one. A hyperactive precordium is a clinical finding in cardiac conditions where there is high volume overload (e.g. left-to-right shunts or severe valvular regurgitation).

Auscultation

The cardiovascular examination itself often begins with auscultation of the apex beat and of the heart sounds. In the newborn the apex beat may be auscultated with a stethoscope placed over the 4th–5th intercostal space in the mid-clavicular line. Experienced practitioners may choose to auscultate and listen for any deviation from the normal heart sounds heard as a result of the closure of the cardiac valves. Murmurs are caused by turbulent blood flow through abnormal connections or an obstruction to flow. Approximately 30% of children with murmurs have structurally normal hearts; these murmurs are referred to as innocent or ejection murmurs. Murmurs are graded 1–6 according to how loud they are and if there is a thrill present (Table 5.2).

A thrill is a palpable murmur and is always abnormal. The location of the thrill can be indicative of certain conditions, for example, a thrill in the upper left sternal border may indicate pulmonary stenosis. Fever or anxiety will cause tachycardia and this should be considered when evaluating if the rate is appropriate for the child's age. A pulse which is faster on inspiration and slower on expiration

Table 5.2 Grading of cardiac murmurs

Grade	
1	Barely audible with auscultation
2	Soft sound but easily audible with auscultation
3	Moderately loud but not accompanied by a thrill
4	Loud and associated with a thrill
5	Audible with the stethoscope barely on the chest
6	Audible with the stethoscope off the chest

Source: adapted from Park 2010.

(sinus arrhythmia) is also common in children and not an indication of cardiovascular compromise.

Palpation

Palpation of the major pulses will enable the practitioner to assess cardiac output through the volume of the pulse and perfusion. The brachial pulse is usually the first choice to palpate in infants and the radial pulse in older children. The pulse should be palpated for 1 minute using the second and third fingers, taking care not to apply excess pressure which may occlude the artery. The carotid, femoral, dorsalis pedis and posterior tibia should also be assessed, noting the volume, which may vary from bounding to diminished or absent, as well as the rate and regularity. The pulses should be compared in the upper and lower extremities and from right to left.

The infant/child should be examined for any signs of oedema, including the presence of hepatomegaly, which is symptomatic of cardiac failure. The oedema may be central, generalised, gravitationally dependent or restricted to the peripheries. In infants who are predominantly in the supine position oedema may be periorbital. In addition, it may be worse at certain times of the day and may indent and leave the imprint of fingers if touched (pitting oedema).

A central capillary refill time is a good reflection of perfusion and can be assessed by pressing a finger on the sternum for 5 seconds, releasing and then timing how long it takes for the blanched area of skin to return to normal colour.

Comparing core and peripheral temperatures will generate similar data providing the child has not been in a cold environment. These can either be measured with a temperature probe in the nasopharynx and one attached to the child's foot, or simply by feeling the child's head and feet and comparing the difference. This is not a reliable measure and should be used with caution, in conjunction with other components of the assessment.

Blood pressure assessment

Non-invasive blood pressure (NIBP) is usually measured from one of the child's arms, but the NIBP in all four limbs should be checked at the initial assessment, especially in newborns, as four limb blood pressure recordings are used as one of the diagnostic criteria for coarctation of the aorta. Ideally, the child should be sitting quietly with the midpoint of their arm at the level of their heart but this is clearly dependent not only on the age of the child but also their clinical condition. The cuff should cover two-thirds of the length of the upper arm and the bladder within the cuff should encircle 80–100% of the child's arm.

Additional assessment points

Urine output can be a good indicator of renal perfusion, which in turn reflects the adequacy or otherwise of cardiac output. Normal urine output values are age-dependent, and cumulative values of less than the anticipated volume based on the expected norms may indicate inadequate cardiac output and/or renal dysfunction. It is common practice to calculate the expected urine output over a 4-hour period and then match this to actual output:

- Newborn and infants up to 1 year: 1.5–2 ml/kg/hr.
- Toddler: 1.5 ml/kg/hr.
- Older child: 1 ml/kg/hr during adolescence.
- Adult: 1 ml/min.

If the child has central venous access, a central venous pressure (CVP) can be transduced and this value will reflect right ventricular preload and right ventricular function, which are important determinants of cardiac output. Similarly, if the child has pulmonary artery or left atrial lines in situ, information can be gained about right ventricular afterload, left ventricular preload and left ventricular function.

The child's respiratory condition should be noted as cardiac function and respiratory function are strongly linked. Any compromise in cardiac output will result in an increased respiratory rate to in an attempt to maintain oxygen delivery to the tissues. Left ventricular failure and the associated high pulmonary venous pressures will increase pulmonary interstitial fluid causing the lungs to be less compliant, resulting in increased respiratory effort and rate.

Congenital heart disease

Congenital heart disease occurs in 5–8/1000 live births and is the most common congenital condition in newborns (Billet et al. 2008; Knowles et al. 2005). A chromosome abnormality is present in 5–8% of babies with congenital heart disease (www.ipch.org/DiseaseHealthInfo/Health Library). It has been suggested that 40–50% of children with Trisomy 21 have a congenital heart lesion and children with DiGeorge syndrome have a higher incidence of outflow tract anomalies such as tetralogy of Fallot and interrupted aortic arch. Approximately 50% of children with an interrupted aortic arch will have DiGeorge syndrome (www.emedicine. medscape.com/article/896979-overview) and the presence of a heart lesion should prompt genetic screening as this can be significant in the child's initial management (e.g. the need for irradiated blood products) as well as ongoing care. Other influencing factors clearly exist as only one of monozygotic twins may have a congenital heart lesion.

As children with congenital heart lesions reach adult age and go on to become parents themselves it is becoming evident that there is a higher incidence of congenital heart disease in children of parents who themselves have a congenital heart lesion. The incidence is slightly higher in children born to mothers with a congenital heart lesion at 2.5–18%, than children born to fathers with a congenital heart lesion, at 1.5–3% (Park 2010).

There are also established links between maternal health and the incidence of congenital heart disease, with a higher incidence associated with maternal rubella, diabetes and phenylketonuria. Children born to mothers who have rubella during the first 8 weeks of pregnancy have a higher incidence of pulmonary stenosis and maternal diabetes causes an increased incidence of between 10 and 20% for lesions such as a ventricular septal defect (VSD) and transposition of the great arteries (TGA), as well as cardiomyopathy (Park 2010). Some anti-epileptic medications, smoking, alcohol and illegal drugs are also known to adversely affect foetal cardiac development.

Diagnosis of congenital heart disease

With advances in foetal screening programmes, the antenatal diagnosis of congenital heart disease is improving, although it only remains around 50% of the total number of infants receiving a diagnosis and requiring intervention in the first year of life (Central Cardiac Audit Database 2010).

For infants who have not received an antenatal diagnosis, postnatal diagnosis is based primarily on clinical presentation, chest X-ray (CXR) and echocardiography (ECHO). Advances in the technical quality of ECHO machines (e.g. colour flow mapping and Doppler echocardiography) have made accurate diagnosis, and therefore treatment planning, more effective.

Hyperoxia test

The hyperoxia or nitrogen washout test is helpful in trying to distinguish between cardiac and respiratory causes of cyanosis in the newborn when there is no access to other diagnostic tools such as ECHO. It works on the assumption that if there is right-to-left shunting, as in cyanotic heart disease, no amount of oxygenation in the pulmonary circulation will alter the desaturating effect of the shunt. However, if there is a pulmonary defect causing cyanosis, this may be corrected by increasing the inspired oxygen.

The test is carried out by placing the infant in 100% oxygen for 10 minutes. If the infant remains cyanotic after this period, the cyanosis is said to be secondary to cyanotic heart disease. This test is not a guarantee of diagnosis and there are exceptions – severe respiratory disease may result in persistent cyanosis even in 100% inspired oxygen. Furthermore, the test is not without risk as placing an infant with a duct-dependent lesion in 100% oxygen may cause a degree of ductal closure and this may be harmful to the infant.

Pulse oximetry

The use of pulse oximetry as a diagnostic tool is currently under evaluation in a trial in UK maternity units. Results of the completed trial are expected in 2012 but preliminary results suggest that it may be a useful routine additional tool in newborn assessment; however, this is also related to the increased detection of diseases other than congenital heart disease and is therefore not advocated as a single assessment tool (Ewer et al. 2011).

Sequential segmental cardiac analysis

Segmental cardiac analysis describes cardiac anatomy by identifying how the various structures relate to each other and the characteristics of those relationships. The technique was first used by Shinebourne et al. (1976) and has since been refined, notably by Anderson and colleagues (1984) and Anderson and Girish (2009).

The heart is described in a sequential manner focusing on:

- The arrangement of the atrial chambers.
- The junction between the atria and the attached ventricle.
- The atrioventricular (AV) valve.
- The ventricular topology.
- The ventricular–arterial junction and the morphology of the valves.
- The arterial relations.

Finally, a description of any abnormalities can be made. The terms used in sequential analysis are detailed in Table 5.3.

Atrial morphology

The right and left atria are structurally different and it is these morphological variants that determine which chamber is a morphological right atria and which is a morphological left atria rather than their position on the right or left side of the heart. The main difference is the size and shape of

Table 5.3 Terms used in sequential analysis

Term	Meaning
Morphology	Structure of an organism.
Situs	Place or position:
	Solitus – in the usual or normal position.
	Inversus – opposite to usual position.
Ambiguous	Not clearly related to one side or the other.
Inversus	Mirror image.
Concordance	In harmony or agreement.
Discordance	Not in agreement, disharmony.
Dextrocardia	Heart is right-sided.
Levocardia	Heart is left-sided.
Mesocardia	Heart is in the midline position.

the atrial appendage: the right atrial appendage is large, has a wide connection to the atria and is a broad-based triangle in shape; in contrast the left atrial appendage is small and tubular, with a narrow connection to the atria. In situs solitus the morphological right atrium is to the right of the heart and the morphological left atrium is to the left. Alternatively, the atria may be transposed into a mirror image of the situs solitus arrangement with the morphological right atrium on the left of the heart and the morphological left atrium on the right of the heart. Finally, the child may have right atrial isomerism where both atria are morphological right atria, or left atrial isomerism where both atria are morphological left atria.

Atrioventricular (AV) connections
There are three possible variables when describing AV connections.

Each atria connects to an underlying ventricle: This is the most common type of AV relationship and will result in a right-sided and a left-sided AV connection. If a morphological right atrium connects to a morphological right ventricle and a morphological left atrium connects to a morphological left ventricle, then this is described as AV concordance. This can be true with either a situs solitus or a mirror image atrial arrangement.

If a morphological right atrium connects with a morphological left ventricle and vice versa, then this is described as AV discordance. In solitude this statement does not clarify whether it is the atrial or the ventricular arrangement which is abnormal and further explanation of the

ventricular topology is required. Description of ventricular topology is also required if the child has atrial isomerism.

The AV valve may or may not be normal but this does not affect the description of the AV connection.

There is a univentricular AV connection: The right- and left-sided atrial chambers may be connected to the same ventricle; this is known as a double-inlet ventricle. There may be two distinct AV valves or one common one but, as before, this does not affect the description of the connection.

Either the right- or the left-sided AV connection is absent: There is an absence of any potential communication between the atrial chamber and the underlying ventricle. This is known as an absent atrioventricular connection and is distinguished from an atretic AV valve.

The atrioventricular (AV) valve
Only if there are completely separate right- and left-sided AV connections with completely separate right- and left-sided AV valves should the terms tricuspid and mitral valve be used. Then the valve associated with the right ventricle can be referred to as the tricuspid valve and the valve associated with the left ventricle as the mitral valve.

Valves may be patent, imperforate, straddling, overriding or one common structure instead of two separate structures.

Either the right- or left-sided AV valve may be imperforate, which means that the valve structure is present but not patent, or it may be that the valve leaflets are fused, but the important factor is that there is the potential for communication between the atria and the ventricles. Straddling and overriding valves are also structurally different. A straddling valve is defined as one in which the papillary muscles and chordae tendineae (the tension apparatus) arise from the ventricular myocardium on both sides of the septum, whereas with an overriding valve it is the annulus which is situated over both sides of the septum. A common valve is one that controls both right and left AV connections and it may straddle and/or override.

Ventricular topology
There are three main components to the structure of each ventricle: the inlet, which extends from the AV junction to the distal tension apparatus; the apical trabecular component; and the outlet. The most obvious structural difference is seen in the apical trabeculations which are coarse within the right ventricle but fine within the left. Additionally, within the morphological right ventricle the AV valve has chordal attachments to the septum, whereas within the

morphological left ventricle the AV valve has no septal attachments.

The relationship between the ventricles can be further defined as being of right or left-handed topology. A structurally normal heart has right-hand ventricular topology and this describes the way in which the palmar surface of the right hand could be placed on the septal surface of the morphological right ventricle with the thumb positioned above the inlet component (tricuspid valve) and the fingers above the outlet component (pulmonary artery) and the wrist covering the apical area. The left hand would then fit in comparable fashion on the left ventricle. In situations of AV discordance the additional description of ventricular topology can clarify whether it is the atria or the ventricles which are abnormally situated.

The ventricular–arterial (VA) junction and the morphology of the valve

The connection between the ventricle and the artery that arises from it should be described before comment is made about the presence, absence or integrity of any valve.

Four possible types of VA connection may be found:

- The pulmonary artery arises from a morphological right ventricle and the aorta from a morphological left ventricle. This is described as a concordant VA connection.
- The pulmonary artery arises from a morphological left ventricle and the aorta from a morphological right ventricle. This is described as a discordant VA connection.
- Both arteries arise from the same ventricle. This is described as a double-outlet connection or ventricle.
- There is only one artery arising from a ventricle or over-riding both ventricles. This is described as a single outlet and it may be that there is a common arterial trunk (persistent truncus arteriosus) which gives rise to the coronary arteries, the pulmonary arteries and the aorta and has a single truncal valve. Both the vessel and the valve override the right and left ventricles. Alternatively, there may be a pulmonary artery with aortic atresia or an aorta with pulmonary atresia. In both cases there is no potential exit from the opposing ventricle in distinction from there being an imperforate pulmonary or aortic valve.

The valve may be patent or imperforate. There can only be a common valve if there is a single common artery. VA valves cannot be described as straddling as they have no distinct tension apparatus, but they can be described as overriding. This would be when the valve annulus is situated over both sides of the septum and the vessel receives blood from both ventricles.

The arterial relations

The positioning of the pulmonary artery and aorta is described in relation to the positioning of the pulmonary and aortic valve. This is a 'stable base' from which the vessels should spiral around each other, usually reflecting normal concordant VA connections. If the vessels are in parallel, then the VA connection is usually discordant or double-outlet. The terms used to describe the valve positions are right or left, anterior or posterior and side by side.

The structure of the normal heart can be described as:

- Situs solitus.
- A–V concordance.
- Correct ventricular architecture.
- V–A concordance.
- Posterior aorta.
- Levocardia.
- No malformations/malformations present.

(Abdulla et al. 2004; Carvalho et al. 2005;
Craatz et al. 2002).

Categorising cardiac lesions

Congenital heart lesions are difficult to classify due to the many complicated variations that are seen even within one diagnostic term, however it is common for them to be classified according to the area of the heart affected and the direction of any shunting of blood caused by the defect. Blood will always flow or shunt from areas of high pressure to areas of low pressure. A defect of the ventricular septum will therefore result in a left-to-right shunt as pressures in the left ventricle are higher than those in the right. To generate a right-to-left shunt and cyanosis there has to be either persistent high pulmonary vascular resistance or a right-sided obstruction or stenosis of the tricuspid valve, the right ventricular outflow tract or the pulmonary artery causing the right-sided pressures to be abnormally high.

Accordingly, broad diagnostic classifications are acyanotic or cyanotic heart lesions. This is determined by whether any shunt is predominantly left to right (acyanotic), with oxygenated blood from the left side of the heart being shunted back to the right side, or right to left (cyanotic), with desaturated blood from the right side of the heart shunting to the left side of the heart and perfusing the systemic circulation. Subdivisions can then be generated according to any changes in pulmonary blood flow, which may be increased, decreased or variable, and any obstructions to outflow. In addition, there are lesions that affect the heart generally, such as cardiomyopathy or congenital arrhythmias or obstructive lesions. Lesions in this

Table 5.4 Normal intracardiac pressures and saturations

Chamber/Vessel	Pressure (mmHg)	Saturation (per cent)
Right atrium	Mean 2–8	65–75
Right ventricle	Systolic 15–20	65–75
	Diastolic 2–8	
Pulmonary artery	Systolic 15–20	65–75
	Diastolic 5–10	
	Mean 15	
Left atrium	Mean 5–10	95–100
Left ventricle*	Systolic 100–140	95–100
	Diastolic 5–10	
Aorta*	Systolic 100–140	95–100
	Diastolic 60–80	

*Denotes a value that varies according to age and figures given relate to adult values.

group will increase the work of the heart, especially the left ventricle, leading to left ventricular hypertrophy, for coarctation of the aorta or aortic stenosis and right ventricular hypertrophy for pulmonary stenosis. As there are no abnormal connections between systemic and pulmonary circulations there is no shunting of blood.

An understanding of normal intracardiac pressures and saturations, as listed in Table 5.4, helps to clarify the direction of shunting when a cardiac lesion is present.

Common management strategies

Prostaglandin

Prostaglandin is a potent arterial vasodilator which as well as dilating the ductus arteriosus causes general vasodilation. This may lead to hypotension so close monitoring of the infant's cardiovascular status is required. Prostaglandin has also been associated with apnoeas and respiratory depression and if they occur, these side-effects may require respiratory support with CPAP or intubation and ventilation.

There are two types of prostaglandin currently used in the United Kingdom: Prostaglandin E1 (Alprostadil) and Prostaglandin E2 (Dinoprostone). Both are detailed in the British National Formulary for Children (2011–12) and use is determined by local policy and practice. Prostaglandin should be given as a continuous IV infusion and the delivery of the drug should not be interrupted. Additional IV

access will therefore be required for maintenance fluids and any other IV bolus drugs the child is prescribed.

Modified Blalock–Taussig (BT) shunt

A modified BT shunt is performed through a thoracotomy incision and is a closed procedure. Synthetic or allograft tissue is used to create a conduit between the subclavian artery and a branch of the pulmonary artery. If the aorta is left-sided, the conduit is usually inserted between the right subclavian artery and the right pulmonary artery. The diameter of the shunt will be determined by the size of the child, the volume of blood required to flow through the shunt and the length of time the shunt needs to stay in place before being upgraded or removed.

Following a modified BT shunt there is the potential of shunt blockage during the immediate postoperative period. A heparin infusion is usually maintained until enteral feeds are established when regular oral aspirin should be commenced to sustain mild anti-coagulation and promote patency of the conduit. Volume boluses may also be required to support the child's blood pressure and maintain adequate flow through the conduit. The infant's arterial saturations will usually be in the region of 70–80%. Close monitoring of the infant's oxygenation is important as poor shunt flow will be indicated by decreasing saturations and an increasing metabolic acidosis. Patency of the conduit can be confirmed by auscultation when a shunt murmur should be heard, or by cardiac ECHO examination.

Glenn procedure

A Glenn shunt involves removing the distal end of the superior vena cava (SVC) from the right atrium and anastomosing it to the right pulmonary artery. If the right pulmonary artery is still attached to the main and left pulmonary artery, blood from the SVC will perfuse both the right and the left lungs. This is termed a bi-directional Glenn and is the most common type of Glenn surgery. Alternatively, if the right pulmonary artery is resected from the main and left pulmonary artery and the resected end is over-sown, blood from the SVC will only perfuse the right lung. This is a classic Glenn.

For the Glenn shunt to provide effective pulmonary blood flow it is important that the child has low pulmonary vascular resistance as the driving force for pulmonary blood flow is now the SVC pressure. To achieve optimum Glenn flow the child should ideally be extubated within the first few hours postoperatively as spontaneous breathing generates lower pulmonary pressures than positive pressure ventilation. Volume boluses may be required to maintain a high preload, which will result in a high central venous pressure and good systemic venous return from the head and upper body, the source of the pulmonary blood flow. The child will be nursed in a head raised or sitting position to optimise venous return from the head and upper body and maximise flow through the Glenn. A heparin infusion will be commenced in the early postoperative period until enteral feeds are established, when oral aspirin will be commenced to reduce the risk of the shunt clotting. The child's arterial saturations will usually be in the region of 70–80%. Close monitoring of the child's oxygenation is important as poor shunt flow will be indicated by decreasing saturations and an increasing metabolic acidosis. Patency of the conduit can be confirmed by auscultation when a shunt murmur should be heard, or by cardiac ECHO examination.

Total caval pulmonary connection (TCPC) (Fontan procedure)

The original Fontan procedure involved connecting the right atrium to the pulmonary artery and using it as the source of pulmonary blood flow. Complications with right atrial distension, atrial dysrhythmias and compromised Fontan flow have led to modifications to this procedure. Although not technically the same as the original Fontan, the terms TCPC and (modified) Fontan are often used interchangeably. The aim of the surgical procedure is to separate systemic and pulmonary circulation, resulting in a child who is no longer cyanosed but has arterial saturations of at least 90%.

Usually the TCPC or Fontan will be preceded by a Glenn shunt where the SVC is attached to the right pulmonary artery in order to increase pulmonary blood flow. In a TCPC/Fontan the Glenn shunt is left in place and the inferior vena cava (IVC) is also attached to the right pulmonary artery so that all systemic venous return is now directed directly to the pulmonary circuit and the remaining single ventricle is only supporting systemic circulation.

The procedure can be further categorised as an internal or external TCPC/Fontan. An internal TCPC/Fontan involves diverting the IVC flow through a tunnel within the right atrium and then attaching the superior portion of the tunnel to the underside of the right pulmonary artery. An external TCPC/Fontan involves the construction of a conduit from the transected IVC around the outside of the right atrium to the underside of the right pulmonary artery.

TCPCs/Fontans may also be fenestrated. This is when a window or opening is left between the tunnel or conduit and the right atrium. If pulmonary blood flow becomes congested then the TCPC/Fontan circuit will offload via the fenestration to the right atrium. This will mean that the child's arterial saturations will drop as desaturated blood is again mixing with the systemic flow, but it also means that when pulmonary vascular resistance is high and pulmonary blood flow is reduced systemic output is maintained as the blood that shunts through the fenestration maintains preload of the systemic ventricle. In addition, the avoidance of pulmonary venous congestion reduces the incidence and duration of pleural effusions. If necessary, the fenestration can be closed at cardiac catheter, although in some children it occludes naturally.

Early postoperative extubation is aimed for, as the self-ventilating child has lower pulmonary pressures than when receiving positive pressure ventilation and this will facilitate flow through the TCPC/Fontan circuit. Volume boluses may be required to maintain a high preload, a high central venous pressure and good systemic venous return as it is the systemic venous return that is generating the pressure for pulmonary blood flow. Postoperatively the child will be nursed in a head-raised or sitting position, with their legs elevated to optimise systemic venous return and maximise flow through the TCPC/Fontan. A heparin infusion should be commenced in the early postoperative period until enteral feeds are established when oral aspirin or warfarin will be commenced to reduce the risk of the shunt clotting.

Cardiopulmonary bypass

Cardiopulmonary bypass is an extracorporeal circuit which is used to maintain circulation and gas exchange during open heart surgery. Open heart surgery refers to any operation where one of the chambers of the heart needs to be surgically opened for the surgery to be performed. In order to achieve this, the blood flow must be diverted away from the operative field to ensure the surgeon has a relatively blood-free and static view. A combination of cardiopulmonary bypass and circulatory arrest may be required.

Closed heart surgery refers to an operation which focuses on the vessels arising from the heart and to complete this surgery the heart does not need to be opened. Examples of closed heart surgical procedures include coarctation repair, ligation of a patent ductus arteriosus, or completion of a Blalock–Taussig shunt.

Cardiopulmonary bypass is established by inserting venous drainage cannula in either the right atrial appendage or the SVC and the IVC. The venous blood is then pumped through an oxygenator where CO_2 is removed and oxygenation occurs. The blood will then be pumped through a heat exchanger which is used to maintain the child's core temperature before being filtered and returned via a cannula in the ascending aorta. The blood that is drained into the bypass circuit does not flow through the child's heart and lungs. The circuit is responsible for maintaining gas exchange and cardiac output and to achieve this pump flows will normally be 100–120ml/kg/min, but can be up to 200ml/kg/min. It should be acknowledged that the venous drainage cannula will never be 100% efficient at catching all the venous return so there will always be a small residual volume of blood within the child's heart and lungs.

To maintain patency of the bypass circuit the child's circulating volume must be anti-coagulated. To achieve this, heparin boluses will be given and the activated clotting time (ACT) will be maintained at around 400 seconds. At the end of the bypass period the heparin will need to be reversed by administering protamine.

In order to provide the surgeon with a motionless operative area the heart needs to be arrested. This is achieved by instilling cold cardioplegia solution into the aortic root so that it perfuses the coronary arteries. Typically, cardioplegia contains large doses of both potassium and magnesium which, combined with hypothermia, induce asystole. Top-up doses are needed approximately every 20 minutes to maintain arrest and the aorta will have been cross-clamped to prevent systemic infiltration of the cardioplegia solution.

The required hypothermia is achieved through a combination of topical cooling of the child with the use of ice packs and core cooling by using the heat exchanger within the bypass circuit to reduce the temperature of the child's blood. Hypothermia is used to reduce the metabolic rate and decrease the tissue's oxygen requirement. Deep hypothermia is a core temperature of 18–22°C and is required for long, complex, open heart procedures, however most surgery will be performed under moderate hypothermia (a core temperature of 30–32°C).

As blood cools it naturally becomes more viscous and more likely to clot. To counteract these undesirable effects the child is given additional volume to dilute the circulation and reduce the viscosity. This is referred to as haemodilution and decreases the formation of micro-emboli which may impair renal and/or cerebral blood flow. Haemodilution is not without complications. The priming solution used in the bypass circuit plays an important role in haemodilution given the relatively low circulating blood volume of newborns and infants compared to that of adults. The prime volume may be as much as three times the actual blood volume of the neonate. As a consequence, the effects of haemodilution are markedly enhanced in neonates compared with adults, as evidenced by decreased levels of plasma protein, coagulation factors and haemoglobin. This increases organ oedema, coagulopathy and transfusion requirements. The use of modified ultrafiltration (MUF) as part of the bypass process helps remove inflammatory mediator-rich fluid from the patient and bypass circuit and aims to reduce the impact of some of the effects detailed (Allen et al. 2009).

Postoperative management of the child after open cardiac surgery

A child undergoing open cardiac surgery will be exposed to two separate but interdependent processes which can cause significant harm (Table 5.5):

- Cardiopulmonary bypass (CPB).
- Cardioplegia, which is the use of extreme cold and induced hyperkalaemia to preserve the myocardium, which paralyses the muscle fibres and reduces the oxygen/metabolic demands of individual myocytes.

These two processes have significant effects on all the major body systems and anticipation of the consequences of the procedure are part of the essential postoperative management of the infant or child.

General postoperative management principles

Timely assessment of the infant or child, identification of problems and prompt intervention improve outcomes. On receiving the infant or child back from theatre, it is essential that the following information is elicited:

- Type of lesion.
- Any previous cardiac surgery.
- Aim of the current procedure – correction, palliation or shunt.
- Post-repair anatomy.
- Bypass statistics (e.g. times/use of MUF).
- Intra-operative problems.

Most postoperative complications will result from primary cardiovascular instability, which will in turn impact on all other systems, but given the possible effects of bypass, consideration should also be given to the other major systems: respiratory, gastrointestinal, haematological, renal and CNS.

Table 5.5   Potential systemic effects of cardiopulmonary bypass

Body system	Effects and care considerations

Pulmonary	• Impaired oxygen uptake as a consequence of increased pulmonary capillary permeability leading to pulmonary oedema.
	• Decreased lung compliance secondary to:
	  – loss of surfactant production due to epithelial cell dysfunction and insufficient alveolar distension to activate surfactant release
	  – pulmonary oedema
	  – mechanical trauma to the lung tissue
	  – hypoperfusion of the lung increasing V/Q mismatch.

Cardiovascular	• Systemic hypotension related to fluid shifts.
	  – Haemodilution reduces colloid oncotic pressure.
	• Systemic hypotension related to altered capillary permeability.
	  – Bypass causes endothelial damage which triggers the release of vasoactive mediators.
	• Systemic hypertension related to peripheral vasoconstriction caused by hypothermia, increased catecholamine release, increased renin secretion/increased angiotensin II levels.
	  – Increases afterload and therefore myocardial oxygen demands.
	• Activation of platelets through contact with pump circuit causes the release of a vasoconstrictor known as thrombaxane-A_2
	• Potential/actual haemorrhage.

Renal	• Increased release of renin (relative hypoperfusion) and increased levels of angiotensin II resulting in vasoconstriction.
	• Increased levels of ADH.
	• Release of atrial natriuretic peptide (ANP).
	  – Inhibits release of aldosterone.
	  – Stimulates excretion of sodium.
	  – Promotes vasodilation.
	• Increased release of aldosterone which results in increased retention of sodium and water and the excretion of potassium.
	All of these will result in oliguria/anuria.

CNS	• Macro- and micro-emboli (air, particles, aggregated blood cells). • Systemic anti-coagulation leads to increased risk of haemorrhage. • Inadequate cerebral blood flow. • Raised ICP secondary to impaired cerebral venous drainage – SVC obstruction. Total circulatory arrest (TCA) The body is cooled by the CPB pump to enable it to withstand no blood flow. The heart is stilled with cardioplegia and the pump is turned off (pump catheters are removed), or the child receives very low flow bypass support during procedure (pump catheters remain in situ). The length of TCA and child's core temperature determine the possible neurological consequences (Barry et al. 2010). *Between 18 and 20 °C* Between 40 and 60 minutes of TCA is possible with minimal risk of ongoing deficits, but studies have cited 11–20% of patients suffering postoperative seizures with variable neurological sequelae demonstrated during long-term follow-up (Goldberg et al. 2007; Markowitz et al. 2007; Wypij et al. 2003).

(Continued)

Table 5.5 (*Continued*)

Body system	Effects and care considerations

Endocrine	• Elevated adrenaline levels – redistribution of blood flow and peripheral vasoconstriction.
	• Increased noradrenaline levels.
	• Hyperglycaemia:
	    – Impaired insulin release.
	    – Peripheral insulin resistance.
	    – Increased glycogenolysis.
	    – Alterations in glucose transport across cell membranes.
	• Hypoglycaemia.
	• Centrally mediated increases in core body temperatures related to increased basal metabolic rate and decreased cardiac output.
	• Elevated levels of glucocorticoids, increased breakdown of fats and proteins (possible acidosis). Can also result in sodium or water retention and potassium excretion.

Inflammatory response	In response to the instigation of bypass the body will mount a generalised inflammatory response to the perceived threat.
	The response is mediated by the release of bradykinin and complement, the effects of which include:
	• Increased capillary permeability.
	• Vasodilation.
	• Leucocyte activation:
	    – Causes disruption of the lung endothelium allowing fluid to shift into the interstitial spaces.
	    – Triggers the postoperative rise in core body temperature.
	• Stimulates the production of histamine and leukotrienes by the mast cells which may further depress myocardial function

Cardiovascular system

This may be related to the heart itself or be a consequence of poor cardiac performance (Table 5.6) and can be attributed to any or all of the following:

• Myocardial dysfunction.
• Dysrhythmias.
• Inadequate tissue perfusion.

Pulmonary hypertension

Pulmonary hypertension is defined as a mean pulmonary artery pressure of >25 mmHg or a systolic pulmonary artery pressure of >35 mmHg. In infants and children with high pre-operative pulmonary blood flow there is a significant risk of postoperative pulmonary hypertension as a consequence of the changes in the muscular (middle layer) of the pulmonary artery in the face of increased and or turbulent pulmonary blood flow or blood flow under relatively high pressure into the pulmonary circuit. Infants and children at particular risk for postoperative pulmonary hypertension can be identified and divided into four broad

categories based on their cardiac disease and the mechanisms responsible for pulmonary hypertension:

1. Increased pulmonary vascular resistance.
2. Increased pulmonary blood flow with normal pulmonary vascular resistance.
3. A combination of increased pulmonary vascular resistance and increased blood flow.
4. Increased pulmonary venous pressures.

The mechanisms involved in the triggering of pulmonary hypertension post-cardiac surgery are multifactorial and are not solely dependent on the child's diagnosis. The effects of cardiopulmonary bypass (Table 5.5),which produces endothelial injury within the pulmonary vasculature and may generate a transient elevation in PVR, are thought to be significant in pulmonary hypertension alongside contributing factors such as impaired nitric oxide production, increased release of endothelin and the inflammatory response to cardiopulmonary bypass, which all increase the possibility of hypoxia-induced increased pulmonary vascular resistance (Taylor and Laussen 2010).

Table 5.6 Cardiovascular complications post-cardiac surgery

Complication	Notes and considerations
Myocardial dysfunction	The myocardium is very sensitive and responds adversely to being handled. There is usually a period of relative stability (between 4 and 8 hours postoperatively) after which the effects become apparent. An awareness of pre-operative cardiac function is important. Myocardial dysfunction may be indicated by ECG abnormalities or increasing pressures such as the LAP or RAP rising above 12mmHg or the CVP above 15–18mmHg (unless high CVP is necessary). Interventions to stabilise or improve myocardial function include: • Prevention of hypoxia and acidosis. • Prevention of hyperthermia. • Prevention or correction of electrolyte imbalance.
Dysrhythmias	Any number of rhythm disturbances may manifest in the postoperative period depending on which part of the conduction pathway has been disturbed. Management strategies include: • Optimisation of blood gases. • Optimisation of electrolytes (potassium, calcium and magnesium). • Check of the position of any intracardiac catheters and central venous lines. • Use of temporary pacing. • Use of cooling.
Inadequate tissue perfusion	May be a consequence of inadequate preload caused by fluid volume deficit, or excessive afterload caused by increased SVR, increased PVR, or both. Management strategies include: • Judicious fluid replacement to ensure adequate intravascular volume. • Careful monitoring of drain losses and urine output. • Use of milrinone to offload ventricles. • Use of vasoactive medications.

Pathophysiology of pulmonary hypertensive crisis

A pulmonary hypertensive crisis can occur if the PA pressure rises to or above systemic pressures. The pathophysiology of pulmonary hypertension in the postoperative period includes not only the increased PVR and elevated PA pressures but also the physiological consequences of RV pressure overload and ventricular dysfunction (Figure 5.9).

Postoperative assessment

This may include the provision of a pulmonary artery (PA) line placed at time of surgery, although this will be based on an individual surgeon's preferences and their use has become less frequent in the last few years. In the absence of a PA line, assessment of pulmonary artery pressures can be undertaken through the use of cardiac ECHO. Clinical signs of pulmonary hypertension in the absence of direct PA pressure monitoring are systemic hypotension, acute desaturations with a corresponding decrease in PaO$_2$ and decreased lung compliance (reduced tidal volumes on the ventilator or difficulty in eliciting chest wall movement with manual hyperinflation in the presence of a patent ETT). The presence of acidosis, hypercapnia and hypoxia may all precipitate an episode of pulmonary hypertension, therefore caution should be exercised when undertaking routine cares such as ETT suctioning.

Management of pulmonary hypertension

The primary aim of management strategies is twofold: first, to reduce the PA pressures; and second, to support right ventricular function, preventing a pulmonary hypertensive crisis.

• Maintain effective analgesia and sedation to avoid the infant/child becoming distressed.
• Use of muscle relaxants if clinically unstable.
• Use of inhaled nitric oxide therapy 5–20ppm to reduce pulmonary vascular resistance (see Chapter 4). The use of inhaled nitric oxide inhibits the production of endothelium-derived relaxing factor (EDRF) and it can be difficult to wean the child from low-dose nitric therapy after a period of time. In these cases, caution

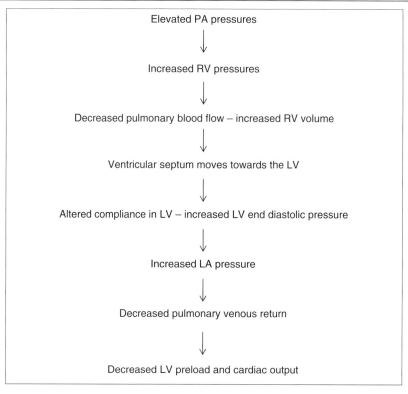

Elevated PA pressures

↓

Increased RV pressures

↓

Decreased pulmonary blood flow – increased RV volume

↓

Ventricular septum moves towards the LV

↓

Altered compliance in LV – increased LV end diastolic pressure

↓

Increased LA pressure

↓

Decreased pulmonary venous return

↓

Decreased LV preload and cardiac output

Figure 5.9   Pathophysiology of right ventricular dysfunction post-cardiac surgery.

should be taken to avoid a rebound increase in pulmonary pressure after discontinuation of therapy. Consideration should be given to use of other pulmonary vasodilators such as sildenafil (or more rarely phenoxybenzamine) to assist with the transition.
- Use of dopamine and milrinone to support RV function.

Pulmonary hypertensive crisis

In the event of an acute deterioration first-line actions are:

- Hand-ventilating the infant/child with a FiO_2 of 1.0 (plus nitric oxide if already receiving therapy), aiming for a normal to slightly low $PaCO_2$ (vasodilatory effect).
- Bolus of analgesia and sedative agents.
- Bolus dose of muscle relaxants.
- Increase in level of inotropic support.

Respiratory complications

Common postoperative respiratory complications include:

- Atelectasis.
- Depressed cough reflexes; secretion clearance impaired.
- Pulmonary oedema and impaired gas exchange.
- Pleural effusion.
- Haemothorax, chylothorax, pneumothorax.

The management of these complications is detailed in Chapter 4. Cardiovascular surgery is the most common cause of acquired diaphragmatic palsy secondary to phrenic nerve damage which occurred in between 0.28 and 5.6% of children included in four studies published since 2005 (Talwar et al. 2010). The clinical signs of diaphragmatic palsy include an inability to wean from ventilatory support or dependency on non-invasive support such as nasal CPAP, as well as a CXR finding of a right or left hemi-diaphragm. The management of these infants/children remains a discussion point in the published literature, however surgical plication of the diaphragm is often the suitable treatment, particularly in the infant population, given the importance of the diaphragm in their breathing patterns.

Gastrointestinal complications

Major complications are unusual post-cardiac surgery in the older and young child, however there is a significant risk of necrotising enterocolitis (NEC) in the neonatal population, both pre- and postoperatively.

Neonates and NEC

NEC is one of the commonest gastrointestinal emergencies in the newborn and although the highest mortality is associated with the most premature infants, there is still a significant associated mortality in the term infant, particularly in infants with cyanotic heart disease or duct-dependent lesions with reduced lower body perfusion (e.g. coarctation of the aorta). The pathogenesis of NEC is uncertain, however there are a number of contributory factors (see Chapter 8 for the management priorities).

Infants and older children care considerations:

- Auscultate for bowel sounds – palpate abdomen.
- Nasogastric tube placed to relieve dilation which is common.
- Monitor feed absorption and tolerance.

Neurological complications

Potential postoperative complications are often difficult to assess in the first few hours post-surgery due to the use of analgesic/sedative agents and muscle relaxants and some complications such as vocal cord palsy will not manifest until the infant is extubated. A careful, detailed neurological assessment is important to rule out events such as:

- Paraplegia secondary to spinal cord ischaemia (after coarctation of the aorta repair).
- Vocal cord paralysis secondary to ligation of a patent ductus arteriosus or shunt insertions.
- Thromboembolic events secondary to bypass.
- Haemorrhage secondary to systemic anticoagulation.

Haematological complications

These usually occur as a consequence of the effects of systemic anticoagulation and the extracorporeal bypass circuit. They include:

- Haemolysis resulting from pump trauma.
- Irreversible platelet deactivation – platelets are usually transfused at the end of surgery prior to the child coming off bypass.
- Heparin used for anticoagulation prevents the formation of anti-thrombin III and increases the risk of haemor-

rhage. Heparin is reversible by the administration of protamine.

Any child with a low cardiac output state (e.g. seen 4–6 hours postoperatively secondary to myocardial dysfunction) is at increased risk of developing disseminated intravascular coagulopathy (DIC).

Infectious complications

These are relatively rare, but there is always a risk of surgical wound infection secondary to microorganism entry as well as the potential for systemic infection secondary to the presence of multiple invasive monitoring lines and/or a urinary catheter, as well as localised infections (e.g. lower respiratory tract infections).

Acyanotic heart lesions

Atrial septal defect (ASD)

Anatomy

An ASD results from an error during atrial septation at weeks 4–6 of gestation. The most common type of ASD is a secundum ASD and this occurs if there is inadequate growth of the septum secundum or excessive reabsorption of the septum primum. It results in an opening in the centre of the atrial septum. Failure of the septum primum to meet the endocardial cushion results in an ASD low in the atrial septum, referred to as a primum ASD, and it may be associated with mitral valve anomalies. A defect high in the atria close to the insertion of the SVC is referred to as a sinus venosus ASD and may be associated with anomalous pulmonary venous drainage.

Altered haemodynamics

Blood will shunt from left to right through the ASD as pressure is higher in the left atrium than the right atrium. The volume of the shunt will be low as the pressure within the atria is low and the pressure gradient between the left and right atria is minimal.

Clinical presentation

A child with an ASD will typically be asymptomatic in early childhood due to the low volume of the left-to-right shunt. If the defect is undiagnosed, the child may develop signs of tachypnoea, dyspnoea and crepitus on auscultation, all associated with increased pulmonary blood flow. Rarely, signs of right ventricular dysfunction, such as hepatomegaly, may be evident.

On examination a murmur will be heard and chest X-ray may reveal increased pulmonary vascular markings.

Management

ASDs can be closed with a septal occlusion device during a cardiac catheter procedure or, if the defect is large, they may require stitch or patch closure during open heart surgery.

Transient atrial dysrhythmias are potential postoperative complications specific to an ASD.

Ventricular septal defect (VSD)

Anatomy

A VSD results from an error during ventricular septation at weeks 4–8 of gestation. The majority of VSDs are membranous (or peri-membranous), which means they are located in the upper portion of the septum. Muscular VSDs are located lower in the ventricular septum.

Altered haemodynamics

Blood will shunt from left to right through the VSD as pressure is higher in the left ventricle than the right ventricle. The volume of the shunt will depend on the size of the defect and the pressure gradient between the left and right ventricles. However, even a small defect will generate turbulent flow, which will be heard on auscultation. The left-to-right shunt will increase the volume load within the right ventricle and will result in increased pulmonary blood flow. This will be more pronounced with a larger VSD.

Clinical presentation

If the VSD is small, the child may be relatively asymptomatic. Symptoms will be more prevalent with larger defects or with increased time before diagnosis and will include tachypnoea, dyspnoea and rhonchi or crepitus on auscultation, all associated with increased pulmonary blood flow. These symptoms may result in feeding difficulties and faltering growth.

On examination a murmur will be heard and CXR may reveal increased pulmonary vascular markings.

Management

Small defects may close spontaneously. Larger defects, or those where the child is symptomatic, require stitch or patch closure via a right trans-atrial approach during open heart surgery. Potential postoperative complications include:

- Heart block or bundle branch block which may occur if the VSD was located close to the conduction pathways.
- Pulmonary hypertension may occur if the VSD was large and/or closed late.

Persistent ductus arteriosus (PDA)

Anatomy

The ductus arteriosus connects the pulmonary artery and the aorta. It is a normal part of foetal circulation, but should start to close within hours of birth, with full closure achieved within the first 7–10 days of life. The main stimulus for the ductus arteriosus to remain patent in postnatal circulation is hypoxia and as such a persistent ductus arteriosus may be seen in premature babies who have a degree of lung disease. PDA may also occur in conjunction with congenital rubella syndrome, Down's syndrome or a cyanotic heart lesion.

Altered haemodynamics

Blood will shunt left to right from the high pressure aorta to the low pressure pulmonary artery. The volume of the shunt and the subsequent increase in pulmonary blood flow will depend on both the diameter and length of the ductus arteriosus and the pressure gradient between the aorta and pulmonary artery. As pulmonary pressures continue to reduce in the initial postnatal period the volume and the significance of the ductal shunt may increase.

Clinical presentation

If the PDA is small, the child may be relatively asymptomatic. Symptoms will be more prevalent with larger defects and are more significant in premature babies with chronic lung disease. The increased pulmonary blood flow from the left-to-right shunt will result in tachypnoea, dyspnoea and rhonchi or crepitus on auscultation. A widened pulse pressure may also be noted as pressure within the aorta is poorly maintained during diastole as blood 'runs off' from the aorta to the low-pressure pulmonary artery.

On examination a murmur will be heard and CXR may reveal increased pulmonary vascular markings.

Management

The first-line approach for closure of a PDA in a premature baby is with the intravenous administration of indomethacin, which inhibits prostaglandin synthesis and therefore promotes ductal constriction and closure.

If medical management is unsuccessful or the child presents beyond the effective time frame, closure may be achieved through use of an occlusion device at cardiac catheter. Large PDAs may be unsuitable for insertion of an occlusion device and need to be ligated during closed heart surgery through a thoracotomy incision. Potential postoperative complications following thoracotomy and ligation of the ductus arteriosus include:

- Bleeding.
- Ligation of the wrong vessel (left pulmonary artery or aorta).
- Laryngeal or phrenic nerve damage.

Atrio-ventricular septal defect (AVSD)

Anatomy

The endocardial cushion is involved in the closure of the atrial septum, the ventricular septum and in the formation of the tricuspid and mitral valves, all between 4–8 weeks of gestation. Failure of correct development of the endocardial cushion can result in abnormalities to the valves and/or the atrial septum and/or the ventricular septum.

An AVSD (also known as an endocardial cushion defect or an atrio-ventricular canal) can be categorised as complete, partial or transitional depending on the components involved. A complete AVSD includes a common AV valve which straddles both the right and left ventricles, an ostium primum ASD and a VSD. A partial AVSD usually involves an ostium primum ASD and a cleft mitral valve and a transitional AVSD has some, but not all, of the components of a complete AVSD.

Altered haemodynamics

For a child with a complete AVSD the presence of a common, incompetent AV valve will mean that there will always be significant regurgitation from the left ventricle to the left atrium with the associated increase in pressure causing pulmonary venous congestion and a left-to-right atrial shunt. There will be further left-to-right shunting through the ventricular component of the septal defect resulting in volume loading of the right side of the heart and a significant increase in pulmonary blood flow. The pulmonary hypertension that results from both the increased pulmonary blood flow and the pulmonary congestion caused by the high left atrial pressures can cause irreversible damage to the pulmonary vasculature. Early, effective management is therefore crucial.

For a child with a partial AVSD the altered haemodynamics will be determined by the severity of the mitral incompetence. If the mitral regurgitation is only mild, then the increase in pressure within the left atrium will be minimal and the child will present similarly to a child with an isolated ostium primum ASD. If the mitral incompetence is moderate to severe, then the regurgitation and subsequent volume loading of the left atrium will increase the volume of the left-to-right atrial shunt. Additionally, the increased left atrial pressure will impede flow from the pulmonary circulation to the left atrium, resulting in pulmonary venous congestion.

The altered haemodynamics, and hence the symptoms exhibited by a child with a transitional AVSD, will be determined by the size of the left-to-right shunt at ventricular level and the severity of regurgitation through the AV valve.

Clinical presentation

A child with a complete AVSD will present early in infancy with symptoms of congestive heart failure. These will be related to the pulmonary congestion caused by the increased left atrial pressures and to the increased pulmonary blood flow, which results from the large left-to-right ventricular and atrial shunts.

A child with a partial AVSD may be relatively asymptomatic if the mitral valve is only mildly incompetent. Symptoms will be more obvious if the AV regurgitation is more severe and will reflect pulmonary congestion and congestive heart failure.

On examination a murmur will be heard and CXR may reveal increased pulmonary vascular markings.

Management

Pre-operatively, any congestive heart failure will be managed with diuretics. Captopril may also reduce left ventricular afterload and improve left ventricular function. Complete, partial and transitional AVSDs will require open heart surgery for their repair. The septal defects will be patched and the AV valve will be repaired to make it as efficient as possible. Valve replacements in the young tend to be avoided because of the need for frequent up-sizing as the child grows and the increased operative risks associated with frequent surgeries. Potential postoperative complications include:

- Pulmonary hypertension and pulmonary hypertensive crisis. The management strategies discussed in the generic postoperative cardiac care section should be employed.
- Increased risk of heart block following repair of an AVSD related to any oedema or trauma close to the location of the atrio-ventricular node. This is usually transient and the child may require temporary epicardial pacing until the oedema resolves and normal conduction returns. Permanent trauma to the conduction tissue may necessitate insertion of a permanent pacing system.

Repair of the AV valve will never be fully effective and any residual regurgitation can cause ongoing problems with poor forward flow from the left ventricle and left ventricular failure. The use of drugs to reduce afterload, such as intravenous milrinone and subsequently oral cap-topril, are useful in optimising left ventricular function and cardiac output.

Coarctation of the aorta

Anatomy

Coarctation of the aorta refers to a narrowing of the lumen of the aorta and results from abnormalities in aortic arch development at 5–8 weeks of gestation. Most commonly, the narrowing occurs between the origin of the left subclavian artery and the insertion of the ductus arte-riosus; this is referred to as a pre-ductal coarctation. Alter-natively, the narrowed segment may be at the site of insertion of the ductus arteriosus (a juxta-ductal coarcta-tion), or after the insertion of the ductus arteriosus (a post-ductal coarctation).

There are two main theories relating to the aetiology of coarctation of the aorta: the haemodynamic theory and the ductal tissue theory (reviewed by Raeside 2009).

The haemodynamic theory suggests that the coarctation results from abnormal flow in the aortic arch with blood in the ascending aorta streaming to the head and upper body and blood from the ductus arteriosus flowing into the descending aorta with little flow across the aortic isthmus between the subclavian artery and the ductus arteriosus. Coarctations are associated with lesions such as ventricular septal defects or bicuspid aortic valves and the decreased ascending aortic flow associated with these defects lends weight to the theory that reduced flow across the aortic isthmus contributes to the formation of a coarctation.

The ductal tissue theory suggests that ectopic ductal tissue within the aorta creates a thickened tunica media and intima, which reduces isthmic flow. Flow is then further compromised as additional constriction occurs with ductal closure.

The haemodynamics, signs and symptoms, management and postoperative complications are different for a pre-ductal coarctation compared to a post-ductal or juxta-ductal coarctation. They will therefore be discussed separately.

Pre-ductal coarctation of the aorta

Altered haemodynamics: Oxygenated, high-pressure blood flow from the left ventricle will flow as normal into the ascending aorta and perfuse the head and upper body via the brachiocephalic artery, the left common carotid artery and the left subclavian artery. However, little of this oxy-genated, high-pressure flow will cross the coarctation to perfuse the descending aorta and the lower body. Desatu-rated, low-pressure blood flow from the right ventricle will flow as normal into the pulmonary artery. However, some of this desaturated blood will shunt right to left across the patent ductus arteriosus to the low-pressure, relatively empty descending aorta. This means that the head and upper body are perfused by a high-pressure oxygenated blood flow while the lower body is perfused by a low-pressure desaturated blood flow. When the ductus arterio-sus closes, typically at 7–10 days of life, perfusion of the lower body is further compromised.

Clinical presentation

Typically, the infant with a pre-ductal coarctation of the aorta will present collapsed with a metabolic acidosis at 7–10 days of age as the ductus arteriosus closes and the already present signs and symptoms intensify.

Assessment will reveal a differential cyanosis: normal saturations in both arms but saturations of 65–75% in the lower limbs. Similarly, blood pressure will be higher in the arms than the lower limbs and palpation of pulses will identify that femoral pulses will be weak and delayed com-pared to brachial or axillary pulses. This reflects that the left ventricle is delivering oxygenated high-pressure blood to the head and upper body but the weaker right ventricle is delivering desaturated blood, via the ductus arteriosus, to the lower body. The difference in blood pressure is referred to as relative hypertension and there needs to be a systolic variance of over 20 mmHg for it to be considered significant.

The low-pressure, desaturated perfusion of the lower body will fail to meet the oxygen requirements of the tissues and the subsequent anaerobic metabolism and pro-duction of lactic acid produces a metabolic acidosis. This will become more evident as the duct closes and the infant will become tachypnoeic and tachycardic with poor periph-eral perfusion, reduced urine output and a decreased con-sciousness level as a consequence.

Management

If the infant presents collapsed, then appropriate resuscita-tion must be provided, although ultimately suspicion of a duct-dependent cardiac lesion and commencement of a prostaglandin infusion are needed to dilate the ductus arte-riosus and improve systemic perfusion.

Once the infant has stabilised, systemic perfusion has been optimised and any metabolic acidosis has resolved or reduced as far as is possible, surgery will be required.

Surgery is via a thoracotomy incision and is closed heart procedure. The aorta is clamped on either side of the coarc-tation, the narrowed segment of aorta is resected and an end-to-end anastomosis performed. Alternatively, a subclavian flap repair may be used, in which the left subclavian artery is isolated and divided distally. The vessel is then opened longitudinally with extension of the incision on to the aorta. The subclavian artery flap is then folded down over the area of aortic narrowing and sutured into place.

Postoperative complications are related to decreased perfusion of the lower body both preoperatively and intra-operatively when the aorta is cross-clamped.

- Spinal cord ischaemia can lead to paralysis, so it is important to assess the infant's legs for movement and strength as soon as possible in the postoperative period. For this reason, the use of muscle relaxants is usually avoided.
- An ischaemic bowel can lead to poor tolerance of feeds, a distended abdomen and potentially necrotising entero-colitis. Enteral feeds should nevertheless be commenced early in the postoperative period once bowel sounds are heard but regular assessment of their tolerance must occur.

Hypertension can also be a problem postoperatively and this is thought to be related to imbalances in sympathetic activity, increased baroreceptor sensitivity and/or an increase in circulating renin and angiotensin (Gargiulo et al. 2008). The hypertension is usually transient and can be managed with intravenous infusions of a vasodilator, such as sodium nitroprusside.

Post-ductal and juxta-ductal coarctation of the aorta

Altered haemodynamics

When the area of coarctation is at the site of, or distal to, the insertion of the ductus arteriosus, systemic blood ejected from the left ventricle is obstructed from perfusing the lower body by the coarctation, and blood from the right ventricle is unable to perfuse the lower body as the coarctation is distal to the insertion of the ductus arteriosus. As this situation exists from 5–8 weeks gestation, collateral circulation will develop from above the coarctation to below it and systemic perfusion will be via these collateral vessels. Blood flow to the lower body will be at a lower pressure and pulses slightly delayed when compared to the upper body due to the restricted flow through the collateral vessels.

When the infant is born the ductus arteriosus will close as normal at 7–10 days of age, however systemic perfusion is not compromised as in pre-ductal coarctation because of the collateral flow.

Clinical presentation

Children with a post-ductal or juxta-ductal coarctation will usually present later than those with a pre-ductal coarctation, even into their teenage or adult years. They may have relatively subtle signs such as frequent headaches or epistaxis related to upper body hypertension. Investigation into hypertension may be ongoing and anti-hypertensive therapy may have been commenced prior to diagnosis of a post- or juxta-ductal coarctation. If upper and lower limb blood pressures are taken, a difference in the systolic pressure will be seen and this is indicative of aortic coarctation. Further examination will reveal weak, delayed lower body pulses and the child may have a history of complaining of cold feet. A CXR in an older child may demonstrate rib notching, which is a defect caused by the collateral vessels affecting rib growth. Auscultation reveals a systolic or continuous murmur, usually heard in the left infraclavicular area and under the left scapula. An ejection click may signify an associated bicuspid aortic valve which is present in about 85% of cases. A thrill or hum due to flow in aberrant collateral vessels may be present over the chest or abdominal wall. Occasionally post- or juxta-ductal coarctations will present within the first few weeks or months of life, with signs of left ventricular failure, pulmonary congestion and dyspnoea.

Management

As with the pre-ductal diagnosis, surgery is required to resect the area of coarctation and the method of repair is essentially the same. Potential postoperative complications are usually related to spinal cord ischaemia, as with the preductal repair, or to hypertension. Hypertension in this group may be challenging as it will be long established and therefore prolonged anti-hypertensive therapy may be necessary.

Long-term effects of coarctation of the aorta

While the majority of infants and older children will have a successful primary repair, long-term follow-up is necessary as there are a number of complications which may manifest in later life. The principal problems are a re-coarctation, aneurysm formation around the site of surgical repair, persistent hypertension and/or the development of premature coronary and cerebrovascular disease.

Aortic stenosis

Anatomy

Aortic stenosis is a lesion which obstructs outflow of the left ventricle. It can be valvular, supravalvular (above the valve) or subvalvular (below the valve).

The normal aortic valve consists of three cusps and develops between 6 and 9 weeks of gestation. Valvular aortic stenosis is caused by an abnormality of this process which results in a unicuspid or bicuspid valve, or a valve in which the commissures are fused. This results in anything from mild to severe valvular stenosis and an associated left ventricular hypertrophy which is proportional to the degree of the stenosis.

Supravalvular aortic stenosis can be caused by the presence of a fibrous membrane, by an hourglass deformity with a narrow segment of restricted lumen size or by a more extensive section of narrowing. The stenosed area is usually distal to the coronary artery ostia, but occasionally there may be some coronary artery malformation, particularly on the left.

Subvalvular aortic stenosis can be caused by the presence of a fibrous membrane, a narrow fibromuscular ring or a more extensive fibromuscular narrowing of the left ventricular outflow tract (LVOT). Subvalvular aortic stenosis usually develops over a period of time and presentation during infancy is rare. Abnormalities of the aortic and mitral valve can occur as their function becomes restricted by the evolving fibromuscular tissue. Aortic regurgitation increases as the pressure gradient over the LVOT increases and the subsequent aortic regurgitation exacerbates the volume loading of the left ventricle.

Altered haemodynamics

In severe neonatal aortic stenosis cardiac output is limited and deoxygenated blood will shunt right to left across the ductus arteriosus into the relatively empty, low-pressure aorta. The left ventricle will become volume-loaded and distended as it fails to empty effectively and signs of left ventricular failure and pulmonary congestion will be evident.

Mild aortic stenosis can produce essentially no haemodynamic changes, although increasing aortic incompetence as the degree of stenosis evolves can result in signs of left-sided failure.

Clinical presentation

Severe aortic stenosis results in reduced cardiac output, poor coronary artery perfusion and myocardial ischaemia. As the duct closes at 7–10 days of age systemic perfusion is compromised and the child will present collapsed with a metabolic acidosis, tachycardia, hypotension, tachypnoea and signs of increased respiratory effort, such as intercostal recession. Peripheral pulses will be poor in all limbs in contrast to a child with a pre-ductal coarctation

who will have weaker pulses in their legs compared to their arms.

Mild aortic stenosis may be reasonably well tolerated and is often asymptomatic, although a systolic murmur can be heard on auscultation. Children may have a history of syncope and chest pain on exertion, or report a history of avoiding exercise.

Management

If the infant presents collapsed, then appropriate resuscitation must be provided, although as with any suspicion of a duct-dependent cardiac lesion, commencement of a prostaglandin infusion is needed to dilate the ductus arteriosus and improve systemic perfusion.

The infant/child may require inotropic support to optimise their systemic perfusion and reduce or resolve any metabolic acidosis. A balloon aortic valvuloplasty at cardiac catheter will be performed to dilate the obstructed area, hopefully without creating a significantly regurgitant valve. Occasionally, this will be ineffective or unsuitable and a surgical valvotomy will be required. Ultimately, these children usually require an aortic valve replacement.

The child with mild aortic stenosis diagnosed by the presence of a murmur usually requires no initial management but close follow-up to monitor the progress of the evolving stenosis. Surgery is considered as left ventricular function deteriorates. Complications post-balloon aortic valvuloplasty or a surgical valvotomy include aortic valve regurgitation. Other complications of a balloon valvuloplasty include myocardial perforation or dysrhythmias, but overall the potential risks of balloon valvuloplasty are similar to those of conventional surgery.

Cyanotic heart lesions

Tetralogy of Fallot

Anatomy

This defect consists of four coexisting lesions: pulmonary stenosis (usually infundibular), right ventricular hypertrophy, a ventricular septal defect (VSD) and an overriding aorta. These are thought to result from malformation of the pulmonary conus at 4–8 weeks of gestation. The pulmonary conus contributes to the formation of the pulmonary infundibulum and ventricular septation and subsequently affects the positioning of the aorta. The right ventricular hypertrophy is a consequence of the pulmonary stenosis.

Altered haemodynamics

The altered haemodynamics are essentially determined by the degree of pulmonary stenosis and the size of the VSD.

The extent of the pulmonary stenosis can vary from mild and relatively insignificant to pulmonary atresia.

The child with severe pulmonary stenosis or pulmonary atresia will have greatly reduced pulmonary blood flow. Pressure within the right ventricle will be high because of the obstructed right ventricular outflow tract and will result in a right-to-left shunt across the VSD. The aorta is displaced to the right and receives deoxygenated blood from the right ventricle as well as blood from the left ventricle, which will also have lower than normal oxygenation due to the right-to-left shunt across the VSD. Consequently, deoxygenated blood perfuses the systemic circulation resulting in cyanosis.

Blood will also shunt left to right across the ductus arteriosus from the high pressure aorta to the lower pressure pulmonary artery. If the pulmonary stenosis is severe or there is pulmonary atresia, this will constitute the main source of pulmonary blood flow. Children with pulmonary atresia may also develop multiple aorto-pulmonary collateral arteries (MAPCAs) for pulmonary blood flow.

The child with only mild or relatively insignificant pulmonary stenosis will not have the same increase in right ventricular pressure as is seen with severe pulmonary stenosis or pulmonary atresia. Consequently, there may be minimal right-to-left shunting through the VSD and the child may only become cyanosed when crying or on exertion.

The degree of pulmonary stenosis will worsen with time as the pulmonary infundibulum becomes more hypertrophied. A child who was relatively asymptomatic at birth may become progressively more cyanosed as the pulmonary blood flow decreases, the right ventricular pressure increases and the right ventricular hypertrophy develops.

Children with Fallot's may also experience hypercyanotic spells (commonly referred to as 'spelling episodes' or 'tet spells') in which there is intermittent worsening of right ventricular outflow tract obstruction (RVOTO) through infundibular spasm. This results in an acute and potentially fatal decrease in pulmonary blood flow. Clinical signs of a hypercyanotic spell are agitation and or increasing distress, tachypnoea, worsening cyanosis and potential syncope.

Clinical presentation

The infant with severe pulmonary stenosis or pulmonary atresia will present with cyanosis, hypoxia, tachypnoea and metabolic acidosis, all of which will become more evident as the ductus arteriosus constricts. These children will need early definitive surgery or a modified Blalock–Taussig shunt followed by definitive repair.

If the pulmonary stenosis is mild, then the child may initially be relatively asymptomatic. As the infundibular pulmonary stenosis worsens the symptoms will become more evident and the child will become more cyanotic and dyspnoeic, and will demonstrate poor feeding and faltering growth. Clubbing of the fingers and toes, a symptom associated with chronic hypoxia, may also be observed. A murmur will be heard on auscultation.

The right ventricular hypertrophy will be identifiable on CXR as a boot-shaped heart and the lungs will appear oligaemic, reflecting the decreased pulmonary blood flow due to the pulmonary stenosis.

Management of hypercyanotic spells

- Oxygen administration to improve cyanosis and as a pulmonary vasodilator.
- Sedation (fentanyl) to reduce the child's distress and therefore reduce tachypnoea.
- Volume to improve cardiac output.
- Positioning – either the child will squat or can be placed in a knee–chest position. It is thought that this position increases peripheral vascular resistance and so increases pressure in the left side of the heart, reduces the right-to-left shunt at ventricular level and subsequently increases pulmonary blood flow.
- Medications:
  - Propranolol – relaxes the infundibular muscle, thus reducing the RVOTO and improving pulmonary blood flow.
  - Phenylephrine – increases systemic vascular resistance therefore reduces the right-to-left shunt through increased left ventricular pressure.

If the infant or child is experiencing an increased number of hypercyanotic episodes, urgent referral for surgical repair is usually indicated.

Management

Infants with severe pulmonary stenosis or pulmonary atresia who present during the neonatal period will need early surgical intervention. A decision will be made whether to perform a definitive surgical repair or to insert a modified Blalock–Taussig (BT) shunt.

The modified BT shunt is largely considered to be a lower-risk surgical procedure than the open heart surgery required for a definitive repair. It can be a useful palliative procedure to alleviate symptoms and improve pulmonary blood flow, particularly in children of low birth weight for whom the complications of cardiopulmonary bypass can be significant. If a modified BT shunt is performed, then the child will return for elective removal of the shunt and definitive repair at a later stage.

For children with mild pulmonary stenosis definitive surgical repair is usually planned for 4–6 months of age. This involves open heart surgery, resection of the hypertrophied right ventricular muscular infundibulum, patch enlargement of the right ventricular outflow tract and closure of the VSD.

Potential postoperative complications

Following a modified BT shunt the child's arterial saturations will usually be in the region of 70–80%, for, while the shunt has improved the volume of pulmonary blood flow, the right-to-left shunt at ventricular level, the pulmonary stenosis and the overriding aorta remain. Close monitoring of the child's oxygenation is important as poor flow through the modified BT shunt will be indicated by decreasing saturations and an increasing metabolic acidosis. Patency of the conduit can be confirmed by auscultation, when a shunt murmur should be heard, or by cardiac ECHO examination.

Following definitive repair of tetralogy of Fallot there is invariably some degree of right ventricular failure. Function can be optimised by using volume boluses to maintain an adequate preload. Much of the surgical repair focuses on the area close to the site of atrio-ventricular node and rhythm disturbances such as junctional ectopic tachycardia (JET) or heart block may occur. Active cooling measures may be required to maintain normothermia or mild hypothermia, thus reducing the risk of tachydysrhythmias. Administration of IV amiodarone may also be useful in the management of episodes of JET. The child will have temporary epicardial pacing wires in situ postoperatively and atrio-ventricular sequential pacing may be required to facilitate conduction and optimise cardiac output.

The poor right ventricular function results in elevated right-sided heart pressures. As a consequence of this pleural effusions are a common postoperative complication. Pleural drains may need to be inserted and may remain in situ for an extended period of time. In addition, the infant/child may develop ascites secondary to venous engorgement due to increased right atrial pressure.

Tricuspid atresia

Anatomy

The tricuspid valve should form from the endocardial cushion tissue and the myocardium at 4–8 weeks of gestation. Failure can result in an absent or imperforate tricuspid valve and tricuspid atresia. The right ventricle is poorly developed (hypoplastic) as a result of the lack of flow from the right atrium and the pulmonary artery is also relatively hypoplastic for the same reasons. Most children with tricuspid atresia will also have a patent foramen ovale or an ASD and a small VSD.

Altered haemodynamics

Venous return entering the right atrium is unable to flow through to the right ventricle and the subsequent increase in right atrial pressure will force the foramen ovale to remain open if there is no ASD. Blood will shunt right to left at the atrial level through the foramen ovale or the ASD and then mix with the oxygenated blood in the left atrium before flowing through to the left ventricle. Some of the blood from the left ventricle will flow as normal into the aorta and a small volume will shunt left to right through the VSD and perfuse the pulmonary artery and the lungs. The volume of the ventricular shunt is limited as the small right ventricle and the narrow pulmonary artery produce a high resistance to flow and elevated right ventricular pressures. Pulmonary blood flow will be enhanced by a left-to-right shunt across the ductus arteriosus from the high pressure aorta to the lower pressure pulmonary artery. If the child does not have a VSD, then this left-to-right shunt across the ductus arteriosus will be the sole source of pulmonary blood flow. The child will be cyanosed as the right-to-left atrial shunt will result in some deoxygenated blood from the right side of the heart perfusing the aorta.

Clinical presentation

Infants with tricuspid atresia usually present within the first few days of life with significant cyanosis, tachypnoea, a metabolic acidosis and a murmur. The cyanosis will be more evident as the ductus arteriosus constricts and pulmonary blood flow is limited. Signs of left ventricular failure, such as poor cardiac output and pulmonary congestion, will be evident because of the volume overloading of the left ventricle. If the foramen ovale or ASD is small and/or restrictive, then the ensuing right atrial engorgement will produce signs of systemic venous congestion. A CXR will have decreased pulmonary vascular markings and show an enlarged heart.

Management

If the infant presents in a collapsed state, appropriate resuscitation must be provided according to current Resuscitation Council guidelines, although ultimately, as with any suspicion of a duct-dependent cardiac lesion, commencement of a prostaglandin infusion is needed to dilate the ductus arteriosus and improve the pulmonary blood flow.

The infant will usually need intubating, ventilating and the support of inotropes to stabilise their condition, optimise pulmonary blood flow and resolve or reduce the metabolic acidosis. A three-stage univentricular heart repair will then be planned. The first of these stages is a modified BT shunt and this will be performed within the first few days of presentation. The modified BT shunt will establish improved and reliable pulmonary blood flow and enable the infant to be discharged home until the second stage of surgery, which is a takedown of the modified BT shunt and insertion of a Glenn shunt. This is usually performed between 6 and 9 months of age. The final stage of the repair, a total caval pulmonary connection (TCPC) or Fontan, will be performed when the child is 2–3 years of age or when clinically indicated.

Potential postoperative complications

Specific complications relating to the modified BT shunt, the Glenn or the TCPC/Fontan are discussed earlier in the chapter and are applicable to the postoperative care of children with tricuspid atresia.

Transposition of the great arteries (D-TGA)

Anatomy

Between weeks 3 and 4 of gestation the truncus arteriosus should divide into the pulmonary artery and the aorta. Failure of the truncal ridges to spiral and septate the truncus arteriosus normally can result in displacement of the pulmonary artery so that it arises from the left ventricle and posterior to the aorta which arises from the right ventricle. This is D-TGA and the child will often have a patent foramen ovale, a patent ductus arteriosus and sometimes a VSD.

Altered haemodynamics

Systemic venous return enters the right atrium and the right ventricle as normal, but is then ejected into the aorta and recirculates around the body, returning to the right atrium. Oxygenated blood in the left atrium enters the left ventricle as normal, but is then ejected into the pulmonary artery and recirculates around the lungs, returning to the left atrium. Initially, right atrial pressures are higher than normal as the right side of the heart is supporting the systemic circulation. This tends to keep the foramen ovale open and there is usually a bi-directional shunt through it. The initial high pulmonary vascular resistance also forces a shunt from the pulmonary artery to the aorta and some oxygenated blood will perfuse the systemic circulation. As the pulmonary vascular resistance falls this shunt changes

and becomes predominantly from the aorta to the pulmonary artery. The now increased pulmonary blood flow volume loads the left atrium and the atrial shunt changes from bi-directional to predominantly left to right. It is this left-to-right atrial shunt which is now providing some oxygenated blood for the systemic circulation. If a VSD is present, blood will shunt from right to left at the ventricular level, as systemic pressure is higher than pulmonary pressure. This further increases pulmonary blood flow, increases left atrial volume and pressure, and increases the left-to-right atrial shunt.

Clinical presentation

The infant with D-TGA and an intact ventricular septum usually presents within the first few hours of birth. As the ductus arteriosus starts to constrict, the volume of the aorta to pulmonary artery shunt is reduced and this subsequently reduces the left atrial volume load and the left-to-right atrial shunt. As this is the only source of systemic oxygenation the reduced left-to-right atrial shunt will result in severe cyanosis, hypoxia, tachypnoea and a metabolic acidosis. Signs of biventricular failure may also be evident as the right ventricle struggles to provide the strength of flow necessary for the systemic circulation and the left ventricle and left atrium are over-distended due to the aorta to pulmonary artery ductal shunt. A murmur may be heard, reflecting the shunt through the patent ductus arteriosus.

If the infant has a D-TGA with a VSD, then symptoms will be similar to those described above although the infant may present slightly later and with less cyanosis as the right-to-left ventricular shunt will maintain volume loading of the left atria and the left-to-right atrial shunt even as the ductus arteriosus starts to constrict.

Management

The primary aim of initial management is to create a communication between the two circulations, which may be achieved initially through the maintenance of a patent ductus arteriosus with an intravenous prostaglandin infusion. Once the infant has been resuscitated and stabilised, an atrial balloon septostomy needs to be performed under cardiac ECHO guidance to establish adequate atrial mixing and sufficient oxygenated systemic flow to reduce or resolve the metabolic acidosis. Intubation, ventilation and inotropic support may also be required to achieve this. The infant will then need an arterial switch procedure which is electively performed at 7–14 days of age, although the infant's clinical condition will also influence the timing of surgery.

An arterial switch is an open heart procedure in which the aorta and the pulmonary artery are transected above the semilunar valves and repositioned in the anatomically correct position. The coronary arteries must also be detached from the base of the aorta as it arises from the right ventricle and then reinserted into the base of the aorta when it is re-implanted on the left ventricle. This is the technically challenging and delicate part of the procedure. The surgery is electively performed during the first couple of weeks of life as there is concern that beyond this time frame the pulmonary pressures drop significantly and the left ventricle adjusts its pressures accordingly. The left ventricle may then struggle to maintain systemic output when the aorta is attached to it. Similarly, there will be increased problems with pulmonary hypertension postoperatively if the right ventricle has to support the systemic circulation for a prolonged period as it will be generating too high a pressure for the newly attached pulmonary artery.

Potential postoperative complications

Infants are at risk of pulmonary hypertension post-arterial switch repair because of the increased pulmonary blood flow in the preoperative period. Other complications may be related to kinking or spasm of the re-implanted coronary arteries and this can compromise flow of oxygenated blood to the myocardium and lead to myocardial ischaemia. This will be evident on the infant's ECG as ST elevation and is usually associated with signs of poor cardiac output. Use of vasodilators, (e.g. glyceryl trinitrate – GTN), can help to relax the coronaries and improve myocardial blood flow.

Cardiac output may also be compromised postoperatively as the left ventricle, which has adjusted to pumping blood around the low-pressure pulmonary system, now has to increase its effort and generate the pressures required to perfuse the systemic circulation. Vasoactive drugs may be required to support the left ventricle during this period.

Truncus arteriosus

Anatomy

Between weeks 3 and 4 of gestation the truncus arteriosus should divide into the pulmonary artery and the aorta. Failure of the truncal ridges to spiral and septate the truncus arteriosus normally can result in persistence of the truncus arteriosus into postnatal life. This common vessel arises from both ventricles, and coronary, pulmonary and systemic vessels arise from it. A VSD is always present and there is a single truncal valve. Truncus arteriosus can be further categorised (I–IV) according to the configura-

tion in which the pulmonary arteries arise from the truncal vessel.

Altered haemodynamics

Blood from both ventricles is ejected via the truncal valve into the common truncal artery. The volume of blood perfusing either the pulmonary or systemic circulations is determined by the pulmonary and systemic pressures. In the initial post-delivery phase pulmonary pressures are relatively high and systemic pressures relatively low. The systemic circuit will be well perfused at the expense of pulmonary flow and while having an adequate blood pressure the infant's saturations will be extremely low due to the minimal pulmonary blood flow. Over the next 48 hours pulmonary pressures will gradually fall and pulmonary blood flow will improve, resulting in the child having increased saturations but a lower blood pressure. The challenge for medical care is to balance the infant's circulation by manipulating pulmonary pressures in order to maintain adequate pulmonary blood flow and reasonable saturations while also having an adequate systemic flow and a reasonable blood pressure. Poor systemic flow and excessive pulmonary flow will result in 'wet' lungs and a combined respiratory and metabolic acidosis due to compromised gas exchange and poor tissue perfusion; too much systemic flow and poor pulmonary flow will result in a metabolic acidosis due to hypoxia.

Clinical presentation

Infants will usually present within the first few days of life with cyanosis. Signs of congestive heart failure will become more pronounced after the first 48 hours as pulmonary pressures start to fall.

Management

The aim of pre-operative management is to balance the flow between the pulmonary and systemic circulation to reduce or minimise any acidosis and mitigate any congestive heart failure.

If a metabolic acidosis, which is the result of excessive pulmonary blood flow and diminished systemic flow, develops, the infant needs to be intubated and ventilated on settings which maintain the $PaCO_2$ at values which are the high side of normal (40–45 mmHg/5.3–6.0 kPa) The effect of this will be to produce pulmonary vasoconstriction, restrict pulmonary blood flow and so increase systemic blood flow. If this is insufficient to balance the circulation, the infant may need to be ventilated using a hypoxic gas mix. This is achieved by infiltrating nitrogen into the inspiratory gases to give a $FiO_2 < 0.21$. Again, the net effect is to cause pulmonary vasoconstriction, restrict pulmonary blood flow and increase systemic blood flow. Vasoactive drugs and/or diuretics may also be needed to manage any congestive heart failure which is present.

Surgical management involves open heart surgery and resection of the pulmonary arteries from the truncal vessel. A valved conduit is then inserted from the right ventricle to the pulmonary arteries. The VSD is also closed.

Potential postoperative complications

Postoperative management strategies should be aimed at preventing or minimising pulmonary hypertensive episodes and optimising cardiac output.

Total anomalous pulmonary venous drainage (TAPVD)

Anatomy

TAPVD results from an abnormality during foetal cardiac development in which the pulmonary veins errantly do not connect to the left atrium. It can be categorised into one of three types:

- Supracardiac – the pulmonary veins connect to the SVC, which then drains into the right atrium.
- Cardiac (intracardiac) – the pulmonary veins connect to the right atrium via the coronary sinus.
- Infracardiac (infradiaphragmatic) – the pulmonary veins connect to the ductus venosus and drain through the liver to the IVC, which in turn connects to the right atrium. There is an increased incidence of obstruction to pulmonary venous drainage in the infracardiac TAPVD as flow through the aberrant pulmonary veins is often restricted as it passes through the muscular diaphragm.

Infants with a TAPVD will always also have a patent foramen ovale or an ASD.

Altered haemodynamics

Oxygenated blood in the pulmonary veins, which should flow to the left side of the heart, is redirected via the anomalous pulmonary connection to the right side of the heart. It will mix with venous blood either in the SVC or IVC (depending on the anomalous connection) before draining to the right atrium. The resulting volume loading of the right atrium will increase right atrial pressures and force a right-to-left shunt through the ASD or foramen ovale. There will also be an increased volume of flow from the right atrium through to the right ventricle and the pulmonary artery and this will lead to pulmonary hypertensive changes if surgery is not timely.

The infant's cardiac output is determined by the volume of the right-to-left atrial shunt as this is the only source of filling for the left ventricle.

If the pulmonary venous drainage is obstructed, which most commonly occurs in infracardiac TAPVD but can occur in any category, the infant will present with profound and life-threatening cyanosis. The pulmonary venous obstruction causes pulmonary congestion and increased right-sided pressures. The right-to-left atrial shunt will be predominantly poorly saturated venous blood as there is minimal forward flow of oxygenated blood through the obstructed pulmonary veins. Consequently, systemic oxygenation is massively compromised producing life-threatening hypoxia.

Clinical presentation

The infant presentation is largely determined by the degree of obstruction to the pulmonary veins (Table 5.7).

Management

For infants with an obstructed TAPVD who present collapsed and shocked, management aims to improve pulmonary blood flow and drainage from the pulmonary veins to the right side of the heart in order that the right-to-left atrial shunt can then fill the left side of the heart and improve the cardiac output. Strategies such as high rate and tidal volume ventilation are used to keep the $PaCO_2$ on the low side of normal (35 mmHg/4.6 kPa) and the PaO_2 as high as is possible to counteract the pulmonary vasoconstriction associated with acidosis. A prostaglandin infusion may help to keep the ductus arteriosus patent and allow some

Table 5.7 Clinical presentation of TAPVD

Unobstructed	Obstructed
Presentation normally between 3 months and 2 years of age. Clinical signs:	Presentation normally in first few days of life and most common with infra-cardiac type. Clinical signs:
• Repeated LRTIs.	• Central cyanosis.
• Dyspnoea.	• Cough/dyspnoea.
• Moderate increased work of breathing.	• Tachypnoea.
• Mild cyanosis present during feeding and/or crying.	• Marked increased work of breathing.
• FTT.	• Pulmonary oedema.
• Hepatomegaly.	• Poor peripheral pulses.
	• Hepatomegaly.

shunting of venous blood from the pulmonary artery to the aorta. While this may help to improve systemic blood flow, the systemic saturations will remain low and the metabolic acidosis associated with poor cardiac output and poor oxygen delivery to the tissues may persist. Vasoactive drugs may be used to manipulate the child's cardiac output, but ultimately the obstruction to pulmonary drainage cannot be managed medically and early surgical intervention is vital.

If the TAPVD is unobstructed, surgery will be planned as a semi-elective procedure. This involves open heart surgery and resection and re-implantation of the anomalous pulmonary arteries to the left atrium.

Potential postoperative complications

Pulmonary hypertension is likely in the postoperative period and preventative measures should be taken to avoid any acute episodes.

Kinking or stenosis of the re-implanted pulmonary veins can cause obstruction to pulmonary drainage and haemodynamic instability related to poor left-sided filling and poor cardiac output, combined with pulmonary congestion. A cardiac ECHO will demonstrate pulmonary venous obstruction and further surgical management may be required.

Hypoplastic left heart syndrome (HLHS)

Anatomy

HLHS refers to a collection of anomalies associated with the development of the left side of the heart. The mitral valve, which should form from the endocardial cushion tissue and the myocardium at 4–8 weeks of gestation, is either absent or atretic. As a consequence of the restricted flow through the valve in utero the left ventricle is poorly developed and unable to support systemic circulation. The aortic valve is narrowed, absent or atretic and the aorta itself is hypoplastic, all due to the restrictive mitral valve. Infants with HLHS will also have an ASD.

Altered haemodynamics

At birth, oxygenated blood from the lungs returns to the left atrium as normal, however, the abnormalities of the mitral valve, the left ventricle, the aortic valve and the aorta mean that little of this blood flows forward through the left side of the heart and into the aorta. Consequently, left atrial pressures are higher than normal and oxygenated blood shunts left to right through the ASD. This oxygenated blood will then mix with venous blood in the right side of the heart, enter the pulmonary artery and some of it will shunt right to left from the pulmonary artery across

the ductus arteriosus to the aorta. The blood that shunts across the ductus arteriosus, combined with the minimal flow from the left ventricle to the aorta, constitutes the infant's systemic blood flow.

Within the first 48 hours of birth the infant's pulmonary vascular resistance continues to fall and the ductus arteriosus starts to constrict which affects the haemodynamics of the infant with HLHS. As the pulmonary pressures fall less blood shunts right to left across the ductus arteriosus to the aorta and more blood from the pulmonary artery will flow preferentially into the low-pressure pulmonary circuit. This increase in pulmonary blood flow results in a decrease in systemic blood flow and although the infant's saturations will be improved they will be poorly perfused, have a poor cardiac output and develop a metabolic acidosis. The challenge of medical management is to balance the infant's circulation so they have adequate pulmonary blood flow and saturations and an adequate systemic blood flow and blood pressure. To achieve this balanced circulation medical management will aim to manipulate the pulmonary vascular resistance.

Additionally, as the ductus arteriosus constricts, the reduction in systemic blood flow is significant and the compromised cardiac output will lead to collapse, shock and a profound metabolic acidosis.

Clinical presentation

HLHS is often diagnosed antenatally at a routine scan as the heart does not have four clearly identifiable chambers. In this situation the infant's management will be structured and planned from the moment of delivery.

If there is no antenatal diagnosis, the infant will usually present soon after birth as the pulmonary pressures fall and the infant's circulation becomes unbalanced and/or as the ductus arteriosus starts to constrict and the systemic perfusion is significantly compromised. The infant will often present obtunded, cyanosed, pale and poorly perfused with feeble pulses and a poor cardiac output. They may be tachypnoeic with sternal recession or be gasping and at the point of cardio-respiratory arrest.

Management

If there is an antenatal diagnosis, then the infant's parents will receive support and counselling regarding the treatment options. As the long-term surgical survival rates are relatively low with actuarial survival rate after staged reconstruction being 70% at 5 years, termination of pregnancy or palliative care on delivery will be offered as treatment options alongside surgical repair (Syamasundar Rao 2011). If the parents opt for surgical repair, the infant's care will be closely managed from the point of delivery. A prostaglandin infusion will be commenced to maintain ductal patency and the infant will preferably be nursed self-ventilating in air. A cardiac ECHO will be performed to confirm diagnosis and also to clarify the size of the ASD and the ductus arteriosus. Close monitoring of the infant's respiratory status and cardiac output is essential in order that any signs of increased pulmonary flow and poor cardiac output (tachypnoea, increased respiratory effort, increased crepitus on auscultation, cyanosis, poor peripheral perfusion and decreased blood pressure) can be responded to immediately.

If the infant's circulation becomes unbalanced as the pulmonary pressures fall, then it will be necessary to intubate and ventilate the infant on settings which maintain the $PaCO_2$ at values which are the high side of normal (40–45 mmHg/5.3–6.0 kPa). The effect of this will be to produce pulmonary vasoconstriction, restrict pulmonary blood flow and so increase systemic blood flow. If this is insufficient to balance the circulation, the infant may need to be ventilated using a hypoxic mix (see management of Truncus Arteriosus).

The prostaglandin infusion may need to be increased if the ductus arteriosus is not widely patent and vasoactive drugs may also be needed to improve ventricular function and cardiac output.

If the infant presents obtunded or arrested, prompt resuscitation is vital and survival depends on early suspicion of a duct-dependent cardiac lesion, cardiac ECHO to confirm the diagnosis and manipulation of the child's circulation. Any profound or prolonged acidosis may result in multiorgan failure and compromise the infant's survival.

Once stabilised a three-stage surgical repair (the Norwood procedure) is recommended. This aims to establish the right ventricle as the systemic pumping chamber and re-route pulmonary blood flow so that it arises from the SVC and IVC.

The first stage involves open heart surgery and is ideally performed within the first week of life. The ductus arteriosus is ligated and an atrial septectomy is performed to allow unrestricted mixing at atrial level. The distal end of the main pulmonary artery is detached from the pulmonary artery branches and the main pulmonary artery trunk is then used to enlarge the hypoplastic aortic trunk. This means that a mixture of oxygenated and de-oxygenated blood from both ventricles is now ejected into the new 'aorta' and perfuses the body. A modified Blalock–Taussig shunt is then inserted to provide pulmonary blood flow.

Alternatively, a hybrid procedure for interim management of HLHS can be performed. The first two parts are usually performed through interventional radiology and consist of:

- Enlargement of the septal defect.
- Stenting of the ductus arteriosus to maintain patency.

The purpose is to enable the right heart to pump blood more easily around the body reducing the stress on the RV. The third part of the hybrid procedure is a PA band, which is usually carried out at the same time in hybrid catheter suites.

The second stage of surgery involves removal of the modified BT shunt and insertion of a Glenn shunt; this is usually performed at 6–9 months of age. The final stage of the repair, a total caval pulmonary connection (TCPC) or Fontan, will be performed when the child is 2–3 years of age, or when clinically indicated.

Potential postoperative complications

Bleeding can be a significant problem in the immediate postoperative period and this is related to the extensive suture lines required to anastomose the pulmonary trunk and the hypoplastic aorta which are then exposed to systemic pressures.

Specific complications relating to the modified BT shunt, the Glenn or the TCPC/Fontan are discussed earlier and are applicable to the postoperative care of children with HLHS. Long-term planning for the child and family should include the potential need for cardiac transplantation as well as the effects on the quality of life for the child and their family.

Extracorporeal membrane oxygenation (ECMO)/extracorporeal life support (ECLS)

In the UK, ECMO/ECLS services are provided by a small number of supra-regional centres for all age groups, and as such are a highly specialised service provision. There is an expectation, however, that all paediatric cardiac surgical centres should be able to offer 'rescue support' to children who are unable to come off cardiopulmonary bypass.

In addition to providing cardiac support, ECMO may be used in the management of primary respiratory failure (e.g. meconium aspiration in the neonate), while ECLS may be used in the management of septic shock in children who are refractory to conventional therapies.

The standard criteria for ECMO/ECLS are:

- Acute severe, reversible respiratory failure.
- Inability to wean from CPB after correcting anomaly or providing surgical interventions.

- Underlying disease process treatable or reversible.
- High predicted mortality with conventional therapy.
- Child otherwise has good prognosis, neurological and other organ function is intact or recoverable.

Exclusion criteria for ECMO/ECLS support

All children:

- Chronic lung disease.
- Severe neurological deficits.
- Malignancy.
- Underlying irreversible disease.
- Mechanical ventilation >10 days.

Neonates:

- Birth weight < 2kg and gestational age < 35 weeks.

ECLS for cardiac support

ECLS is not a cure for underlying disease processes but is a mechanical support system which allows time for the damaged heart (and/or lung tissue) to heal while resting them from the damaging effects of mechanical ventilation or vasoactive drugs.

The role of ECLS post-cardiac surgery is to:

- Maintain tissue perfusion.
- Maintain tissue oxygen delivery.
- Prevent cardiac distension.
- Minimise myocardial work.

As well as being used to support children who are unable to come off CPB, ECLS is used to support children who have had witnessed cardiac arrests or those with cardiomyopathy awaiting cardiac transplant (Extra Corporeal Life Support Organisation 2009). These children are supported on veno-arterial (VA) ECLS.

Advantages of VA ECLS

- Supports both cardiac and pulmonary function.
- Provides rapid patient stabilisation.
- Safer during haemodynamic deterioration.

Disadvantages of VA ECLS

- Potential for arterial emboli.
- Low or non-pulsatile flow.
- Lower myocardial oxygen delivery.
- Possible carotid ligation.

Cardiovascular considerations

Cardiac performance on ECLS can be optimised by maintaining a higher preload and a lower afterload status. There will always be some native cardiac output from the patient and to achieve full gas exchange, approximately 80% of the cardiac output must be diverted to the oxygenator. Blood flow through the ECLS circuit is calculated in terms of normal cardiac output and 'full flow' is achieved at flows of 100 ml/kg/min (normal cardiac output 120 ml/kg/min).

Children on VA support will have a flattened systolic/ diastolic waveform due to the non-pulsatile ECLS pump flow. This becomes more flattened as the level of ECLS support is increased and more blood is drained from the right side of the heart, therefore it is important to observe MAP on VA ECLS. There may on occasion be a more pulsatile waveform present on the arterial line trace, because blood from the bronchial blood network returns to the left ventricle filling the heart.

There should always be an ECG trace on the monitor even on full flows and no ECG means that either the leads are not attached or the child is in asystole.

If the heart is not ejecting or is ejecting poorly because of myocardial stun, the BP is determined only by pump flow and vascular tone. If the heart has the ability to eject, adding volume will increase BP but at the cost of myocardial strain.

The pump is load-sensitive, therefore anything that increases resistance in the circuit will decrease the circuit flow. This includes the patient's vascular system and a sudden change in flow at the same driving pressure (pump speed in RPMs) should alert practitioners to a change in the system resistance.

Weaning from ECLS

Children should remain on ECLS for the minimum length of time necessary and removal of ECLS should occur when there is evidence of improvement, recovery or a complication that will cause irreversible loss of function. In cardiac surgical centres offering 'rescue' ECLS post-cardiotomy there should be a clearly documented plan (discussed with the parents) detailing the number of days of support the child will be offered. Rescue ECLS post-cardiotomy is a short-term support, designed to rest the stunned myocardium only and myocardial function should have recovered within 3–5 days post-surgery.

Weaning generally involves decreasing pump flows over a period of time until 'idling' flow has been achieved and ventilatory support and inotropic support are increased as ECLS support is decreased.

Weaning failure is indicated by:

- LAP > 10 mmHg – indicative of poor left ventricular function.

- Adrenaline infusion at > 0.2 mcg/kg/min.
- Ventilation – PIP/PEEP > 30/10.
- Lactate > 4.

If the child fails to wean from support, then ideally a period of 48 hours of rest on full support should be given before another attempt is made. In some children, however, where the fail was borderline and myocardial function has improved significantly, further weaning attempts are often made within 24 hours.

Rhythm disturbances and temporary pacing

Rhythm disturbances can be the primary cause of illness (e.g. SVT, LQT syndrome) or secondary to the illness itself (e.g. cardiac surgery, electrolyte imbalance). There are three main types of significant dysrhythmia/arrhythmia, classified as:

- Bradyarrhythmias.
- Tachyarrhythmias.
- Collapse rhythms.

ECG (Figure 5.10)

ECG review – questions to ask

- Has the surface ECG changed?
- What is the rate – too fast/too slow?
- Is the rate regular or irregular?

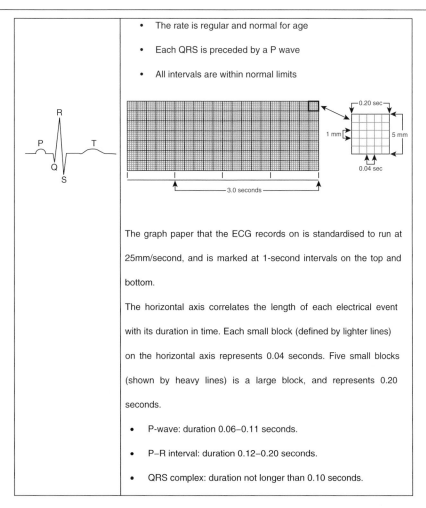

The graph paper that the ECG records on is standardised to run at 25mm/second, and is marked at 1-second intervals on the top and bottom.

The horizontal axis correlates the length of each electrical event with its duration in time. Each small block (defined by lighter lines) on the horizontal axis represents 0.04 seconds. Five small blocks (shown by heavy lines) is a large block, and represents 0.20 seconds.

- P-wave: duration 0.06–0.11 seconds.
- P–R interval: duration 0.12–0.20 seconds.
- QRS complex: duration not longer than 0.10 seconds.

Figure 5.10 Normal ECG trace.

- Are the QRS complexes narrow or broad?
- Is shock absent or present?

Bradyarrhythmias

These are rhythms where the rate is slower than normal and consequently cardiac output may be compromised. If the child is shocked, full cardiopulmonary resuscitation must be commenced. Where possible the cause of the dysrhythmia (e.g. hypoxia) should be identified and treated. Drug therapy may be indicated to restore a normal heart rate and rhythm. Pacing may also be a useful management strategy to maintain output on a temporary or permanent basis depending on the cause of the dysrhythmia.

Sinus bradycardia (Figure 5.11)

- Rate is regular but slow for age or clinical condition.
- P-wave precedes each QRS.

Junctional rhythm (Figure 5.12)

The rhythm is initiated by junctional tissue surrounding the SA node rather than the node itself.

- P-waves often absent, but if present are dissociated from QRS.

- QRS is normal, indicating normal conduction from AV junction onwards.

  Causes: SA node damage (sick sinus syndrome)

Heart block

Occurs when there is disruption to the normal conduction pathway.

  Causes:

- Post-cardiac surgery, which may be temporary or permanent due to oedema or damage to the conduction pathway.
- Can occur congenitally–complete heart block.
- Associated with structural anomalies (e.g. left atrial isomerism) which mean there is no SA node.

First-degree heart block (Figure 5.13)

Caused by a conduction delay through the AV node, but all the electrical signals reach the ventricles. This rarely causes any problems.

  On reviewing the ECG:

- Rhythm – regular.
- Rate – normal.
- QRS duration – normal.

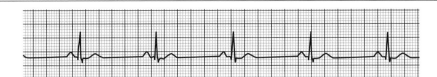

Figure 5.11   Sinus bradycardia.

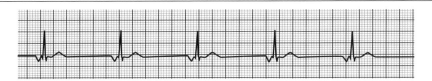

Figure 5.12   Junctional rhythm.

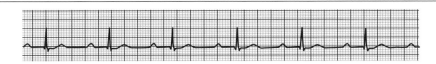

Figure 5.13   First-degree heart block.

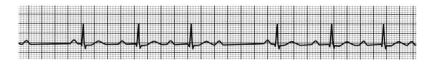

Figure 5.14   Mobitz type I (Wenckebach).

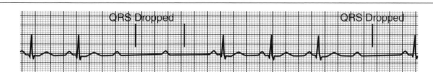

Figure 5.15   Mobitz type II.

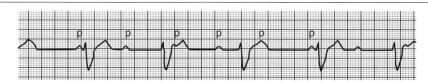

Figure 5.16   Complete heart block.

- P wave – QRS ratio – 1:1.
- P-wave rate – normal.
- P–R interval – prolonged (>5 small squares).

Second-degree heart block

Atrial depolarisation intermittently fails to conduct to the ventricles. There are two types:

- Mobitz type I (Wenckebach).
- Mobitz type II.

Mobitz type II is more worrying as it can progress to complete heart block.

Mobitz type I (Wenckebach) (Figure 5.14)

Some but not all atrial impulses are transmitted to the ventricles. There is progressive lengthening of the PR interval and then a failure of conduction of an atrial impulse.
   On reviewing the ECG:

- Rhythm – regularly irregular.
- Rate – normal or slow.

- QRS duration – normal.
- P wave – QRS ratio – 1:1 for 2, 3 or 4 cycles then 1:0.
- P-wave rate – normal but faster than QRS rate.
- P–R interval – progressive lengthening until a QRS complex is dropped.

Mobitz type II (Figure 5.15)

The atrial impulse fails to pass through the A-V node or bundle of His. This can progress to complete block but this is rare in children.
   On reviewing the ECG:

- Rhythm – regular.
- Rate – normal or slow.
- QRS duration – prolonged.
- P wave – QRS ratio – 2:1, 3:1.
- P-wave rate – normal but faster than QRS rate.
- P–R interval – normal or prolonged but constant.

Complete heart block (Figure 5.16)

There is no P-wave conduction to the ventricles, therefore the heart rate is determined by a slow junctional or ventricular escape pattern.

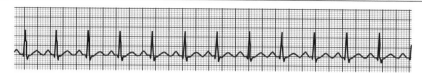

Figure 5.17   Sinus tachycardia.

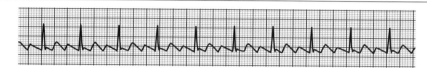

Figure 5.18   Atrial flutter.

On reviewing the ECG:

- Rhythm – regular.
- Rate – slow.
- QRS duration – prolonged.
- P-wave – unrelated to QRS.
- P-wave rate – normal but faster than QRS rate.
- P–R interval – variation.

Tachyarrhythmias

The rate is faster than normal and cardiac output is often compromised for a combination of reasons. Whether the overall rate is fast or slow the time taken for atrial and ventricular contraction is relatively unchanged; what changes is the length of time spent in ventricular diastole. During ventricular diastole the ventricles fill and the coronary arteries are perfused. If the ventricular diastolic time is shortened due to tachycardia, there is less time for ventricular filling, which will result in a reduced stroke volume and reduced cardiac output. There is also less time for the coronaries to perfuse, deliver oxygen to the myocardial tissue and remove waste products of metabolism, such as lactate. In combination with the fast rate which increases myocardial workload and increases myocardial oxygen demand this reduced coronary perfusion will result in myocardial ischaemia and ultimately myocardial infarction and cardiac arrest.

If the child with a tachydysrhythmia is shocked, immediate management is required. Where possible the cause of the dysrhythmia (e.g. fever) should be identified and treated. Drug therapy may be needed to restore a normal rate and rhythm. Over-drive pacing may also be useful to gain control of the heart rate, reduce the heart rate and so improve cardiac output.

Sinus tachycardia (Figure 5.17)

Sinus tachycardia is a normal response to illness, pain and distress:

- Rate is regular but fast for the age of the child.
- P-wave precedes each QRS and the normal conduction pathway is followed.

Atrial flutter (Figure 5.18)

Tissue in the atria is involved in generating the abnormal rhythm and the haemodynamic effects will depend on the ventricular rate.

On reviewing the ECG:

- Rhythm– regular.
- QRS duration – usually normal.
- P-wave – replaced with multiple F (flutter) waves, usually at a ratio of 2:1 (2F–1QRS) but sometimes 3:1.
- P-wave rate – typically around 300 beats/min.
- P–R interval – not measurable.

Atrial fibrillation (Figure 5.19)

Many sites within the atria generate their own electrical impulses leading to irregular conduction of impulses to the ventricles. Once again the haemodynamic effects will depend on the ventricular rate.

On reviewing the ECG:

- Rhythm – irregularly irregular.
- QRS duration – usually normal.

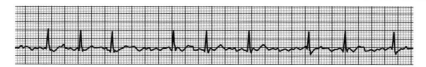

Figure 5.19 Atrial fibrillation.

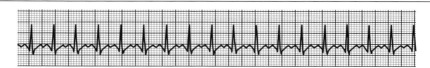

Figure 5.20 Supraventricular tachycardia.

Cardiac output compromised	Cardiac output not compromised
CPR	Vagal manoeuvres: suction, 'diving reflex'
Cardioversion:	Valsalva manoeuvre: coughing, sneezing
• Electrical	Elective cardioversion
• Chemical (adenosine)	Anti-arrhythmics– amiodarone, flecainide
	Ablation if continuing problems with re-entry
	circuit

Figure 5.21 Management of SVT.

- P-wave – not distinguishable as the atria is in continuous motion at a rate >400.
- P–R interval – not measurable.

Supraventricular tachycardia (Figure 5.20 and Figure 5.21)

This is a narrow complex tachycardia or atrial tachycardia which originates in the 'atria' but is not under direct control from the SA node. Impulses are therefore not being generated by the SA node, but come from a collection of tissue around and involving the AV node. SVT can occur in all age groups.

On reviewing the ECG:

- Rhythm – regular.
- Rate – >220 beats/min.

- QRS duration – usually normal.
- P-wave – often buried in preceding T-wave.
- P–R interval – depends on site of supraventricular pacemaker.

Wolff (Wolfe)–Parkinson–White syndrome is a type of SVT which is relatively common in children, affecting 1:1500 (Moss and Allen 2008). It involves an accessory pathway between the atria and the ventricles known as the bundle of Kent.

Junctional ectopic tachycardia (JET)

A malignant rhythm seen in post-cardiac surgery children most significantly associated with AVSD, TCPC, Fallot's, arterial switch and TAPVD repairs. Tissue trauma to the AV node or bundle of His leads to automaticity. As a consequence, ectopic foci emit impulses at a very fast rate (160–260) and conduction is 1:1.Complete AV dissociation occurs with a slower atrial rate. The result of this rhythm is low cardiac output. The duration of JET is normally 2–5 days following surgery.

Management of JET – key principles
- Over-pacing – aim to gain capture and reduce rate.
- Cooling to 35°C – reduces oxygen demands.
- Good levels of sedation.
- Antiarrhythmics – amiodarone.
- Optimal electrolyte levels.
- Inotropes to support cardiac function.

Long QT syndrome (LQTS)

LQTS is a congenital disorder characterised by a prolongation of the QT interval on ECG and a propensity to ventricular tachyarrhythmias. LQTS is known to be caused by mutations of the genes for cardiac potassium, sodium or calcium ion channels, and at least 10 genes have been identified. QT prolongation can lead to polymorphic ventricular tachycardia or torsade de pointes (Figure 5.22), which itself may lead to ventricular fibrillation and sudden cardiac death. Approximately 75% of patients with LQTS have a specific genetic mutation.

The diagnosis of LQTS is mainly based on ECG examination and any clinical history, including family history, which is a key factor. LQTS is defined as a QT interval >0.44 seconds, however 10% of those with LQTS will have a normal QT interval on a routine ECG.

Management of LQTS
- Medical therapy with beta-blockers is considered to be first-line prophylactic therapy. These drugs should be administered to all intermediate or high-risk individuals and considered on an individual basis in low-risk patients (Goldenberg and Moss 2008).
- If episodes continue, some patients will need an internal implantable cardioverter-defibrillator (ICD) fitting.
- Immediate family members should be investigated if not already under review.

Temporary pacing

Pacing can be used in the management of both brady- and tachydysrhythmias and is useful in maintaining coordinated contraction of the myocardium until the cause of the dysrhythmia has been resolved or until a permanent pacing system can be placed. Different systems are available for use as temporary systems (Table 5.8).

Types of pacing mode
Demand pacing

This is also referred to as A-V sequential pacing and it is the most commonly used pacing mode. Demand pacing refers to the ability of the pacing system to sense for atrial activity and to pace the atria only if a native P-wave is not sensed. It will then pause for a set period to allow normal conduction through the AV node before sensing for a QRS impulse. If a QRS impulse is sensed, then the pacing system will not pace the ventricles. If no QRS impulse is

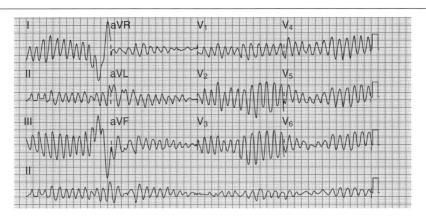

Figure 5.22   Torsade de pointes.

Table 5.8 Different temporary pacing systems

Type of system	Notes and considerations
Epicardial pacing	Temporary pacing system used post-cardiac surgery. Wires are sited on the outer (epicardial) layer of the heart wall: • Atrial wires exit on right of the sternum. • Ventricular wires exit on the left of the sternum. It is imperative that the atrial wires and leads are attached to the atrial connections on the box and the ventricular wires and leads to the ventricular connections as the sensitivity and stimulation thresholds vary in magnitude to account for the larger impulse generated and required by the more muscular ventricular myocardium as compared to the smaller, less muscular atria.
Transvenous pacing	Pacing wire threaded through subclavian or femoral vein to right atria or ventricle. This system requires lower stimulation thresholds than epicardial pacing as the pacing wire is sited within the atrial or ventricle. The diameter of the wires makes it a challenging process in children less than 10 kg but there are reports of successful transvenous pacing in neonates (Pinto et al. 2003) although lead dislodgement, myocardial perforation and thrombi are more of a problem in the smaller child.
Transoesophageal pacing	A flexible pacing catheter is inserted into the oesophagus and advanced until it is at atrial level. A specific box is required as the stimulus current required is higher than that necessary in transvenous or epicardial pacing modes.
External	Thorax pads are placed anteriorly and posteriorly on the child's chest and back. Large stimulation thresholds are required and this is a very short-term pacing mode which is used as a bridge to transvenous/trans-oesophageal pacing.

detected, then the pacing system will pace the ventricles. How much or how little of the system is required to maintain a safe heart rate is determined by the child's underlying dysrhythmia and the settings will be programmed according to the child's needs.

Fixed pacing

In contrast, dual chamber fixed pacing is now never used. In fixed pacing the pacing system is set to stimulate an atrial and/or ventricular impulse regardless of the child's intrinsic rhythm. While fixed atrial pacing has value within the clinical setting, fixed ventricular pacing is rarely used as it can have potentially fatal results. If the pacing box delivers a ventricular impulse on the T-wave of an intrinsic beat, this may induce ventricular tachycardia and the child will require immediate resuscitation.

Over-drive pacing

This is used in the management of tachydysrhythmias which originate above the AV node, such as SVT. The pacing system is initially set to deliver a rate which is faster than the child's intrinsic rate. Once the pacing box 'captures' the atrial rate, the rate can be gradually turned down with the intention that the atria will then follow the pacing stimuli rather than continue to generate an aberrant rhythm.

Pacing modes

The pacing mode will be set in response to the child's intrinsic heart rate and rhythm. For example, a child with a damaged SA node and a sinus bradycardia may need fixed atrial pacing to establish an appropriate atrial rate, but demand ventricular pacing as the native conduction pathways are able to transmit an atrial impulse once it is generated. A child with a damaged AV node may be generating an appropriate intrinsic atrial rate but only some of these impulses may be transmitted through the AV node to the ventricular system. A pacing mode which senses the atrial rate but will pace the ventricles if the impulse is not conducted through the AV node would therefore be appropriate (i.e. demand AV pacing). Most modern pacing systems have the flexibility to be set to complement the

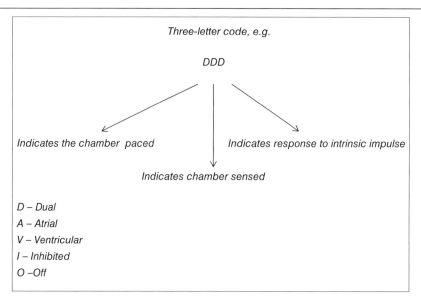

Three-letter code, e.g.

DDD

Indicates the chamber paced   Indicates response to intrinsic impulse

Indicates chamber sensed

D – Dual
A – Atrial
V – Ventricular
I – Inhibited
O –Off

Figure 5.23   Programme settings on demand pacing systems.

child's intrinsic rate and the pacing mode is identified by a three-letter code (Figure 5.23).

The settings on the pacing box will be determined by the child's underlying rhythm and clinical condition. Settings include:

- Mode.
- Rate.
- AV delay.
- Atrial sensitivity (0–10 mV).
- Atrial stimulation (0–17 V).
- Ventricular sensitivity (0–20 mV).
- Ventricular stimulation (0–17 V).

Considerations for practice

Whichever technique is being employed to pace the child it is vital that the practitioner ensures that the values set on the pacing box translate into the appropriate response on the child's heart rate and rhythm. The effect of pacing can be visualised on the child's ECG. Any stimulation from the pacing box is graphed as a vertical line, or pacing spike, on the ECG and should be followed by a P-wave or QRS complex as appropriate. As the origin of the impulse is the tip of the pacing wire rather than the SA or AV node the subsequent complex will have a differing morphology from native complexes and the pacing system-generated QRS complexes will be wider than the normal narrow QRS

complex of the child's native conduction system. If the pacing spike is not followed by an appropriate response, the stimulation threshold may need to be increased. Conversely, if the pacing spikes appear to be competing with intrinsic activity, the sensing threshold may need to be decreased.

It is also important to ensure that all connections are secure and that a spare battery is available for the pacing box. As with any ECG interpretation it is essential to ensure that the electrical activity visualised on the ECG converts into effective myocardial contraction and an adequate cardiac output.

The sensitivity and stimulation thresholds should be checked and adjusted as needed by senior medical staff every day. The longer the temporary pacing wires have been in place the more scar tissue forms around the wire site and a larger stimulation threshold may be required to overcome tissue resistance and induce an electrical response and a contraction.

Acquired heart disease

Although this is less common than congenital heart disease, acquired heart disease in infants and children can lead to significant cardiac dysfunction, morbidity and mortality. Acquired heart disease refers to a group of diseases in which the central feature is involvement of the heart muscle or tissues/vessels within the heart. Diseases within this category include:

Table 5.9 Common pacing modes

Pacing mode	Notes
DDD Both chambers can be paced – the first letter is **D.** Both chambers are being sensed – the second letter is **D.** The pacing box will be inhibited from pacing either the atria or the ventricles if an intrinsic impulse greater than the sensitivity threshold is sensed – the final letter is **D.**	This is one of the most frequently used pacing modes and provides the ability for full AV sequential pacing. Providing the native rate is slower than the set rate of the pacing system, the pacing system will sense for an atrial impulse greater than the set atrial sensitivity threshold. If one is not detected, then the atria will be paced at the set stimulation threshold. If an atrial impulse greater than the sensitivity threshold is detected, then the pacing system will not pace the atria. The pacing box will then sense for a ventricular impulse greater than the set ventricular sensitivity threshold. If one is not detected within the time determined by the set AV delay, then the ventricles will be paced at the set stimulation threshold. If a ventricular impulse greater than the sensitivity threshold is detected then the pacing system will not pace the ventricles.
DVI Both chambers can be paced – the first letter is **D.** Only the ventricles are being sensed – the second letter is **V.** The pacing box will be inhibited from pacing the ventricles if an intrinsic impulse greater than the ventricular sensitivity threshold is sensed. As there is no atrial sensing, the pacing system cannot be inhibited from pacing the atria – the final letter is **I.**	Another frequently used pacing mode which effectively provides fixed atrial pacing and demand ventricular pacing. Providing the native atrial rate is slower than the set rate of the pacing system, the pacing system will pace the atria at the set rate and the set stimulation threshold regardless of any intrinsic atrial activity. This is because the pacing system is not set to sense atrial activity, it is only set to sense ventricular activity – the middle letter is V. The pacing box will then sense for a ventricular impulse greater than the set ventricular sensitivity threshold. If one is not detected within the time determined by the set AV delay, then the ventricles will be paced at the set stimulation threshold. If a ventricular impulse greater than the sensitivity threshold is detected then the pacing system will not pace the ventricles.
AAI Only the atria can be paced – the first letter is **A.** Only the atria are being sensed – the second letter is **A.** The pacing box will be inhibited from pacing the atria if an intrinsic impulse is sensed – the final letter is **I.**	This mode effectively delivers demand atrial pacing but no ability to sense or pace the ventricles. Providing the native atrial rate is slower than the set rate of the pacing system, the pacing system will sense for an atrial impulse greater than the set atrial sensitivity threshold. If one is not detected then the atria will be paced at the set stimulation threshold. If an atrial impulse greater than the sensitivity threshold is detected then the pacing system will not pace the atria. NB: Not all commercially available pacing systems display this mode, but if the pacing system is set to DDD but only the atrial wires are attached, then the child is effectively being paced on an AAI mode.

D – Dual; A – Atrial; V – Ventricular; I – Inhibited; O – Off.

- Acute myocarditis.
- Cardiomyopathies.
- Kawasaki disease.

Acute myocarditis

Acute myocarditis is a generalised myocardial inflammation characterised by lymphocytic infiltration and myocardial necrosis. The clinical presentation varies from subclinical, impaired myocardial function which may be asymptomatic, through mild symptoms with a degree of clinical impairment to severe inflammation, which leads to congestive heart failure, arrhythmias and possible death. Doolan et al. (2004) suggest that 10% of cases of sudden death in young adults could be attributable to myocarditis. Causes of acute myocarditis can be divided into infectious and non-infectious.

Infectious causes

- Any infectious organism, but most commonly found after Coxsackie viral infection
- Other enteroviruses.

Non-infectious causes

- Drugs – doxorubicin, cocaine.
- Chemicals – carbon monoxide.
- Hypersensitivity reactions.
- Autoimmune diseases (e.g. systemic lupus erythematosus).
- Vasculitis.
- Secondary to Kawasaki disease, which causes:
  - Inflammation of the blood vessels.
  - Inflammation of the heart muscle.
  - Aneurysms in arteries which increase the risk of blood clots and heart attacks.

Pathophysiology of acute myocarditis (Figure 5.24)

The time between the onset of inflammation and initial clinical presentation of the disease varies. At a cellular level myocardial necrosis develops within a week of infection. Subsequent inflammatory and immune responses then become primary mediators of clinical disease progression and while the different triggering pathogens may engender slightly different responses within the myocardium, the end point is the same in each case.

Infectious agents cause myocardial damage as a consequence of:

- Direct invasion of the myocardium.
- Production of a myocardial toxin.
- Immune-mediated inflammation of the myocardium.

In viral myocarditis damage of the myocardium is through:

- Direct destruction of the myofibrils.
- Cytotoxic T-cell destruction of myocytes.
- Cell-mediated immunological reaction which destroys the cell.
- Adjacent cells may be destroyed by complement-mediated antibody action.

Clinical presentation (non-specific)

Neonates/infants – usually a sudden onset of illness which rapidly progresses to critical illness:

- Lethargy.
- Fever.
- Tachycardia.
- Respiratory distress/cyanosis.
- Vomiting or poor feeding.

Older children – usually a less rapid onset than that seen in the neonatal population:

- Fever.
- Lethargy.

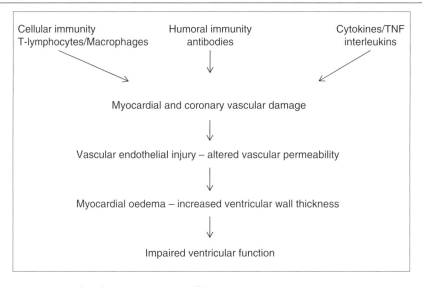

Figure 5.24   Disease progression in acute myocarditis.

- Muscular aches.
- Gastrointestinal disturbances.
- Pharyngitis.
- Meningitis.

Clinical presentation

Specific cardiovascular signs:

- Tachycardia out of proportion to any fever present.
- Poor peripheral perfusion.
- Thready pulses.
- Cool extremities.
- Pallor.
- Diaphoresis.
- Muffled heart sound if pericardial effusion present.
- Severe myocardial dysfunction:
  – Gallop rhythm.
  – High-frequency holosystolic murmur of mitral regurgitation.

Management of acute myocarditis

The primary aim is to support myocardial function and improve cardiac output while managing the underlying cause (if known). General organ support may be required, such as intubation and ventilation if the infant or child is significantly compromised. Anticipating and preventing complications is also key to good outcomes in this clinical scenario. If the symptoms are mild, then treatment of the infective cause and rest are the main priority. If signs of heart failure are evident, then diuretics and fluid restriction may be required.

More severe cases of myocarditis may warrant the use of:

- Vasoactive drugs such as dobutamine and milrinone to optimise cardiac function and cardiac output.
- Anti-arrhythmics to manage any dysrhythmias.
- Steroids, beneficial in reducing inflammation and helping to relieve symptoms, although their effect should be balanced against potential steroid-induced immune suppression.
- Anti-coagulants, often warranted to combat the risk of embolism resulting from sluggish blood flow.

Cardiomyopathy

Cardiomyopathy is a disease of the heart muscle which may be classified into three subtypes:

- Dilated cardiomyopathies.
- Hypertrophic cardiomyopathies.
- Restrictive (very rare in children).

Dilated cardiomyopathy

Dilated cardiomyopathy is the most common type of cardiomyopathy in children (Venugopalan 2010) and is more likely to present during the first year of life than in older children (Towbin et al. 2006). Dilated cardiomyopathy is characterised by dilation of all four cardiac chambers, although it is the left ventricle where this dilation is most pronounced.

In the majority of cases the cause of DCM is idiopathic (www.cardiomyopathy.org). However, dilated cardiomyopathy can be caused by a viral illness, with Coxsackie B being a common pathogen. The viral infection may directly affect the myocardium or trigger an immune response which results in myocardial damage. In 30% of patients an autoimmune process is thought to cause or exacerbate the DCM process (www.c-r-y.org.uk) and 25–50% of DCM cases have a genetic cause (Kimura 2008). The genetic defect is autosomal-dominant so the child of an affected adult has a 50:50 chance of inheriting the condition. Screening of first-degree relatives should be offered if the cause of DCM is found to be genetic as appropriate management and support can then be provided. Infrequently, Barth syndrome, a rare, X-linked genetic disorder of lipid metabolism, or a mitochondrial defect may be the cause of DCM.

DCM is characterised by:

- Increased ventricular volume.
- Ventricular dilation – enlarged, thin-walled ventricles with atrial enlargement.
- Systolic (contractile) dysfunction.
- Stasis of blood with possible thrombus formation.
- Ventricular arrhythmias.
- Signs of congestive heart failure.

Clinical presentation

Children with DCM may be asymptomatic for months even in the presence of systolic dysfunction and ventricular dilation. Severe ventricular dysfunction will precipitate cardiogenic shock with low cardiac output, although occasionally clinical presentation will be ventricular ectopy/syncope.

Management of the child with DCM

- Vasoactive medications – dobutamine and milrinone.
- Anti-failure therapy – diuretics, ACEI, beta-blockers.
- Anti-coagulation – use of heparin/enoxaparin.
- Anti-arrhythmics – amiodarone has been shown to be effective in the management of ventricular dysrhythmias associated with DCM.

- Serial monitoring of cardiac function – may ultimately require cardiac transplantation.

Hypertrophic cardiomyopathy (HCM)

HCM is an autosomal dominant genetic condition which affects approximately 1:500 of the population (Watkins et al. 2008), although not all those who have the condition will be symptomatic. The defective gene causes an abnormality of the sarcomeric contractile proteins which affect myocardial function (www.c-r-y.org.uk/hypertrophic_cardiomyopathy). The children of a parent with the HCM gene have a 50:50 chance of inheriting it.

HCM is typified by ventricular hypertrophy with no obvious cause (Colan et al. 2007) and myocardial disarray – a condition where the myocardial cells, myofibrils and myofilaments are not in parallel but are aligned randomly. This myocardial disarray is thought to interfere with normal conduction pathways and predisposes children with HCM to dysrhythmias, such as atrial fibrillation. A normal left ventricular myocardium is less than 12mm thick; in HCM it will typically be >15 mm (Maron 2002). This myocardial hypertrophy adversely affects both systolic and diastolic function as the stiff muscle relaxes poorly, which impairs filling and also has poor compliance which affects contractility and compromises cardiac output. The high filling pressures cause systemic and pulmonary venous congestion and result in ascites and peripheral oedema as well as respiratory difficulties and pulmonary oedema. The defect is present from birth, but it is usually from adolescence to early adulthood that the hypertrophy evolves. The enlargement or hypertrophy always affects the left ventricular myocardium and may sometimes affect the right ventricular myocardium. Hypertrophy of the ventricular septum may also be present and this, in combination with the left ventricular hypertrophy, may result in obstruction of the left ventricular outflow tract. If the mitral valve is also involved, hypertrophy of the valve leaflets results in mitral incompetence.

There are four recognisable patterns to the hypertrophy present in HCM (Table 5.10).

Clinical presentation (Table 5.11)

Table 5.11 Clinical presentation of HCM according to age

Infants	Older children
Tachypnoea	Usually asymptomatic
Tachycardia	Exercise intolerance
Poor feeding	Dyspnoea
Congestive	Chest pain
heart failure	Systolic murmur on examination in 40% of patients
	Audible 3rd and 4th heart sounds

Table 5.10 Patterns of hypertrophic cardiomyopathy

Asymmetric septal hypertrophy with no obstruction	The upper region of the ventricular septum becomes thickened and encroaches into both the right and left ventricles but does not affect flow from the left ventricle to the aorta.
Asymmetric septal hypertrophy with obstruction	The upper region of the septal wall becomes thickened and intrudes into the left ventricular outflow tract, narrowing the gap between the ventricular septum and the mitral valve, restricting flow from the left ventricle to the aorta and compromising cardiac output. The obstruction creates turbulent blood flow which can be heard as a murmur on auscultation and the restricted movement of the mitral valve results in mitral incompetence.
Symmetrical or concentric hypertrophy	The hypertrophy is evenly spread throughout the ventricle and can cause obstruction to the left ventricular outflow tract by narrowing the gap between the ventricular septum and the mitral valve. The obstruction compromises cardiac output and creates turbulent blood flow which can be heard as a murmur on auscultation and the restricted movement of the mitral valve results in mitral incompetence.
Apical hypertrophic cardiomyopathy	In approximately 10% of patients with HCM the hypertrophy is focused around the apical area of the ventricles. This produces a small left ventricular cavity but no obstruction to the outflow tract. Symptoms include palpitations and syncope related to dysrhythmias and a murmur if the hypertrophy is causing outflow tract obstruction.

Management of the child with HCM

Medical treatment is often with beta-blockers or calcium antagonists:

- Beta-blockers aim to decrease the speed at which the left ventricle contracts and the more controlled contraction results in less outflow tract obstruction.
- Calcium antagonists improve left ventricular relaxation and filling, reducing left ventricular end diastolic pressure and relieving some of the symptoms of pulmonary congestion as well as reducing myocardial ischaemia.
- Fluid restriction, electrolyte management and diuretics are also key therapies in controlling the degree of heart failure.
- Anti-arrhythmics should be used with care as the majority have a negative inotropic effect, so ECG and invasive blood pressure monitoring will be required if they are to be incorporated into the treatment regime.
- Implantable pacemakers or defibrillators may be required to manage dysrhythmias effectively if anti-arrhythmics prove insufficient.

If there is concern about stasis and possible clot/thrombus formation due to the low cardiac output, anti-coagulation may also be required.

On occasion, the surgical option of a myectomy may be advised. This involves resecting the left ventricular outflow tract in an attempt to relieve the obstruction and improve cardiac output. An evolving alternative to surgical myectomy is the relatively new procedure of alcohol ablation. Under ECHO or cardiac catheter guidance a small amount of absolute alcohol is injected into the coronary artery which supplies the upper portion of the ventricular septum to induce a controlled infarction / of the hypertrophied septum in order to remodel the left ventricular outflow tract. In severe HCM a cardiac transplant may be required.

Restrictive cardiomyopathy

Restrictive cardiomyopathy describes a disease process characterised by an increased stiffness of the myocardium which subsequently causes increased ventricular pressures and restricted ventricular filling. It is the rarest of the cardiomyopathies and may be idiopathic or caused by endomyocardial fibrosis or cardiac amyloidosis where abnormal proteins are deposited in the heart tissue (www .cardiomyopathy.org). The heart is not obviously enlarged, although there may be some increase in myocardial thickness due to the amyloidosis. Systolic function often remains good, but cardiac output is compromised as the high diasto-lic pressures restrict ventricular filling and reduce the end diastolic ventricular volume and so compromise the stroke volume. Symptoms include signs of pulmonary and systemic congestion as well as lethargy and weakness. Emboli are a common complication, as are dysrhythmias.

Management of restrictive cardiomyopathy

Effective treatment is challenging as the aim is to enhance ventricular relaxation only during diastole, most drug therapies will affect ventricular tone throughout the whole cardiac cycle causing the unwanted result of reduced cardiac output. Current therapy includes cautious use of diuretics and anti-arrhythmics to manage any rhythm disturbances. Anti-coagulation may be required if there is a risk of emboli formation. Ultimately, transplantation may be the only management strategy if myocardial function is severely compromised.

Kawasaki disease

Kawasaki disease (KD; also known as acute febrile mucocutaneous syndrome) is a febrile illness of childhood. It is a self-limited acute vasculitic syndrome of unknown aetiology but thought to be an immunological response to an infective organism (Pinna et al. 2008). It mainly affects children between 6 months and 4 years of age, with a peak incidence at around 1 year. It is more common in children of Japanese and to a lesser extent Afro-Caribbean ethnicity than in Caucasian children, which has led to suggestions that there may be a genetic predisposition to disease development (Burns et al. 2005). The diagnosis of classic KD requires a persistent fever with a duration of 5 or more days, together with a combination of four of the following signs:

- Changes in extremities which include desquamation, oedema and or erythema.
- Bilateral non-exudative conjunctivitis.
- Polymorphous rash.
- Changes in the lips or oral cavity (strawberry tongue).
- Cervical lymphadenopathy.

Cardiovascular implications of KD

Initially, there is a microvasculitis of medium-sized muscular arteries which triggers an immunological activation. This results in cytokine-induced changes in the vascular endothelium which makes it susceptible to lysis by antibodies. The vasculitic changes can be divided into four stages (Table 5.12).

More general cardiovascular implications include:

Table 5.12 Vasculitic stages of Kawasaki disease

Stage	Vasculitic changes
Stage 1 1–2 weeks after the onset of illness	Acute perivasculitis (inflammation of a perivascular sheath and surrounding tissue) and vasculitis of microvessels such as arterioles, capillaries and venules. Inflammation of the intima, externa and perivascular areas of large and medium-sized arteries. Vascular oedema and localised leucocyte and lymphocyte infiltration. Aneurysms not present at this stage.
Stage 2 2–4 weeks after onset of illness	Reduced inflammation in small arteries and veins and micro-vessels compared to stage 1, but there is continued inflammatory changes in all layers of the medium-sized arteries with focal vasculitis – oedema/necrosis and fibrotic changes. Aneurysms with thrombi and stenosis seen in medium-sized arteries, most significantly the coronary arteries.
Stage 3 4–7 weeks after onset of illness	Subsidence of inflammation in small arteries and veins and micro-vessels. Granulation (formation of healed tissue structures) in the medium-sized arteries due to concealed intimal thickening.
Stage 4 More than 7 weeks after onset of illness	No acute inflammation present in the vessels but in the medium-sized arteries there is continued scar formation (continued intimal thickening with stenosis), aneurysm development and thrombi formation due to narrowed lumen.

- Myocarditis, which usually develops within 3–4 weeks and is associated with white cell infiltration and oedema of the conduction system and myocardial muscle fibres.
- Valvular inflammation and coronary artery dilation.
- Development of coronary artery aneurysms as a consequence of the changes to the vascular endothelium.

Management of the child with Kawasaki disease

Only a few children with KD require intensive care, although some may require high dependency care in the very acute presentation phase. The treatment of KD is essentially through the instigation of supportive measures, however two specific interventions are indicated:

- Administration of intravenous gamma globulin (IVIG) to reduce the formation of aneurysms. IVIG is most effective when given in the first 10 days of illness (i.e. from the onset of fever) and the result is dose-dependent. Current UK guidelines advocate the use of an IVIG dose of 2 g/kg as a single infusion over 12 hours. If there is no improvement, a second dose may be considered (Wood and Tulloh 2009).
- High-dose aspirin to reduce thrombi formation. There is considerable discussion as to the efficacy of aspirin therapy in KD and a review concluded that there was insufficient evidence to determine whether it should continue to be used (Baumer et al. 2006). As a consequence,

it is still currently used in the management of most children with KD.

Pharmacology (Appendix 1)

To optimise cardiovascular function, preload, afterload, contractility and fluid balance can be managed by using a combination of drug therapies, fluid restriction and fluid administration.

Vasoactive drugs

Catecholamines and sympathomimetics

The majority of vasoactive drugs used in paediatric intensive care are positive inotropes (i.e. they increase cardiac contractility), however, many drugs also optimise cardiac output by manipulating heart rate or systemic vascular resistance and it is a combination of these effects that will produce the best function from a failing cardiovascular system.

The cardiovascular system is predominantly regulated by the autonomic nervous system, which consists of the sympathetic and parasympathetic systems. The parasympathetic nervous system consists of long preganglionic neurons which arise from the sacral region of the spinal cord between S_2 and S_4 and synapse with relatively short postganglionic neurons that terminate close to or within the effector tissues; hence parasympathetic stimulation produces a localised response (McCorry 2007). The parasympathetic nervous system releases acetylcholine as its neurotransmitter, the fibres are described as cholinergic fibres and the effects of parasympathetic stimulation are to reduce the heart rate and blood pressure and promote digestion and excretion.

In contrast, the sympathetic nervous system consists of short preganglionic neurons which arise between segments T_1 and L_2 of the spinal cord. Each preganglionic neuron may synapse with up to 20 postganglionic fibres (McCorry 2007). The result is that stimulation of just one sympathetic neuron elicits a response in many organs and tissues. Other preganglionic neurons synapse directly with the adrenal medulla stimulating the release of the catecholamines noradrenaline and adrenaline into the blood stream from where they will have a global effect. Preganglionic nerve fibres of the sympathetic system are cholinergic fibres as they have the ability to release acetylcholine, as do the postganglionic sympathetic fibres that innervate the sweat glands. However, most postganglionic nerve fibres of the sympathetic system are adrenergic fibres and release noradrenaline. Drugs that elicit sympathetic stimulation are referred to as sympathomimetics and the majority of sympathomimetics come from the class of drugs known as catecholamines.

The effect of the neurotransmitters and the circulating catecholamines is determined by specific receptors on the cell membranes within the effector tissues. Acetylcholine binds with muscarinic receptors and can produce either an excitatory or an inhibitory effect depending on the tissue in which they are located. Stimulation of muscarinic receptors in the myocardium is inhibitory and results in a decreased heart rate, while stimulation of muscarinic receptors in the lungs is excitatory and results in smooth muscle contraction and bronchoconstriction.

Noradrenaline and adrenaline are the main neurotransmitters of the sympathetic nervous system and stimulate adrenergic receptors. These can be divided into alpha$_1$ (α_1), alpha$_2$ (α_2), beta$_1$ (β_1) or beta$_2$ (β_2) receptors.

Alpha$_1$ receptors are found in the smooth muscle of the peripheral vasculature and the bronchi. Stimulation produces vasoconstriction of both veins and arteries and increased myocardial contraction. This will result in increased blood pressure, decreased urine output and decreased blood flow to the skin and splanchnic vessels.

Alpha$_2$ receptors are found on postganglionic neurons, and stimulation reduces the amount of noradrenaline released, resulting in vasodilation and decreased heart rate. Alpha$_2$ stimulants are not frequently used in the clinical setting.

Beta$_1$ receptors are the predominant adrenergic receptor of the heart. Stimulation results in an increase in heart rate, contractility and AV conduction velocity. The clinical response is an increase in cardiac output.

Beta$_2$ receptors are found in smooth muscle and stimulation results in relaxation of the smooth muscle producing vasodilation and bronchodilation. Their main clinical use is as a bronchodilator to relieve the bronchospasm associated with asthma.

Dopaminergic receptors are also components of the sympathetic nervous system and are found in the myocardium and the renal, coronary and intestinal blood vessels. Stimulation of these receptors produces vasodilation; coronary vasodilation will enhance oxygen delivery to the myocardium and renal vasodilation will improve the glomerular filtration rate and help to maintain a good diuresis.

Knowledge of the physiology of the autonomic nervous system allows drugs to be selected according to their specific clinical response: an α_1 agonist will increase the child's blood pressure through vasoconstriction in contrast to a β_1 agonist, which will increase blood pressure through increasing heart rate and contractility.

Considerations for practice

With the exceptions of dobutamine and milrinone and, in emergencies, dilute dopamine, all vasoactive drug infusions are preferably given via a central line. It is the individual practitioner's responsibility to have the knowledge relating to the management and care of central access (according to local policy) and the potential complications associated with both long- and short-term central lines.

Most vasoactive medications have extremely short half-lives and this dictates the need to administer them by continuous infusion. The infusion should never be paused or interrupted, and syringes should be changed smoothly and efficiently. If volume or other bolus drugs are required, they must always be administered on a separate line to the vasoactive drug infusions. It is essential that the practitioner has knowledge of the compatibility of vasoactive drugs to ensure their safe administration and is familiar with the effects and side-effects of any drug therapy used.

Phosphodiesterase inhibitors

These drugs block the action of the phosphodiesterase enzyme and consequently increase the levels of active cyclic adenosine monophosphate (cAMP) and cyclic guanosine monophosphate (cGMP). The effect is to enhance cardiac output by improving diastolic relaxation, improving contractility and decreasing vascular resistance. The resultant increase in stroke volume and afterload reduction is useful in optimising output in severe left ventricular failure or reducing pulmonary hypertension and optimising right ventricular function.

Angiotensin converting enzyme (ACE) inhibitors

These drugs prevent the conversion of angiotensin I to angiotensin II, a potent vasoconstrictor which therefore reduces afterload and blood pressure. In addition, the reduced amount of angiotensin II means that less aldosterone is produced by the adrenal cortex and so less water and sodium are retained by the kidney, whilst potassium is excreted. This fluid loss further contributes to the reduction in blood pressure. If the child is receiving diuretics as well as ACE inhibitors, they should not be given at the same time as the combined fluid and potassium loss could lead to cardiovascular instability. ACE inhibitors are useful in the management of hypertension and also in improving left ventricular function and cardiac output.

Beta-blockers

This class of drugs work by blocking catecholamine-induced increases in heart rate and contractility and so induce a slower rate and a decrease in contractility. An adverse effect can be bronchoconstriction which results from blockage of β_2 receptors.

Calcium channel blockers

These drugs inhibit the influx of calcium ions across the cellular membrane in smooth and cardiac muscle. The effect is to reduce contractility, slow conduction within the heart and cause arteriolar dilation. This then reduces cardiac output and also blood pressure.

Nitrates

These dilate coronary arteries, systemic arteries and veins through the production of nitric oxide. They decrease both preload and afterload and so reduce myocardial oxygen demand while simultaneously improving coronary blood flow and oxygen delivery.

Considerations for practice

To ensure the therapy is safely delivered and the child's response is accurately assessed, continuous monitoring of the child's ECG, invasive blood pressure, CVP and arterial saturations are required. If invasive blood pressure monitoring is not available, then a cuff blood pressure should be checked frequently, for example every 5 minutes or more if the child's condition is unstable or critical. Attention should be paid to the child's urine output, with hourly measurements recorded. Central and peripheral tempera-

ture monitoring, combined with visual assessment of the child's perfusion, will add to the overall evaluation of the child's cardiac output. Poor cardiac output will also be demonstrated by blood gas results that show a metabolic acidosis. Careful evaluation of the child's vital signs will indicate whether vasoactive drugs, volume administration, or a combination of both therapies, is required to improve output. Cardiac ECHO, if readily available, may be useful in providing information about the heart's contractility and volume status.

Volume and diuretics

While the child's systemic vascular resistance and so their afterload can be manipulated through the use of vasodilators and vasoconstrictors, the child's circulating volume and therefore their preload can also be manipulated through the use of diuretics and fluid administration.

If the child has a poor cardiac output due to a decreased circulating volume, a volume bolus is necessary to improve the cardiac output. Whether crystalloid solutions such as 0.9% sodium chloride or colloid solutions such as 4.5%/5% human albumin solution (HAS) is used for the volume bolus is much discussed in the literature (Perel et al. 2007) and clinical practice varies. Whichever type is used, the quantity given remains crucial. In cardiac arrest the Resuscitation Council (UK) recommends 20 ml/kg aliquots in combination with appropriate CPR and drug therapy. However, in situations where the child's cardiac output is compromised, 10 ml/kg aliquots of volume, with frequent evaluation of their effectiveness, are recommended. The speed and mode of administration will vary with the urgency of the situation. If the child's blood pressure has gradually declined over the period of a few hours, then the volume bolus can be administered via an infusion pump or syringe driver over a period of 20–30 minutes. If the child's blood pressure has fallen precipitously, the volume can be drawn up in a 50ml syringe and delivered as an immediate bolus.

Consideration for practice

If only peripheral access is available, then the gauge of the cannula may determine the speed of volume administration and care should be taken not to cause extravasation of the cannula.

In contrast, a child who has a poor cardiac output due to right or left ventricular failure may benefit from diuretic therapy to minimise the amount of systemic and/or pulmonary oedema resulting from the poor cardiac function. A loop diuretic such as furosemide is usually the drug of first choice. This works by inhibiting the reabsorption of sodium and therefore water from the ascending limb of the loop of

Henle. The excess water excretion results in excess potassium also being excreted and potassium supplementation may be required and/or concomitant treatment with a potassium-sparing diuretic, such as spironolactone. Spironolactone has only a weak diuretic action. It is an aldosterone receptor antagonist and causes the collecting duct to excrete sodium and water while retaining potassium.

Anti-arrhythmic medications

Anti-arrhythmic drugs (Table 5.13) are classified according to their mode of action and the ion channels which they affect.

Circulatory failure

The management of the child with circulatory failure as a consequence of cardiac arrest is detailed in Chapter 2. This section focuses on the child in shock and multi-system failure.

Shock

Shock is a clinically diagnosed condition that results from many aetiologies. It can damage any and all tissues and organ systems in the body. Delay in recognising the shocked child and prompt intervention may result in a progression from compensated reversible shock to widespread multi-system organ failure and death. Associated morbidity may be widespread and involve all the major body systems leading to renal failure, hepatic failure with metabolic derangements, diffuse intravascular coagulation (DIC), acute respiratory distress syndrome (ARDS), cardiac failure and death (Schwarz 2011). There are different types of shock, however probably the major challenge for the intensive care practitioner is the infant or child who presents in cardiogenic shock or with septic shock.

Shock may be classified based on the pathways involved in the process (Table 5.14). These mechanisms are not mutually exclusive and as the shock process progresses all three pathways will be involved.

Table 5.13 Anti-arrhythmic medications

Drug	Effect	Side-effect
Adenosine	Class V Causes a temporary atrioventricular (AV) nodal conduction block Interrupts re-entry circuits that involve the AV node	Severe bradycardia Chest pain Dyspnoea Dizziness Nausea
Amiodarone	Class III – prolongs phase 3 of the cardiac action potential Slows the intrinsic rate of the SA node Slows AV conduction Prolongs the AV refractory period and QT interval Slows ventricular conduction	Hypokalaemia Bradycardia Pulmonary toxicity
Atenolol	Class II – beta-blocker (selective) Selectively blocks β_1 receptors, slowing heart rate and decreasing contractility Decreases renin secretion	Bradycardia Hypotension
Esmolol	Class II Blocks β activity	
Labetalol	Class II – beta-blocker Blocks α and β receptors, slowing heart rate, decreasing contractility and reducing vasoconstriction	Fatigue Headache Ventricular arrhythmias
Lignocaine	Class IB Decreases the refractory period and the automaticity of the Purkinje fibres Suppresses ventricular dysrhythmias	Seizures Heart block Hypotension
Propranolol	Class II – beta-blocker (non-selective) Blocks the action of adrenaline on β_1 and β_2 receptors Depresses renin secretion	Bradycardia Hypotension Bronchospasm

Two key points about shock:

- Shock results from an inability or failure of the cardio-vascular system to deliver adequate amounts of essential nutrients, especially oxygen, to meet the metabolic needs of the cells, or there is impaired use of essential cellular substrates despite adequate delivery.
- There is inadequate removal and therefore a build-up of the by-products of cellular metabolism which are harmful to the cells.

Table 5.14   Classification of shock

Primary mechanism involved	Example
Decreased oxygen content (decreased oxygen binding to haemoglobin)	Dissociative, e.g. carbon monoxide poisoning Acute respiratory failure with hypoxaemia
Decreased flow (inadequate circulating volume or pump failure)	Hypovolaemic shock Cardiogenic shock
Distributive (decreased oxygen extraction)	Anaphylactic shock Sepsis Neurogenic shock

Compensatory mechanisms

Compensatory mechanisms arise from stimulation of the sympathetic nervous system (SNS) and are either hormonal (Figure 5.25) or neural responses. The combination of these two pathways leads to the physiological responses seen in the initial or triggering event. The release of adrenaline and noradrenaline enables a number of the major organ systems to increase their performance:

- The heart rate increases.
- The force of cardiac contraction increases.
- Coronary arteries dilate to maximise oxygen delivery which is essential for sustained myocardial performance.
- Blood vessels in the skeletal muscles dilate.
- The blood flow to the mesenteric circulation and the skin is diverted to the central organs to maintain adequate perfusion.
- Smooth muscle in the airways relaxes to accommodate larger tidal volumes.

Uncompensated shock

In the presence of inadequate cellular oxygen delivery (DO_2) metabolism switches from aerobic to anaerobic which is an inefficient method of producing the adenosine triphosphate (ATP) necessary to maintain adequate energy

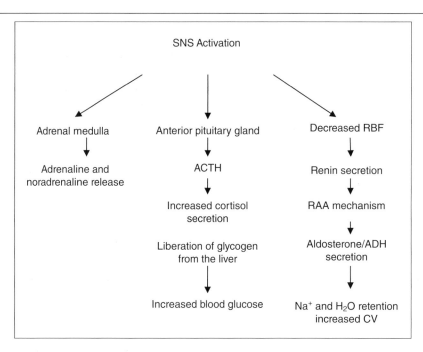

Figure 5.25   Hormonal compensatory responses.

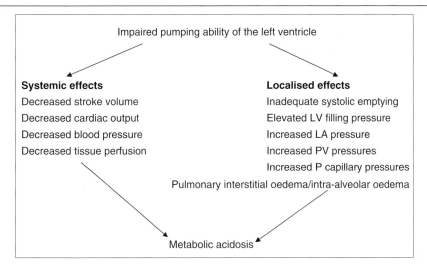

Figure 5.26 Pathophysiology of cardiogenic shock.

for the cell. DO_2 is defined as the amount of oxygen delivered to the tissues of the body per minute. DO_2 depends on cardiac output, which is the amount of blood pumped per minute and the arterial oxygen content of the blood being delivered blood (CaO_2).

DO_2 may be defined as:

$$DO_2 \text{ (ml } O_2/\text{min)} = CaO_2 \text{ (ml } O_2/\text{l blood)} \times \text{cardiac output (l/min)}$$

The CaO_2 depends on how much oxygen-carrying capacity there is available in terms of the haemoglobin (Hb) content of the blood and will depend on how much oxygen the patient's Hb contains, defined as the arterial oxygen saturation (SaO_2). Eventually, anaerobic cellular metabolism is no longer able to generate enough energy to maintain cellular homeostasis which leads to the disruption of the cell membrane ionic pumps, accumulation of intracellular sodium with an efflux of potassium, and accumulation of cytosolic calcium. The cell swells, the cell membrane breaks down and cell death ensues. Widespread cellular death will result in multi-system organ failure with dysfunction of the myocardium which decreases cardiac output to the point of cardiac standstill.

Cardiogenic shock

Cardiogenic shock occurs as a consequence of the failure of the heart to deliver the required substrates and oxygen to the tissues. The majority of presentations in neonates or children are secondary to congenital or acquired heart disease. Other causes include persistent rhythm distur-

bances or, very rarely, myocardial infarction/myocardial contusion. The pathophysiology of cardiogenic shock is outlined in Figure 5.26.

Clinical presentation

- Tachycardia.
- Hepatomegaly.
- Cardiac gallop rhythm.
- Cardiac murmurs.
- Precordial heave.
- Cardiomegaly on chest radiography.
- Cardiac hypertrophy on cardiac ECHO.
- Jugular venous distension.
- ECG abnormalities.
- Decreased skin perfusion.
- Diminished peripheral pulses.
- Mottled, pale appearance.
- Pulmonary oedema/increasing O_2 demands.
- Altered level of consciousness.

Management of cardiogenic shock

The management priorities for the child in cardiogenic shock are mainly focused on supporting myocardial performance and identifying the underlying cause (with appropriate treatment interventions).

- Respiratory support may be necessary to maximise oxygen availability and reduce the body's oxygen demands.
- Cardiovascular support will be required in the form of vasoactive medications to support myocardial function

and reduce ventricular afterload. Other medications such as anti-arrhythmics may be required, depending on the underlying cause. Correction of electrolyte imbalances, in particular potassium, calcium and magnesium, to optimise cardiac performance. The myocardium dislikes being acidotic therefore careful attention to the underlying acid base environment is also important.

- Nutritional support – early enteral feeding to maximise calorific intake wherever possible, however if the infant or child is unable to tolerate enteral feeds, parenteral nutrition may be required.
- Renal support – the use of diuretics is indicated to reduce any pulmonary oedema and prevent additional strain on the myocardium from fluid overload. Rarely, more intensive renal support such as peritoneal dialysis or continuous renal replacement therapy (CRRT) is needed if there is significant renal dysfunction.
- Pain management –stress or anxiety may exacerbate cardiac symptoms by inducing a tachycardia. Careful consideration of which sedative/analgesic agents are used is important to prevent any cardiovascular side-effects.

Sepsis and multi-organ dysfunction

The spectrum of sepsis ranges from microbial invasion of the bloodstream or intoxication with early signs of circulatory compromise, including tachycardia, tachypnoea, peripheral vasodilation and fever (or hypothermia), to full-blown circulatory collapse with multi-organ system failure and death (Santhanam and Tolan 2011). The consensus statement definitions of the terms used to describe the sepsis spectrum are detailed in Table 5.15; however, practitioners need to be aware of the associated normal values determined for heart rate and respiratory rate within the definitions which can be found within the full guideline.

Common causes of sepsis in children

Neonatal sepsis and sepsis in the older child differ in terms of cause. Common causes of sepsis in neonates are:

- Group B β-haemolytic streptococcus.
- *Escherichia coli* (*E. coli* K1 strain).
- Coagulase negative staphylococcus (Levene et al. 2008).

Common causes of sepsis in children are:

- *Neisseria meningitidis* (meningococcal disease).
- *Streptococcus pneumoniae* (pneumococcus).
- *Staphylococcus aureus*.
- Varicella.

Table 5.15 Definitions of the sepsis spectrum

Category	Criteria for application
Systemic inflammatory response (SIRS)	The presence of at least two of the following four criteria, one of which must be abnormal temperature or leucocyte count: • Leucocyte count elevated or depressed for age. • Tachycardia – above expected value for age in the absence of external stimuli or persistent over a period of ½–4 hours (or for children under the age of 1 year bradycardia with a heart rate 10% less than the expected mean value for age. • Temperature of >38.5°C or <36°C. • Mean respiratory rate above normal for age or mechanical ventilation for an acute process not related to underlying neuromuscular disease or the receipt of general anaesthesia.
Infection	A suspected or proven (by positive culture, tissue stain or polymerase chain reaction test) infection caused by any pathogen, or a clinical syndrome associated with a high probability of infection. Evidence of infection includes positive findings on clinical examination, imaging or laboratory tests (e.g. white blood cells in a normally sterile body fluid, perforated viscus, chest X-ray consistent with pneumonia, petechial or purpuric rash, or purpura fulminans).
Sepsis	SIRS in the presence of, or as a result of, suspected or proven infection.
Severe sepsis	Sepsis plus one of the following: cardiovascular organ dysfunction, acute respiratory distress syndrome; or two or more other organ dysfunctions.
Septic shock	Sepsis and cardiovascular organ dysfunction.

(adapted from Goldstein et al. 2005).

Table 5.16   Examples of the mediators of sepsis and MODS

Mediator	Source	Actions
Histamine	Mast cells, basophils, platelets	Vasodilatation Increased vascular permeability
Cytokines (interleukin, e.g. IL1, tumour necrosis factor)	Macrophages, lymphocytes	Vasodilatation Fever Attract leucocytes
Nitric oxide	Endothelial cells, macrophages, platelets	Vasodilatation
Leukotrienes	All white blood cells (leucocytes)	Vasoconstriction Bronchospasm Increased vascular permeability
Prostaglandins	All white blood cells (leucocytes), platelets, endothelial cells	Most cause vasodilatation but Thromboxane A2 (TXA2) causes vasoconstriction
Complement system	Cascade of inactive plasma proteins	White cell (leucocyte) activation Phagocytosis Certain components cause increased vascular permeability and vasodilatation
Platelet-activating factor	All white blood cells (leucocytes), platelets, endothelial cells	Platelet aggregation and degranulation Vasodilatation Increased vascular permeability Leucocyte adherence

Source: Thibodeau and Patton 2007; Tortora and Derrickson 2009; Trzeciak and Rivers 2005.

The pathophysiology of sepsis and multi-organ dysfunction is very complex and still not completely understood. As a consequence detailed discussion is outside the scope of this text. The key contributor to the development of MODS is thought to be mediator release and the host response to the presence of these mediators. It is the amplification of these responses and the inability of the body to stop their production which contributes to the MODS process and to the severity of the illness (Proulx et al. 2009). Mediators are released as a normal protective host response to endothelial damage, ischaemia and reperfusion injury. Examples of some of the mediators are detailed in Table 5.16.

The main pathophysiological changes are:

- Deranged cellular and metabolic function secondary to inadequate oxygen and essential substrate delivery to the tissues.
- Myocardial dysfunction and depressed cardiac contractility.
- Endothelial injury.
- Increased vascular permeability/capillary leak.
- DIC.

Arachidonic acid (AA) is a normal constituent of all cell membranes (except red blood cells). Cytokines, catecholamines, neuroendocrine responses, tissue hypoxia and/or endotoxins all liberate AA from the cell membrane and AA can be metabolised via two pathways, each of which contributes to the production of mediators such as Thromboxane A2, prostaglandins E2 and D2 and leukotrienes. The effects of AA metabolism are increased capillary permeability, platelet dysfunction and altered blood flow with organ ischaemia.

Myocardial dysfunction

Depression of myocardial performance is a relatively early finding in severe sepsis/septic shock and may be attributed to:

- The presence of a severe metabolic acidosis/hypoxia and/or metabolic derangement which affects myocardial contractile performance.
- Circulating endotoxins which may directly suppress myocardial function. (Endotoxins are released when gram-negative bacteria are released and are known to be a stimulus for mediators in MODS.)

- Activation of coagulation and inhibition of anti-coagulation factors.
- The release and circulation of myocardial depressant factors in sepsis having a direct effect on myocardial contractility.

Endothelial injury and increased vascular permeability/capillary leak

Damage to capillary endothelium leads to the inability to maintain its normal functions of anticoagulation and vasoregulation. The presence of different mediators causes changes in the tight junctions of the capillary wall which are small spaces between the individual cells which can increase in size in response to activation of the inflammatory/immune responses to allow the migration of platelets, macrophages and other essential components of repair to reach a site of tissue injury/damage. Widening of these gaps allows other components, such as plasma proteins, to be lost from the intravascular space and as a consequence of loss of oncotic pressure; water is also lost to the interstitial and extracellular spaces.

The dominance of pro-coagulant activity leads to thrombin formation and fibrin deposits which causes obstruction to blood flow and ischaemia within the microvasculature.

Disseminated intravascular coagulation

Coagulopathy is an associated marker of critical illness in the intensive care setting, however the severity of the disorder varies widely and is difficult to predict (Morley 2011). Disseminated intravascular coagulation (DIC) is characterised by a systemic activation of the blood coagulation system, which results in the generation and deposition of fibrin, leading to microvascular thrombi in various organs and contributing to the development of multi-organ failure. Consumption and subsequent exhaustion of coagulation proteins and platelets, due to the activation of the coagulation system, may induce severe bleeding complications, although micro-clot formation may occur in the absence of severe clotting factor depletion and bleeding. DIC, therefore, results in bleeding and intravascular thrombus formation, which can lead to tissue hypoxia, multi-organ dysfunction and death (Levi and Ten Cate 1999) (Table 5.17).

Several simultaneously occurring mechanisms play a role in the pathogenesis of DIC. The main pathways that lead to fibrin deposition are tissue factor-mediated thrombin generation and dysfunctional ant-coagulant mechanisms, such as the anti-thrombin system and the protein C system, which lack the ability to balance the level of thrombin

generation. A third pathway, in addition to enhanced fibrin formation, is impaired fibrin removal due to depression of the fibrinolytic system (Levi 2008; Morley 2011).

Meningococcal disease

Neisseria meningitidis is a major infectious cause of childhood death in developed countries. The mortality rate remains around between 5 and 10% (Pollard et al. 2007). It appears that some of the effects identified in the previous section are significantly worse in children with meningococcal disease than in those with sepsis with a different causative pathogen.

- Myocardial performance in meningococcal disease is worse than in other forms of gram-negative sepsis. Lower cardiac output, despite maintaining higher filling pressures, has been demonstrated in clinical studies and prolonged decreased ventricular function has been determined by sequential ECHOs. In addition, persistent tachycardias are more evident in meningococcaemia (Baines and Hart 2003). Interleukin 6 (IL6) has been identified as possibly a significant factor causing myocardial depression in meningococcemia (Pathan et al. 2005). Empirically, it is noted that similar levels of inotropic support produced less notable effects in meningococcaemia than in those with other forms of gramnegative sepsis. Low calcium concentrations are found in meningococcal disease with either ionised or total hypocalcaemia. It is thought to be related to intracellular redistribution of calcium rather than calcium chelation. In adult studies, correction of hypocalcaemia increased arterial pressure without increasing cardiac output, while in animal studies the administration of calcium increased mortality. The clinical significance of this is that calcium supplementation is advocated for refractory hypotension but not otherwise.
- Disturbances of clotting factors and modulators as well as fibrinolytic components and their modulators are clearly demonstrated in meningococcaemia. Formal coagulation tests usually indicate markedly prolonged INR (>3), but there is a tendency towards thrombosis. In addition, activation of protein C (inhibits activated clotting factors) is impaired (Baines and Hart 2003).
- Inducible nitric oxide synthase produced in response to inflammation produces 1000-fold as much as the usual endothelial-derived relaxant factor (EDRF) form. High nitric oxide metabolite levels have been noted in both meningococcal disease and other forms of sepsis and relate to disease severity in meningococcaemia. The clinical significance relates to the over-production of

Table 5.17 Systemic effects of sepsis and multi-organ dysfunction

Body system	Changes in sepsis and multi-organ dysfunction
Pulmonary	The lungs present a large surface area of endothelium and cellular damage will rapidly lead to vasoconstriction, increased capillary permeability and the development of pulmonary oedema. Damaged pulmonary endothelium activates the cascade of cellular protein and biochemical mediators which serve to heighten both the immune response and the inflammatory response.
Hepatic	The liver has many essential functions in the maintenance of normal metabolism and homeostasis. Impaired hepatic function may lead to: • Altered carbohydrate metabolism. • Altered glycogen storage. • Altered blood glucose homeostasis. • Impaired deamination of amino acids for energy production. • Impaired conversion of ammonia to urea. • Decreased plasma protein synthesis. • Increased rate of oxidation of fatty acids for ATP production may lead to formation of metabolic acidosis. • Decreased capacity to detoxify/secrete/excrete drugs and/or hormones.
Cardiac	A persistent poor cardiac output state emerges as a consequence of: • Persistent vasoconstriction. • Release of myocardial depressant factor. • Systemic acidosis.
Gastrointestinal	The GI tract has a high metabolic rate and is exceptionally sensitive to hypoxia and or ischaemia; equally, there is a tendency to bleeding into the GI tract. With GI tract dysfunction the feedback mechanisms for carbohydrate metabolism are lost and a process of auto-cannibalism occurs. The release of lysosomal enzymes causes extensive local tissue damage which contributes to the continued activation of the host responses. Insulin production and glycogen storage are impaired.
CNS	In the presence of decreased cerebral blood flow, the cerebral metabolic demands are not met and there is increased tissue ischaemia. Toxic mediators, such as false neurotransmitters, are released and affect cell-to-cell communication.
Renal	Occurs frequently in paediatric patients and is thought to be related to acute tubular dysfunction caused by hypoperfusion, the presence of immune mediators, vaso-active therapies and antibiotics. Impaired renal function will lead to: • Alteration in acid base balance. • Alteration in clearance of urea. • Alteration in electrolyte balance. • Decreased chemical detoxification. • Reduced haematopoiesis (stimulation of the production of red cells).
Haematological	There is increased component consumption through sustained immune function stimulation, however there is a decrease in the availability of cellular components due to decreased bone marrow function.

Source: Barry et al. 2010; Brierley et al. 2009; Carcillo 2003; Naran et al. 2010; Proulx et al. 2009.

nitric oxide, lowering arterial pressure as a consequence of vasodilation, which impairs cardiac contractility.

Management of sepsis

In 2002, a campaign entitled Surviving Sepsis® was launched in a bid to reduce the mortality and morbidity rates associated with sepsis. Guidelines were published in 2004 and again with updates in 2008. As the guidelines are reviewed and updated on a regular basis when new evidence emerges, the algorithm is not provided here and practitioners should refer to the Surviving Sepsis® website for the current version of the guidelines at the time of reading (www.survivingsepsis.org/guidelines).

The most recent guidelines highlight that when compared to adults with sepsis, children are more like to require:

- Proportionally larger quantities of fluid.
- Inotrope and vasodilator therapies.
- Hydrocortisone for absolute adrenal insufficiency.
- ECMO for refractory shock.

The recommendation in the 2008 guidelines is for the early use of inotrope support through peripheral access until central access is attained (Brierley et al. 2009).This has resulted in a significant change in practice.

Key interventions for cardiovascular support in the first hour after presentation

- Aggressive fluid resuscitation (up to 60 ml/ kg or more if needed) within the first 15 minutes of presentation with either 0.9% sodium chloride, Hartmann's solution, Ringer's lactate or colloid such as 4.5/5% human albumin solution (HAS).
- For fluid refractory shock (no/minimal response to fluid given in first 15 minutes) inotropes should be instituted – recommendations are for adrenaline or dopamine with noradrenaline suggested if the child is vasodilated on presentation.
- Early placement of central access.

Other significant immediate interventions include:

- Respiratory support to maximise oxygen availability and reduce oxygen demand.
- Correction of coagulopathies – use of platelets, FFP/cryoprecipitate to address the disturbances in the child's coagulation status.
- Treatment of the underlying cause, e.g. a broad-spectrum third-generation Cephalosporin until the source of infection or pathogen is identified.

- Correction of electrolyte imbalances, in particular potassium, calcium and magnesium, to optimise cardiac performance and maintain cellular metabolic processes.
- Correction of hypoglycaemia (if present) to avoid potential neurological effects and maintain carbohydrate source of energy for the cells.
- The ongoing management of the child with sepsis and or multi-organ dysfunction is determined by the severity of dysfunction in each of the body systems. Mechanisms for supporting their function are detailed in the relevant chapters.

Current research studies

There are two studies (of many) currently underway in paediatric intensive care which may add important evidence in the management of the child with sepsis/multi-organ dysfunction.

Use of steroids

Steroid use has been shown to improve outcome in children with meningitis and their use is advocated in this group. Studies have shown that critically ill adults requiring catecholamine infusions had a reduction in the duration of infusion time when given steroids, but improvements in mortality are still not clearly demonstrated and there remains significant debate in the published literature within the adult field (Vincent 2008). There is evidence of adrenal insufficiency in children with meningococcaemia; however, there is no direct evidence regarding the use of steroid replacement therapy in children with meningococcal sepsis (Branco and Russell 2005). A multi-centre trial is currently underway in PIC in the United Kingdom which aims to establish an evidence base for current empirical practice, based on individual centres or medical practitioners' opinion and experience.

Hyperglycaemic control

There is evidence that uncontrolled hyperglycaemia is detrimental to the outcome of children with meningococcal sepsis (Day et al. 2008) and this finding is mirrored in studies undertaken in the adult intensive care population. In the United Kingdom, a multi-centre trial randomised controlled trial of tight hyperglycaemia control with the use of insulin (the CHiP Study) completed its recruitment phase in August 2011 and publication of results is awaited.

Conclusion

This chapter has provided an overview of the developmental anatomy and physiology, considered assessment of cardiac function and reviewed some of the major abnormalities of cardiac structure, disease, rate and rate and rhythm.

Appendix 5.1 A summary of vasoactive drugs, the adrenergic receptor stimulated the physiological response and side-effects

Vasoactive drug	Physiological effect	Side-effects
Adrenaline/epinephrine *Catecholamine*	α_1 – vasoconstriction β_1 – increased heart rate, contractility and AV conduction velocity	Tachycardia Increased afterload due to vasoconstriction Increased O_2 consumption due to increased afterload Splanchnic constriction
Amlodipine *Calcium channel blocker*	Primarily acts on the smooth muscle in arterial walls Dilates coronary and systemic arteries and so reduces blood pressure	Headache Oedema
Atropine *Anticholinergic*	Blocks vagal stimulation of the SA node Increases AV conduction	Tachydysrhythmias Blurred vision Dry mouth
10% calcium gluconate *Electrolyte*	Increased contractility Enhanced ventricular automaticity	Dysrhythmias, especially if given with digoxin Vasodilation and hypotension if administered too rapidly Diaphoresis Nausea and vomiting Severe irritation and necrosis with extravasation, avoid peripheral administration
Captopril *Angiotensin converting enzyme (ACE) inhibitor*	Prevents vasoconstriction Decreased water and sodium retention	Dizziness Tachycardia Hypotension
Dobutamine *Synthetic catecholamine*	Predominantly β_1 – increased heart rate, contractility and AV conduction velocity Some β_2 – vasodilation and bronchodilation	Hypertension Tachycardia
Dopamine *Catecholamine*	Low dose (1–5 mcg/kg/min): Dopaminergic – coronary, renal and intestinal vasodilation Moderate dose (5–10 mcg/kg/min) β_1 – increased heart rate, contractility and AV conduction velocity High dose (>10 mcg/kg/min) α_1 – vasoconstriction	Ventricular dysrhythmia Tachycardia Vasoconstriction
Esmolol *Beta-blocker*	Blocks β_1 receptor activity – decreased heart rate, contractility and AV conduction velocity	Bradycardia/asystole Hypotension
Glyceryl trinitrate (GTN) *Nitrate*	Low dose: Venodilation High dose: Venous and arterial vasodilation	Tachycardia or bradycardia Hypotension Headache

(Continued)

Vasoactive drug	Physiological effect	Side-effects
Isoprenaline *Synthetic catecholamine*	β_1 – Increased automaticity of SA node and enhanced AV conduction velocity β_2 – Vasodilation and bronchodilation	Tachycardia Palpitations Pulmonary oedema Headache
Labetolol *Beta-blocker*	Anti-hypertensive α_1 blockade – results in vasodilation β_1 blockade – decreased heart rate and contractility and prolonged AV conduction time result in decreased cardiac output and decreased blood pressure	Hypotension Nausea Dizziness Hepatic dysfunction Bronchospasm caused by β_2 blockade
Milrinone *Phosphodiesterase inhibitor*	Increases intracellular cyclic AMP which results in increased cardiac contractility and vasodilatation	Ventricular dysrhythmias and SVT Hypotension Long half-life so effects continue after the infusion has stopped
Nifedipine *Calcium channel blocker*	Primarily acts on the smooth muscle in arterial walls Dilates coronary and systemic arteries and so reduces blood pressure	Headache Oedema
Noradrenaline/norepinephrine *Catecholamine*	α_1 – vasoconstriction Some β_1 – increased heart rate and contractility	Bradycardia Increased myocardial workload and O_2 consumption due to increased afterload Hepatic and mesenteric ischaemia due to vasoconstriction
Sildenafil *Phosphodiesterase inhibitor*	Enhances the effect of inhaled nitric oxide therapy Reduces pulmonary vasoconstriction and right ventricular afterload	Headache Dizziness Visual disturbances Flushing
Sodium nitroprusside (SNP) *Nitrate*	Anti-hypertensive Breaks down to release nitric oxide which causes arterial and venous vasodilation through relaxation of vascular smooth muscle	Hypotension Abdominal pain Decreased platelet aggregation Cyanide toxicity and methaemoglobinaemia – more likely at infusion rates of >10 mcg/kg/min. Treatment is with IV methylene blue

References

Abdulla R, Blew GA, Holterman MJ. 2004. Cardiovascular embryology. Pediatric Cardiology, 25:191–200.

Allen M, Sundararajan S et al. 2009. Anti-inflammatory modalities: their current use in pediatric cardiac surgery in the United Kingdom and Ireland. Pediatric Critical Care Medicine, 10(3):341–5.

Anderson RH, Becker AE et al. 1984. Sequential segmental analysis of congenital heart disease. Pediatric Cardiology, 5(4):281–7.

Anderson RH, Girish S. 2009. Sequential segmental analysis. Annals of Pediatric Cardiology, 2:24–35.

Baines PB, Hart CA. 2003. Severe meningococcal disease in childhood. British Journal of Anaesthesia, 90(1):72–83.

Barry P, Morris K, Ali T (Eds). 2010. Paediatric Intensive Care. Oxford: Oxford University Press.

Baumer JH, Love SJ et al. 2006. Salicylate for the treatment of Kawasaki disease in children. Cochrane Database of Systematic Reviews, 4:CD004175.

Billett J, Cowie MR et al. 2008. Comorbidity, healthcare utilisation and process of care measures in patients with congenital heart disease in the UK: cross-sectional, population-based study with case–control analysis. Heart, 94:1194–9.

Blackburn ST. 2007. Maternal, Fetal and Neonatal Physiology: a clinical perspective. St Louis, MO: Saunders.

Branco RG, Russell RR. 2005. Should steroids be used in children with meningococcal shock? Archive of Diseases of Childhood, 90:1195–6.

Brierley J, Carcillo JA et al. 2009. Clinical practice parameters for hemodynamic support of pediatric and neonatal septic shock: 2007 update from the American College of Critical Care Medicine. Critical Care Medicine, 37(2):666–88.

Burns JC, Shimizu C et al. 2005. Genetic variations in the receptor-ligand pair CCR5 and CCL3L1 are important determinants of susceptibility to Kawasaki disease. Journal of Infectious Diseases, 192(2):344–9.

Carcillo JA. 2003. Pediatric septic shock and multiple organ failure. Critical Care Clinics, 19:413–40.

Carvalho JS, Ho Y, Shinebourne EA. 2005. Sequential segmental analysis in complex congenital cardiac abnormalities: a logical approach to diagnosis. Ultrasound Obstetrics and Gynecology, 26:105–11.

Central Cardiac Audit Database. 2010. www.ccad.org.uk

Colan SD, Lipshultz SE et al. 2007. Epidemiology and cause-specific outcome of hypertrophic cardiomyopathy in children. Circulation, 115:773–81.

Craatz S, Kunzel E, Spanel-Borowski K. 2002. Classification of a collection of malformed human hearts: practical experiences in the use of sequential segmental analysis. Pediatric Cardiology, 23:483–90.

Day KM, Haub N et al. 2008. Hyperglycemia is associated with morbidity in critically ill children with meningococcal sepsis. Pediatric Critical Care Medicine, 9(6):636–40.

Doolan A, Langlois N, Semsarian C. 2004. Causes of sudden cardiac death in young Australians. Medical Journal of Australia, 180:110–12.

Ewer AK, Middleton LJ et al. on behalf of the PulseOx Study Group. 2011. Pulse oximetry screening for congenital heart defects in newborn infants (PulseOx): a test accuracy study. The Lancet, 378(9793):785–94.

Extracorporeal Life Support Organization. 2009. ELSO General Guidelines. www.elso.med.umich.edu/Guidelines.html.

Gargiulo G, Napoleone CP et al. 2008. Neonatal coarctation repair using extended end-to-end anastomosis. Multimedia Manual of Cardiothoracic Surgery, 0328:2691.

Goldberg CS, Bove EL et al. 2007. A randomized clinical trial of regional cerebral perfusion versus deep hypothermic circulatory arrest: outcomes for infants with functional single ventricle. Journal of Thoracic and Cardiovascular Surgery, 133(4):880–7.

Goldenberg I, Moss AJ. 2008. Long QT syndrome. Journal of the American College of Cardiology, 51(24):2291–300.

Goldstein B, Giroir B, Randolph A. 2005. International pediatric consensus conference: definitions of sepsis and organ dysfunction in paediatrics. Pediatric Critical Care Medicine, 6(1):2–8.

Kimura A. 2008. Molecular etiology and pathogenesis of hereditary cardiomyopathy. Circulation, 72(Suppl. A):A38–48.

Kirby ML. 2007. Cardiac Development. Oxford: Oxford University Press.

Knowles R, Griebsch I et al. 2005. Newborn screening for congenital heart defects: a systematic review and cost-effectiveness analysis. Health Technology Assessments, 9(44). www.hta.ac.uk.

Levene MI, Tudehope DI, Sinha S. 2008. Essential Neonatal Medicine (Fourth Edition). Oxford: Blackwell Publishing.

Levi M. 2008. The coagulant response in sepsis. Clinics in Chest Medicine, 29(4):627–42.

Levi M, Ten Cate H. 1999. Disseminated intravascular coagulation. New England Journal of Medicine, 341(8):586–92.

Markowitz SD, Icbord RN et al. 2007. Surrogate markers for neurological outcome in children after deep hypothermic circulatory arrest. Seminars in Cardiothoracic and Vascular Anesthesia, 11(1):59–65.

Maron BJ. 2002. Hypertrophic cardiomyopathy. Circulation, 106:2419–21.

McCorry LK. 2007. Physiology of the autonomic nervous system. American Journal of Pharmaceutical Education, 71(4):78–88.

Morley SL. 2011. Management of acquired coagulopathy in acute paediatrics. Archives of Diseases in Childhood. Education practice edition, 96:49–60.

Moss AJ, Allen HD. 2008. Heart Disease in Infants, Children, and Adolescents (Volume 1, 7th edition). Philadelphia: Lippincott.

Naran N, Sagy M, Bock KR. 2010. Continuous renal replacement therapy results in respiratory and hemodynamic beneficial effects in pediatric patients with severe systemic inflammatory response syndrome and multiorgan system dysfunction. Pediatric Critical Care Medicine, 11(6):737–40.

Nydegger A, Bines JE. 2006. Energy metabolism in infants with congenital heart disease. Nutrition, 22(7–8):697–704.

Park MK. 2010. The Pediatric Cardiology Handbook (4th edition). Philadelphia: Mosby Elsevier.

Pathan N, Williams EJ et al. 2005. Changes in the interleukin-6/soluble interleukin-6 receptor axis in meningococcal septic shock. Critical Care Medicine, 33(8):1839–44.

Perel P, Roberts I, Pearson M. 2007. Colloids versus crystalloids for fluid resuscitation in critically ill patients. Cochrane Database of Systematic Reviews, 4.

Pinna GS, Kafetzis DA et al. 2008. Kawasaki disease: an overview. Current Opinion in Infectious Diseases, 21(3):263–70.

Pinto N, Jones TK et al. 2003. Temporary transvenous pacing with an active fixation bipolar lead in children: a preliminary report. Pacing Clinical Electrophysiology, 26(7 Pt 1):1519–22.

Pollard AJ, Nadel S et al. 2007. Emergency management of meningococcal disease: eight years on. Archive of Diseases of Childhood, 92(4):283–6.

Proulx F, Joyal JS et al. 2009. The pediatric multiple organ dysfunction syndrome. Pediatric Critical Care Medicine, 10(11):12–22.

Raeside L. 2009. Coarctation of the aorta: a case presentation. Neonatal Network, 28(2):103–13

Santhaman S, Tolan RW. 2011. Pediatric Sepsis. emedicine. medscape.com/article/972559-overview.

Schwarz AJ. 2011. Shock in Pediatrics. emedicine.medscape. com/article/1833578-overview.

Shinebourne EA, Macartney FJ, Anderson RH. 1976. Sequential chamber localisation – logical approach to diagnosis in congenital heart disease. British Heart Journal, 38:327–40.

Steltzer M, Rudd N, Pick B. 2005. Nutrition care for newborns with congenital heart disease. Clinics in Perinatology, 32(4):1017–30.

Syamasundar Rao. 2011. www.emedicine.medscape.com/article/890196-followup.

Talwar S, Agarwala S et al. 2010. Diaphragmatic palsy after cardiac surgical procedures in patients with congenital heart. Annals of Pediatric Cardiology, 3(1):50–7.

Taylor MB, Laussen PC. 2010. Fundamentals of management of acute postoperative pulmonary hypertension. Pediatric Critical Care Medicine, 11(2):S27–S29.

Thibodeau GA, Patton KT. 2007. Anatomy and Physiology (6th edition). Missouri: Mosby Elsevier.

Tortora GJ, Derrickson BH. 2009. Principles of Anatomy and Physiology (12th edition). Vol. 2: Maintenance and Continuity of the Human Body. Asia: John Wiley and Sons.

Towbin JA, Lowe AM et al. 2006. Incidence, causes, and outcomes of dilated cardiomyopathy in children. JAMA, 296:1867–76.

Trzeciak S, Rivers EP. 2005. Clinical manifestations of disordered microcirculatory perfusion in severe sepsis. Critical Care, 9 (suppl. 4):S20–S26.

Venugopalan P. 2010. Dilated Cardiomyopathy. www. emedicine.medscape.com/article/895187-overview.

Vincent J-L. 2008. Steroids in sepsis: another swing of the pendulum in our clinical trials. Critical Care, 12(2):141.

Watkins H, Ashrafian H, McKenna WJ. 2008. The genetics of hypertrophic cardiomyopathy: teare redux. Heart, 94:1264–86.

Wood LE, Tulloh RMR. 2009. Kawasaki disease in children. Heart, 95:787–92.

Wypij D, Newburger JW et al. 2003. The effect of duration of deep hypothermic circulatory arrest in infant heart surgery on late neurodevelopment: the Boston Circulatory Arrest Trial. Journal of Thoracic and Cardiovascular Surgery, 126(5):1397–1403.

Further reading

Antman E. 2007. Cardiovascular Therapeutics: a companion to Braunwald's heart disease? Philadelphia: WB Saunders.

Biewer ES, Zürn C et al. 2010. Chylothorax after surgery on congenital heart disease in newborns and infants – risk factors and efficacy of MCT diet. Journal of Cardiothoracic Surgery, 5(127).

Bizzarro, M, Goss I. 2005. Inhaled nitric oxide for the postoperative management of pulmonary hypertension in infants and children with congenital heart disease. Cochrane Database of Systematic Reviews, 19:CD0050055.

Dadvanda P, Rankin R et al. 2009. Descriptive epidemiology of congenital heart disease in Northern England. Paediatric and Perinatal Epidemiology, 23:58–65.

Guven MA, Carvalho J et al. 2003. Sequential segmental analysis of the heart: a malformation screening technique. Artemis, 4(3):21–3.

Mahlea WT, Lundined K et al. 2004. The short-term effects of cardiopulmonary bypass on neurologic function in children and young adults. European Journal of Cardiothoracic Surgery, 26:920–5.

Ungerleider RM. 1998. Effects of cardiopulmonary bypass and use of modified ultrafiltration. Annals of Thoracic Surgery, 65(6 Suppl):S35–38

Yates AR, Dyke PC et al. 2006. Hyperglycemia is a marker for poor outcome in the postoperative pediatric cardiac patient. Pediatric Critical Care Medicine, 7(4):351–5.

Chapter 6
CARE OF THE INFANT OR CHILD IN RENAL FAILURE

Ben Harvey[1] and Doreen Crawford[2]

[1] Paediatric Intensive Care Unit, Sheffield Children's Hospital, Sheffield, UK
[2] School of Nursing and Midwifery, Faculty of Health and Life Sciences, De Montfort University, Leicester, UK

Introduction

This chapter considers the basic embryology and anatomy and physiology of the kidney then reviews the pathophysiology, diagnosis and treatment of renal failure in children. The chapter focuses on the management of acute and chronic renal failure where it relates to children's intensive care.

Terminology

The term acute renal failure is now being replaced by the less restrictive term acute kidney injury (AKI) (Phillips-Anderoli 2009) in line with the changing and increasing population of children who now present with AKI in association with multi-organ failure (MOF) or other system failure instead of isolated primary renal failure. There are many definitions of AKI in children, all with their own difficulties, however the following is useful: 'sudden loss of the kidney's ability to maintain fluid and electrolyte homeostasis and an inability to excrete the solute load' (Davies et al. 1994).

Embryological development of the kidney is complex and staged. At birth the kidney function is still immature (Table 6.1).

Anatomy and physiology of the kidney

The normal mature kidneys are paired structures located at the rear of the abdominal cavity in the retroperitoneal cavity. Each kidney receives blood from the renal arteries and drains into the renal veins. The kidneys have several functions and regulatory roles. They are essential in maintaining homeostatic balance with the regulation of electrolytes, maintenance of acid base balance and management of blood pressure by maintaining the salt and water balance.

The functional unit of the kidney is the nephron and this contains the glomeruli which are modified capillaries and serve as a filter of blood, removing waste, which is excreted in urine (Figure 6.1). The rate of filtration can be measured (Table 6.2).

The kidneys also have a regulatory function and conserve water, glucose and amino acids by selective reabsorption according to need. The kidneys also produce a range of hormones and enzymes (e.g. calcitriol, erythropoietin and renin).

At the point of birth the kidney is relatively immature and conserves water poorly. This is an important consideration when administering drugs to neonates and young children (European Medicines Agency 2004). The immature

Paediatric Intensive Care Nursing, First Edition. Edited by Michaela Dixon and Doreen Crawford.
© 2012 John Wiley & Sons, Ltd. Published 2012 by John Wiley & Sons, Ltd.

Table 6.1   Summary of the embryological development of the kidney

Focus	Timing	Function
Stage 1 Pronephroi	Appear ~21 days	Located in cervical region. Non-functioning, main structures degenerate by day 25 but ducts remain to be utilised by mesonephroi.
Stage 2 Mesonephroi	Appear ~28 days	Elongated structures that utilise duct remnants; they contain primitive tubules and glomeruli. Blood is delivered to these structures and urine is produced. Act as functioning interim kidneys. Degeneration occurs at 10 weeks gestation but some tubules and ducts remain. In the male: Tubules → efferent ductules of the testes. Ducts → epididymis, ductus deferens and ejaculatory duct. In the female: Ducts mostly disappear. Tubules retained near uterus and broad ligament.
Stage 3 Metanephroi	Starts development early in week 5	These originate from two embryonic sources which develop in partnership to form the functioning definitive kidneys: 1. Metanephroric diverticulum → ureter, renal pelvis, calices, collecting tubules. 2. Metanephric blastema → creates the nephrons, the basic functional unit of the kidney (the glomerular apparatus – a capsule which surrounds the glomeruli – a knot of blood capillaries, tubules and collecting duct). As the nephrons continue to grow during foetal life the tubules continue to elongate, forming the proximal tubule, the loop of Henle (LOH) and the distal tubule. In week 10 the ends of distal tubules connect and join to form the collecting tubule or duct. The metanephroi produces urine from weeks 11–13 onwards.
Ongoing internal development	By week 15 Weeks 10–32	Medulla and cortex visible as two distinct regions, both areas fully formed by 36 weeks gestation. Glomerular apparatus, proximal and distal tubules are found within the cortex Collecting ducts and LOH grow down into the medulla. Length increases after birth which increases kidney size. Numbers of nephrons increase during foetal life until birth when full complement in place. Postnatal glomeruli also increase in size, so rates of excretion increase progressively.
Location		The location of each set of kidneys alters primarily due to the rapid growth of the tail section of the embryo which gives the impression of the kidneys migrating upwards during foetal life. Alongside this ascent, the kidneys undergo a 90° rotation to face the midline.

Table 6.1 (*Continued*)

Focus	Timing	Function
Blood supply		External structures alter; ureters increase in length to provide the route to the bladder for urine storage, the origin of the blood supply shifts. The first source is the common ileac artery, but as the embryo grows flow is derived from new branches off the aorta. Ultimately, all previous blood supply routes degenerate as the renal arteries become the key supply route. Once blood is delivered to the kidney the renal arteries progressively subdivide delivering blood into the glomerular capsule via the afferent arteriole where simple filtration takes place. Blood flows away from the glomeruli via the efferent arterioles which become the peritubular capillaries surrounding the tubules in the cortex, so allowing selective reabsorption, tubular secretion. Ultimately, the peritubular capillaries drain into the renal vein and blood flows away from the kidney. All these vessels have thin, semi-permeable walls to allow movement of solutes and electrolytes to and from the blood and nephron.

Source: Dixon et al. 2009, adapted from Chalmley et al. 2005; Hockenberry et al. 2003; Lote 2000; Moore and Persaud 2003.

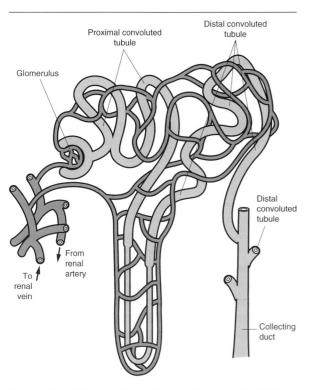

Figure 6.1 The nephron. From Dixon et al. 2009.

Table 6.2 Glomerular filtration rate

Age	Rate
Preterm (28 weeks gestation)	$10\,ml/min/1.73\,m^2$
Term	$20\,ml/min/1.73\,m^2$
Adult	$80–120\,ml/min/1.73\,m^2$

developmental factors are significant in increasing the risk of developing AKI in children under 1 year. A shorter loop of Henle and reduction in functional ability compared to adults have a number of effects:

- Reduction in ability to concentrate urine.
- Inability to excrete sodium.
- Alteration of water reabsorption.
- Altered excretion of hydrogen ions.
- Reduced reabsorption of bicarbonate ions.

These factors make water balance and acid base balance control in metabolic acidosis more difficult. The reduced ability to control blood flow and cardiac output also causes potential damage in the younger child. The kidneys initially receive approximately 15% of cardiac output, but once mature this increases to 25%. Renal blood flow (RBF) is autoregulated and determined by the renal perfusion pressure (RPP) divided by the renal vascular resistance (RVR). This in turn is affected by the afferent and efferent arterioles in the glomeruli being constricted and dilated. Autoregulation allows the blood flow to the kidney to be constant even with large fluctuations of RPP. In infants the mean arterial pressure (MAP) is lower than in maturity, therefore the RBF is lower, making autoregulation effective in a much narrower range of MAP. Immature kidneys cannot cope with even small changes in blood pressure. This is compounded in the neonatal period by the increased levels of renin in this population, thought to be a mechanism to prevent excess sodium loss as the kidneys grow and the subsequent increase in GFR that take place. One of the effects of elevated renin levels is a decrease in cortical blood flow, thus further reducing the kidney's ability to compensate for small reductions in blood pressure.

Renal pathology (Table 6.3)

Insults to the kidney will have a number of effects which, if not reversed, may lead to acute tubular necrosis (ATN). Once ATN has developed, improvement to renal perfusion will not enhance urine output until the ATN has resolved, and this may take from days to weeks. The processes of ATN include vasoconstriction, desquamation of cells from the renal tubule leading to cast formation and impediment to flow in the tubule. This in turn may generate back-

leakage of glomerular filtrate out of the renal tubule. Neutrophils will also adhere to ischaemic endothelial tissue, which in turn causes damage and further inflammation.

AKI can be broken down into three broad categories: pre-renal, intrinsic renal and post renal (obstructive) uropathies.

Prerenal

Prerenal injury is caused by hypoperfusion from reduction in intravascular volume and/or hypoxia. In children this is usually associated with maldistribution of fluid associated with septic shock. However it can also be due to cardiac failure or shock from acute dehydration (Shaheen et al. 2007). If the hypoperfusion is short-lived and the kidneys are physiologically normal, restoration of intravascular volume will lead to speedy reversal of AKI. However, if it persists, a number of mechanisms come into play to avoid further intrinsic renal damage. Initially, dilation of renal arterioles takes place in an attempt to maintain glomerular blood flow. Prostaglandin generation is also associated with hypoperfusion; vasodilatory effects are designed to increase renal perfusion. There is some suggestion that these processes are impeded or reversed with the use of a number of targeted drug therapies used in animal models, but their clinical use has not yet been fully evaluated (Knoderer et al. 2008; Kohda et al. 1998; Landoni et al. 2007; Marthur et al. 1999).

Intrinsic

While there are many diseases that can cause intrinsic renal injury, only the causes likely to lead to treatment in PICU are discussed in this chapter with the notable exception of haemolytic uraemic syndrome (HUS), which can vary in severity, and extreme forms of which can lead to admission to PICU.

The intrarenal category includes all physiological events directly affecting kidney tissue structure and function. This may be the end-point of prerenal failure, particularly with hypoxic or ischaemic injury. Intrarenal injury is characterised by cell damage from ischaemia after hypoperfusion or direct damage of nephronic cells from drugs, toxins or swelling. Whatever the cause, the outcome is cell death and apoptosis. Cell debris then obstructs the tubule, further compounding the damage to the tubule. If the process continues and is severe, acute tubular necrosis (ATN) will develop. This can be entirely reversible depending on the length and type of injury. The child in PICU is particularly at risk because of the need to use nephrotoxic agents in life-threatening conditions in association with multiorgan failure.

Table 6.3 Summary of diseases associated with types of renal failure

Type	Cause
Prerenal	Hypovolaemia from any cause, including sepsis, cardiac failure, renal vein or artery thrombosis, persistent foetal circulation, cardiac bypass and dehydration including D&V.
Intrinsic	Toxins, therapeutic agents, tumour lysis syndrome, hypoxia and birth asphyxia, haemolytic uraemic syndrome (HUS), glomerulonephritis, infections, massive rhabdomyolysis (e.g. following massive crush injury or electric shock).
Postrenal (obstructive)	Urethral, ureteric obstruction, including blocked urinary catheter, kidney stones, tumours.

Postrenal (obstructive)

Anything that reduces or obstructs flow from the urine-collecting duct to the exit of the bladder can cause AKI. Varying damage is caused by back-pressure on the kidneys. Postrenal AKI is rare in PICU, but should not be ruled out, primarily because it can be caused by urethral obstruction from posterior urethral values. Ureteric obstructions can include kidney stones or tumours. Always ensure a urinary catheter is not blocked by flushing it with 1 ml/kg 0.9% sodium chloride.

Although there are three classic classifications of renal failure in PICU, the causes can be attributed to a number of factors rather than one discrete event. The aim of treatment is to prevent further damage and treat complications of AKI. AKI in the PICU population accounts for about 2.5% of admissions (Shaheen et al. 2007).

Signs of acute kidney injury and useful tests in children

A good history may reveal that the child has suffered from bloody diarrhoea, proteinuria or another disease, making the child seriously unwell. Examples of the underlying causes include meningococcal sepsis, diarrhoea and vomiting, thermal injury, malaria, Weil's disease/leptospirosis, tumour lysis, HUS or traumas such as crush injuries, electrocution and birth asphyxia. To date there are no specific biomarkers for AKI, but a number of physiologically indicators. Table 6.4 lists indicators that may be useful. Urea and creatinine are variable markers with a huge normal range, depending on age, disease process and level of physical activity. Severe renal impairment may be present with normal creatinine in children with little muscle bulk. Urea may be low in fluid overload or where liver failure is present.

It is essential to catheterise the patient when an AKI is suspected because of the need to assess urine output and effects of treatment. Urinary biochemistry may be useful in interpreting the type of AKI (Table 6.5). However, this cannot be used once diuretics have been initiated and acute fluid resuscitation has taken place.

Other tests, such as urinalysis for blood protein, casts and MC&S (microscopy, culture and sensitivities) are also required.

Acute treatment (Table 6.6)

Treatment priorities are:

- Restoration of circulating blood volume.
- Treatment of electrolyte disturbances.
- Nutrition.
- Prevention of complications.

Restoration of circulating volume

The judicious use of fluid restriction with accurate fluid balance in renal failure will prove useful. Very careful reassessment of fluid status should be made after 5 or 10 ml/kg boluses of fluid have been given. Ideally, the fluid that most closely resembles that being lost should be used. However in practice, at least initially, the use of 0.9% sodium chloride or 4.5% human albumin solutions are used. After initial restoration of circulating blood volume with fluid boluses it may be necessary to restrict the child to infusing a calculation based on the child's urine output plus insensible losses to avoid fluid overload. This is impractical in the ITU because of the use of inotropes, sedation and the need for nutrition. In these cases the early use of renal replacement therapy (RRT) is essential as there is evidence that fluid overload is a significant factor in mortality in children treated with RRT (Goldstein et al. 2004). It should be remembered that in AKI symptoms can be due to acute intravascular water loss as well as fluid overload and the child's inability to handle solutes and

Table 6.4 Indications of AKI

	Newborn	Children
Urine output	<1 ml/kg/hr >4 ml/kg/hr without diuretics	<0.5 ml/kg/hr >7 ml/kg/hr without diuretics
Urea	>10 mmol/l	>20 mmol/l
Creatinine	>50	>90 micromol/l
Metabolic acidosis	Usually in conjunction with other signs of renal insufficiency	
Hb/platelets	Low Hb and platelet count with raised urea and creatinine, suspect HUS	

Table 6.5 Indications of types of AKI from urinalysis

	Urinary sodium (mmol/l)		Osmolarity (osm/kg)	
	Neonate	Child	Neonate	Child
Prerenal	>20	>10	>400	>500
Renal	>40	>40	<400	<400

Table 6.6 Treatment for electrolyte disturbance

Electrolyte	Level	Effects	Treatment
Raised potassium	>6 mmol/l	Peaked T-waves, widening QRS, asystole Effects extenuated by acidosis	Nebulised salbutamol: 2.5 mg < 25 kg, 5 mg > 25 kg PR calcium resonium: 2.5 ml < 1 year, 5 ml 1–5 years, 10 ml > 5 years IV calcium gluconate 10% 0.5–1 ml/kg slow bolus IV sodium bicarbonate 1–2 mmol/kg IV over up to 30 mins *8.4% bicarbonate should be further diluted before peripheral infusion IV salbutamo l4 ng/kg over 15 mins*
Low potassium	2.5–3 mmol/l	Ventricular disturbance, including ventricular fibrillation	Replace potassium orally or IV (with care)
Low sodium	>118 mmol/l	Intravascular fluid loss	Fluid restriction and replacement with 0.9% saline Treatment with RRT
Extremely low sodium	<118 mmol/l	Cerebral irritation and damage	Bolus of 3% saline to raise sodium to 125 mmol/l over at least 2 hours; calculation = 125 − serum sodium × kg × 0.6 = mmol of sodium to be given Treatment with RRT if oliguria and low sodium do not improve
Raised sodium	>155 mmol/l	Cerebral irritation, fitting, coma. Cause may be from sodium retention or water loss	High dose furosemide slow bolus If sodium retention is the problem, reduction in sodium input by using 0.45% saline to replace insensible loss Control of total body water, correction using RRT‡
Raised phosphate	Above 1.7 mmol/l or 2.0 mmol/l in neonates	Raised PO_4 will cause a drop in serum calcium see below	Restrict phosphate intake in feed/TPN Oral phosphate binders (often impractical in PICU) Treat with RRT. Usually other biochemical disturbances will have necessitated RRT at this point
Low calcium	Ionised calcium below 1 mmol/l	Cardiac arrest, effects potentiated by raised potassium	IV calcium gluconate 0.1 mg/kg over at least 30 mins Also give above dose if sodium bicarbonate is needed because calcium will drop as acidosis corrects
Metabolic acidosis	pH < 7.30, bicarbonate < 20 mmol/l	Cardiac failure and further acidosis, vasoconstriction and raised lactate Calcium will drop as acidosis corrects	IV sodium bicarbonate to raise bicarbonate above 18 mmol/l, 1 mmol/l/kg infusion over 30 min. Or, correction using formulary 18-serum bicarbonate × 0.5 × kg = amount to be infused over at least 1 hour. 8.4% bicarbonate should be further diluted before peripheral infusion

*PR calcium resonium should not be given if there is a risk of NEC or other bowel damage, as it can cause constipation and if it stays in the gut potassium will potentially leak back into the circulation. Salbutamol will very effectively push potassium back into the cells out of the circulation; however, this is only a temporary measure which buys time for the instigation of RRT or return of urine output. Calcium gluconate and bicarbonate work by reducing the effects of acidosis.

‡Correction of sodium should always be at a rate that will not induce speedy changes in serum osmolality and subsequent cerebral fluid shifts associated with that.

maintain acid base balance. Therefore, fluid balance and fluid resuscitation will always need to be considered as first-line treatment. However, strict assessment of fluid balance, where practical, including accurate weighing for fluid trends, should take place. It is also essential to consider insensible loss carefully. The insensible loss can be calculated as $330 \, ml/m^2/day$ or $10 \, ml/kg/day$. All forms of insensible loss should be taken into account, including increases from raised temperature, thermal injury, phototherapy and chylothorax.

Nutrition in AKI is essential to hasten recovery, prevent catabolism and reduce the need to control metabolic abnormalities. Suitable nutrition may avoid the need for RRT. However, in PICU where RRT is instigated for fluid balance or metabolic control, space for nutrition can be generated with ease. This is particularly important when dealing with a critically ill child who has a large calorific need. Nutrition should be managed with a dietician to maximise calories without additional protein. Where specialist renal feeds are not available, combinations of nutritional supplements and feed fortifiers will have to be handmade. These are often strange combinations which are complicated to make up.

Prevention of complications

AKI has the potential to cause anticoagulation with platelet dysfunction, hypertension, fluid overload, gastrointestinal bleeding, immunocompromise and reduced ability to handle drugs and toxins. In addition, children who require intensive care will usually need multiple invasive lines and catheters. The need to adhere to strict infection control measures is essential. Full blood count, platelets, coagulation and biochemistry, including phosphate, magnesium, calcium and liver function tests, must be checked urgently if AKI is suspected or known to be involved. Frequency of repeated samples depends on the patient's response, but it is essential to check levels when potentially dangerous or in assessing response to treatment, rather than hope for the best. Most blood gas machines now measure corrected calcium, sodium and potassium on small sample sizes, which can be very useful.

One of the effects of AKI, particularly with fluid overload, is hypertension and potentially a hypertensive crisis. Hypertension should be treated with nifedipine then labetalol, at a rate starting at $0.5 \, mg/kg/hr$, up to a maximum $3 \, mg/kg/hr$ (Barry et al. 2010). Sodium nitroprusside (SNP) can then be used. SNP is a very potent vasodilator and will potentially lower blood pressure very quickly. It does, however, have a short half-life so once switched off, blood pressure (BP) will recover. It is essential to protect SNP from the light and change it regularly as it degrades into cyanide. The SNP infusion rate is $0.5 \, mcg/kg/hr$ with a maximum of $8 \, mcg/kg/hr$ (Barry et al. 2010). Furosemide should only be used if the patient is not intravascularly fluid-depleted. It is essential to reduce the pressure at a controlled rate to avoid organ damage and prevent permanent neurological disability.

Because of the varying length of hypertension before treatment in PICU, BP should be reduced by 25% in the first 8 hours and then reduced to normal over the next 16–48 hours, that is to say the aim is to return blood pressure to expected values relative to age over a 48-hour period using a two-stage approach (Barry et al. 2010).

Renal protection measures

Low-dose dopamine (2–5 mcg/kg/min) has been demonstrated to dilate renal arteries and increase renal blood flow in animal studies. For some years low-dose dopamine was standard treatment in the PICU to generate this renal perfusion effect; however, it has largely been abandoned because of lack of evidence of improved renal function in clinical practice.

The use of furosemide infusions has gained some ground as an avoidance strategy for RRT and as a way of increasing urine output to stop re-instigation of RRT. Again there is no evidence to support this; anecdotally, the ability to control fluid balance may be useful in the avoidance of RRT. However, it is essential to remember that furosemide will work only when there is cortical blood flow. As it is also nephrotoxic its use should not continue if it does not have an effect.

Drug metabolism and excretion

The kidneys are responsible for the elimination of many drugs and their metabolites. This is through the process of glomerular filtration of drugs and active renal secretion. As glomerular filtration rate (GFR) drops in renal failure, drug removal becomes less efficient. Normal GFR is $120 \, ml/min$ per $1.73 \, m^2$. There are various calculations for estimating GFR; however they are difficult to interpret when diuretics and fluid resuscitation have been administered.

Changes to electrolytes, body water and uraemia will increase the effects of centrally acting drugs because of changes to the blood–brain barrier and to the distribution and amount of body water and therefore drug distribution.

There are further points to consider in renal failure especially when RRT is involved, these are detailed in Table 6.7.

Renal excretion is the active removal of a drug and its metabolites by cells sensitive to drugs in the tubule. Many

Table 6.7   Characteristics of drugs

Drug factor	Implication for the child with impaired renal function
Molecular weight	Molecular weight refers to the size of the drug molecule and will theoretically affect a drug's removal. Most drugs, however, are small enough to fit through the semi-permeable membrane which forms the capillaries in the Bowman's capsule. Once through into the tubule some drug may be reabsorbed along with water back into the peritubular capillaries. Eventually, the unabsorbed drug will pass into the collecting duct and be carried to the bladder. In RRT all non-protein and fat-bound drugs will be filtered with increasing efficiency as treatment rate goes up. Adding dialysate flow to CVVH will increase the efficiency of drug removal.
Protein binding	Protein binding is one of the most important factors as drugs that are protein-bound (e.g. albumin) will not be filtered with the glomerular filtrate. Once unbound, the free drug may be removed. This is potentially highly significant in children who are critically ill as at least 50% of them will be hypoalbuminaemic and 25% will be severely hypoalbuminaemic. In addition, acidosis affects protein binding; this may lead to more unbound drug being available while having unchanged drug levels on drug assay.
Water solubility	Water solubility is the ability of a drug to dissolve in water. Drugs that are highly water soluble will be likely to be removed by glomerular filtration.
Volume of distribution	Volume of distribution depends on where the drug is likely to disperse through the body. Drugs with a high volume of distribution will be less available for glomerular filtration. Volume of distribution is often changed by fluid overload in renal failure.

drugs have metabolites that are removed by the kidneys after initial metabolism in the liver.

Practical drug dosing

Ideally, known nephrotoxic agents should be avoided; however, this may be impossible in PICU. Dose or dose interval may have to be changed. Generally, loading doses should not be changed. As GFR improves or worsens, changes in dosage will have to be reassessed. When drug assays can be performed they should be done to aid decision-making on dosing and effects. Drugs with short half-lives, inotropes and inodilators should not have changes made to prescription as they are usually not affected by renal function.

Aminoglycosides, gentamicin, amikacin and tobramycin should be used with extreme caution in AKI in PICU. They are nephrotoxic and ototoxic and these risks are increased in renal failure. The effects are caused by reduction of intravascular volume, use of diuretics and hypokalaemia/magnesia, particularly in neonates. To reduce clinical incidents many units prescribe individual dosage of these agents rather than a course. This allows for individual consideration of the infant's needs.

For gentamicin dosing Barry et al. (2010) and Rees et al. (2007) suggest the drug levels be monitored frequently but that the daily dosing schedule be replaced by a divided dosing regimen where 2.5–3.5 mg/kg be given when there is renal impairment. This should be reviewed if the child's infection was not responding to management. Vancomycin will be removed by CVVH/DF, which is more efficient at drug removal than other forms of RRT, especially when using high-volume treatments. Vancomycin trough levels should be performed to determine dose schedule. Liposomal amphotericin B is considerably less nephrotoxic than conventional amphotericin and therefore dose adjustment is usually not necessary. Cephalosporin and penicillin will also need dose-adjustment.

Morphine and midazolam metabolites are removed by active renal secretion. Reduction in dose by up to 50% will usually be appropriate with full assessment of effects and sedation scoring. Some centres routinely change regimes from morphine to fentanyl once RRT is instigated.

The electrolyte content of drugs also needs to be considered in AKI (e.g. drugs with high sodium content such as Gaviscon and 4.5% human albumin solution).

Drug dosing in AKI and RRT is a highly complex, imprecise area. The advice of a specialist pharmacist should always be sought as well as up-to-date literature (BNFc 2011–12; Patzer 2008)

Long-term follow-up

Long-term follow-up from AKI has until now been restricted to children with primary renal injury. It was thought that those who survived multi-organ failure would recover normal renal function. Some studies (Kist-van Holthe et al. 2002; Polito et al. 1998; Slack et al. 2005) suggest a need for long-term follow-up in those children.

Specific renal diseases that may present in PICU

Haemolytic uraemic syndrome (HUS)

The syndrome is characterised by haemolytic anaemia with raised urea and creatinine, and low platelet count. Verotoxins are usually released after a diarrhoeal illness and cause a number of problems within the circulation. The toxins attack the endothelial cells in the kidney and brain; in addition, the breakdown of red cells and platelet aggregation partially or totally occlude blood supply in the kidneys. Usually, though not exclusively, this is associated with exposure to *E. coli* 0157, but can have a number of other causes. In most cases bloody diarrhoea is the first sign of illness although occasionally no diarrhoea is present and HUS may be the underlying pathology. While there is no specific treatment for HUS other than supportive management, RRT is often necessary to manage severe electrolyte disturbance and fluid imbalance. Occasionally, children develop severe cerebral irritation and cerebral bleeds, and this often necessitates intensive care for neurological protection and airway management. In these patients the use of plasma exchange has been found to be useful, possibly because of the removal of the toxin, but the process is not well understood. The use of all extracorporeal techniques in acute HUS can be challenging because of the tendency of circuits to clot owing to the large clumps of red cells and platelets occluding the circuit filters.

Strict barrier nursing is essential when dealing with cases of HUS because of the ease of transfer to staff and relatives. There are well-documented cases of fatalities in health care workers. In HUS blood film and stool culture will be helpful.

Nephrotic syndrome

This occurs when the glomeruli become permeable to albumin. If unchecked the oncotic pressure can drop to a point where intravascular fluid is lost from the circulation. Acute treatment usually involves infusion of 20% albumin followed by furosemide. Occasionally, intravascular losses

will cause very significant pulmonary oedema and ventilation may be required. It is then usually necessary to perform fluid removal with haemofiltration.

Hepatorenal syndrome

This is renal failure secondary to hepatic failure. It should be considered when children with liver failure show signs of kidney insufficiency. Children may well be hypovolaemic despite the appearance of ascites. It is essential to replace intravascular volume if the central venous pressure (CVP) is low; however, CVP must not be raised above 10 mmHg because of the risk of further liver damage.

Tumour lysis syndrome (TLS)

Tumour lysis occurs when tumours that are sensitive to chemotherapy are treated causing dead cells and cell debris to be released into the blood. Uric acid and calcium phosphate potentially precipitate in the renal tubules causing AKI. Large amounts of potassium will also be released, causing potentially life-threatening hyperkalaemia. Acute RRT may be necessary to treat symptoms in TLS. It may be avoided with aggressive fluid management, diuresis and possibly the use of rasburicase and allopurinol (Ahn et al. 2011; Sood et al. 2007).

Transplant

Kidney transplant patients are not routinely admitted to PICU unless undergoing a more complex procedure, including liver and kidney transplant or have comorbidity that requires intensive monitoring or ventilation. General principles will be discussed.

It is vital to ensure good communication between teams caring for these children, with coordination of ward rounds to include all the senior medical staff.

Immunosuppression is one of the most important aspects of immediate post-transplant care to avoid acute rejection of the transplanted kidney. The therapy causes significant immunocompromise and strict adherence to reverse-barrier nursing protocols is essential. Where practical the child should be nursed in a cubicle or at the very least away from other infectious children. Combinations of monoclonal antibodies that inhibit CD50, calcineurin inhibitors and corticosteroids are used to achieve immunosuppression and local protocols should be strictly adhered to, including the use of drug levels to assess dose effectiveness. Some of these agents (e.g. cyclosporine) are cytotoxic and the usual precautions should be taken. Tacrolimus and cyclosporine both interact with many drugs causing increased or decreased effect and nephrotoxicity. Of particular note in the PICU are: amphotericin, vancomycin, aminoglycosides, fluconazole, erythromycin, chloramphenicol, rifampicin, nifedipine, cimetidine, phenytoin, phenobarbitone and carbamazepine (Rees et al. 2007). This is not an exhaustive list and before administering any new agents to children on anti-rejection therapy the current British National Formulary for Children (BNFc) should be consulted.

Important postoperative factors include the need to be scrupulous about fluid balance and monitoring the function of kidney graft with the fluid allowance, including a calculation for urine replacement initially millilitre for millilitre to avoid dehydration. Other considerations are the risk of urine leakage from the ureteric anastomosis site. Urine leakage may be detected by an improvement in biochemistry without adequate urine output, although pain and swelling can also be a clue. The leak can be confirmed with ultrasound and will require surgical intervention to rectify it. Blood clots can restrict and occlude the transplanted kidney's blood supply. Most centres overcome this with the use of heparin or aspirin and this can lead to bleeding problems postoperatively. Often, kidneys are transplanted from much older donors; consequently, a higher blood pressure than physiological normal for the child will be needed to 'drive' the new kidney.

Renal replacement therapies

Renal replacement therapy (RRT) has in important role in PICU.

Acronyms

Continuous veno-venous haemofiltration (CVVH) is a substitute for haemodialysis. There are different types and they all come under the general term renal replacement therapy. There has been an increase in the use of CVVH, CVVHD (continuous veno-venous haemodialysis) and CVVHDF (continuous veno-venous haemodiafiltration) in the last decade, with the availability of automated machines and paediatric tubing, filters and software. However, peritoneal dialysis (PD) still has a place. Choice of therapy should be based on advantages and disadvantages (Table 6.8), as well as experience with the setup, what the continuing treatment options are and the availability of each method.

Peritoneal dialysis

PD is not suitable for every child as there are a number of contraindications (Table 6.9). However, it is still widely used as a renal replacement therapy for children outside the specialist renal units. PD may be used, for example, during the postoperative phase of a cardiac patient, where the placement of a PD catheter can be done under direct visualisation.

Peritoneal catheter access

The best form of access is obtained by either laparoscopic surgical or percutaneous insertion of a tunnelled double-cuffed catheter, with antibiotic cover. Ideally, these should not be used for 2 weeks; however, in the PICU the need for acute biochemical control will circumvent this. There are 'blind' insertion acute peritoneal dialysis catheters, which can be used in an emergency; however these do have an increased complication rate, in particular bowel perforation, leakage, mechanical obstruction and infection. As

Table 6.8 Advantages and disadvantages of different therapies

Therapy	Advantages	Disadvantages
Peritoneal dialysis	Circulatory stable	Potential respiratory compromise
	No anticoagulation	Infection
	Can be used in infants <2 kg	Catheter placement
	Technically easy	Less efficient
	Less resource-intensive	Moderate fluid volume control
CVVH/CVVHD/ CVVHDF	Efficient	Access
	Circulatory stable after initial connection	Clotting/bleeding problems
	Efficient fluid balance control	Platelet consumption
	'Evil humour removal'	Electrolyte disturbance, e.g. $Ca^{2+}/Mg/PO_4$
		More technical
Intermittent haemodialysis	Drug removal	Access
	Toxin removal	Can cause severe circulatory instability
	Quick	Water supply needed
	Very efficient removal of wastes	Dedicated operator

Table 6.9 Contraindication and requirements for PD

Contraindications	Essential requirements
Diaphragmatic hernia	Peritoneal access
Omphalocoele	Dialysis fluid
Gastroschisis	A delivery system
Possibility of intra-abdominal catastrophe (necrotising enterocolitis in most circumstances)	incorporating timer and measuring device
Recent abdominal surgery	Fluid warmer
Multiple adhesions	
Peritonitis	
Presence of VP shunt	

Table 6.10 Cycles of PD

Cycle	Time (min)	Comment
Fill	10	
Dwell	30–60	Reduce cycle time if fluid removal is the main aim.
Drain	10	Continue drain if fluid is draining.

with all practical procedures experience reduces the risk of complications.

Dialysis fluid and kinetic principles

In PD the peritoneum acts as the semi-permeable membrane, allowing diffusion, convection and osmosis to play a role. The dialysis fluids use glucose as the main osmotic agent. The higher the glucose concentration, the greater the fluid removal. However, due to absorption of glucose this can lead to hyperglycaemia, thus the glucose concentration should be as low as possible to achieve the required fluid removal.

The dialysate is buffered with bicarbonate or lactate. In general there has been a trend to using bicarbonate solutions in PICU, as they can be used in liver failure and lactic acidosis and reduce infusion pain. Because of bicarbonate's instability with calcium all bicarbonate-based fluids need to mixed before use and usually have a 24-hour expiry. Observation for calcium precipitation should always take place.

The dialysate fluid can be used as an effective method of temperature control. The fluid is normally heated to 37°C; however, a lower temperature provides an extremely effective central cooling.

Tubing and connections

These are straightforward and come in sterile packaging. They are simply a means of connecting the dialysis fluid to a burette then to the catheter via a three-way tap, with the third connection to a waste bag fitted with a measuring device. They must be managed aseptically at all times. Luer lock connecters are preferable as they are more secure.

Cycles time and fluid volumes (Table 6.10)

Volumes: The starting fill volume should be 10–15 ml/kg, which can be increased to 30 ml/kg if no leaks occur. Maximum volumes of 50 ml/kg can be used. The larger the volume the more diffusion can occur and thus increased efficiency of the dialysis. However, the larger the volume the more likely it is that there will be respiratory and cardiovascular instability and exit site leakage.

There are automated machines to simplify the process of cycling. However, these cannot perform fill volumes below 100 ml and so they are unsuitable for newborns. Neonates have a very varied response to dwell times. Paradoxically, the reverse of what is physiologically expected may sometimes be the case.

Cross-flow: In situations where large volumes in the abdomen cannot be tolerated it is possible to insert two PD catheters. One can be used to fill and the other to drain. The fill volumes are the same; however it is infused and drained continuously over 1 hour.

Additives to peritoneal dialysis fluid: PD fluid can be added to if necessary, in particular with heparin, to prevent fibrin deposits (be aware of systemic absorption especially in neonates), antibiotics to prevent or treat peritonitis and potassium to prevent hypokalaemia. PD is efficient at removing potassium, therefore close monitoring of levels is essential. All additions to bags must strictly comply with infection control measures because of the increased risk of peritonitis.

Peritonitis

Peritonitis is one of the most important complications of PD as it can be life-threatening. The standard symptoms of pain, fever and cloudy PD fluid do not have to be present. Examples of antimicrobials that can be added to the PD fluid are shown in Tables 6.11 and 6.12. Because of the changing nature of the problem, drug choice should adhere to local policy based on bacterial sensitivities. There should be case-specific discussion with the pharmacist and microbiologist.

Table 6.11   Example regimen in PD

MRSA status	Management
MRSA negative	Load with tobramycin (16 mg/l) and cefuroxime (500 mg/l). Subsequent maintenance doses as prescribed examples provided below. Dwell time 6 hours.
MRSA positive	Load vancomycin (500 mg/l) and cefuroxime (500 mg/l). Subsequent maintenance doses as prescribed. Dwell time 6 hours.

Table 6.12   PD fluid additives and dose

Therapeutic agent	Suggested dosage
Cefuroxime	125 mg/l
Vancomycin	30 mg/l
Ceftazidime	125 mg/l
Teicoplanin	20 mg/l
Cefazolin	125 mg/l
Tobramycin	8 mg/l
Heparin	Max. 500 units/l
Potassium	Max. 5 mmol/l; standard 4 mmol/l

Drug levels initially at 48 hours

Total treatment duration is 2 weeks, except for *Staphylococcus aureus* and *Pseudomonas* which should be 3 weeks. If infection persists or recurs, catheter removal may be necessary.

Fungal peritonitis can occur with few signs and often necessitates catheter removal and fluconazole treatment.

Where prophylaxis is the aim, cefuroxime at 125 mg/l is often the first choice.

Catheter leakage

This is more common in the acute PD catheters and it greatly increases the likelihood of infection.

- Use occlusive dressings if possible.
- Apply pressure dressing to site. Remember to weigh prior to application in neonates, to allow calculation of fluid balance.
- Purse string suture around catheter.
- Consider a new catheter if leakage continues.

(See Table 6.13.)

Continuous venous-venous filtration and haemodialysis (CVVH and CVVHDF) (Figure 6.2 and Figure 6.3)

Kinetic principles

Haemofiltration is the removal of plasma water by filtration of the blood. Blood runs through the filter which has fibres made of semi-permeable membranes.

Filtration occurs because of the pressure gradient inside the filter (blood) and outside the filter (ultrafiltration). Because plasma water has molecules dissolved in it those that are small enough to fit through the filter are also removed. This is called convection. Electrolytes, acids and some wastes are filtered; proteins, red cells, clotting components and immunoglobulin are not. The filtered fluid is then replaced with a physiological, 'normal' replacement fluid either pre- or post-filter. If replaced pre-filter a higher solute clearance is obtained at the cost of using more replacement fluid. Because of distribution of solutes through the intra- and extracellular compartments, the volume of filtration is related to total body water. This correlates to approximately half of body weight to achieve adequate solute and electrolyte removal. With no pre-dilution this equates to 25 ml/kg/hr; with pre-dilution it equates to 30 ml/kg/hr. Dose rate is an approximation at best, so staff should not be too concerned if exact rates cannot be achieved for technical reasons.

The addition of haemodialysis is achieved by using counter-current flow of dialysis fluid through the haemofilter, leading to a diffusion gradient and therefore dialysis. Diffusion is a two-way process so, while molecules that are at a high concentration in the patient's blood diffuse out, molecules that are at a high concentration in the dialysate fluid diffuse into the blood. The flow rates are limited compared to intermittent HD-limiting clearance, but are still more efficient than haemofiltration on its own.

Essentials for running therapy

- Patient access.
- Blood filter.
- Blood pump.
- Replacement/dialysis fluid.
- Fluid warmer.
- Anticoagulation.

Venous access

In most cases double lumen lines are used, but occasionally two single lines can be used in cases of low flow rate or low weight. In general, the bigger the cannula the better (Table 6.14). However, even with a large cannula, there can be flow problems and these can often be improved

Table 6.13 Troubleshooting PD

Problem	Cause	Solution
No/reduced flow on drain	Clamped or kinked lines or catheter	Unclamp or unkink lines.
	Fibrin blockage	Flush catheter with heparin and 0.9% sodium chloride *never aspirate*. Add heparin to bags.
	Position of catheter obstructing drain	Reposition patient. Some positions can be counterintuitive.
	Fluid may have fully drained straight into drain bag because drain line not clamped	Clamp drain line clamp. Perform one cycle with no dwell time, observing closely for signs of over-filling.
More fluid removal required	Increase strength of dialysis fluid	Use higher-strength glucose bag. Try mixing of two strengths rather than going straight to a higher strength.
	Decrease dwell times	Shorten the length of time the dialysate stays in the patient. This can increase the fluid removal but can also have an effect on solute removal.
	Increase fill volumes	Increasing the amount of fluid going into the patient (max. 50 ml/kg) can sometimes increase fluid removal but should be done cautiously. This will also increase the solute removal.
Too much fluid being removed	Decrease the glucose concentration	Use a weaker strength bag if using pre-made. Try mixing two strengths.
	Lengthen the dwell time	Leaving the dialysate in the patient for longer will remove less fluid.
More clearance of waste and electrolytes required	Urea	Longer dwell times are required to remove more urea.
	Potassium	Shorter dwell times are required to remove more potassium. Continuous dialysis can cause hypokalaemia, requiring the addition of potassium to the PD fluid.
	Sodium	Sodium should be lowered slowly to avoid any adverse effects. 1 mmol/hr is a safe reference to use. Very hypernatraemic patients should have additional sodium chloride added to the dialysate to avoid lowering levels too quickly.
	Calcium	Pre-made solutions are available with different calcium concentrations (range 0–1.75 mmol/l).
	Creatinine	Creatinine is not removed very efficiently during short-dwell peritoneal dialysis. It is, however, a useful indicator of kidney function and should be observed in the acute setting for any improvement.
Pain on infusion	Internal position of catheter	Tidal dialysis can be tried in order to keep a pool of fluid in the peritoneum to float the catheter. Change patient position. Reposition catheter (acute only).
	Intra-abdominal pressure	Reduce fill volume. Try cross-flow dialysis.
	Air under diaphragm	Normally corrects over 30 minutes. Analgesia. Try cross-flow dialysis.
Pain on outflow	Internal position of catheter	As for pain on infusion.
Breathlessness	Intra-abdominal pressure	Reduce fill volume. Cross-flow dialysis.
	PD fluid migrating into chest via a diaphragmatic hole	Drain fluid, stop PD and convert to an alternative therapy.

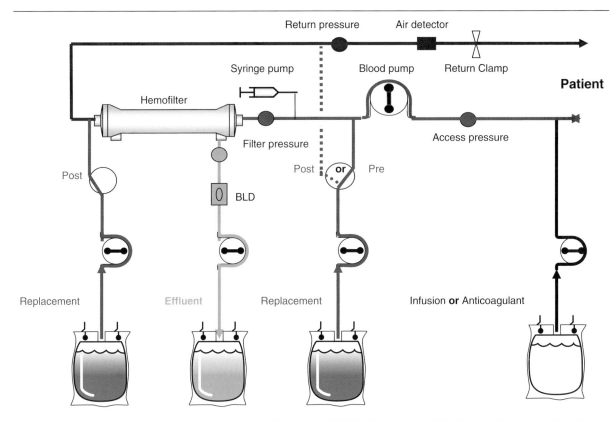

Figure 6.2 Continuous venous-venous haemofiltration (CVVH). Based on 2005 Prismaflex manual, with kind permission from HospalGambro.

by rotation, slight retraction of the cannula or swapping venous/arterial connections. If at all possible a 5 Fg cannula should be avoided as flow is severely limited due to its diameter. Insertion can be made more successfully with ultrasound guidance.

Blood filter

The best filter partly depends on the machine used. In general, the filter surface area should not exceed the patient's and the total circuit volume should be < 10% of the patient's circulating blood volume. Exceptions can be made, in particular when using extracorporeal life support.

Filter materials vary between manufacturers. Non-surface-treated AN69 membranes are pH-sensitive and their use with low pH primer has been associated with the bradykinin release syndrome (Brophy et al. 2001). Anyone starting filtration should be aware of the possible side-

effects of the filter membranes. Polysurphone, poly-etheilesurphone and surface treated ST-AN69 membranes do not cause bradykinin release. There are small-scale studies and contradictory evidence on which membrane is most appropriate in AKI (Gasche and Pascual 1996; Gastaldello et al. 2000). While polysulfophone and polyethylsulfophone appear to be the most bio-compatible, anecdotally ST-AN69 may have circuit preservation properties, possibly because of heparin bonding on initial prime of the filter.

To prime the filter and circuit, follow local guidelines. Priming can be started before the catheter is inserted, as even with modern machines this is time-consuming.

Most manufacturers recommend changing the circuit after 72 hours. However, this is based on the likelihood of blood pump raceway rupture at adult blood pump speeds. Because of the risks associated with circuit change in small children and slower blood pump speeds some centres run beyond 72 hours, without problems (Ali et al. 2006).

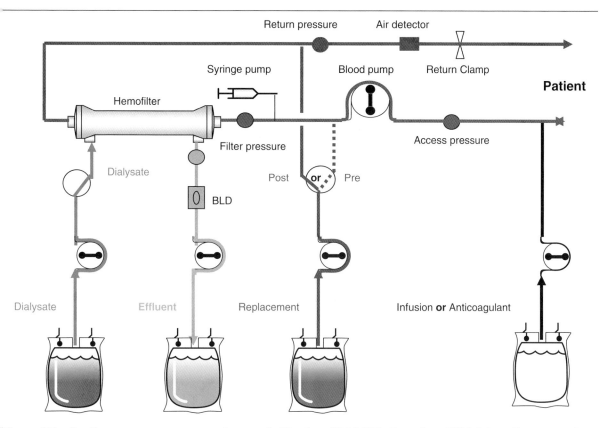

Figure 6.3 Continuous venous-venous haemodiafiltration (CVVHDF). Based on 2005 Prismaflex manual, with kind permission from HospalGambro.

Table 6.14 Weight to cannula size

Weight (kg)	Size (Fg)
<3	5
3–10	6.5
10–20	8
20–50	11
>50	>12

Fluid pump control

Volumatic pumps were used in the past but were highly inaccurate and mostly have been replaced with fully automated machines. These have the additional advantages of error control and data-gathering. These machines must be configured to allow slow pump speed and fluid handling in children. Where volumetric pumps are used, especially in ECMO, recorded fluid may be inaccurate because of highly positive and negative circuit pressures and effective pump control systems that are designed to work at atmospheric pressure. This means it is essential to use secondary measuring devices to avoid hypo- or hypervolaemia if using this type of system. At all times monitor and treat the patient's clinical fluid status.

Replacement/dialysate fluid

Fluid can be buffered with lactate or bicarbonate. In PICUs bicarbonate has become the first choice as lactic acidosis is often the reason for instigating renal replacement therapy and lactate handling in newborns is unpredictable because of liver immaturity. The concentration of electrolyte needs to be taken into account and sometimes changed to meet clinical need. Fluid content is therefore governed by compatibility and ion and cation balance such as adding sodium if the patient is extremely hypernatraemic (Na > 160) to reduce the speed of sodium reduction. Most fluids have low magnesium concentrations of 0.5 mmol/l and additional IV magnesium boluses will be needed. Currently no commercial fluid contains phosphate, and HF will efficiently remove phosphate. IV phosphate can be given or added to replacement fluid bags at a concentration of 1 mmol/l. If using potassium acid phosphate each mmol of phosphate is associated with 1 mmol potassium. Sodium glycerophosphate does not contain additional potassium and maybe a safer alternative. Because calcium and bicarbonate are unstable, all bicarbonate fluids need to be mixed before use. Clinically, if there is a rapid fall in the patient's bicarbonate or calcium with the instigation of RRT, bag mixing should be checked. Warming bicarbonate fluid can causes CO_2 production and calcium carbonate deposits in the warming coil. Automated machines now have degassing chambers which should be checked and emptied hourly. Heater coils should be checked for calcium deposits and changed when necessary.

Temperature control

Patient cooling can be dramatic, especially in newborns. Machines have a blood warmer or fluid-warming attachments which ensure the blood returning to the body is at the correct temperature. Additional patient heating devices may have to be used. The filter can be wrapped in tin foil or bubble wrap, and this provides a surprisingly effective reduction in heat loss.

Anticoagulation

Heparin, sodium citrate and prostaglandins are all effective anti-coagulation techniques. In the United Kingdom heparin remains the mainstay of anti-coagulation. Low molecular weight heparin has not been used to any great extent in children in the United Kingdom because of its longer half-life and unpredictable reversibility with protamine sulphate.

If using heparin, a loading dose of up to 50 units/kg may be used, followed by a continuous infusion to achieve activated clotting times (ACT) of 1.2–1.8 normal or aPPT ratios of 1.2–1.5 times the respective baseline. Infusion rates of up to 30 units/kg/hr are used (Strazdins et al. 2004). It should be noted that heparin only works when enough anti-thrombin 3 and protein C are present; therefore, when patients are consuming clotting factors, heparin may become more effective once coagulation products have been replaced, e.g. with fresh frozen plasma (FFP). Platelet count and use of other anti-coagulants should be taken into account when using heparin and the dose reduced accordingly. Risk of bleeding with heparin in surgery will have to be decided on a case-by-case basis; however, neurosurgery precludes the use of heparin. Heparin-induced thrombocy-

topenia (HIT) is a very rare side-effect. It normally manifests after secondary large exposure to heparin with a drop in platelets of 50% in approximately 5 days after exposure. HIT is both pro- and anti-coagulatory with a risk of clotting large vessels. If HIT is suspected, alternative anti-coagulation is essential and the advice of a haematologist must be sought. ACT measurements are system and bottle specific so care should be taken to check standard reference ranges using ACT systems.

In North America and increasingly in Europe sodium citrate is commonly used. This works by chelating ionised calcium prior to filtration. Calcium is then infused after filtration. Many of the newer machines have an automated function to achieve this and show some promise in the safe delivery of citrate anti-coagulation.

Prostacyclin (epoprostenol) can also be used, although if used alone it reduces circuit life. It has been used in combination with heparin with more success; however, it can cause profound hypotension. For epoprostenol rates of 5–7 ng/kg/min are used (Strazdins et al. 2004). There is some debate as to whether it is better infused into the patient or the circuit to obtain maximum effects. Boluses should be avoided because of the potential for hypotension. Standard coagulation tests are not affected by epoprostenol, so the circuit must be observed closely for clot formations.

Treatment starting parameters

Table 6.15 is a guide to initiating treatment; however, these will be tailored to individual needs and in the light of patient experience. When treatment is for metabolic disease, sepsis or drug removal, high-volume treatment is necessary. In high-volume treatment dramatic effects on electrolyte balance can occur, thus regular review of potassium, phosphate, calcium, sodium and pH is essential. Replacement and dialysate rates of up to 120 ml/kg/hr have been used (Harvey et al. 2005; Westrope and Morrison 2006). However, while replacement is low efficiency, dialysate should be increased more slowly because of the potential for speedy changes in electrolytes, and waste level causes large intravascular fluid shifts and the potential for dangerous cerebral fluid shifts.

Start of treatment

At the start of treatment there is often a period of hypotension. Potential causes are the inflammatory response to the circuit, transient reduction in serum inotrope levels as well as the increase to the total circulating volume or haemodilution.

Table 6.15 Initial parameters for pre-filter replacement fluid

	Flow	Action
Exchange/ replacement/ turnover rate	30 ml/kg/hr standard starting point	Approximately half of body weight will be exchanged in 24 hours taking into account 25% lost to pre-dilution.
Blood flow	6–9 ml/kg/min	This is at least 10 times filtration rate to prevent excessive haemoconcentration in the filter.
Dialysate flow rate	20 ml/kg/hr	Maximal efficacy is achieved at 2–3 times the blood flow rate.
Fluid loss	Customise to patient need	This is the net fluid loss through haemofiltration and will depend on patient need. It is difficult to achieve a negative balance of more than 5–10% of the patient's actual body weight in 24 hours.

Troubleshooting (Table 6.16)

Circuit pressures are measured in mmHg and reflect the flow and resistance to flow within the circuit. Measured pressures vary between different manufactures and filters, so close attention to these details is necessary when running circuits. Arterial pressure is always negative as the blood pump is sucking blood out of the patient. Different manufacturers describe pressures differently: arterial = access pressure; venous = return pressure

At all times protect the patient from air embolism and blood loss. When troubleshooting, it may be safer to disconnect from the patient and recirculate. Always flush the access if this is being done. Circuits should be spiked onto a small bag of 0.9% sodium chloride and use a partly open three-way tap, or ideally a connector with two or three taps to generate arterial and venous pressure and avoid continuous circuit alarms.

Intermittent haemodialysis

IHD is highly efficient dialysis and is useful for drug, toxin and metabolite removal. IHD is often associated with a high degree of cardiovascular instability in the critically ill child and therefore it has a limited place in PICU. It should only be performed in centres were dedicated staff are available.

There may be a rebound effect from highly efficient removal of drugs from the vascular space and redistribution into the circulation from extra vascular spaces. Some centres have used IHD for initially removal of drugs/toxins and switch to CVVHDF after initially treatment.

Haemoperfusion

Haemoperfusion uses activated charcoal cartridges with a large surface area placed in an extracorporeal circuit as an absorbent to remove toxins. It has been used historically for toxin and drug removal, but is technically difficult because of absorption of anti-coagulant and glucose. Its use is now been superseded by other more reliable methods of drug removal including plasmafiltration and the Molecular Adsorbent Recirculation System (MARS). Potentially double filtration plasma fractionation may have a number of advantages over plasmafiltration, however there are currently no data concerning its use in the PICU.

Plasmafiltration (PF)

Plasmafiltration uses a plasma filter in an extracorporeal circuit. Plasma filters have large holes which allow molecules up to and including albumin size to be removed. This necessitates the use of replacement fluid which includes human albumin and often clotting factors.

PF removes antibodies in immune-mediated disease, albumin-bound drugs and has been employed in some centres in cases of sepsis, although this use remains unproven and controversial (Iwai et al. 1998; Reeves et al. 1999). However, in the authors' clinical experience it has had some startlingly beneficial effects. When attempting to remove antibodies or drugs a number of treatments may be necessary because of further production of antibodies or redistribution of drug. Multiple treatments will cause significant immune compromise.

Treatment guide for standard PF

- Blood pump speed 5–9 ml/kg/min.
- Circuit size as CVVH.
- Treatment 100ml/kg exchange to exchange 2 plasma volumes.
- Treatment time no less than 4 hours.

Table 6.16 Troubleshooting extracorporeal therapies

Problem	Cause	Solution
Excessively negative arterial pressure	Clamp/kinked line Catheter up against the vessel wall Arterial line/access clotting	Unclamp/kink line. Swap lines so arterial connects to venous side of catheter. Check clotting and increase anticoagulation if necessary. Aspirate and flush access.
Positive arterial pressure	Disconnection or patient coughing	Clamp lines and reconnect if no air in circuit or wait for coughing to stop.
Excessively positive venous pressure	Clamp/kinked line Venous line/access clotting	Unclamp/unkink line. Bedside clotting check and increase anticoagulation if necessary.
Low/negative venous pressure	Disconnection Low flow in small patients	Clamp lines and reconnect if no air in circuit. Partially occlude venous line to generate higher venous pressure.
Rise in TMP/filter pressure rising	Filter/circuit clotting Ultrafiltrate too high for filter/blood flow rate	Check no clamps on ultrafiltrate line or bag. Check filtration fraction below 25%. Increase pre-dilution percentage. Check maximum ultrafiltrate for filter size. Stop circuit if filter is clotted.
Air detector	Air in venous line May also be caused by circuit clotting	Remove air. If large amounts are present, take patient off and flush access with saline. Recirculate circuit and remove air while patient isolated. Find source of air.
Blood leak	Blood in ultrafiltrate Viscous ultrafiltrate, associated with liver failure Air in blood leak detector Air detector out chamber Dirty mirror on detector	Stop treatment if real blood leak. Continue if possible but filter likely to clot off. Seek liver opinion. Remove air from blood leak detector find cause. Put blood leak detector back into position. Clean mirror.

- Replacement fluid ratio's 67% albumin, 33% FFP or Octaplas.
- Beware of dropping ionised calcium. Calcium is removed PF and FFP contains citrate, which chelates calcium. Life-threatening arrhythmias have been reported, particularly when performing treatments at fast rates.
- No fluid removal while on PF.
- Anticoagulation is the same as in CVVH although considerably higher rates of continuous infusion may well be necessary. ACT range 1.5–2 times normal.
- Plasma filters have a lower maximum trans-membrane pressure, which means higher blood pump speed may cause rupture of the membrane.

Conclusion

This chapter has briefly considered the anatomy and physiology of the kidney, then provided a summary of the diagnosis and treatment of renal failure in children. The chapter focused on the management of acute and chronic renal failure where it related to children's intensive care. This is not an exhaustive review of the renal replacement strategies or a comprehensive prescription of care for these children. The care of children with renal failure is complex and swiftly changing, so it is important to keep up to date.

References

Ahn YH, Kang HJ et al. 2011. Tumour lysis syndrome in children: experience of last decade. Hematol Oncol. 24 June. doi: 10.1002/hon.995. Epub ahead of print.

Ali F, Basu R, Lane J. 2006. Hemofiltration Circuit Use Beyond 72 Hours in Pediatric Continuous Renal Replacement Therapy. Presentation at the Paediatric Continuous Renal Replacement Therapy Conference, Zurich, Switzerland.

Barry P, Morris K, Ali T (Eds). 2010. Paediatric Intensive Care. Oxford: Oxford University Press.

British National Formulary for Children (BNFc). 2011–12. bnfc.org/bnfc.

Brophy P, Mottes T et al. 2001. AN-69 membrane reactions are pH-dependent and preventable. American Journal of Kidney Diseases, 38(1):173–8.

Davies M, Evans J, McGonigle R. 1994. The dialysis debate: acute renal failure in burns patients. Burns, 20(1):71–3.

Dixon M, Crawford D et al. 2009. Nursing the Highly Dependent Child or Infant. Oxford: Wiley-Blackwell.

European Medicines Agency. 2004. Discussion paper on the impact of renal immaturity.

For paediatrics: www.ema.europa.eu/docs/en_GB/document_library/Scientific_guideline/2009/09/WC500003807.pdf.

Gasche Y, Pascual M. 1996. Complement depletion during haemofiltration with polyacrilonitrile membranes. Nephrology Dialysis Transplantation, 11(1):117–19.

Gastaldello K, Melot C et al. 2000. Comparison of cellulose diacetate and polysulfone membranes in the outcome of acute renal failure. A prospective randomized study. Nephrology Dialysis Transplantation, 15(2):224–30.

Goldstein SL, Somers MJG, et al. 2004. The Prospective Pediatric Continuous Renal Replacement Therapy (ppCRRT) Registry: design, development and data assessed. International Journal of Artificial Organs, 27(1):9–14.

Harvey B, Hickman C et al. 2005. Severe lactic acidosis complicating metformin overdose successfully treated with high-volume venovenous hemofiltration and aggressive alkalinization. Pediatric Critical Care Medicine, 6(5):598–601.

Iwai H, Nagaki M, Naito T. (1998) Removal of endotoxin and cyctokines by plasma exchange in patients with acute hepatic failure. Critical Care Medicine, 26(5):873–6.

Kist-van Holthe J, Goedvollk C et al. 2002. Prospective study of renal insufficiency after bone marrow transplantation. Pediatric Nephrology, 17(12):1032–7.

Knoderer C, Leiser J et al. (2008) Fenoldopam for acute kidney injury in children. Pediatric Nephrology, 23(3):495–8.

Kohda Y, Chiao H, Star R. 1998. A melanocyte stimulating hormone and acute renal failure. Current Opinion in Nephrology and Hypertension, 7(4):413–17.

Landoni G, Biondi-Zoccai G, Tumlin J. 2007. Beneficial impact of fenoldopam in critically ill patients with or at risk for acute renal failure: a meta-analysis of randomized clinical trials. American Journal of Kidney Disease, 49(6):56–68.

Marthur VS, Swan SK et al. 1999. The effects of fenoldopam, a selective dopamine receptor agonist, on systemic and renal hemodynamics in normotensive subjects. Critical Care Medicine, 27(9):1832–7.

Patzer L. 2008. Nephrotoxicity as a cause of acute kidney injury in children. Pediatric Nephrology, 23(12):2159–73.

Phillips-Anderoli S. (2009) Acute kidney injury in children. Pediatric Nephrology, 24(2):253–63.

Polito C, Papale MR, LaManna AL. 1998. Long-term prognosis of acute renal failure in the full term newborn. Clinical Pediatrics (Phila), 37(6):381–6.

Rees L, Webb N, Brogan P (Eds). 2007. Paediatric Nephrology. Oxford: Oxford University Press.

Reeves J, Butt W et al. 1999. Plasmafiltration in Sepsis Study Group: Continuous plasmafiltration for sepsis syndrome. Critical Care Medicine, 27(10):2096–104.

Shaheen I, Harvey B et al. (2007) Continuous venovenous hemofiltration with or without extracorporeal membrane oxygenation in children. Pediatric Critical Care Medicine, 8(4):362–5.

Slack R, Hawkins KC et al. 2005. Long-term outcome of meningococcal sepsis-associated acute renal failure. Pediatric Critical Care Medicine, 6(4):477–9.

Sood A, Burry L, Cheng K. (2007) Clarifying the role of rasburicase in tumour lysis syndrome. Pharmacotherapy, 27(1):111–21.

Strazdins V, Watson A, Harvey B. 2004. Renal replacement therapy for acute renal failure in children: European guidelines. Pediatric Nephrology, 19(2):199–207.

Westrope C, Morrison G. 2006. High volume haemofiltration (CVVH) in the management of neonates with hyperammonaemia. Poster presentation PCRRT conference, Florida, USA.

Chapter 7
CARE OF THE INFANT OR CHILD WITH ACUTE NEUROLOGICAL DYSFUNCTION

Michaela Dixon

Paediatric Intensive Care Unit, Bristol Royal Hospital for Children, University Hospitals Bristol NHS Foundation Trust, Bristol, UK

Introduction

This chapter describes the developmental aspects of the nervous system, reviews neurological assessment and provides an overview of some of the major conditions which may be seen in the PICU.

Infants and children with acute neurological dysfunction of any aetiology account for around 11% of all paediatric intensive care admissions (PICANet 2011). Admission may be necessary as a consequence of primary neurological injury (e.g. traumatic brain injury), secondary to generalised systemic illness (e.g. sepsis) or as a consequence of failure in other body systems (e.g. hepatic encephalopathy). Seizures are one of the most common reasons for children presenting to the Emergency Department (Davis et al. 2005) and prompt management is important in reducing, where possible, the potential for long-term impairment. Status epilepticus remains an important cause of both mortality and morbidity in those children with underlying seizure disorders, while head injury is the single most common cause of death in children aged between 1 and 15 years. Traumatic brain injury is a primary insult about which little can be done, however if the child survives the initial insult their outcome is often determined by the severity of secondary insults relating to hypoxia and or hypotension. Once again, prompt, targeted management is important in potentially improving outcomes.

Embryological development of the neurological system

The developing nervous system appears in week 3 of gestation which is a period of general rapid embryonic development. Around day 18 there is differentiation of the three primitive germ layers into:

- Ectoderm.
- Mesoderm.
- Endoderm.

The ectoderm gives rise to the CNS, the brain and the spinal cord as well as other structures, including the skin. It starts as a plate of cells known as the neuroectoderm which folds to form the neural tube (Table 7.1). The upper two-thirds of the neural tube (the rostral end) are the area from which the brain develops, while the lower third (the caudal end) ultimately gives rise to the spinal cord.

There are three types of cells in the primitive neural tube:

Paediatric Intensive Care Nursing, First Edition. Edited by Michaela Dixon and Doreen Crawford.
© 2012 John Wiley & Sons, Ltd. Published 2012 by John Wiley & Sons, Ltd.

Table 7.1 Development of the primitive brain

Time	Detail of development
Week 4	Before complete fusion of the neural tube, the upper portion of the neural tube develops three fluid-filled enlargements or vesicles which are the beginnings of the primitive brain. These three primary vesicles are: • Forebrain or prosencephalon • Midbrain or mesencephalon • Hindbrain or rhombencephalon *Closure of the neural tube* Fusion or complete closure of the neural tube occurs within week 4 of gestation. The process of fusion begins in the centre of the tube, moving in an upward direction (towards the future brain) first and then about 2 days later downwards to complete closure. The canal through the middle of the complete neural tube will become the ventricular system of the brain and the central canal of the spinal cord. A failure of the tube to close completely at this point leads to neural tube defects. If the closure is not complete at the caudal end of the tube, congenital malformations affecting the spinal cord will develop (e.g. spina bifida occulta or a myelomeningocele). If the closure is not complete at the rostral or cranial end, then congenital malformations affecting the brain will develop (e.g. anencephaly).
Week 5	The vesicular region has undergone several flexures and changes and the embryonic brain consists of five secondary vesicles: Prosencephalon divides into the telencephalon and the diencephalon. Mesencephalon remains unchanged. Rhombencephalon divides into the metencephalon and the myelencephalon. Cranial nerve nuclei start to appear in the brain stem.
Week 6	Further differentiation and development of the five secondary vesicles refines the developing brain into the identifiable components seen in the adult brain. This is completed by the end of the week 6. Telencephalon – cerebral hemispheres/basal ganglia. Diencephalon – thalamus/hypothalamus/pineal gland. Mesencephalon – midbrain. Metencephalon – pons/cerebellum. Myelencephalon – medulla oblongata. The cavities within the vesicles develop into the ventricles of the brain.

Source: Levy, Koeppen and Stanton 2006: Neill and Knowles 2004; Tortora and Derrickson 2009.

- The outer layer, known as the marginal layer which develops into the white matter of the nervous system.
- The middle layer, known as the mantle layer which develops into the grey matter of the nervous system.
- The inner layer, known as the ependymal layer which forms the lining of the ventricles.

The neural crest, which is a mass of cells arising from the neuroectoderm, separates from the neural tube and gives rise to:

- Spinal nerves and posterior root ganglia of the spinal nerves.
- Ganglia of the cranial nerves.
- Ganglia of the ANS.
- Adrenal medulla.

Brief overview of neuroanatomy and physiology

The nervous system consists of two major divisions:

- The peripheral nervous system (PNS).
- The central nervous system (CNS).

The CNS consists of both the brain and the spinal cord, and is the principal integrator of sensory input and motor output. The CNS is capable of evaluating incoming information and formulating responses to changes that threaten the homeostatic balance.

The brain is one of the largest organs of the body, weighing around 1.3 kg when fully grown. The brain of an average adult is made up of approximately 1000 billion neurones and makes approximately 20% of the body's oxygen demands. Because the brain and spinal cord are both delicate and vital, nature has provided them with two protective coverings. The outer covering consists of bone: cranial bones encase the brain; vertebrae encase the spinal cord. The inner covering consists of three distinct membrane layers known as the meninges.

The meninges

These are three layers covering the brain and the spinal cord. The outermost is the dura mater which is made of strong white fibrous tissue. Owing to its proximity to the cranial vault it also serves as the inner periosteum of the cranial bones. The dura mater has three important inward extensions:

- Falx cerebri – this projects downward into the longitudinal fissure to form a partition between the two cerebral hemispheres (falx means sickle and refers to the curving sickle shape of this partition as it extends from the roof of the cranial cavity).
- Falx cerebelli – this is a sickle-shaped extension that separates the two halves, or hemispheres, of the cerebellum.
- Tentorium cerebelli – this separates the cerebellum from the cerebrum (tentorium means tent and refers to the tent-like covering over the cerebellum).

The arachnoid mater, a delicate, cobweb-like layer, lies between the dura mater and the pia mater, or innermost layer of the meninges.

The transparent pia mater adheres to the outer surface of the brain and spinal cord and contains blood vessels.

There are several spaces between and around the meninges known as the epidural, subdural and subarachnoid spaces.

The epidural ('on the dura') space is immediately outside the dura mater but inside the bony coverings of the spinal cord. It contains a supporting cushion of fat and other connective tissues. Around the brain, because the dura mater is continuous with the periosteum on the inside face of the cranial bones, there is no epidural space normally present.

The subdural ('under the dura') space is between the dura mater and arachnoid mater. The subdural space contains a small amount of lubricating serous fluid.

As its name suggests, the subarachnoid space is under the arachnoid mater and outside the pia mater. This space contains a significant amount of cerebrospinal fluid.

Spinal anaesthesia

This is induced by injecting small amounts of local anaesthetic into the cerebrospinal fluid (CSF). The injection is usually made in the lumbar spine below the level at which the spinal cord ends (L2).

Epidural anaesthesia

The segmental nerves in the thoracic and lumbar region contain somatic sensory, motor and autonomic (sympathetic) nerve fibres. The introduction of anaesthetic agents produces a regional anaesthesia.

The ventricles

The four, fluid-filled spaces within the brain are the ventricles. Two of them, the lateral (or first and second) ventricles, are located one in each hemisphere of the cerebrum. The third ventricle is little more than a thin, vertical pocket of fluid below and medial to the lateral ventricles. The fourth ventricle is a tiny, diamond-shaped space where the cerebellum attaches to the back of the brainstem. The fourth ventricle is simply a slight expansion of the central canal extending up from the spinal cord.

Cerebrospinal fluid (CSF)

Further protection of the brain and spinal cord against injury is provided by a cushion of fluid both around the organs and within them called cerebrospinal fluid. CSF, which is produced by the ependymal cells in the ventricles and from a collection of capillaries known as the choroids plexus, is a clear, colourless liquid which contains proteins, glucose, urea and salts. CSF is responsible for delivering nutritive substances filtered from the blood to the cells in the brain and spinal cord, as well as removing waste products and toxic substances. This is achieved through the constant circulation of CSF through the subarachnoid space around the brain and spinal cord, as well as the ventricles themselves. The cerebrospinal fluid does more than simply provide a supportive, protective cushion; it is also a reservoir of circulating fluid which, along with blood and the brain monitors for changes in the internal environment – for example, changes in the carbon dioxide (CO_2) content of CSF trigger homeostatic responses in the respiratory control centres of the brainstem which help regulate

Table 7.2 Cranial nerves and their primary functions

	Cranial nerve	Function controlled
I	Olfactory	Sensory – smell
II	Optic	Sensory – vision
III	Oculomotor	Motor – all eye muscles except those served by IV and VI
IV	Trochlear	Motor – superior oblique muscle
V	Trigeminal	Sensory – face, sinuses and teeth
		Motor – muscles of mastication
VI	Abducens	Motor – external rectus muscle
VII	Facial	Motor – facial muscles
VIII	Vestibulocochlear	Sensory – inner ear
IX	Glossopharyngeal	Motor – pharyngeal musculature
		Sensory – posterior part of the tongue, tonsil and pharynx
X	Vagus	Motor – heart, lungs, bronchi and gastrointestinal tract
		Sensory – heart, lungs, trachea, pharynx, larynx, gastrointestinal tract and external ear
XI	Accessory	Motor – sternocleidomastoid and trapezius muscle
XII	Hypoglossal	Motor – muscles of the tongue

the overall CO_2 content and pH of the body. CSF is reabsorbed through the arachnoid villi in the sagittal sinus and is absorbed as quickly as it is formed. At any one time there is between 80 and 150 ml of CSF within the entire CNS.

Cranial nerves

There are 12 pairs of cranial nerves, the functions of which are detailed in Table 7.2.

The brain

There are four principal parts to the brain (Table 7.3):

- Brain stem (medulla oblongata, pons, midbrain).
- Cerebrum.
- Cerebellum.
- Diencephalon (hypothalamus, thalamus, pineal gland).

The blood–brain barrier

The blood–brain barrier exists to protect the brain cells from harmful substances and pathogens. The barrier is not a physical barrier as such, but a combination of the presence of tight junctions in the endothelial cells of the capillaries and the presence of a basement membrane around the capillaries.

The blood–brain barrier is selectively permeable to certain substances, including:

- Water.
- Oxygen and carbon dioxide.
- Glucose.

- Alcohol.
- Anaesthetic agents.

The blood–brain barrier is essentially impermeable to proteins and most antibiotics. Trauma, certain toxins and inflammation can cause a breakdown of the blood–brain barrier.

Neurological assessment

Neurological assessment in the critically ill child is a challenging part of critical care nursing as many factors may affect the child's neurological function, including the child's underlying cognitive maturation, the effects of sedative or analgesic agents, the consequences of systemic critical illness, as well as the psychological effects of intensive care. Neurological assessment is important because it is the only guide to neurological function in children who are unable to communicate due to age or cognitive ability, and prevention of secondary insult is vital in improving morbidity (and mortality) in children with primary brain injury.

The immaturity of the infant's neurological system is very evident, as is their subsequent growth and development. The major portion of brain growth occurs in the first year of life, along with completion of the myelination of brain and nervous system. Motor function maturation proceeds in a cephalocaudal direction and is a succession of integrated milestones. Brain growth continues up to 15 years of age. There are a number of primitive reflexes

Table 7.3   Principal parts of the brain and their functions

Structural components	Anatomy and summary of the functions
Brain stem	
Medulla	The medulla is continuous with the spinal cord, beginning at the foramen magnum and extending to the inferior border of the pons. The white matter of medulla contains all the sensory (ascending) tracts and all the motor (descending) tracts which extend between the spinal cord and the rest of the brain. Some of the white matter forms bulges on the anterior aspect of the medulla, which are known as pyramids. These contain the corticospinal tracts that run from the cerebrum to the spinal cord. Just above junction of medulla and spinal cord, decussation of the pyramids occurs. This is where 90% of axons in the right pyramid and 90% of axons in the left pyramid cross to their respective opposite pathways. This explains why the right side of the brain controls the left side of the body, and vice versa. The medulla also contains several nuclei which are masses of grey matter where neurons form synapses with each other. A number of these nuclei control essential functions including: • Cardiovascular centre responsible for controlling the rate and force of the heartbeat and diameter of blood vessels. • Medullary rhythmicity area which is responsible for adjusting the basic rhythm of breathing. • Other nuclei which are involved in coordinating vomiting, coughing, swallowing, sneezing and hiccups. The posterior part of medulla contains nuclei associated with the sensations of touch, conscious proprioception and vibration Additionally the medulla contains nuclei associated with five pairs of cranial nerves: • Vestibulocochlear (VIII) • Glossopharyngeal (IX) • Vagus (X) • Accessory (XI) • Hypoglossal (XII)
Pons	The pons (bridge) lies directly above the medulla and anterior to the cerebellum. It consists of both nuclei and tracts and the primary function is to act as a bridge connecting various parts of the brain. Signals for voluntary movements originate in the cerebral cortex and are relayed through pontine nuclei into the cerebellum. Pneumotaxic area – (pontine respiratory group PRG) The PRG antagonises the apneustic centre, cyclically inhibiting inspiration. The PRG limits the burst of action potentials in the phrenic nerve, effectively decreasing the tidal volume and regulating the respiratory rate. Absence of the PRG results in an increase in depth of respiration and a decrease in respiratory rate. Apneustic area The apneustic centre of the lower pons appears to promote inspiration by the stimulation of the neurons in the medulla oblongata providing a constant stimulus.
Midbrain	The midbrain extends from the pons to the diencephalon and contains both tracts and nuclei. The cerebral aqueduct passes through the midbrain connecting the third ventricle above it with the fourth ventricle below. • The anterior part of midbrain contains a pair of tracts called the cerebral peduncles which contain the axons of the corticospinal/ corticopontine and corticobulbar motor neurones. These transmit nerve impulses from the cerebrum to the spinal cord/pons and medulla.

- The posterior part of the midbrain (the tectum) contains four rounded elevations which are reflex centres for certain visual and auditory responses and the movement of the eyes, head and neck to facilitate these responses.

The midbrain also contains nuclei known as the substantia nigra. These are large, darkly pigmented nuclei that produce dopamine which is responsible for subconscious muscle movement.

The midbrain contains the nuclei associated with two pairs of cranial nerves

- Oculomotor (III)
- Trochlear (IV)

Reticular formation

The reticular formation (RF) is a broad area which extends from the upper part of the spinal cord throughout the brain stem into the lower part of the diencephalon. Clusters of neuronal cell bodies (grey matter) interspersed among small bundles of myelinated axons (white matter) are found throughout the brain stem and form the RF. These neurones have both sensory and motor functions.

Reticular Activating System (RAS)

Composed of sensory axons which project to the cerebral cortex, the RAS helps maintain consciousness and is active when we are awakened from sleep. The RAS is also responsible for helping regulate muscle tone (degree of contraction in normal resting muscles)

Cerebrum

The cerebrum is known as the 'seat of intelligence'. The right and left halves of the cerebrum are known as cerebral hemispheres and are separated by the falx cerebri. The hemispheres are connected internally by the corpus callosum which is a broad band of white matter (containing axons). Each hemisphere consists of:

- An outer rim of grey matter.
- An internal region of cerebral white matter.
- Grey matter nuclei deep within white matter.

Absence of the corpus callosum may be indicative of Aicardi syndrome.

Each hemisphere can be further subdivided into four lobes: frontal, parietal, temporal and occipital.

- The central sulcus separates the frontal lobe from the parietal lobe.
- The precentral gyrus, which lies immediately in front of the central sulcus, contains the primary motor area of the cerebral cortex.
- The postcentral gyrus, which is located immediately posterior to the central sulcus, contains the primary somatosensory area of the cerebral cortex.

Basal ganglia

Within each cerebral hemisphere are three nuclei collectively termed as the basal ganglia.

Basal ganglia receive input from the cerebral cortex and provide output to the motor parts of the cortex via the medial and ventral group nuclei of the thalamus. In addition, the basal ganglia have extensive pathways which connect to each other.

The major function of the basal ganglia to is to help regulate the initiation and termination of movements as well as controlling subconscious skeletal muscle contraction.

(Continued)

Table 7.3 (Continued)

Structural components	Anatomy and summary of the functions
Cerebellum	The cerebellum occupies the inferior and posterior portions of the cranial vault. It resembles a butterfly in shape with a central constricted area known as the vermis and lateral lobes which are the cerebellar hemispheres. Each hemisphere consists of lobes which are separated by deep and distinct fissures. The superficial layer of the cerebellum is the cerebellar cortex consisting of grey matter. Lying under the grey matter is the white matter, which lies in tracts known as arbor vitae. Buried within the white matter lie the cerebellar nuclei, which give rise to axons carrying impulses from the cerebellum to other brain structures and the spinal cord. Three paired cerebellar peduncles attach the cerebellum to the brain stem. Each of the peduncles carry different sets of information, e.g. • Inferior cerebellar peduncle – sensory information from the vestibular apparatus of the inner ear to the cerebellum. The primary function of the cerebellum is to evaluate how well movements initiated by the motor areas of the cerebrum are being carried out. Feedback signals are relayed to the motor areas of the cerebral cortex via the thalamus/red nuclei to correct abnormal movements. The cerebellum is also the main area for the regulation of balance and posture. Abnormalities within the cerebellum will lead to disorders of speech patterns and ataxias.
Diencephalon	The hypothalamus is responsible for the maintenance of the body's homeostatic balance. It achieves this through undertaking a number of roles: • Control of the autonomic nervous system. • Production of hormones which act on the pituitary gland (see Table 7.4). • Regulation of emotional and behavioural patterns. • Regulation of eating and drinking. • Control of body temperature. • Regulation of circadian rhythms and states of consciousness. The epithalamus consists of the pineal gland and habenular nuclei. • The pineal gland secretes melatonin, which contributes to the promotion of sleep and is thought to assist with the regulation of the body's biological clock. • The habenular nuclei are involved in olfaction, especially emotional responses to familiar smells such as perfume, aftershave and home cooking. The thalamus lies above the midbrain and contains nuclei which serve as relay stations for sensory impulses travelling to the cerebral cortex. The thalamus is also responsible for the crude appreciation of pain, temperature and pressure, as well as being involved in the mediation of some motor activities.

Source: Levy et al. 2006; Tortora and Derrickson 2009.

Table 7.4 Hormones secreted by the hypothalamus and the area of the pituitary gland affected

Anterior pituitary	Posterior pituitary
Thyrotrophin releasing hormone (TRH)	Vasopressin (ADH)
Gonadotrophin releasing hormone (GnRH)	Oxytocin
Growth hormone releasing hormone (GHRH)	These travel via the neurons to the posterior pituitary where they are
Corticotrophin releasing hormone (CRH)	released directly into the blood
Somatostatin	stream.
Dopamine	
These are released into the blood and travel to the capillary bed in the anterior pituitary gland where they trigger the release of other hormones.	

present in the infant which disappear over the first few months of life. The absence of these reflexes in the newborn, or their presence after the first year of life, is a cause of concern and merits further investigation.

- Palmar grasp (birth): disappears by 3 months.
- Plantar grasp (birth): disappears by 9 months.
- Moro reflex (birth): disappears by 6 months.
- Placing (4 days): disappearance variable.
- Stepping (0–8 weeks): disappears before walking.
- Fencing (2–3 months): disappears by 6 months.

Consideration for practice

The plantar reflex (also known as the Babinski response), the presence of which is an abnormal finding in the older child or adolescent, is an unreliable reflex test in younger children who have yet to start walking and will be present in infants under the age of 1 year as a normal finding. A positive Babinski response means that when the sole of the foot is stroked in an upward motion, the toes will fan out rather than the foot flexing at the ankle and the toes curling inwards as would be expected.

The bones of the cranial vault are incompletely fused at birth, with the marginal gaps between them connected by membranous tissues. This facilitates a reduction in the skull size during the passage down the birth canal. The gaps between the bones are known as fontanelles and through a gradual process of ossification of the mem-

branes, the gaps close in the first two years of life. The anterior fontanelle lies in the midline between the frontal and parietal bones and will close between 18 months and 2 years of age. The posterior fontanelle, which lies between the parietal and occipital bones, usually closes within the first two months of life.

A rapid assessment tool, advocated for use primarily for the first assessment of a critically unwell infant or child (e.g. in the Emergency Department or in an emergency situation) is the AVPU scale. This very simple tool assesses the child's responsiveness, which is good indicator of general cerebral perfusion, however it does not provide the same depth of information regarding the function within the CNS so the infant or child with primary neurological dysfunction (traumatic or non-traumatic) should also be assessed using the appropriate GCSS (National Institute for Health and Clinical Excellence [NICE] 2007).

The most frequently used tool for neurological assessment used in critical care is the Glasgow Coma Scale Score (GCSS or GCS) which was originally developed in 1974 by Teasdale and Jennett for use in the adult population. The GCSS is divided into three sections– eye-opening response, verbal response and motor response – with a final score ranging from 3 to 15. The total score achieved is reflective of CNS functioning, with patients achieving low scores having decreased functioning. There have been a number of adaptations of the tool since its introduction and for the under 4 year olds, the modified Glasgow Coma Scale Score, adapted to take into account pre-verbal children, is now used. In addition, the James adaptation (JGCS), which includes a grimace score rather than a verbal score for intubated children (Tatman et al. 1997), ensures that this group of children can also be assessed fully.

One of the keys to effective assessment is validation of an individual practitioner's findings with the other healthcare professionals involved in the child's care to avoid irregularities in scoring based on subjective interpretation of the criteria applied within each section. Many centres have produced their own version of the GCSS/modified GCSS incorporated into printed observation charts such as that detailed in Figure 7.1, which allows for continuity of recorded observations in the child whose clinical condition changes (e.g. the child who either requires intubation or is successfully extubated).

Pupillary assessment of size, shape and reactivity is an important component of a neurological assessment.

Considerations for practice

- Pupil size can be influenced by poisons such as opiates (pinpoint) or tricyclic anti-depressants (dilated).

ADDRESSOGRAPH LABEL	Modified Paediatric Coma Score
Name:	Adapted by Tatman, Warren, Powell, Whitehouse & Noons 1997, Birmingham Children's Hospital NHS Trust
Date of Birth:	**Coma Score (Infant - < 4 yrs)**
Hospital No:	Ward Area: ....
Ward / Hospital:	Patient's Weight: .... in kilograms (kg)
	Patient's Height: .... in centimetres (cm)

		DATE:		
		TIME:		

NEURO OBSERVATIONS:

COMA SCALE				
	Eyes Open	Spontaneous	4	
		To verbal stimuli	3	
		To painful stimuli	2	
		No response to painful stimuli	1	
		Eyes closed – swelling / bandages	C	
	Best Motor Response	Obeys commands or normal spontaneous movements	6	
		Localises to painful stimuli or withdraws to touch	5	
		Withdraws to painful stimuli	4	
		Abnormal flexion to pain	3	
		Abnormal extension to pain	2	
		No response to pain	1	
		Not applicable	NA	
	Best Verbal OR Grimace Response — Verbal	Alert, babbles, coos, words / sentences to normal ability	5	
		Less than usual ability or spontaneous irritable cry	4	
		Cries inappropriately	3	
		Occasionally whimpers &/or moans	2	
		No response	1	
		Silent or mute	S	
		Intubated	T	
	Grimace	Spontaneous normal facial / oro-motor activity	5	
		Less than usual spontaneous ability or only response to touch stimuli	4	
		Vigorous grimace to pain	3	
		Mild grimace to pain	2	
		No grimace to pain	1	
		Not applicable	NA	
		Total Coma Score (out of 15)		

PUPIL SCALE IN mm

1mm	2mm	3mm	4mm	5mm	6mm	7mm	8mm	9mm
•	•	●	●	●	●	●	●	●

PUPIL	Right	Size	
		Reaction	
	Left	Size	
		Reaction	

+ = Reaction   - = No Reaction   S = Sluggish   C = Eyes Closed

LIMB MOVEMENTS	Arms	Normal power	
		Mild weakness	
		Severe weakness	
		Spontaneously	
		Painful stimuli	
		No response	
	Legs	Normal power	
		Mild weakness	
		Severe weakness	
		Spontaneously	
		Painful stimuli	
		No response	

Record right (R) and left (L) separately if there is a difference between the 2 sides.   P = Paralysed   # = Fracture

COMA SCORE GUIDELINES

- Painful stimuli should be created by applying central pressure for no longer than 30 seconds (i.e. sternal or supraorbital pressure).
- Score NA (not applicable) when there is for example brainstem, cervical spine cord or neuromuscular junction (neuromuscular block) impairment.
- Score C for eyes closed by swelling or bandage.
- Use Grimace score if there is no verbal (audible) response, i.e. if silent (S) or intubated (T).

Figure 7.1 Neurological observation chart for the under fours incorporating the grimace score. Reproduced with permission from Bristol Royal Hospital for Children.

- Unequal pupils can indicate a unilateral lesion.
- Unilateral dilated pupil may be indicative of 3rd nerve compression on the same side or a subdural haematoma.
- Reactivity – sluggish pupil reactions may occur due to sedation.
- Administration of adrenaline and/or atropine during resuscitation may lead to abnormal pupillary reactions (e.g. dilated, seemingly unreactive pupils in the immediate post-event period).
- The use of dilating drops for ophthalmological examination, in cases of suspected non-accidental injury, may cause abnormal findings (e.g. dilated unreactive pupils). Cyclopentolate drops, which are a parasympathetic antagonist, act by paralysing the iris sphincter muscle. This will both make the pupil larger and paralyse the muscle involved in focusing of the lens. The effects of cyclopentolate may last for up to 24 hours.
- Fixed and dilated pupils in the absence of the above factors indicate brain stem death/herniation.
- Congenital or acquired conditions may produce effects that influence pupil reactions, for example:
  – Coloboma: this is an uncommon, congenital condition characterised by a unilateral or bilateral partial iris defect.
  – Horner's syndrome: results from an interruption of the sympathetic nerve supply to the eye characterised by the classic triad of miosis (constricted pupil), the presence of a partial ptosis and loss of hemi-facial sweating (anhidrosis).

Other clinical parameters which should be incorporated as part of neurological assessment include:

- Heart rate, blood pressure, respiratory rate and pattern.
- Assessment for the presence of photophobia.
- Assessment for the presence of neck stiffness (meningism).
- Assessment of fontanelles – bulging anterior fontanelles may be indicative of volume overload or meningitis.
- Glucose – hypoglycaemia will lead to decreased levels of consciousness and possible coma.
- PaO_2 and $PaCO_2$ levels – hypoxia and hypercapnia both affect the child's level of consciousness.
- Core temperature – hypothermia will lead to altered level of consciousness and in neonates may lead to irregularities in respiratory pattern, periods of apnoea and bradycardia.

Causes of decreased conscious level in children are multifactorial, however coma in children is caused by diffuse metabolic insult in 95% of cases and by structural lesions in the remaining 5% (Advanced Paediatric Life Support 2011). Causes include:

- Head injury.
- Space-occupying lesions.
- Seizures.
- Infection.
- Metabolic causes, such as diabetic ketoacidosis, hypernatraemia, fulminant hepatic failure.
- Vascular lesions.
- Hypoxic, ischaemia, encephalopathy (HIE), post-cardiorespiratory failure.
- Administration of anaesthesia and/or sedative agents.
- Accidental or deliberate ingestion of toxins (e.g. alcohol and/or drugs).

Central nervous system infections

Bacterial meningitis

This is less common than viral meningitis but bacterial meningitis has a reported overall mortality of 10–30% worldwide (Levine et al. 2010). Up to 10% of children affected will suffer permanent neurological impairment such as hearing loss, memory loss or altered mood patterns.

The causative pathogens vary with age although there are some common causes across the age range seen in children's care (Table 7.5).

Table 7.5 Age-related bacterial causes of meningitis

Age group	Common causative pathogens
Newborn (up to 3 months)	Group B streptococcus *E. coli* Listeria *Haemophilus influenzae* type B (uncommon)
Infants/young children	*Neisseria meningitidis* (meningococcal infection) *Streptococcus pneumoniae* (pneumococcal infection) *Haemophilus influenzae* type B
School-age children	*Neisseria meningitidis* (meningococcal infection) *Streptococcus pneumoniae* (pneumococcal infection)

Pathophysiology of bacterial meningitis

Bacteria will either reach the subarachnoid space transported in the blood or may directly reach the meninges in patients with a parameningeal focus of infection, such as abscesses in the epidural or subdural spaces. Once the bacteria are established in the subarachnoid space, a host inflammatory response is triggered by bacterial cell wall products produced as a result of bacterial lysis. This response is mediated by the stimulation of specific cells within the brain parenchyma which respond as macrophages would and produce cytokines and other inflammatory mediators. This cytokine activation then initiates several processes that ultimately cause damage in the subarachnoid space, culminating in neuronal injury and cell death through apoptosis. As a consequence of the infective processes and the responses invoked there is swelling and proliferation of the endothelial cells in the local arterioles and the veins causing obstruction of flow through these vessels. This results in an increase in intracellular sodium and intracellular water. The development of cerebral oedema further compromises cerebral circulation, which can result in increased intracranial pressure. Increased secretion of antidiuretic hormone resulting in the syndrome of inappropriate antidiuretic hormone secretion (SIADH) occurs in most patients with meningitis, which causes further retention of free water. These factors contribute to the development of either focal or generalised seizures.

Pathophysiology of neonatal meningitis

Bacteria from the maternal genital tract can colonise the foetus after the rupture of membranes and specific bacteria, such as *Group B streptococci (GBS)*, enteric gram-negative rods, and *Listeria monocytogenes* can reach the foetus via placental transfer and cause infection. Newborns can also acquire bacterial pathogens from their surroundings, and several host factors facilitate a predisposition to bacterial sepsis and meningitis. Bacteria reach the meninges via the bloodstream and cause inflammation. After reaching the CNS, bacteria spread from the longitudinal and lateral sinuses to the meninges, the choroid plexus and the ventricles. Inflammation of the meninges and ventricles produces a polymorphonuclear response alongside an increase in cerebrospinal fluid (CSF) protein content and an increased utilisation of glucose in CSF. Inflammatory changes and tissue destruction in the form of empyema and abscesses are more pronounced in gram-negative meningitis. Thick inflammatory exudate causes blockage of the aqueduct of Sylvius and other CSF pathways, resulting in both obstructive and communicating hydrocephalus.

Clinical presentation

The clinical signs of bacterial meningitis develop over a relatively short period, normally within a few hours. Early signs are very similar to those found in viral meningitis, although the relative rapidity of their development may give a clue to a bacterial cause.

Clinical signs may be divided into non-specific and specific signs (Table 7.6).

Considerations for practice

The presence of a non-blanching petechial rash is indicative of septicaemia and must be acted on immediately. Children may also present with coagulopathies, which again required prompt intervention.

Management of the child with bacterial meningitis

Priorities of care for this group of children are geared towards treating the symptoms and, where possible, preventing complications, such as cerebral oedema or cerebral abscesses.

Table 7.6   Clinical signs of bacterial meningitis

Non-specific signs	Specific signs
Lethargy and/or drowsiness Irritability and poor handling in the neonate Poor feeding Nausea and/or vomiting Fever Headache	Bulging fontanelles in infants Light sensitivity/photophobia Neck stiffness (may not be evident in infants) Decreased level of consciousness Seizures or other focal neurological signs Positive Brudzinski's or Kernig's signs. These are physical signs of meningeal irritation which can be elicited when the spinal cord is stretched or flexed. They may be absent in the younger child. • Brudzinski's sign is the involuntary flexion of the legs in response to the child's head and neck being lifted or flexed. • Kernig's sign is positive when the leg is bent at the hip and knee to a 90° angle and subsequent extension in the knee is painful leading to resistance.

- The main treatment priority is the administration of appropriate IV antibiotics according to the sensitivity of the organism involved. Once samples have been obtained broad spectrum therapy can be given until results are available.
- The use of steroids is advocated in the management of bacterial meningitis, with the drug of choice usually being dexamethasone. However, its use is not recommended in infants under 3 months of age or if more than 12 hours has passed since the administration of the first dose of antibiotics (NICE 2010).
- Lumbar puncture is contraindicated in children who are demonstrating signs of possible raised intracranial pressure as the sudden release of pressure could cause herniation of the brainstem. It is also contraindicated in the presence of a coagulopathy or cardiovascular instability. A CT scan may be required to determine the presence of cerebral oedema in these children.
- Fluid and electrolyte management – fluid restriction reduces the risk of the child developing cerebral oedema. Maintaining electrolytes within normal limits can prevent fluid shifts and reduce the risk of the child developing cerebral oedema. Increased cellular activity increases the metabolic demands for glucose and other nutrients, and as hypoglycaemia may cause seizures in children, it is essential that the serum blood glucose levels are maintained within normal limits.

Complications of bacterial meningitis
- Hearing loss.
- Subdural effusions (particularly associated with pneumococcal meningitis).
- Cerebral abscesses, which will require surgical drainage.
- Seizures.
- Hydrocephalus.

Viral meningitis

This is the most common cause of meningitis; most cases are relatively mild and seldom fatal. Viral meningitis does not usually result in septicaemia and the risk of complications is minimal in contrast with the bacterial form of the disease. It is extremely rare for a child with viral meningitis to warrant intensive care admission; indeed, few children will merit hospital admission at all.

Common causes include adenoviruses, herpes viruses, Epstein–Barr virus and, more rarely, the mumps virus. Clinical signs usually develop over a period of days, although they may have an acute onset (uncommon) but

are rather non-specific and mimic those seen in a flu-type illness.

Viral encephalitis

Encephalitis is a much rarer form of neurological illness than meningitis and refers to a more generalised inflammation of the brain tissue as well as possible involvement of the meninges. Encephalitis is normally viral in origin although bacterial and fungal-associated encephalitis can develop. The exact infective mechanism is virus-specific, with some being transmitted by human contact while others may occur as a consequence of insect or tick bites. Viral encephalitis can be primary (where virus is present in the CNS) or post-infection, due to immunoallergic mechanisms. More than 150 viruses have been implicated in the pathogenesis of encephalitis; however, because of limitations with diagnostic testing, causative factors of more than 50% of cases remain unknown (Yao et al. 2009).

Frequently identified viral strains responsible for encephalitis include:

- Herpes simplex virus (HSV) types 1 and 2.
- Epstein–Barr virus (EBV).
- Cytomegalovirus (CMV) (more common in immune-compromised children).
- Varicella zoster virus (VZV) (more common in immune-compromised children).
- Paramyxovirus family:
  – Measles.
  – Mumps.
- Togavirus family:
  – Rubella.
  – Human herpes virus 6.
  – Arbovirus (transmitted by tick bite).
  – Rabies (transmitted by animal bite).

Pathophysiology of viral encephalitis

The virus usually replicates outside the CNS and gains entry through the blood or by travelling along neural and olfactory pathways. Once the virus has crossed the blood–brain barrier it enters the neural cells, causing significant disruption in their functioning. As a consequence of viral infection, perivascular congestion, haemorrhage and significant inflammatory responses occur which affect the grey matter disproportionately to the white matter. Localised pathology occurs as a result of neurone cell membrane receptors found only in specific portions of the brain. An example is the herpes simplex virus (HSV), which targets the inferior and medial temporal lobes in particular.

Clinical presentation

- Fever.
- Uncharacteristic behaviour.
- Confusion and/or altered level of consciousness.
- Seizures.
- More focal neurological signs may be noted at initial presentation or they may become apparent as the illness progresses. These signs will be determined by the specific area(s) of the brain affected and will therefore vary from child to child.

Management of the child with encephalitis

Management of encephalitis is essentially supportive and follows the major principles detailed in the management of bacterial meningitis.

As the cause is normally viral in origin, the use of antibiotics is limited but aciclovir therapy should be continued until there is either confirmation of the viral organism involved or there has been exclusion of the HSV as the cause.

HSV is one of the least common causes of encephalitis but it can have devastating consequences if not managed correctly, with a mortality rate of >70% if untreated and ongoing neurological impairment in many of the children who survive. It may occur either as a primary infection or due to reactivation of latent infection, especially in the neonatal population. Clinical presentation is normally associated with a history of fever and malaise, in addition to which there may have been disturbances of memory or behaviour. The illness progresses with reduced levels of consciousness and seizures which are often focal and ongoing. HSV causes necrotic lesions, typically in the temporal lobes, but these can be widespread and even involve the brainstem. There is raised ICP and papilloedema in approximately 15% of cases and these children will require intensive care management (see Raised intracranial pressure).

Approximately 40% of children who survive will have long-term adverse consequences (Tunkel et al. 2008):

- Minor to major learning disabilities.
- Memory impairment.
- Neuropsychiatric abnormalities.
- Epilepsy.
- Fine motor control deficits.
- Dysarthria.

Acute disseminating encephalomyelitis (ADEM)

ADEM is an uncommon presentation of an inflammatory demyelinating disease which affects only a small number of children each year in the United Kingdom. The onset of ADEM usually occurs in the wake of either a clearly identifiable febrile prodromal illness or an episode of immunisation (although there remains considerable discussion in the literature about the strength of the evidence which supports this) and in association with encephalopathy of varying degrees, which is one of the differential diagnostic criteria distinguishing ADEM from multiple sclerosis (Dale and Branson 2005).

Clinical presentation

- Abrupt onset of lethargy and irritability.
- Altered level of consciousness.
- Behavioural changes.
- Fever.
- Headache.
- Focal or generalised signs of neurological dysfunction:
  - Focal or generalised seizures.
  - Ataxia.
  - Cranial nerve palsies.
  - Hemiparesis.

Management of the child with ADEM

Management is focused on reducing the inflammatory processes through the use of steroids and, in cases of refractory or relapsing disease, plasma exchange and the provision of IV immunoglobulin therapy. Intensive care support is matched to the individual child's needs, some of whom may require intubation and ventilatory support due to inadequate airway protective mechanisms or rapid deterioration in their clinical condition (Barry et al. 2010).

The prognosis is good for the majority of children, with full recovery occurring within weeks. Current acute mortality rates in the published literature are thought to be around 2% or less and mortality is most usually associated with children who have either fulminant cervical transverse myelitis or cerebral oedema. There is an increased risk of the child developing MS as a consequence of experiencing ADEM, with long-term figures being estimated at anywhere between 6 and 25% (Rust 2010; Wingerchuk 2006).

Guillain-Barré syndrome (GBS)

Classic GBS is a demyelinating neuropathy associated with ascending weakness, however there are a number of well-documented clinical variants. Among these are acute inflammatory demyelinating polyradiculoneuropathy, which is the most widely recognised form in Western countries, with variants known as acute motor axonal neuropathy (AMAN) and acute motor-sensory axonal neuropathy

(AMSAN) also being well recognised (Andary 2011). The most common presentation is characterised by an acute monophasic, non-febrile, post-infectious illness manifesting as ascending weakness and areflexia. Sensory, autonomic and brainstem abnormalities may also be seen during the child's clinical course (Chibber 2011).

Clinical presentation
- Abnormal gait.
- Progressive, symmetrical muscle weakness.
- Pain.
- Dysaesthesia (abnormal sensations such as a burning sensation).
- Autonomic instability resulting in orthostatic hypotension (secondary to standing upright), hypertension, pupillary dysfunction, sweating abnormalities and sinus tachycardia.
- Respiratory weakness leading to respiratory failure (in severe cases).
- Bulbar muscle weakness (in severe cases).

There are a number of stages in the disease process from the onset (1–2 weeks before becoming acutely unwell) through to acute presentation (for up to 2 weeks, with progression of symptoms during this phase), then a plateau phase before reaching recovery or the resolution phase. Just as symptoms develop in an ascending order, recovery occurs in descending order; therefore the last symptoms to develop should be the first to show signs of improvement.

Management of the child with GBS
As with the management of ADEM, the management of GBS is aimed at controlling symptoms and providing intensive care interventions such as ventilatory support (if required). Very few children require intensive care support; however, they may well need to be admitted for close observation if they have significant cardiovascular changes associated with autonomic instability.
Treatment strategies include:

- Regular assessment of respiratory function (4–6 hourly).
- Intubation and mechanical ventilation if respiratory failure present.
- Provision of IV immunoglobulin (IVIG) therapy over the first 3–5 days after acute presentation.*
- Use of plasma exchange for refractory disease.*
- Management of pain and or dysaesthesia with the use of agents such as gabapentin.
- Early physiotherapy to minimise the effects of immobility.

*There is an evidence base for the use of both IVIG and plasma exchange in the management of GBS with reported reductions in recovery time of as much as 50% (Miller 2011). There is no significant difference in terms of recovery demonstrated to date between the use of IVIG and plasma exchange in managing children or adults with GBS therefore most centres will use IVIG as a first-line intervention, given its ease of administration in comparison to plasma exchange. Similarly, there is no evidence to suggest that this combination of therapies administered together improves recovery rates (Hughes et al. 2010).

Seizure disorders
Seizure disorders in children are an extremely complex group of clinical presentations, the majority of which will not be addressed in this text. Rather, this section focuses on the care of the child presenting in the intensive care unit in status epilepticus (SE).

Basic pathophysiology of seizures
The brain has over 10 million neurones the function of which is to transmit information from cell to cell. This is achieved by the presence of chemical messengers which make the cells more or less excitable. During episodes of super-excitability, many cells will fire together and the brain activity at a cellular level becomes out of control. A single burst of excessive activity is known as an epileptic spike discharge and groups of these discharges, which are uninhibited or uncontrolled, will lead to epileptic fits or seizures.

Classification of seizures
There is a myriad of seizure types, but they can usually be classified as:

- Generalised – these arise over a wide area of the brain and affect both sides of the body from the beginning.
- Partial/focal – these arise from a specific focus in the brain and may be either simple or complex. These seizures may also develop into generalised seizures if they persist.

Acute causes of seizures
There is no identifiable cause in 50% of seizures. However, clinical conditions predisposing the infant or child to seizures include:

- Febrile convulsions.
- Toxic ingestion – poisons or alcohol.

- Metabolic disorders.
- Pre-existing seizure disorder – sub-therapeutic serum levels of anticonvulsants or concomitant illness.
- Trauma – head injury or birth trauma.
- Cerebral pathology – tumours, bleeds or abscesses.
- Systemic disturbances – sepsis, hepatic or renal failure.

Neonatal seizures

Most healthy babies display startle-like movements or fine tremors when stimulated or during active sleep, however seizure activity is usually unstimulated. Due to the immaturity of the neonate's brain, clinical signs of seizure activity may well be subtle and can therefore be missed. This is particularly applicable in the pre-term population (Lissauer and Clayden 2007). The causes of neonatal seizures differ slightly from those for children, although there are some common causes:

- Metabolic causes – hypoglycaemia, hypo-/hypernatraemia, hypocalcaemia, inborn errors of metabolism.
- Hypoxia.
- Hypoxic-ischaemic encephalopathy (HIE).
- Drug withdrawal (from maternal source).
- Kernicterus (condition in which bilirubin is deposited in brain tissue as a consequence of jaundice).
- Intracranial haemorrhage.
- Congenital infections – Group B streptococcus, hepatitis B and C, HSV, cytomegalovirus (CMV).

As noted, the clinical signs may be subtle in this age group, therefore frequent assessment of the neonate is essential if there are concerns about the possibility of seizure activity. Of concern are:

- Movement of the mouth in either a chewing motion or lip smacking.
- Grimacing.
- Deviation of the eyes or staring.
- Increased tone in one or more limbs.
- Hiccups not associated with feeds.

More general clinical signs include:

- Tachycardia.
- Tachypnoea.
- Bradycardia.
- Apnoeas.
- Posturing (abnormal flexion or extension of the limbs).

Children presenting in the intensive care unit with SE may well already be receiving anti-epileptic drugs (AEDs). Medications will vary according to type and presentation of seizures and the individual child's response to treatment strategies. Common anti-convulsants recommended for use in the management of seizure disorders in infants and children include (www.nice.org.uk/CG020):

- Phenobarbitone (used in infants <1 month).
- Phenytoin.
- Sodium valproate.
- Gabapentin.
- Carbamazepine.
- Lamotrigine.
- Clobazam.
- Keppra (levetiracetam).
- Topiramate.

Status epilepticus (SE)

SE is defined as a prolonged seizure lasting more than 30 minutes or recurrent seizures within a 30-minute period during which the infant or child does not regain consciousness. Such seizures are life-threatening and may result in permanent neurological injury. There can also be significant haemodynamic consequences of prolonged seizure activity which also contribute to potential long-term damage (Figure 7.2). The continued firing of the neurons increases the metabolic demands of the cerebral cells which eventually exceed the available nutrients leading to possible cell death.

SE can be subdivided into convulsive or non-convulsive presentations. As the name suggests, non-convulsive SE may be difficult to diagnose in the absence of any overt convulsive movements, therefore EEG studies are often required for a confirmed diagnosis to be made.

Management of the child in SE

The immediate aim of treatment is to control the seizure activity to reduce the potential for further harm. Adherence to published national guidelines, such as those from the Advanced Paediatric Life Support manual, will provide a step-by-step approach.

Immediate steps
- Airway.
- Breathing.
- Circulation.
- Administration of anti-convulsants (1–4) over a defined period of time (30 minutes).

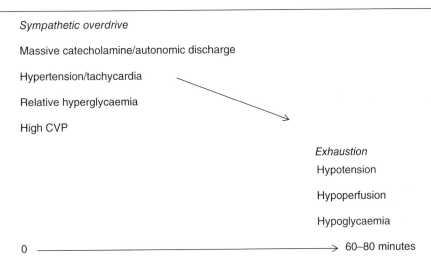

Figure 7.2 The haemodynamic effects of prolonged seizures.

1. IV lorazepam or rectal diazepam.
2. Rectal paraldehyde (if available).
3. IV phenytoin (or IV phenobarbitone if already on phenytoin).
4. If no relief from seizure activity after 30 minutes may need to consider thiopentone and rapid sequence induction.

Once there is control of seizure activity the management of the child in SE is centred on full neurological assessment and identification of the cause, which can be treated where indicated.

Investigations
- Lumbar puncture (contraindicated if there is a suspicion of raised intracranial pressure).
- EEG.
- CT scan.
- History from parents may be useful in those children with pre-existing seizure disorders as well as those with a first presentation.

Fluid management

Fluid restriction to two-thirds of usual requirements reduces the risk of the child developing cerebral oedema, although this may depend on the cause of the seizures. Electrolytes should be reviewed to ensure that serum sodium levels in particular are within normal range. Hypo- / hypernatraemia may be a precipitating factor for seizure activity.

Temperature management

Fever increases cellular metabolic demands and the use of available glucose and oxygen supplies, therefore the maintenance of normothermia is beneficial in reducing the demands placed on the body. Hyperthermia can be a contributory factor for seizure activity in some children.

Spinal cord injuries

Spinal cord injury is an uncommon presentation in children with this age group accounting for between 1 and 10% of all cases in published studies worldwide (Hagen et al. 2011; Muzumdar and Ventureyra 2006). Injuries may occur through a number of different mechanisms as a consequence of excessive acceleratory or deceleratory forces. Patterns of injury are different in children from those seen in adults as the spinal column in the young is very elastic and flexible compared with the older age group. There are more spinal cord injury without radiological abnormality (SCIWORA) and pure ligamentous injuries in children under the age of 10 years and more fracture subluxations in the over 10 age group. Similarly, there is a higher incidence of cervical spine fractures in adolescents than in the young child. Thoracolumbar and lumbar injuries are primarily lesions of adolescence.

Injury may be seen as a consequence of:

- Hyperextension (e.g. C2 fractures).
- Deformation.
- Hyperflexion.

- Axial loading (e.g. C1 fractures, which are very rare in children).
- Excessive rotation.

SCIWORA describes an acute spinal cord injury and may result in varying degrees of sensory or motor deficit, or both, without evidence of vertebral fracture or misalignment on plain X-rays and/or CT scans (Sidram et al. 2009). It is predominantly a presentation of childhood; however there are reported cases from the adult population. The possibility of SCIWORA is the key rationale for maintaining C-spine immobilisation in children until there is the chance to undertake a complete clinical examination, although practice varies. MRI scans may be useful to demonstrate the presence of haemorrhage or oedema in the cord and these findings are related to the overall prognosis for the child. MRI findings of either complete cord transection or the presence of major areas of haemorrhage within the cord are indicative of a very poor prognosis while the presence of minor haemorrhage or oedema alone offers a better outcome (Barry et al. 2010).

Clinical presentation (Table 7.7)

Clinical presentation will depend on the site of injury and whether it is complete or partial (Chapter 9).

Management of a child with spinal cord injury

Management of a child with spinal cord injury will be determined by its site and the relative stability of the injury. It is likely that a child with a complete C-spine fracture/injury higher than C3 will not survive the primary injury causing event as this type of injury will cause respiratory arrest. Cord injury around C3–C5 will cause respiratory insufficiency secondary to disruption of the impulses to the phrenic nerve responsible for movement of the diaphragm. These children will require long-term ventilatory support. Unstable injuries put the child at risk of secondary spinal cord injury, therefore immobilisation is necessary through the use of a halo traction system for C-spine injuries or a plaster jacket for mid-thoracic through to lumbar injuries. Surgical intervention, such as spinal fusion or surgical decompression, may be indicated if there is continued injury instability, misalignment or bone fragments or large clots are pressing on the spinal cord.

Steroids

Steroids are thought to moderate and reduce the effects of secondary injury to the spinal cord and studies have shown limited but significant improvement in the neurological

Table 7.7 Clinical signs of spinal cord injury

Cervical injury	Thoracic injury
When spinal cord injuries occur in the cervical area, symptoms can affect the arms, legs and middle of the body. The symptoms may be unilateral or bilateral.	When spinal injuries occur at a thoracic spine level, symptoms mainly affect the lower body.
• Respiratory failure.	• Loss of normal bowel and bladder control.
• Loss of normal bowel and bladder control (may include constipation, incontinence, bladder spasms).	• Numbness.
	• Sensory changes.
	• Spasticity (increased muscle tone).
• Numbness.	• Pain.
• Sensory changes.	• Weakness, paralysis.
• Spasticity (increased muscle tone).	
• Pain.	
• Weakness, paralysis.	

Injuries to the cervical or high thoracic spinal cord may also result in blood pressure problems, abnormal sweating and trouble maintaining normal body temperature secondary to autonomic dysfunction.

outcome of adult patients treated within 8 hours of injury (Bracken 1999, updated 2007). While there is no established evidence base for their use in children, it is currently advocated in this population.

Cerebrovascular events

The incidence of cerebrovascular events or strokes in children is rare but there is an associated risk in children with certain underlying conditions such as:

- Sickle cell disease.
- Cerebral vascular abnormalities:
  – AV malformations.
  – Aneurysms.
- Cerebral infections.
- Congenital heart disease:
  – Cyanotic lesions with induced polycythaemia.
  – Post-cardiopulmonary bypass.

These events may be thrombotic, embolic or haemorrhagic in nature and require urgent treatment. The management priorities are the same as the general management strategies detailed for a child with raised intracranial pressure, while the underlying cause of the stroke will require tailored intervention depending on the type of event and the child's overall clinical condition.

CNS and brain tumours

Brain and CNS tumours (malignant and non-malignant) are the second most common group of cancers in children, accounting for a quarter of all childhood cancers. In the United Kingdom, brain tumours occur in about 5/100 000 of children between the ages of 0 and 9 years meaning around 300 children are diagnosed each year. Tumours may be broadly classified based on their location within the brain/CNS and will either be supratentorial (involving the cerebral hemispheres and structures above the tentorium cerebelli) or infratentorial (involving the brainstem and structures below the tentorium cerebelli). The majority of tumours (70–80%) are infratentorial.

Types of tumour

The largest subgroup is the astrocytoma, which can be diagnosed at any time throughout childhood. They account for around 43% of all brain and CNS tumours in children. These tumours can be further classified according to the speed at which they grow – grade 1 is the slowest-growing type and grade 4 is the fastest-growing type. About three-quarters (76%) of astrocytomas are diagnosed as low-grade and around 15% classified as high-grade.

The second most common subgroup is the intracranial and intraspinal embryonic tissue tumours, which account for around 19% of all childhood brain and CNS tumours. The majority of these are primitive neuroectodermal tumours (PNETs) and about 73% are medulloblastomas. PNETs occur most frequently in younger children (Cancer Research UK 2008; Packer et al. 2008).

Management of the child with a brain or CNS tumour

Management strategies will be determined by the type, location and grade of tumour. Surgical removal, chemotherapy, radiotherapy, or a combination of these interventions, will be required. Intensive care management will focus on symptom management and facilitation of any of the interventions. (For further details of the management of the child with an oncological diagnosis see Chapter 11.)

Raised intracranial pressure

The brain occupies a rigid container (the skull) with a fixed volume (once the fontanelles have closed). It shares the space with the two other components which together make up the contents of the intracranial vault:

- Brain (80%).
- Cerebrospinal fluid (10%).
- Blood (10%).

Intracranial pressure (ICP) is defined as the pressure exerted by the three components against the inside of the skull. Given the presence of the open fontanelles in the under 2 year olds, the intracranial pressure is lower in the infant and rises once the fontanelles close, gradually increasing until it reaches the normal values expected in the adult.

Normal ICP depends on age, body posture and level of activity. The normal ICP value in a healthy adult ranges between 7 and 15 mmHg. In term infants, values between 1.5 and 6 mmHg are considered normal, whereas in children values between 3 and 7 mmHg are cited (Steiner and Andrews 2006).

As the volume of the brain parenchyma cannot be adjusted, normal ICP is maintained primarily through a balance between CSF production and CSF absorption. At any one time there is between 80 and 150 ml of CSF within the CNS. In addition, autoregulation of cerebral blood flow helps maintain adequate constant cerebral perfusion, with the blood flow volume being regulated through a tight coupling of cerebral metabolism with regional blood flow. Cerebral blood vessels have the ability to change diameter to maintain constant flow regardless of the mean arterial pressure. These two mechanisms help to maintain intracranial pressure within normal limits on a day-to-day basis.

According to the Monro–Kellie hypothesis, an increase in the volume of one of the three components will cause ICP to rise unless there is proportional reduction in the volume of one of the other two components. The ability of the brain to accommodate changes in the intracranial volume is achieved by two properties:

- Elastance – relates to the stretchiness of the intracranial compartments.
- Compliance – the ability to tolerate an increase in volume without a corresponding increase in pressure.

If the brain develops poor compliance and high elastance owing to pathological processes, it will no longer have further elastic properties. Once it is stretched to its maximum and there is a subsequent increase in the volume of the intracranial vault (tissue, blood or CSF), there will be increased intracranial pressure.

Cerebral perfusion pressure (CPP)

CPP is the driving pressure required to maintain effective cerebral blood flow to meet cellular metabolic demands (in conjunction with autoregulation). If the pressure within the intracranial vault rises due to pathological processes, then the pressure required to drive blood up towards the cerebral circulation increases. CPP is calculated by subtracting the ICP value from the mean arterial pressure (MAP) and to measure CPP accurately invasive monitoring of both MAP and ICP is required. There is considerable discussion in the literature regarding the required CPP in children and various values are suggested, for example in Chambers et al. (2006) the CPP critical threshold values determined for children aged 2–6, 7–10 and 11–15 years were 48, 54, and 58 mmHg respectively. A later study, however, suggested that a CPP of more than 50 mmHg was the minimum required to support cerebral function (ages 6 months–12 years) with preferred CPP values of >60 mmHg in the under 2 year olds and >70 mmHg in the over 2 year olds (Shetty et al. 2008).

Definition of raised ICP measurements
- Normal: <10 mmHg.
- Abnormal: sustained level >15 mmHg.
- Moderate: 21–40 mmHg.
- Severe: >40 mmHg.

Causes of raised ICP
- Trauma.
- Tumours – primary and secondary.
- Hypoxia – ischaemic encephalopathy.
- Hypermetabolic states – seizures and hyperpyrexia.
- Metabolic disorders – liver failure, DKA and severe hypoglycaemia.
- Infection – encephalitis and meningitis.
- Vascular – subarachnoid haemorrhage and infarction.

Measurement of intracranial pressure

There are a number of sites where an ICP monitor can be placed (Table 7.8). ICP pulse waveforms are generated from a pressure wave transmitted through the cardiovascular system into the tissues within the intracranial cavity including the choroid plexus, where CSF is produced (Arbour 2004). The ICP monitoring waveform has a flow of three upstrokes (P) in one wave:

- P1 (percussion wave) represents arterial pulsation.
- P2 (tidal wave) represents intracranial compliance.
- P3 (dicrotic wave) represents aortic valve closure.

Table 7.8 Sites for ICP monitor placement

Device/Site	Advantages	Disadvantages
Intraventricular catheter	Gold standard of accuracy. Allows for sampling of CSF. Allows ICP control through CSF drainage. Inexpensive.	Most invasive. Sometimes difficult to cannulate the ventricle. Catheter can be occluded by blood or tissue. Needs repositioning of transducer level with change in head position. Potential source of infection.
Subarachnoid bolt/ screw	Quickly and easily placed. Does not invade brain. Allows sampling of CSF. May have lower infection rate.	Catheter can be occluded by tissue or blood. Needs to be recalibrated frequently.
Subdural, epidural catheter	Least invasive. Easily and quickly placed.	Increasing baseline drift over time, therefore accuracy and reliability are questionable. Does not provide CSF sampling.
Fibreoptic probe/ catheter	Can be placed in the subdural, subarachnoid, intraventricular or intraparenchymal spaces. Easily transported. Minimal artefact and drift. High resolution of waveform.	Cannot be recalibrated after it is placed, unless a ventriculostomy is used simultaneously for reference. Damage to or break in the cable makes it unusable.

Source: adapted from Zhong et al. 2003.

In a normal compliant brain, the highest peak or upstroke is seen in P1 with the upstroke of P2 being lower than P1 and P3 should show lowest upstroke. If the upstroke of P2 is equal to or higher than P1, then significant intracranial pressure is present (Czosnyka and Pickard 2004).

The management of the child with raised ICP is detailed in the management of the child with traumatic brain injury.

Traumatic brain injury (TBI)

One million people attend Emergency Departments in the United Kingdom every year with some degree of head injury, half of whom (500 000) are children <16 years of age, however only 5% of these are deemed to be severe (Dunning et al. 2006). Severe traumatic brain injury is an important contributor to morbidity as well as mortality in children. Children are more susceptible to severe TBI due to pliable skull bones, weak cervical musculature and proportionally bigger head mass to body ratio (Walker et al. 2009). In children aged 4 years or less, between 30 and 50% of traumatic brain injury is caused by a fall or is inflicted by a carer. Overall mortality in children is lower than in adults with TBI, 2.5% vs. 10.4% (Sookplung and Vavilala 2009), however morbidity is generally more significant in children due to the vulnerability of the immature brain and enhanced mechanisms of cellular destruction. In the infant population with inflicted TBI there are usually associated repeated injury patterns and episodes as well as delay in seeking treatment, which lead to a significant degree of hypoxic–ischaemic injury seen less commonly in adult TBI. This has implications for some of the proposed cellular changes associated with children.

Traumatic brain injury involves two separate but interrelated processes: the primary injury which causes direct disruption to the brain parenchyma, and the secondary injury, characterised by a cascade of biochemical, cellular and molecular events resulting in further injury to the brain tissue (Martin and Falcone 2008; Walker et al. 2009).

Primary brain injury may be caused by any or a combination of:

- Cerebral lacerations.
- Cerebral contusions – may be coup (damage to tissue directly below the point of injury) or contrecoup injuries (damage to tissue on the opposite side of the brain to the initial point of injury).
- Dural sac tears.
- Diffuse axonal injuries.
- Concussion.
- Intracranial haemorrhage.
- Subarachnoid haemorrhage.

- Extradural or subdural haematoma.
- Intraventricular haemorrhage.
- Basal skull fractures.

Depressed skull fractures

A depressed skull fracture is defined as displacement of the inner table of the skull by more than one thickness of the bone. Most depressed fractures are simple and the dura remains intact underneath the depressed segment. However, up to 30% are associated with a dural laceration or tear.

Basal skull fractures

Signs of a basal skull fracture include evidence of blood or cerebrospinal fluid leaking from the ear or nose, Battle's sign, haemotympanum, facial crepitus or serious facial injury. Children with basal skull fractures are at increased risk of developing meningitis and are especially vulnerable to infection with *Streptococcus pneumoniae*, therefore consideration should be given to the administration of the pneumococcal vaccine in these children.

Traumatic axonal injury (TAI)

TAI encompasses a broad spectrum from mild to severe traumatic brain injury. The extent and distribution of TAIs depend on the injury severity and they may be classed as either focal or diffuse. Primary traumatic axonal injury occurs within three hours of injury with secondary axonal injury developing after this time. Secondary axonal injury is part of the continuum of secondary brain injury.

Pathophysiology of axonal injury

The different layers of the brain move at different rates because each layer has a different density. The axons can therefore end up being stretched, sheared, twisted or compressed as a consequence of the time delay between the movements of the layers. The injury involves reactive swelling at the axonal site which leads to:

- Loss of control of ionic flux.
- Compaction of the neurofilaments.

This process obstructs axonal transport and causes further damage along the length of the axon. The flow of ions and fluid into the axon causes it to swell, which in turn leads to the destruction of the neurolemma (a thin layer of cells, called Schwann cells which myelinate the axon). The axon then separates in the area of the swelling. The end of the axon (the distal portion) that is furthest from the cell body disintegrates and the remaining portion of the axon also dies.

Secondary brain injury

There are thought to be a number of pathways which contribute to the development of secondary brain injury, including:

- Ischaemia.
- Continuation of axonal injury.
- Inflammation and regeneration.
- Secondary cerebral swelling due to vasogenic and cytotoxic cerebral oedema.

Post-traumatic ischaemia

Early post-traumatic hypoperfusion is thought to be very relevant to outcome and there is a relatively short time frame early post-injury in which measures may be effective. Causes of post-injury ischaemia may be related to the presence of hypotension and hypoxaemia or to a loss of regulatory control within the cerebral circulation (Table 7.9). This loss of regulatory control is thought to be more significant in children aged <4 years (Freeman et al. 2008).

Neuronal excitotoxicity

Excitotoxicity is the process through which cells are damaged by excitatory amino acids such as glutamate (normally a neurotransmitter). Glutamate, when present in large volumes, causes cell death as a consequence of altered cellular metabolism. Glutamate exposure may lead to disruption of the normal influx and efflux of calcium in

the cells as well as causing a sodium- dependent neuronal swelling. These processes lead to cell death. The mechanisms involved in this process are extremely complex and outside the scope of this text but this is an area which is the subject of continuing research in the management of TBI in children.

Brainstem death

Advances in intensive care provision in the 1980s and early 1990s meant that patients who would have previously not survived their initial illness and injury now did so, however this led to a number of severely brain-damaged patients being supported with mechanical ventilation in both paediatric and adult intensive care. The current position is that there is no statutory definition of death in the United Kingdom (Gallimore 2006; Niranjan and Duffy 2008) and this was one of the factors in the development of the brainstem death criteria. The satisfactory application of these criteria ensures that where there is no hope of functional recovery, treatments which are not in the patient's best interests may be withdrawn. Brainstem death has been accepted in the United Kingdom as the death of an individual since 1976 (Inwald et al. 2000).

The situation for children is less clear cut and currently the consensus of opinion in the United Kingdom is that brainstem death criteria may not be used in infants less than 2 months of age (Niranjan and Duffy 2008), while in the United States the criteria may be applied to infants from 7 days of age if two separate EEG recordings have been made (Koszer 2010). For infants less than 37 weeks of gestational age the concept of brainstem death is deemed to be inappropriate. The most recent publication from the Academy of Royal Colleges (2008) offers a comprehensive code of practice concerning the diagnosis of death.

Brainstem death is defined as the irreversible cessation of brainstem function. Whether induced by intracranial events or the result of extracranial phenomena, such as hypoxia, it will produce this clinical state; therefore, irreversible cessation of the integrative function of the brainstem equates with the death of the individual and allows the medical practitioner to diagnose death (Academy of Royal Colleges 2008).

Three criteria must be fulfilled before testing may be considered (Table 7.10).

Brainstem death tests

The tests should be undertaken by two senior clinicians, one of whom is usually the consultant involved in the child's care. The tests examine cranial nerve function,

Table 7.9 Causes of post-traumatic ischaemia in the development of secondary brain injury

Causes of hypotension and hypoxaemia	Loss of regulatory control
Ischaemia secondary to blood loss and hypotension. Hypoxia from inadequate ventilation caused by loss of respiratory drive. Hypoxia from airway obstruction or thoracic trauma. Ischaemia from poor cerebral perfusion secondary to raised intracranial pressure.	Loss of vasodilatory response to nitric oxide, prostaglandins and c-AMP. Loss of endothelial nitric oxide production. Elaboration of vasoconstriction mechanisms.

Table 7.10 Pre-existing criteria for consideration of brain stem death

1. There must be an identifiable pathology causing irremediable brain damage. This may be intra- or extracranial in origin.
2. The patient must be deeply unconscious and the following factors accounted for:
   (a) Hypothermia must be excluded as the cause of unconsciousness and the patient's core temperature should be >34 °C.
   (b) There should be no evidence that the patient's state is due to depressant drugs. This refers to narcotics, hypnotics and tranquillisers as well as neuromuscular blocking drugs. A careful drug history is required, while drug levels and antagonists may need to be used.
   (c) Potentially reversible circulatory, metabolic and endocrine disturbances must have been excluded as the cause of the continuing unconsciousness. Some of these disturbances may occur as a result of the condition rather than the cause and these do not preclude the diagnosis of brain stem death.
3. The patient must be apnoeic, needing mechanical ventilation. This condition must not be secondary to the effect of sedative drugs or neuromuscular blockade. This may require testing with a nerve stimulator to show intact neuromuscular transmission. Alternatively, demonstration of tendon reflexes can also demonstrate intact transmission.

Table 7.11 Brainstem death testing criteria

	Test	Cranial nerves tested
Pupillary response to light	Pupils must be fixed in diameter and unresponsive to incident light.	II, III
Corneal reflex	There must be no corneal reflex when a soft piece of material (usually cotton wool) is passed gently over the cornea.	V, VII
Vestibulo-ocular reflexes	There must be no eye movements following the slow injection of at least 50 ml of ice cold water over 1 minute into each external auditory meatus (the normal reflex is deviation of the eyes away from the side of the stimulus). Injury or pathology may prevent this test being performed on both sides – this does not invalidate the test.	VIII, III
Motor response	No motor responses in the cranial nerve distribution should occur as a result of stimulation of any somatic area. No limb movement should occur in response to supra-orbital pressure.	V, VII
Gag reflex	No gag reflex should be present in response to posterior pharyngeal wall stimulation with a spatula.	IX
Cough reflex	No cough or other reflex should occur in response to bronchial stimulation by a suction catheter being passed down the ETT.	X
Respiratory drive/ effort	No respiratory movements should occur in response to disconnection from the ventilator. This tests the stimulation of respiration by $PaCO_2$, which should be allowed to rise to 50 mmHg (6.65 kPa) and needs to be confirmed by arterial blood gases. Hypoxia should be prevented by pre-oxygenation and insufflation of oxygen through a tracheal catheter.	

brainstem function and respiratory drive (Table 7.11). While there is no specific timeframe identified which needs to be left between the two sets of tests, consideration must be given to the needs of the child's parents and wider family and a balance sought between completing the process and their need to spend time with the child. If the child fulfils each of the individual test criteria, then they have fulfilled brain stem death criteria.

Once the child has fulfilled the criteria, a discussion should be held with the child's parents about the possibility of organ donation. It is the responsibility of the senior staff (nursing or medical) involved in the child's care to notify the Specialist Nurse for Organ Donation or Clinical Lead for Organ Donation prior to the tests being carried out, so that any possible exclusion criteria for organ donation have been identified and staff are fully prepared for any questions the parents may have. These discussions should be held away from the clinical setting wherever possible. It is imperative that any religious and or cultural practices are taken into account when approaching parents for discussion regarding either brainstem death testing or organ donation. It is also important that these two subjects are not raised in the same discussion with parents unless they raise the subject themselves at that point. The fulfilment of brainstem death criteria does not automatically mean that the child is suitable for organ donation or that parents will wish to consider it (see Chapters 16 and 17).

Management of the child with TBI

The management of TBI in children is based on the 2003 'Guidelines for the acute medical management of severe traumatic brain injury in infants, children, and adolescents' published in *Pediatric Critical Care Medicine*. The key priorities of management are focused on:

- Maintaining good oxygenation.
- Maintaining effective circulation.
- Preventing intracranial hypertension, but
- Maintaining cerebral perfusion pressure (CPP).
- Maintaining glucose intake to meet demands but avoiding hyperglycaemia.
- Preventing or controlling seizures.

Ventilation management of child with traumatic brain injury

The purpose of intubation and mechanical ventilation in the child with severe TBI is threefold:

- To maintain a safe patent airway (loss of airway protective reflexes likely).

- To ensure delivery of maximal FiO_2, thus reducing the effects of hypoxia within the cerebral vasculature.
- To allow for the manipulation of $PaCO_2$, which can be important in preventing cerebral vasoconstriction or vasodilation, both of which may have detrimental effects on the cerebral vasculature and cerebral perfusion.

Hypoxia within the cerebral vasculature will induce vasodilation as the vessels attempt to maintain adequate cellular oxygen delivery. This will increase total cerebral blood flow and in situations where autoregulation is no longer intact will lead to increased intracranial pressure. Maintaining a normal PaO_2 will negate this potential action.

The relationship between hyperventilation and outcome is not clearly proven in paediatric studies (Curry et al. 2008). The evidence base suggests that hyperventilation can reduce CBF to potentially ischaemic levels and episodes of severe hypocarbia lead to worse outcomes (within 48 hours). In adult studies aggressive hyperventilation ($PaCO_2 < 30\,mmHg/4\,kPa$) has been shown to produce worse outcomes in TBI survivors.

The use of PEEP in children with TBI is sometimes considered controversial, given the potential effects of impeding venous drainage from the cerebral circuit due to the increased intrathoracic pressures generated, however this risk needs to be balanced against the risks associated with atelectasis and increased ventilation perfusion mismatching associated with low PEEP ventilation strategies which may contribute to post-injury hypoxia. Most clinicians recommend the use of normal PEEP values (4–$6\,cmH_2O$).

Temperature management

Hyperthermia

There are no published data for paediatrics, but adult studies have demonstrated that hyperthermia should be avoided in severe traumatic brain injury. Hyperthermia is related to:

- Increased cerebral metabolic demands.
- Increased inflammatory responses.
- Increased excitotoxicity.
- Increased cell death.

Induced hypothermia

It has long been accepted practice that induced hypothermia is a useful adjunct in the management of TBI in children although there has been wide variance in the levels of hypothermia induced. A multi-centred international

RCT in 2008 compared induced moderate short-term hypothermia to the maintenance of normothermia with children being randomised to either normothermia (37°C) or induced hypothermia (32.5°C for 24 hours). This second group were then rewarmed to 37°C (±0.5°C), i.e. the temperature that the normothermia group were maintained at throughout. Key findings from the study were:

- At 6 months, 31% of the patients in the hypothermia group, as compared with 22% of the patients in the normothermia group, had an unfavourable outcome.
- There were 23 deaths (21%) in the hypothermia group and 14 deaths (12%) in the normothermia group.
- There was more hypotension and more vasoactive agents were administered in the hypothermia group during the rewarming period than in the normothermia group.
- Lengths of stay in the ICU and in the hospital and other adverse events were similar in the two groups.

The study concluded that in children with severe traumatic brain injury, hypothermia therapy initiated within 8 hours after injury and continued for 24 hours does not improve the neurological outcome and may increase mortality (Hutchison et al. 2008).

The findings caused further discussion and current research is focused on the hypothesis that modified protocols with a shorter time from the accident to the start of active cooling, longer cooling and rewarming time and better control of blood pressure and intracranial pressure may be beneficial for TBI patients (Grände et al. 2009).

Hyperosmolar therapy

This refers to the use of hypertonic saline and or mannitol.
Mannitol can reduce the ICP in two ways:

- It reduces blood viscosity by increasing the water content, which in turn decreases the blood vessel diameter in the cerebral circulation. This occurs as a result of cerebral blood flow (CBF) autoregulation. This reflex vasoconstriction means that while CBF is maintained, actual blood volume and therefore ICP is reduced. The effects last for approximately 1 hour and for it to be successful intact autoregulation mechanisms are necessary.
- As an osmotic diuretic, mannitol removes water gradually from the brain parenchyma into the circulation. This is a relatively slow-acting therapy and lasts for up to 6 hours. Consideration needs to be given to the fact that mannitol can accumulate in the injured brain tissue and

can cause reverse osmotic shift. The blood–brain barrier needs to be intact for mannitol to exert its effects in this way.

Hypertonic saline

Hypertonic saline (3% or 5% saline) works primarily as an osmotic diuretic and as such gradually removes water from the brain parenchyma and returns it to the circulation. Maintaining a higher than normal serum sodium level also contributes to water remaining in the intravascular compartment rather than moving into the brain tissue. In addition, hypertonic saline is thought to exert other positive attributes, including:

- Restoration of normal cellular resting membrane potential.
- Inhibition of inflammatory responses at a cellular level.
- Stimulation of atrial natriuretic peptide release.
- Enhanced cardiac output.

Seizure control

Early post-traumatic seizures (EPTS) occur within the first week of injury and complicate the management of the child by increasing the ICP and cerebral metabolic demands and may cause hyperthermia. Phenytoin prophylaxis has been shown to reduce the incidence of EPTS in adults, however there is no evidence base for its use in children (Barry et al. 2010). In addition, its use does not prevent the subsequent development of an ongoing seizure disorder (epileptogenesis). The use of EEG monitoring may be used to detect subtle seizure activity.

Sedation

There is no consensus in the literature about the type of sedation that should be used in the management of TBI and there are often local differences in preference.

It is estimated that 21–42% of children with severe TBI will develop intractable raised intracranial pressure despite medical and surgical management (Adelson et al. 2003) and studies have suggested that high-dose barbiturates such as thiopentone are effective in lowering ICP in certain children with refractory intracranial pressure. The use of barbiturates may cause myocardial depression, leading to an increased risk of hypotension. Therefore, these children often require the use of increased inotropic support and/or fluid resuscitation to maintain a good MAP. In addition, continuous EEG monitoring is necessary to monitor the effects of such therapies, with the primary aim being to achieve 'burst suppression'. (Burst suppression is indicated by isoelectric activity with intermittent spikes of high voltage activity which is indicative of a significant reduction in cerebral metabolic activity.)

Decompressive craniotomy and craniectomy

Decompressive craniotomy is a second-line intervention used to gain control of ICP in the child with a persistent elevated ICP refractory to other interventions such as hyperosmolar therapy, manipulation of $PaCO_2$ and the use of sedatives or muscle relaxants. DC is the removal of a portion of the cranial bone, thus creating free space for the swollen brain parenchyma. There is only one study in children, which suggests that DC may be useful (Sahuquillo 2006), however given the paucity of evidence this procedure is usually reserved for children with extremely high ICP readings. A trial is currently underway in the adult population (the RESCUEicp trial), which may have significance for the older teenagers seen in the paediatric intensive care setting.

Extraventricular drains (EVD)

An EVD is a catheter inserted into the ventricle of the brain and then attached to a closed and sterile system allowing for CSF drainage from the ventricles of the brain. The mechanism for controlling the amount of CSF which may be drained is through controlling the height of the drain chamber. To achieve this, the chamber needs to be level with the foramen of Monro. This can be estimated by the midpoint of a line drawn from the outer corner of the eye to the external auditory canal (or top of child's ear). The CSF then drains by gravity into the collection chamber depending on the ICP and the level the chamber is set at.

Considerations for practice

- When transporting the child with an EVD in situ, the drain should be clamped just prior to the child leaving the centre and should remain clamped for the duration of the journey. A transfer to CT/MRI scan requires the same precautions. Failure to do so may lead to excessive amounts of CSF being drained. Once the child is back in the ICU, the drain should be re-levelled and then unclamped. If there is a significant increase in the child's ICP during transfer, the EVD may be transiently unclamped but it should be clamped again before continuing any significant patient movement.
- Hourly measurements of the CSF drainage are required. The colour of the drainage should be noted and changes identified to the medical staff. If there is no drainage, ensure that the tubing is not clamped or kinked. If there has been a change in the set drain chamber level just prior to the loss of drainage, it maybe that the level that

the drainage chamber has been set at is too high. In this instance it is possible to assess the patency of the drain by lowering the drain chamber to its original position. The drain should then be returned to the required position.

- EVD losses are usually replaced on a like-for-like basis with 0.9% sodium chloride.
- Daily samples of CSF should be sent for MC&S as there is a risk of the child developing ventriculitis if the EVD is in situ for more than 7 days (Barry et al. 2010).
- If there is microbiological confirmation of ventriculitis, intrathecal antibiotics should be administered according to local unit policy.
- Prior to removal of the EVD it is usually clamped for 24–48 hours and a CT scan is undertaken to ensure that there is no evidence of hydrocephalus developing.

General care considerations

- Positioning – to maximise cerebral venous return and minimise the potential for jugular venous obstruction the child should be nursed in the supine position with their head in the midline position. Care should be taken to ensure that ETT fixations (e.g. if using twill tapes that circle the child's neck) do not apply undue pressure on the jugular veins. If possible the bed should be tilted to a 25–30° angle.
- In cases where there have been concerns about the child's C-spine, once this has been cleared the use of a pressure-relieving mattress is advantageous to promote good skin condition and prevent the development of pressure spots. The type of mattress will be determined by local policy guidelines.
- Nutrition – as with any critically ill child, effective nutrition is essential, therefore early enteral nutrition should be started unless there are any clinical contraindications. Enteral feeds may be given either via an oro- or nasogastric tube (if there is suspicion or evidence of a basal skull fracture nasogastric tube placement should not be attempted) or via a naso-jejunal tube. Referral to Dietetic Services should also be made to ensure the child is receiving the required calorific intake to match their demands. Constipation should be avoided in children with raised ICP, therefore consideration should be given to maintaining normal bowel function and the use of osmotic laxatives such as Movicol™ or Lactulose™ may help to achieve this.
- In the child whose ICP is stable, physiotherapy should be instituted as soon as clinically possible to reduce the risk of limb contractures.

Diabetes insipidus

Diabetes insipidus (DI) may be central (neurogenic) or nephrogenic. Central DI is characterised by the decreased secretion of anti-diuretic hormone (ADH, also known as arginine vasopressin, AVP), which gives rise to polyuria by diminishing the ability to concentrate urine. It is this form of DI that is seen post-traumatic brain injury.

Clinical presentation

- Increased serum sodium levels (usually >150 mmol/l).
- Increased free water loss in the urine indicated by a urine osmolality <300 mOsm/l.
- Low urine sodium levels.
- Clinical features of dehydration.

For central (neurogenic) DI, the treatment of choice is the use of DDAVP (1-deamino-8-D-arginine vasopressin), which is a synthetic ADH equivalent. Careful monitoring of the child's fluid balance status and a fluid replacement strategy to ensure that the child does not become further dehydrated is also required.

Conclusion

This chapter has reviewed the anatomy and physiology of the nervous system and considered a range of conditions which may be seen in the intensive care area. Care of the child with a complex neurological condition can be challenging, especially when the progress is uncertain. In many cases the child and family become fairly long-term residents. The reader is asked to remember the holistic dimensions to care and the family.

References

Academy of Royal Colleges, 2008. A Code of Practice for the Diagnosis and Confirmation of Death. www.ics.ac.uk/intensive_care_professional/code_of_practice_08.

Adelson PD, Bratton SL et al. 2003. Guidelines for the acute medical management of severe traumatic brain injury in infants, children, and adolescents. Pediatric Critical Care Medicine, 4(3):S1–S75.

Advanced Life Support Group. 2011. Advanced Paediatric Life Support. 5th edition. Oxford: BMJ Books/Wiley Blackwell.

Andary MT. 2011. Guillain-Barré Syndrome. emedicine.medscape.com/article/315632-overview.

Arbour R. 2004. Intracranial hypertension: monitoring and nursing assessment. Critical Care Nurse, 24:19–32.

Barry P, Morris K, Ali T (Eds). 2010. Paediatric Intensive Care. Oxford: Oxford University Press.

Bracken MB. 1999, updated 2007. Steroids for acute spinal cord injury. Cochrane Database of Systematic Reviews, 2: Art. CD001046.

Cancer Research UK Cancer Statistics. Information for most current year. info.cancerresearchuk.org/cancerstats.

Chambers IR, Jones PA et al. 2006. Critical thresholds of intracranial pressure and cerebral perfusion pressure related to age in paediatric head injury. Journal of Neurology, Neurosurgery and Psychiatry, 77:234–40.

Chibber S. 2011. PediatricGuillain-Barré Syndrome. emedicine.medscape.com/article/1180594-overview.

Curry R, Hollingworth W et al. 2008. Incidence of hypo- and hypercarbia in severe traumatic brain injury before and after 2003 pediatric guidelines. Pediatric Critical Care Medicine, 9(2):141–6.

Czosnyka M, Pickard JD. 2004. Monitoring and interpretation of intracranial pressure. Journal of Neurology, Neurosurgery and Psychiatry, 75:813–21.

Dale RC, Branson JA. 2005. Acute disseminated encephalomyelitis or multiple sclerosis: can the initial presentation help in establishing a correct diagnosis? Archives of Diseases in Childhood, 90:636–9.

Davis MA, Gruskin, KD et al. 2005. Signs and Symptoms in Pediatrics: Urgent and emergent care. Philadelphia: Mosby Elsevier.

Dunning J, Patrick Daly JP et al. on behalf of the Children's Head Injury Algorithm for the Prediction of Important Clinical Events (CHALICE) Study Group. 2006. Derivation of the children's head injury algorithm for the prediction of important clinical events decision rule for head injury in children. Archives of Disease in Childhood, 91:885–91.

Freeman SA, Udomphorn Y et al. 2008. Young age as a risk factor for impaired cerebral autoregulation after moderate to severe pediatric traumatic brain injury. Anesthesiology, 108:588–95.

Gallimore D. 2006. The diagnosis of brainstem death and its implications. Nursing Times, 102(13):28–30.

Grände PO, Reinstrup P, Romner B. 2009. Active cooling in traumatic brain-injured patients: a questionable therapy? Acta Anaesthesiologica Scandinavica, 53(10):1233–8.

Hagen EM, Eide GE, Elgen I. 2011. Traumatic spinal cord injury among children and adolescents; a cohort study in western Norway. Spinal Cord, 49:981–5.

Hughes RAC, Swan AV, van Doorn, PA. 2010. Intravenous immunoglobulin for Guillain-Barré syndrome. Cochrane Database of Systematic Reviews, 6: Art. CD002063.

Hughes RA, Wijdicks EF et al. 2005. Supportive care for patients with Guillain-Barré syndrome. Archives of Neurology, 62(8):1194–8.

Hutchison JS, Ward RE et al. for the Hypothermia Pediatric Head Injury Trial Investigators and the Canadian Critical Care Trials Group. 2008. Hypothermia therapy after traumatic brain injury in children. New England Journal of Medicine, 358:2447–56.

Inwald D, Jakobovits I, Petros, A. 2000. Brain stem death: managing care when accepted medical guidelines and religious beliefs are in conflict. British Medical Journal, 320:1266–8.

Koszer S. 2010. Determination of Brain Death in Children. emedicine.medscape.com/article/1177999-overview.

Levine OS, Jones A et al. 2010. Global status of Haemophilus influenzae type B and pneumococcal conjugate vaccines: evidence, policies, and introductions. Current Opinion in Infectious Diseases, 23(3):236–41.

Levy MN, Koeppen BM, Stanton BA. 2006. Berne and Levy Principles of Physiology, 4th edition. Philadelphia: Mosby Elsevier.

Lissauer T, Clayden G. 2007. Illustrated Textbook of Pediatrics (3rd edition). China: Mosby Elsevier.

Martin C, Falcone RA.2008.Pediatric traumatic brain injury: an update of research to understand and improve outcomes. Current Opinion in Pediatrics,20:294–9.

Miller AC. 2011. Emergent Management of Guillain-Barré Syndrome. medicine.medscape.com/article/792008-overview.

Muzumdar D, Ventureyra EC. 2006.Spinal cord injuries in children. Journal of Pediatric Neurosciences, 1:43–8.

National Institute for Health and Clinical Excellence (NICE). 2007. Head Injury: Triage, assessment, investigation and early management of head injury in infants, children and adults. NICE Clinical Guideline 56.www.nice.org.uk/CG56.

National Institute for Health and Clinical Excellence (NICE). 2010. Bacterial Meningitis and Meningococcal Disease. NICE Clinical Guideline 102. www.nice.org.uk/CG102.

Neill S, Knowles H.2004. The Biology of Child Health: a reader in development and assessment. Basingstoke: Palgrave Macmillan.

Niranjan N, Duffy M. 2008. Brain stem death. ATOTW 115.www.frca.co.uk/Documents/115%20Brainstem%20death.pdf.

Packer RJ, MacDonald T, Vezina G. 2008.Central nervous system tumors. Pediatric Clinics of North America, 55(1):121–45.

Paediatric Intensive Care Audit Network (PICANet). 2011–12. Annual report. www.picanet.org.uk.

Rust RS. 2010. Acute Disseminated Encephalomyelitis. emedicine.medscape.com/article/1147044-overview.

Sahuquillo J. 2006.Decompressivecraniectomy for the treatment of refractory high intracranial pressure in traumatic brain injury. Cochrane Database of Systematic Reviews 1: Art.CD003983.

Shetty R, Singhi S et al. 2008. Cerebral perfusion pressure – targeted approach in children with central nervous system infections and raised intracranial pressure: is it feasible? Journal of Child Neurology, 23(2):192–8.

Sidram V, Tripathy P et al. 2009. Spinal cord injury without radiographic abnormality (SCIWORA) in children: A Kolkata experience. Indian Journal of Neurotrauma, 6(2):133–6.

Sookplung P, Vavilala MS. 2009. What is new in pediatric traumatic brain injury? Current Opinion in Anaesthesiology, 22:572–8.

Steiner LA, Andrews PJD. 2006. Monitoring the injured brain: ICP and CBF. British Journal of Anaesthesia, 97(1):26–38.

Tatman A, Warren A et al. 1997.Development of a modified pediatric coma scale in intensive care clinical practice. Archives of Disease in Childhood, 77:519–21.Witherratum. 1998. Archives of Disease in Childhood, 78:289.

Teasdale G, Jennett B. 1974. Assessment of coma and impaired consciousness: a practical scale. The Lancet, 2:81–4

Tortora GJ, Derrickson BH. 2009. Principles of Anatomy and Physiology, 12th edition, Volume 2: Maintenance and Continuity of the Human Body. Asia: John Wiley and Sons.

Tunkel AR, Glaser CA et al. 2008. The management of encephalitis: clinical practice guidelines by the Infectious Diseases Society of America. Clinical Infectious Diseases, 47(3):303–27.

Walker PA, Harting MT et al. 2009.Modern approaches to pediatric brain injury therapy. Journal of Trauma, 67:S120–S127.

Wingerchuk D. 2006. The clinical course of acute disseminated encephalomyelitis. Neurological Research, 28(3):341–7.

Yao K, Honarmand S et al. 2009.Detection of human herpesvirus-6 in cerebrospinal fluid of patients with encephalitis. Annals of Neurology, 65(2):257–67.

Zhong J, Dujovny M et al. 2003.Advances in ICP monitoring techniques. Neurological Research, 25:339–50.

Chapter 8
CARE OF AN INFANT OR CHILD WITH GASTROINTESTINAL OR ENDOCRINE DYSFUNCTION

Doreen Crawford[1] and Michaela Dixon[2]

[1] School of Nursing and Midwifery, Faculty of Health and Life Sciences, De Montfort University, Leicester, UK
[2] Paediatric Intensive Care Unit, Bristol Royal Hospital for Children,
University Hospitals Bristol NHS Foundation Trust, Bristol, UK

Introduction

This chapter reviews the relevant embryology, anatomy and physiology of the gastrointestinal tract and considers alterations in the normal gastrointestinal function related to some of the more common conditions seen by the children's nurse in areas where intensive care is carried out. The chapter is primarily a surgical one but considers some examples of medical emergencies and management before going on to review abdominal trauma, gut rescue and protection, major elective surgery and some emergencies. The chapter provides an overview of congenital corrective surgery as these infants can be seen in paediatric intensive care units as well as on neonatal units. The management of stress ulceration and paralytic ileus is also considered. Finally, the chapter reviews some of the metabolic and endocrine presentations seen in the intensive care. However, it is acknowledged that the spectrum of metabolic disease is wide and complex, and therefore practitioners should refer to resources specifically written for that speciality for more detailed information.

The gastrointestinal tract is an enormously complex system and this chapter is not an exhaustive review. It focuses on the core principles of the anatomy and physiology of the tract and makes links to the chapter which will consider the importance of fluids, electrolytes and nutrition to a child.

Adequate fluid, electrolyte and nutritional status are essential for growth, development and homeostasis in children. It is crucial that the child in intensive care is adequately hydrated and nourished in order to support their bodily functions and systems during a time of stress and high metabolic demand. The needs of one child may differ greatly from the needs of another, depending on their age and the stage of their illness, disease or condition.

Embryological development of the gastrointestinal tract (GIT)

See Table 8.1.

Overview of the postnatal anatomy and physiology of the gastrointestinal tract

This section presents an overview of the structure and function of the GIT. For a more detailed perspective, practitioners are advised to refer to a detailed anatomy and physiology textbook. The GIT is often referred to as the digestive tract reflecting its function, or the alimentary canal. It is a continuous tubular structure commencing at the mouth and ending with the anus. The oral and pharyngeal structures are shared with the respiratory tract and will

Paediatric Intensive Care Nursing, First Edition. Edited by Michaela Dixon and Doreen Crawford.
© 2012 John Wiley & Sons, Ltd. Published 2012 by John Wiley & Sons, Ltd.

Table 8.1 Embryology and foetal development of the gastrointestinal tract

Gestational age	Development
Weeks 2–3	Gastrulation comes from the Greek word for stomach but is also used to define the trilaminar embryo (this is made up of three layers: the ectoderm, mesoderm and endoderm). A cavity (intraembryonic coelom) forms with a layer of endoderm and mesoderm. This is still in communication with the yolk sac but will extend and grow later to become a continuous tubular structure which will extend from the pharyngeal membrane to the cloacal (meaning sewer) membrane.
Week 4	Three distinct portions can be identified: the foregut, midgut and hindgut. These extend the length of the embryo and outgrowths will contribute different components of the GIT. The large midgut is generated by lateral embryonic folding which 'pinches off' a pocket of the yolk sac. The two coelomic compartments continue to communicate through the vitelline duct. The blood vessels are derived from the vessels which supplied the yolk sac. The terminal expanded part of the hindgut is the embryonic cloaca and this develops a fork-like projection which grows downwards towards the tail.
Weeks 5–6	Lateral folds have given the embryo a cylindrical appearance. The development of the umbilical cord and the regression of the yolk sac reduces the communication between the intraembryonic coelom and the extracoelomic coelom. The foregut, midgut and hindgut are suspended from the posterior abdominal wall by the dorsal mesentery. The portion of the foregut destined to become the stomach is already dilating and rotating. Growth of the stomach is not equal and this results in the curvatures. Migration of the neural crest cells into the colon begins to innervate the walls of the intestine.
Weeks 7–9	Massive growth and differentiation of the liver and heart result in a limited amount of intraembryonic space for the developing midgut loop; therefore this projects and herniates into the base of the umbilical cord where the intestines lengthen and rotate. The proliferations of the epithelial cells which line the gut actually occlude the lumen. The cloaca has now divided into the urogenital sinus and the structure which will become the rectum and anal canal. By the end of week 7 the anal membrane ruptures to form the anal opening. By week 8 there are gastric pits, rugae and smooth muscle in the walls of the stomach.
Week 10	With a relative increase in the size of the abdominal cavity the intestines migrate back into this cavity and the developing peritoneal cavity loses its connections with the extraembryonic coelom. A key step in development is the rotation of the midgut which occurs to place the intestines in the correct abdominal position with its associated mesentery. An increasingly rich blood supply is provided by branches of the superior mesenteric artery.
Weeks 11–20	By week 11 the caecum is in the right iliac fossa and there are villi increasing the surface area of the small intestine. The liver produces bile, which is secreted into the duodenum. Increasing cellular differentiation allows for the unique and specialist histology within the GIT. This is mainly endodermal in origin. Chief structures and parietal cells are present by week 16. The foetus can swallow amniotic fluid stimulating a limited peristalsis. The framework of the GIT is established. All that is required is growth and maturity. The surface mucosa will not mature fully till after birth and exposure to milk.

Source: adapted from Moore and Persaud 2003.

not be considered here. The functions of the GIT are supported by a range of accessory glands and organs.

Basic functions

- Ingestion.
- Digestion and absorption.
- Egestion and elimination.

Ingestion

This is the physical process of taking in food and fluids for processing in the GIT. In sick children this process often has to be supported by the selective use of nasal or oral tubes. Nurses are skilled and accustomed at passing these into the stomach but if the stomach has to be bypassed for any reason these can be passed through the pylorus and placed into the duodenum or the jejunum. If the requirement for support is likely to be long term, then a gastrostomy or a jejunostomy may be performed. These are surgical openings into the stomach or jejunum.

Digestion and absorption

This process is divided into two complementary functions: mechanical digestion and chemical digestion. The result is to process food and fluid into small enough component parts to facilitate absorption across the gastrointestinal membrane and transportation in the circulation. The ultimate stage in these digestive processes is assimilation into the cells to provide the raw materials for metabolism. The function of digestion is supported by peristalsis (a powerful rhythmic sequential unidirectional muscular contraction, propelling gut contents forward). In children who require intensive care there are many reasons why this might not happen normally. There could be altered anatomy with insufficient surface area to absorb required nutrients (e.g. short gut syndrome possibly as a result of surgical resection for necrotising enterocolitis). The surface area may not be compromised but the child's metabolic needs are increased because of their illness. There could be sensitivity or inflammatory conditions impeding the absorption of nutrients or liquid from the gut (e.g. coeliac and Crohn's disease). There could be a physical problem with the gut motility; this may be a result of sedation or related to the GIT itself (e.g. malrotation, volvulus, intussusception causing acute obstruction or Hirschsprung's which may present as a more chronic condition). Alternatively, peristalsis could be dramatically speeded up as a reaction to infection, toxins or irritation causing profound and profuse diarrhoea.

Egestion and elimination

This is the excretion of waste and non-absorbable bulk. Defecation is a painless process and the quantity and content of the stool passed reflects the quantity and content of the diet, the state of the GIT and the general wellbeing of the individual. Bowel patterns change with developmental maturity of the GIT, and bowel habits can vary enormously among individuals. Children requiring intensive care will be unable to evacuate their bowel normally and many of the children with GIT conditions will have a temporary or permanent stoma of some type. There are different types of stoma and the name reflects the area of the GIT involved (e.g. a colostomy is a surgical opening into the colon). Generally speaking the higher up the intestinal tract the more liquid the stool and the child will have a higher requirement for nutritional support.

The formation of the mouth is considered separately as it is closely associated with the airways (Table 8.2).

General care principles

It is essential to have a basic working knowledge of the normal anatomy and physiology as well as the related developmental stages of the mouth as the child in PICU may have impaired functioning or related risks, for example oral intubation impairs the swallowing reflex and the presence and stimulation of an orally placed endotracheal tube can cause excess salivation. This will result in the children's nurse having to make frequent assessment of salivary build-up and decide whether to start oral suctioning, mindful of the fact that this procedure can also cause stimulation which will increase secretions as well as disturb and frighten a lightly sedated child.

The procedure of intubation or the friction caused by the presence of an ETT can cause complications, such as the displacement of loose teeth. The presence of an endotracheal tube interrupts the normal routine of a child's oral hygiene and although there is a paucity of evidence to support good practice, the management of a child in PIC must include consideration of oral hygiene to prevent infection or the risks associated with descending infection resulting in ventilator associated pneumonia (Cutler and Davis 2005; Pobo et al. 2009; Somal and Darby 2006; Wikin 2002) (Chapter 4).

Pre-operative fasting

The RCN guidelines on pre-operative fasting (2005) focus on healthy infants and children and although there is some comparison where major elective surgery is concerned

Table 8.2   Embryology, foetal, early development and maturation of the mouth

Week	Development
Early tissue organisation	The mouth is a derivative of the stomodaeum, an external pit bounded by the over-jutting, primitive nasal region and the early upper and lower jaw projections. Its floor is a thin membrane, where ectoderm and endoderm fuse. By the end of week 3 this membrane disappears and a communication is formed between the future mouth and the future pharynx.
Week 4	The face, head and neck structures are derived from the pharyngeal arches 1 and 2. The pharyngeal arches are derived from endoderm, mesoderm, neural crest and ectodermal cells, which are the precursor materials required to form the specialist tissues and complex organs which will ultimately shape and develop the face. The first pharyngeal arch will form the jaws.
Weeks 6–8	During this period the shape of the embryo's head is formed, expanding rapidly reflecting the tumult of developmental activity going on underneath.
	Five primitive tissue lobes grow: one from the top of the head down towards the future upper lip – the frontonasal prominence; two from the cheeks, which meet the first lobe to form the upper lip – the maxillar prominence; and two from the lower sides, which will form the chin and lower lip – the mandibular prominence. If these tissues fail to meet there will be a birth defect, the severity of which will reflect the location and extent of the failure of fusion.
	Following the fusion of the prominences the palates form to divide the primitive oral cavity into a separate nasal cavity and oral cavity. By day 51 the fusion is completed and the soft palate and uvula are formed by day 53.
	The tongue begins to form at approximately the same time as the palates. It extends from various protuberances on the pharynx floor. The tongue receives material from all four occipital somites reflecting its ultimate complexity for the building up the muscle, connective tissue and the formation of the sensory structures which will ultimately conduct information to influence the perception of taste.
	The salivary glands begin to form around day 44. They arise as ectodermal buds that branch, like the lung buds, into the deeper mesoderm. The endings dilate like alveoli to become the secretory acini (small sacs) and the canal like network which will serve as ducts.
	Towards the latter part of this stage the teeth begin to form with the development of the epithelia lamella parallel to the lip edge. Through interactions between neural crest cells and ectoderm 10 roundish teeth buds appear in the lower and upper jaws which will eventually become the deciduous teeth.
Foetal maturity	By the end of the embryological stages the GIT framework is completed; during foetal life tissues grow, mature and begin to function.
Weeks 12–16	Enamel (the hard tissue that surrounds the deciduous teeth) is formed, around 3–4 months of gestation. The cap of enamel develops from ectodermal tissue, the main mass of the tooth, the dentin and the encrusting cement surrounding the root of the developing tooth differentiate from the mesoderm.
	Towards the latter part of this phase small buds begin to form in the jaws on the oral side. These are the precursors of the permanent teeth.
Birth to 8 years	Development of suck–swallow coordination. Chewing. Primary dentition.
8 to young adult years	Secondary dentition.

(e.g.an infant or child who is fit and well and going to be recovered following surgery on PICU), most pre-operative fasting guidelines now permit the intake of water and other clear fluids up to 2 hours before the induction of anaesthesia for elective surgery in healthy infants and children in order to prevent the risks of excessive pre-operative fasting and enhance the child's wellbeing. The children's nurse needs to be aware that some surgical procedures are lengthy and children may have been fasted for prolonged periods by the time they reach PICU. The same guidelines do not apply to children who have been traumatised and are in a shocked state. In addition, where emergency admissions are concerned, the history of when the infant was last fed or the child last ate may be vague. The decision to proceed with urgent surgery needs to be made in the child's best interests.

There is a high correlation between malnutrition and outcome, yet fasting and feeding practices for children in PIC are not based on good evidence. As there is more evidence available to support the neonatal nurse this can be used to support infant gut management. There is also good quality work informing general intensive care practice and this can be used to support the management of the adolescent and the young person. Where possible appropriate evidence has been cited but there is a distinct gap in the evidence base covering the intermediate age range. Intubation and ventilation can delay the gastric emptying time and this has been associated with increased gastric residual volumes. It is known that morphine administration affects antroduodenal motility as the gastrointestinal motor pattern involved is characterised by antral hypomotility (Bosscha et al. 1998); however, there is little information on normal gastric residual volume in paediatric patients (Babbitt 2007). An awareness of gastric emptying in critically ill children is important as the consequences of this phenomenon have implications for intolerance to enteral nutrition, the range and extent of gastric colonisation and an increased risk of aspiration pneumonia (Heyland et al. 1996; Moreira and McQuiggan 2009). (See Chapter 12 for complex fluid and feeding management.)

Stress ulceration

Stress ulcers of the stomach and duodenum, as well as upper gastrointestinal (UGI) bleeding are well-known complications of critical illness in children who are admitted to a PICU. Calculations of the prevalence of stress ulceration are variable, with the incidence increasing with the duration of stay and there being a correlation with the development of ulceration and risk of mortality. Prophylaxis against stress ulcers is the preferred form of manage-

ment, using a range of strategies, pharmaceutical agents and a variety of dosage and regimens:

- Early feeding.
- Omeprazole.
- Ranitidine.
- Sucralfate.
- Famotidine.
- Amalgate.
- Antacids.

Further work requires to be done to develop good guidance and treatment protocols (Reveiz et al. 2010).

Medical management of acute or life-threatening abdominal conditions

Pancreatitis

Pancreatitis, although uncommon during childhood, is associated with significant morbidity and mortality. This condition is characterised by inflammation of the pancreas, clinical signs of epigastric abdominal pain and elevated serum digestive enzymes. Pancreatitis can be local or diffuse and is classified as acute, chronic, inherited, necrotic or haemorrhagic. Occasionally, pancreatitis is complicated by the formation of a fibrous-walled cavity filled with pancreatic enzymes, termed a pseudocyst (Chang et al. 2011).

Pancreatitis occurs as a consequence of the blockage or disruption of the collecting ducts and damage to the pancreatic acinar cells, which leads to activation and then the release of digestive enzymes. The activated enzymes autodigest the pancreatic parenchyma, causing inflammation and necrosis.

Pancreatitis may follow blunt abdominal trauma, occur as a result of congenital abnormalities in the pancreatic ducts, as a complication following a 'mild' viral ailment or as a serious side-effect of a powerful drug such as asparaginase, a chemotherapy drug. Asparaginase is an enzyme that breaks down protein, but fortunately this is a rare if serious side-effect. Children with cystic fibrosis may develop a chronic pancreatitis. Hereditary pancreatitis is an autosomal dominant disorder with an 80% penetrance, accounting for about 1% of cases (Obideen et al. 2008).

Acute haemorrhagic pancreatitis rarely occurs in children. This is a life-threatening condition with a mortality rate approaching 50% because of shock, systemic inflammatory response syndrome with multiple-organ dysfunction, acute respiratory distress syndrome (ARDS), disseminated intravascular coagulation (DIC), massive gastrointestinal bleeding and systemic or peritoneal infection (Werlin 2003).

Physical examination findings associated with haemorrhagic pancreatitis may include a bluish discoloration of the flanks (Grey Turner sign) or peri-umbilical region (Cullen sign) because of blood accumulation in the fascial planes of the abdomen. Additional signs may include the accumulations of pleural effusions, haematemesis, melaena and coma (Chang et al. 2011; Werlin 2003).

Clinical presentation of acute pancreatitis
- Severe pain located in the epigastric or para-umbilical regions, with the child adopting a foetal position with their knees drawn up to try to relieve this.
- Abdominal distension.
- Presence of abnormal bowel sounds.
- Nausea and vomiting.
- Unexplained fever.
- Unstable serum blood glucose values.
- Elevated pancreatic enzymes.

Treatment

The goal of medical management of acute pancreatitis is to achieve adequate rehydration, analgesia and pancreatic rest and to restore normal metabolic homeostasis. In patients with severe pancreatitis, oral intake is usually restricted and total parenteral nutrition should be initiated within 3 days to prevent catabolism. There is considerable discussion in the literature about the point at which enteral nutrition should be reinstituted, but currently there is no consensus. In cases of intractable vomiting or ileus, a nasogastric tube left to free drain is helpful in promoting intestinal–pancreatic rest by eliminating gastric secretions in the duodenum, the most potent activator of pancreatic secretion. Fluid, electrolyte and mineral imbalances should be corrected urgently. Antibiotic therapy is indicated for systemic infections or sepsis. Acute pancreatitis should resolve in 2–7 days with adequate resuscitation (Benifla and Weizman 2003; Chang et al. 2011).

In chronic relapsing pancreatitis, pancreatic enzyme supplementation, insulin and elemental or low-fat diets are useful adjuncts to maximise the child's nutritional status. For the alleviation of pain, opioids are essentially contraindicated as they can contribute to spasms of the sphincter of Oddi. Advice should be gained from a specialist pain team.

Crohn's disease

Crohn's disease (CD) is an inflammatory bowel disease. It is a chronic condition characterised by repeated exacerbations and periods of remission. It usually involves the small intestine, most often the lower part (the ileum). However, inflammation may also affect the entire digestive tract, including the mouth, oesophagus, stomach, duodenum, appendix or anus. The cause is unknown, however there are several theories. One suggests that a trigger, possibly a microorganism, affects the body's immune system and this results in an inflammatory reaction in the intestinal wall. There is supporting evidence that children with the disease have abnormalities of the immune system, however it is uncertain whether the immune problems are a cause or a result of the disease.

Pharmacological agents used in the management of Crohn's disease

Drug therapy singly or in combination is the first-line approach to management. 5-aminosalicylates (5-ASAs) are a group of compounds that have long-established use in inflammatory bowel disease. However, while sulphasalazine may have a role in the treatment of mild CD, the overall evidence does not support the use of 5-ASA agents for inducing remission in CD (Akobeng 2008).

Antibiotics

Although there is no convincing and reproducible evidence, a number of antibiotics have been tried for the induction of remission in CD. However, the most rigorous available evidence does not support the routine use of antibiotics for the induction of remission in active CD (Akobeng 2008). Immunosuppressive agents such as azathioprine and 6-mercaptpopurine are purine analogues that have demonstrated effectiveness for the treatment of CD and in establishing remission.

Methotrexate

No controlled trials have been performed in children, but a retrospective case note analysis has suggested that methotrexate may be effective and safe for inducing remission in paediatric Crohn's disease (Weiss et al. 2009).

Corticosteroids

Corticosteroids are also effective for inducing remission but may be associated with significant adverse events. Infliximab is recommended for the treatment of patients with severe Crohn's disease who do not respond to conventional management (NICE 2002).

Symptomatic control may be achieved with the management of diet and analgesic regimes. There is interest in probiotic use, although the supportive action of probiotics is as yet not fully understood (Patel and Lin 2010).

Extracorporeal photopheresis for inflammatory bowel disease

Under research and awaiting clinical trials is the procedure called extracorporeal photopheresis. This is when the patient is anticoagulated with heparin and blood is removed from the patient using a two-way circulatory device to provide access to the circulation and allows the circulation to be returned. Once removed the blood is filtered and the white blood cells are separated from the whole blood. These white cells are treated with ultraviolet light and are then returned to the patient where they produce a generalised immune response against the pathogenic T-cell clones that are involved in the pathogenesis of inflammation in Crohn's disease (NICE 2009). Extracorporeal photopheresis is usually carried out over two consecutive days at intervals of 2–4 weeks for about 20 treatment sessions. One ECP session takes about 3–4 hours. The therapy has a number of side-effects and it should only be performed as a last resort and as part of a research programme.

It is rare for these children to be admitted to a PICU unless in a life-threatening condition or to facilitate close postoperative monitoring and management.

Commonalities across gastrointestinal conditions, surgery or major gut insult

Peritonitis

This is inflammation or infection of the peritoneum; the inflammation can be caused by a blood-borne bacterial or fungal infection or be a result of perforation of the gut or digestive organs. It can be seen as a complication in children who are on chronic peritoneal dialysis (Chapter 6), or as a result of blunt trauma causing tears in fragile abdominal organs resulting in the spillage of gut contents into the abdominal cavity. However, it can also be caused by other conditions that allow bacteria, enzymes or bile into the peritoneum from damage to the gastrointestinal or biliary tracts. Examples include pancreatitis, a perforated appendix (the most common), stomach ulcer, Crohn's disease or diverticulitis.

Signs of peritonitis

- Swelling and tenderness in the abdomen with pain ranging from dull aches to severe, sharp pain.
- Pyrexia.
- Anorexia.
- Nausea and vomiting.
- Limited urine output.
- Ileus – silent abdomen, no flatus or stool.

Management of peritonitis

Treatment and management is surgical repair where this was the primary cause and broad spectrum antibiotics. The gut needs to be rested and enteral fluids and feeds re-graded with care. The child needs effective management of pain. Drains are not routinely used in the management of post-surgical intervention in children but these children are at a relatively high risk of intra-abdominal abscesses (van Wijck et al. 2010), so rather than repeated trips to theatre some external drainage of the abscess bed may be considered.

Paralytic ileus

This is a disruption of normal intestinal peristalsis, the natural gastrointestinal motor activity. Paralytic ileus is common following surgery where the gut is handled or the abdominal cavity has been opened, for example, to access the retroperitoneal space for renal surgery. It can also result from certain drugs such as anaesthetics and from major injuries where there has been circulatory impairment and poor perfusion. In children it can also be caused by sepsis. Paralytic ileus causes total constipation, absence of flatus and abdominal distension. Auscultation with a stethoscope will reveal a silent abdomen as there are no borborygmi since the bowel is inactive. Despite treatment and management a small proportion of children go on to develop sub-acute pseudo-obstruction syndromes (Barr 1998).

'Drip and suck'

There is controversy about the requirement for gastric and gut decompression with a nasogastric tube (NGT) in abdominal surgery patients, in many cases it seems to be performed routinely in spite of the absence of good evidence (Moreira and McQuiggan 2009; Williams and Leslie 2004). Dinsmore and colleagues (2004) suggest that it is an unnecessary intervention in most cases. However, if paralytic ileus is present and gastrointestinal secretions are pooling in the stomach and gut loops, aspiration of these is an appropriate nursing action, particularly if the build-up of gastrointestinal secretions could cause vomiting and risk aspiration. In addition, aspiration of these secretions may avoid leakage or spillage through a perforation and their removal may reduce intestinal intra-lumen tension and help protect a new anastomosis. Sometimes the NGT is left on free drainage/siphon drainage. The volumes and character of all aspirated fluids need to be charted and as this is fluid lost to the child, a clear strategy of replacement fluid and electrolytes implemented.

The strategies for managing paralytic ileus are to rest the gut and allow it to recover, to prevent further

complications and to administer sufficient fluids and calories to allow repair, recovery growth and development. In
some cases this will mean long-term parenteral nutrition
(Chapter 12).

Managing gut motility problems, promoting absorption
and preventing long-term sequelae need to be done with
the full involvement of the paediatric dietetic team and
where indicated, the speech and language department. In
self-ventilating small infants or those supported via a tracheostomy there is a need for oral stimulation and non-
nutritive sucking if a good long-term outcome is to be
achieved, as these infants may not have established feeding
by mouth and, where the mouth has been used to access
the airway during intubation procedures, steps need to be
taken to avoid oral aversion, etc. Although controversial,
a strategy of 'kick-starting' the gut may be tried in order
to stimulate it into motility and acclimatise it to holding
volume and absorbing elements. Both Miedema and
Johnson (2003) and Stewart and Waxman (2007) reviewed
additional supportive methods for stimulating gut activity
and although there is a requirement for paediatric evidence
to be built up, ultimately the adoption of prokinetic pharmaceutical support to enhance motility may shorten the
duration of the ileus (Deane et al. 2009).

Necrotising enterocolitis (NEC)

This is primarily a disease of the premature infant and is
the most common gastrointestinal emergency in neonates.
The aetiology is uncertain; however the smaller and sicker
the infant, the greater the risk. Suggested contributing
factors include the immature gastrointestinal anatomy and
physiology. An immature intestinal barrier may permit
bacteria to penetrate the mucosal barrier and trigger an
inflammatory response. Immature biochemical defences
may also be a factor where bacterial overgrowth is permitted and this may attack the bowel wall. Other contributory
factors include hypoxic-ischaemic injury, early feeding
with formula milk, not having breast milk and colonisation
by pathological bacteria (Schnabl et al. 2008).

The epidemiology of NEC is little understood, with
cases seemingly coming in clusters and some infants
succumb who would seem not to have the predisposing
factors of immaturity or a compromised gut because of a
difficult postnatal phase, with serious RDS and early artificial feeding. Gut ischaemia and ileus in older infants and
children can result in a toxic state where prolonged ileus
can allow enteric bacteria to ferment malabsorbed carbohydrates to various gases, producing distension and
increase the intraluminal pressure. This can result in a

vicious cycle where distension of gut loops can further
decrease the mucosal blood flow. The products of fermen-
tation could be toxic to enterocytes and impair the mucosal
barrier function. The inflammatory response can be triggered and the gut walls become very friable. There may be
a risk of perforation and life-threatening peritonitis can set
in.

Neonates with cyanotic heart disease also have a higher
risk of developing NEC. While the pathophysiology of this
is not completely determined, it is thought to be related to
hypoxic injury (secondary to cyanotic heart lesion) to the
immature GIT. NEC is a serious complication and can be
staged based on clinical presentation and radiological findings (Table 8.3).

NEC – strategies for reducing the risk

Neonatologists have developed a strategy where small
amount of 'gut priming' or trophic feeds are given in order
to avert adverse events, although Bombell and McGuire
(2009) conclude that there was insufficient evidence to
justify the practice of withholding or initiating early feeds.
Gut stimulation may also prevent fasting-induced mucosal
atrophy, so preventing bacterial translocation and the risk
of endotoxaemia, mucosal inflammation or sepsis (Premji
and Chessell 2007). It is important to remember that these
'feeds' are not given for nutritional value but to act as a
protective function, and by giving the gut secretions something else to work on, may help prevent mucosal damage.
Patole and de Klerk (2005) note a significant decline in the
incidence of NEC following the implementation of a standardised feeding regime.

Reducing the risk of NEC has resulted in studies which
employ probiotics and there is some evidence of their
effectiveness (Alfaleh et al. 2010). Although there is
emerging support for the use of oral lactoferrin, which is
a normal component of human colostrum, milk, tears and
saliva in enhancing the infant's host defence in the prevention of sepsis, there is, as yet, no evidence that it reduces
the incidence of NEC (Pammi and Abrams 2011).

Preventing mucosal damage is also part of the controversial theory behind the prophylactic prescribing of a
histamine receptor blocker, for example IV ranitidine or
cimetidine. These drugs work by blocking H_2 receptors
found on the cells in the stomach lining. Histamine normally binds to these receptors, causing the cells to produce
stomach acid. Blocking the H_2 receptors, prevents histamine from binding to them. This stops the cells from producing stomach acid which erodes the mucosa, producing
ulceration and occasionally causing major haemorrhage.
However, all drugs have side-effects. Consequently,

Table 8.3 Stages of necrotising enterocolitis

Stage	Impact on the infant
Stage 1 Suspected NEC	Systemic but non-specific signs such as thermal instability, lethargy, apnoea, bradycardia, not being themselves. Feeding intolerance with increasing gastric aspirates and blood in the stool. Abdominal X-ray may be normal. Management: medical as described below and await progression or resolution.
Stage 2(a) Mild NEC	Systemic non-specific signs; unstable, increasing apnoea and bradycardia which may require PICU management. Vomiting, abdominal distension, pain on examination, silent abdomen, frank blood in stool. Abdominal X-ray confirms ileus and local pneumatosis intestinalis. Management: continue medical management and refer for surgical opinion.
Stage 2(b) Moderate NEC	Systemically increasingly unwell with mild acidosis, thrombocytopenia. Abdominal wall oedema and tenderness with or without mass. Abdominal X-ray shows extensive pneumatosis intestinalis, early ascites, with or without intrahepatic portal gas.
Stage 3(a) Advanced NEC	Systemically very unwell with a respiratory/metabolic acidosis, apnoea, hypotension, decreasing urine output, leucopenia and disseminated intravascular coagulation (DIC). GIT: spreading oedema, erythema, induration of the abdomen. Abdominal X-ray shows prominent ascites with or without persistent sentinel loop but no perforation. Consent for surgery and monitor very closely. Transfusion and blood products.
Stage 3 (b) Advanced NEC	Systemically demonstrating clinical deterioration, shock, electrolyte imbalance. Abdominal X-ray shows signs of perforation. Requires urgent surgery.

Source: modified from Bell et al. 1978; Walsh and Kliegman 1986.

Messori and colleagues (2000) recommend the use of H_2 blockers on the basis of symptoms only, as there may be a link with their routine use and atypical pneumonia; and Donowitz and colleagues(1986) note the abnormal gastric colonisation of patients with therapeutically altered gastric acidity by hospital- acquired gram-negative rods.

Medical management of NEC

There is an element of repetition in the strategy for managing NEC medically in common with other intestinal failures:

- Enteral feeding is stopped so the gut is rested.
- NGT placement – this is usually left on free drainage with regular aspiration for gastrointestinal decompression and the infant's comfort.
- Excessive gastric losses may need to be replaced (millilitre for millilitre) with 0.9% sodium chloride +/–

potassium supplementation to avoid the infant becoming hypokalaemic or hyponatraemic.

- PN and complex fluids are titrated to the individual infant's needs (Chapter 12).
- Triple antibiotic therapy, including metronidazole.
- Analgesics.
- Supportive management.
- Minimal handling.

Surgical management of NEC

There is a general reluctance to expose fragile infants to the trauma of surgery; however some who are not recovered by medical means are so sick that surgery becomes their only option for survival (Pierro and Hall 2003). Tepas and colleagues (2010) consider some metrics of metabolic derangement which could be used as indicators to support the clinical decision to intervene surgically.

There are two main surgical options: laparotomy, visual inspection, resection and anastomosis; and the less invasive paracentesis and primary peritoneal drainage. Moss and colleagues (2006) consider one option as having a greater advantage than the other. Other units have used a combination of methods, with the drainage sometimes being used as an interim method to try to stabilise the infant before laparotomy. However Rees and colleagues (2010) did not find that peritoneal drainage improved clinical stability in infants where there was bowel perforation.

If the infant requires a laparotomy, it is difficult to prepare the parents as to how the infant may look following surgery and whether they will have an ileostomy or not. If a single area of bowel is affected and resected and the remainder of the bowel is in good condition, a primary anastomosis may be possible. However, this exposes the infant to the risk of leakage, stricture, fistula or breakdown. More frequently a proximal ostomy and distal mucous fistula are created, which may be reversed once the infant's condition improves.

Vaughan et al. (1996) refined a technique of clipping and closing where necrotic segments of intestine were resected and the transected ends stapled closed. This meant that the infant had to return to theatre 2–3 days later and have a reanastomosis. If all went well, however, these infants did not have a stoma.

Surgeons sometimes have to make some very difficult choices. When less than 25% of the intestinal length is found to be unaffected the choices are restricted. Simple closure results in a very poor outcome and most surgeons opt for patching where they can, drain, hope and wait.

The prognosis is variable in infants with surgically managed NEC and can differ according to the location of the NEC. The infants who had resection for NEC in the large bowel did better than infants who had resection in the short bowel (Zhang et al. 2011). This also had implications for mortality, co-morbidities, length of stay and the cost of the hospital stay.

Short gut syndrome and short bowel syndrome (SBS)

SBS can be defined as a malabsorptive state resulting from a congenital malformation of the gut or occurring after an extensive resection of the small intestine (Sala et al. 2010) or for acquired lesions such as intestinal volvulus resulting in ischaemia (Duro et al. 2008). Regardless of the primary cause, the gut usually compensates by dilating to create more surface area to absorb nutrients. This slows down food transit, can increase the amount of bacteria in situ and can result in potentially life-threatening infections. Where children cannot absorb their nutrients, Parenteral nutrition (PN) will be employed to sustain growth. However, this

places the child at risk of PN-associated complications resulting in more pathology.

Strategies to manage short bowel syndrome

Wherever possible the remaining gut should be put to use and refeeding introduced:

- Parenteral nutrition with vitamin and mineral replacement.
- Careful fluid management.
- Monitor for and manage gastric acid hypersecretion.
- Management of the complexities of malabsorption.
- Management of motility.
- Management of any bacterial overgrowth with appropriate antibiotics.
- Surgical lengthening procedures and transplant.

Some of these children are frequently exposed to a range of medications in the hope of improving the residual gut function. There is a paucity of evidence regarding the application of pro-motility and anti-diarrhoeal medications in patients with SBS and intestinal failure, although they continue to be used (Dicken et al. 2011).

Refeeding collected gut secretions

High stomas located in the jejunum or proximal ileum can result in the production of large quantities of effluent containing unabsorbed nutrients resulting in poor growth and electrolyte imbalance. The neonate is usually dependent on PN until the intestinal adaptation takes place; however PN is associated with significant risk of central line-related sepsis, thrombosis and neonatal cholestasis. Collecting the effluent from the high stoma and refeeding this effluent into the distal mucous fistula uses the absorptive surface of the distal bowel for nutrient absorption, may stimulate mucosal growth, improve intestinal adaptation and prevent atrophy of the distal bowel. This should result in weight gain, reduce the electrolyte imbalance and decrease dependency on PN (Richardson et al. 2006). The procedure is simple to perform and may be done by parents following discharge. However, the effluent has an unappealing character and this strategy needs considerable explanation to the parents to allow them to come to terms with it.

Surgery

SBS has been treated with a surgical process called the Bianchi procedure. During this, the bowel is bisected and one end is sewn to the other. However, the bowel often redilates, leaving patients in the same condition as when they started. Serial transverse enteroplasty has the potential to avoid these difficulties and the procedure involves stapling V shapes into alternating sides of the bowel resulting in a decrease of width and an increase in length (NICE 2007). Research supports an improvement in bowel function and nutrition (Kajia et al. 2009) and it is possible the procedure will become more commonplace and lend itself to other applications (Modi et al. 2007).

Intestinal transplant

This is now a well-recognised alternative treatment strategy for SBS (Grant et al. 2005). Although most will come from cadaveric donation there is an interest and an increase in living related donations (Li et al. 2008). Graft choice depends on the presence of associated liver disease (Duro et al. 2008) as a block graft including liver may be preferred to isolated bowel graft. Although puberty can be delayed in some cases, a functional intestinal graft can result in a normal growth pattern; the exception seems to be in children who remain on high-dose steroids (Lacaille et al. 2007). Post-transplant children require life-long anti-rejection management as the gut is an immune organ harbouring a large amount of immune-competent cells, has a large colony of microorganisms (Braun et al. 2007) and it is particularly vulnerable to the effects of ischaemic injury. This susceptibility to damage will not permit time-consuming HLA matching prior to transplantation (Ruemmele et al. 2006). Although protocols differ (Pirenne and Kawai 2006) anti-rejection management may include starting therapy before the transplant to kill or deplete T- and B-cells which would target the transplanted intestine.

Following transplantation, the immunosuppressive therapy such as tacrolimus and tapered corticosteroid doses (Martingale 2009) continues, although there seems to be controversy regarding the use of steroids (Dazzi et al. 2007). Chronic rejection does not appear to develop insidiously in compliant patients and although rare, late acute rejection may complicate infectious diarrhoea (Lacaille et al. 2007).

Stoma formation and stoma care

A stoma simply means an opening. Paediatric ostomies include any surgically created opening between a hollow organ and the skin connected either directly (stoma) or in the case of gastrostomy with the use of a tube or peg. The following are examples of stoma and are not an exhaustive list:

- Gastrostomy usually created for enteral feeding.
- Duodenostomy usually created for enteral feeding.
- Jejunostomy.

- Ileostomy.
- Proximal colostomies.

In infants and children, stomas are used for various purposes, including access, decompression, diversion and evacuation (Minkes et al. 2008). Most ostomies in children are for temporary use and are typically reversible after a determined period of time, although some medical conditions may dictate the need for a permanent stoma (Minkes et al. 2008). Complications following intestinal diversional (ostomy) surgeries are high (Park et al. 1999) and can present a significant problem to many individuals. It has been estimated that up to 70% of patients with an ileostomy and 43% of those with a colostomy experience complications (Pittman and Rawl 2009).

There are several differences between adult and paediatric ostomies. In adults most stomas are formed in the distal ileum or colon for the treatment of inflammatory bowel disease, malignant conditions or trauma. In infants and children a stoma may be required anywhere along the GI tract because of a range and variety of congenital and acquired conditions. The effects of stoma formation for the infant or child should not be underestimated. They include the impact on the parents, which can affect bonding in the neonatal period, the impact on the family of repeated hospitalisations, which can affect other siblings, and the effects that a stoma may have on the child's physical and emotional development. The physiological impact may affect a child's growth and ability to maintain their own nutritional needs, while the emotional and psychological effects, particularly in the older child or adolescent, require careful management. There is potential for social isolation, with some children being reluctant to attend school or engage with their peer group; referral to a specialist nurse is recommended.

Many stomas in infants and children are undertaken as emergency procedures, however whenever possible a primary stoma site and back-up sites should be selected and marked before surgery. The stoma should be distant from the incision and away from skinfolds, bony prominences and umbilicus. Treating a child with multiple abdominal stomas can be challenging, especially when the anatomy is unclear and the fluid and electrolyte abnormalities are difficult to manage (Minkes et al. 2008).

Small bowel stomas, such as a jejunostomy, ileostomy or a proximal colostomy, have very liquid output and the volumes of effluent may be large. The stoma output can contain enzymes and other bowel contents which have the potential to irritate the skin. Skin irritation, excoriation and infection are among the most common complications with paediatric stomas. To help prevent this, the use of an appropriately fitting stoma appliance is essential. Various styles of appliance are available and there is an increasing range of barrier creams and products to select from.

Major surgery

Indications for major surgery

It is estimated that about 75% of individuals who live with Crohn's disease will require surgery at some point and that 75% of those who have one surgery will need at least one subsequent surgery. Many of these procedures will be minor, however some can be life-threatening. In life-threatening inflammatory bowel disorder, surgery is indicated:

- Where the bowel has become irreparably damaged.
- Where there is necrotic tissue causing toxaemia.
- Where a stricture has formed resulting in obstruction.
- To drain large and deep abscesses.
- To correct defects where there are multiple fistula.

Surgical approaches include conventional laparotomy, minimally invasive surgical techniques or endoscopic procedures. Increasingly, major procedures will be performed using a minimally invasive surgical procedure or an endoscopic surgical approach. However, at present only a few paediatric procedures are routinely offered, or can be performed using the minimally invasive approach. The laparotomy technique is used to expose the majority of the abdominal organs which allows for confirmation or correction of the preoperative diagnosis in a child presenting with an acute abdomen.

Minimally invasive surgery

Jaffray (2005) states that minimal access techniques are sought to perform a range of surgical procedures while avoiding the morbidity of conventional surgical wounds. This was first developed in the mid-1980s and became possible following three technological advances: a system allowing instrumental access into the body cavities; the scaling down of video cameras which provided good visualisation inside the body; and the production of insufflation devices to allow controlled distension of body cavities with gas to provide the surgeon opportunity to see and space to work.

The advantages of minimally invasive techniques include avoiding large wounds and the need to cut through abdominal muscles which results in less pain and the complications of immobility. Less pain facilitates earlier dis-

charge and shorter absences from school. There is also a better cosmetic result and less risk of infection.

Endoscopic approach

This is one of the fastest-growing fields of surgery. The flexible endoscope containing some form of illumination (usually a fibre-optic light source) which also contains a small channel for instruments to enable procedures such as taking biopsies and the retrieval of foreign bodies is appealing and effective for minor paediatric procedures. However, its use is limited owing to the small size of the gut lumen in the infant population.

Further developments in paediatric surgery and the flexibility of endoscopic equipment should allow for expansion of both these approaches in children. Trials underway with animal studies are being carried out to assess the possibilities of a natural orifice endoscopic minimally invasive approach (ASERNIP-S Report 2007).

Congenital corrective surgery

While the majority of infants requiring congenital corrective surgery will be managed in the neonatal intensive care unit, a number of usually full-term infants with potentially life-threatening defects will be managed in the paediatric intensive care setting as a consequence of cot shortages in the neonatal unit. On occasions, units may also need to accommodate pre-term infants and managing these infants can be a challenge as they have different requirements in terms of fluid management strategies, thermoregulation and pain control. In addition, the parents are in a uniquely vulnerable situation as the mother may be unwell herself following delivery and the father may have divided loyalties, having to allocate his time between the sick infant, his partner and any other children.

Tracheoesophageal fistula and oesophageal atresia

Tracheoesophageal fistula is very commonly associated with oesophageal atresia (OA) and therefore the lesions will be discussed together. The abbreviation TOF referring to this condition should not be confused with tetralogy of Fallot which is also referred to as TOF in some sources. TEF is the abbreviation used in the United States for this condition and may minimise confusion.

A tracheoesophageal fistula is a congenital (or occasionally acquired) communication between the trachea and oesophagus, while oesophageal atresia refers to a congenitally interrupted oesophagus. A tracheoesophageal fistula/ OA will occur as a consequence of the failure of the mesenchymal separation of the upper foregut, but there is no fixed time for this to happen. It affects more males than females and between 10 and 40% of infants in the reported series are preterm. Between 35 and 65% of these infants will have associated anomalies such as congenital heart disease, VATER syndrome or VACTERL association (Diaz et al. 2005).

V: Vertebral anomalies or VSD
A: Anorectal malformation
C: Cardiac anomalies (common)
T: Tracheal
E: Oesophageal atresia
R: Renal abnormalities
L: Limb/radial malformation

There are five commonly identified variants of tracheoesophageal fistula +/– OA which are detailed in Table 8.4.

Table 8.4 Variants of tracheoesophageal fistula and OA presentation

Type	Characteristics of lesion
A	OA with distal tracheoesophageal fistula (most common variant)
B	Pure OA with no tracheal involvement
C	Isolated tracheoesophageal fistula with no oesophageal involvement
D	OA with proximal tracheoesophageal fistula
E	OA with both distal and proximal tracheoesophageal fistula (least common variant)

Clinical presentation of TOF/OA
- Choking on first feed.
- Coughing.
- Cyanosis.
- Excessive salivation.
- Aspiration pneumonia.

Chest X-ray findings
- Coiled orogastric tube in the cervical pouch; air in the stomach and intestine.

Pre-operative management

The major aim of preoperative management is to minimise or prevent any pulmonary complications which may occur as a consequence of the aspiration of gastric or oesophageal pouch contents. The infant is kept nil by mouth and nursed in a cot or babytherm on a tilt to ensure that a head-up position is maintained. A Repogle tube (a double lumen, radio-opaque tube) is sited into the blind-end oesophageal pouch, left on low continuous suction and flushed regularly with a small volume (0.5 ml) of 0.9% sodium chloride to maintain patency. Guidelines for the frequency of flushing should be available from the neonatal unit with intervals varying between 15 and 30 minutes. The thickness of secretions will determine how regularly the Repogle tube requires flushing.

Surgical management

The type of surgical approach will be determined by the size of the gap between the two ends of the oesophagus (Table 8.5). A primary repair is possible when there is a small gap and reanastomosis will not cause undue tension on the site of repair when the infant moves. Delayed primary repair may be required if there is a long gap OA

Table 8.5 Management approaches for TOF/OA

Primary repair	Delayed primary repair	Oesophageal substitution
Intubation/ventilation for up to 5 days Head midline and use of muscle relaxants to avoid tension on the suture line Feed via a trans-anastomotic tube (TAT) Barium swallow prior to commencing oral feeds (to check for anastomotic leak)	Gastrostomy Long-term Repogle tube placement/ management Re-imaging to determine growth Use of cervical oesophagostomy and sham feeding will allow infant to develop feeding skills during this time Adequate growth – postoperative care as per primary repair	Management as per delayed primary repair and then surgical approach of: • colonic interposition • gastric tube oesophagoplasty • gastric transposition

(<the distance between six vertebrae) or if the gap is greater than six vertebrae then oesophageal substitution may be necessary.

Colonic interposition

A section of colon is transposed, with its blood supply intact, into the chest where it is joined to the oesophagus and the stomach bridging the gap. The advantages of this procedure are that the size of the graft is of equal diameter to the missing oesophagus and there is no limit to the size of the graft required (Thomas et al. 2009). The associated complications, however, need to be considered carefully:

- The blood supply to the transplanted section of colon is precarious.
- Poor peristalsis can lead to feeding difficulties.
- High incidence of leakage (30%).
- Stricture (narrowing) can occur (20%).
- Redundancy (lack of any muscular activity) can develop in the long term.

Gastric tube oesophagoplasty

A longitudinal segment is taken from the stomach, which is then positioned into the chest and joined to the oesophagus. The advantages include a good blood supply to the graft and the size of the graft is appropriate to the infant or child. Complications again need careful consideration as there is a very long suture line which leads to an increased risk of leakage and a high stricture rate. In addition, there is a significant risk of reflux disease.

Gastric transposition

This is a relatively new procedure in which the whole stomach is freed, mobilised and moved into the chest. The upper end of the oesophagus is then anastomosed to the top of the stomach in the neck (Hirschl et al. 2002). Advantages of this procedure are the lack of a long suture line, which minimises the risk of both leakage and stricture formation. The long-term consequences are not yet clearly identified, however, short-term complications include:

- Poor gastric emptying.
- As the bulk of the stomach is in the chest, respiratory capacity is reduced.
- Reflux can be a problem.
- 'Dumping syndrome' occurs when food enters the intestine relatively quickly and causes sweating, dizziness and diarrhoea and blood glucose imbalances.

Long-term consequences of TOF/OA

- Persistent cough.
- Gastro-oesophageal reflux disease (GORD).
- Recurrent lower respiratory tract infections.
- Strictures.
- Feeding difficulties.

Duodenal atresia

This is the most common foetal atresia, occurring in 1/5 000 births and is associated with Down's syndrome. It is a condition in which a part of the GIT tract from the duodenum to the anus has failed to form correctly and that part of the gut is either completely blocked or is missing altogether. This can result in life-threatening obstruction and the defect can only be corrected surgically.

There are three main types:

- Type I: Obstruction due to a mucosal web with normal muscular wall.
- Type II: Two atretic duodenal ends joined by a short fibrous cord.
- Type III: Complete separation of atretic ends with no connective tissue.

Many cases are now picked up on antenatal scans as a 'double bubble' may appear on scan due to the dilated, fluid-filled stomach and proximal duodenum. Parental counselling, advice and support should be offered at this point to ensure that they are adequately prepared. The pregnancy may be complicated by polyhydramnios owing to the impaired absorption of amniotic fluid by the foetal intestines. The defect may be a single one or complicated by intestinal malrotation and congenital heart disease. Postnatally, it may be suspected by the presence of vomiting within hours of birth. This vomit is most often bilious, although it may be non-bilious because a small number of atresia occurs proximal to the ampulla of Vater. Because the gut is not patent the infant might have a 'hollow'-looking abdomen (scaphoid). An X-ray may demonstrate a gas-filled 'double bubble' which corresponds to the antenatal fluid-filled image and, unless there is perforation, there is no other gas present in the intestine or abdominal cavity.

Pre-operative management

Although the condition is potentially life-threatening it is not an emergency and, if otherwise well, the infant can be left for between 24 and 48 hours before undergoing surgery. The infant must remain nil by mouth and be maintained with IV hydration. An NGT should be passed and the gut aspirated. If prolonged NGT aspiration is necessary or the amounts copious, the IV regime should include replacement of the gastric aspirate with either 0.45% or 0.9% sodium chloride. Prior to surgical repair, the infant's fluid and electrolyte status must be checked.

Surgical management

This has been performed laparoscopically and the techniques are being continually refined (Valusek et al. 2007). However, a laparotomy and a duodenostomy are the most commonly performed procedures. There are a couple of techniques for this and they are used at the surgeon's preference, but essentially they involve opening the duodenum channel along its length and joining it to the next portion of patent intestine, and correcting the duodenal lumen end to end so that a fully open channel exists. Most surgeons place a small trans-anastomotic (TAT) feeding tube to protect the suture line and expedite gut priming; some evidence suggests that toleration of enteral feeds is quicker as a result (Arnbjörnsson et al. 2002). The entire small bowel is carefully explored for other sites of obstruction, the hepatic and pancreatic anatomy is checked and any malrotation corrected.

Postoperative management

During the immediate postoperative phase the infant is usually intubated and ventilated. This maintains the airway and provides adequate oxygenation; it also permits effective analgesia and sedation to be administered and keeps the infant immobile to protect the wound and the TAT tube. Because the gut is extensively handled, a paralytic ileus is expected and the infant must remain on the 'drip and suck' mode of management until some motility returns. Once gut motility has commenced, small enteral feeds, ideally of expressed breast milk, may be commenced. Supporting the mother to express her breast milk and ensuring the future nutrition of the infant in line with World Health Organisation and Department of Health recommendations is a key children's nurse role and the RCN best practice guidelines (2009) can help inform unit policy. Typically, these children are quickly extubated and can be moved to a high dependency area or a cubicle in a children's ward. As it can sometimes take these infants a while to tolerate full feeds, full or fractional PN is maintained via a long line while full enteral feeding is established. This can be established on the children's ward, however this can be a frustrating time for the family as the infant is otherwise well and handles normally. Reverse transfers to the referring hospital may relieve some for the pressure on the family,

however clear PN prescription and feeding re-grade plans have to be in place and suitable follow-up organised.

Colonic atresia

This is rare but life-threatening if left untreated. In colonic atresia, the problems are complete bowel obstruction through which gas and stool cannot pass, the colonic segment above the atresia becomes distended and, if left untreated, leads to perforation (Nielson and Zitsman 2008). Davenport and colleagues (1990) reviewed the incidence of colonic atresia and suggest the following incidence within their sample of population.

- Ascending colon – 28%.
- Transverse colon – 23%.
- Splenic flexure – 25%.
- Descending and sigmoid – 20%.
- Hepatic flexure – 3%.

Treatment

A surgical repair with resection of the atretic component and end-to-end anastomosis is required. In complex cases where there may be multiple atresias or where the repair has been difficult the formation of a temporary stoma may be employed to protect the anastomosis. General postoperative care principles are required to manage the infant, with consideration given to fluid management, electrolyte balance, pain management and the reinstitution of enteral feeding when clinically indicated.

Colonic stenosis

Narrowing of the colon is much more common and frequently occurs following necrotising enterocolitis. In colonic stenosis, the problem is that gas and stool can pass through a narrow area and while the infant is passing milk stools, this may not be noticeable. When the diet changes from breast milk or formula to cereals and solid foods, the stool becomes more formed. This will result in the stenosis becoming symptomatic. The toddler can present with signs of obstruction, distension, feeding intolerance or faltering growth (Nielson and Zitsman 2008).

Gastroschisis

This occurs due to a congenital anterior abdominal wall defect usually to the right of the umbilicus which results in the evisceration of abdominal contents. The incidence of this condition has been increasing, however this may not be a year-on-year trend (Office for National Statistics 2006, 2007) and the risk is not geographically equally distributed (Kilby 2006), with more infants with this defect being born in the north of England and to younger mothers. Advances in neonatal care, total parenteral nutrition, surgical confidence and technique have all improved the prognosis and 90% of affected babies now survive. Long-term prognosis is also positive as late mortality following the infant year is rare and usually unrelated to the primary defect (Davies and Stringer 1997). Complications from the original defect requiring prolonged hospital management or further corrective intervention may result from the condition of the bowel at birth, prolonged paralytic ileus, malrotation, malabsorption, adhesions or abnormal bowel habit.

Diagnosis is usually made antenatally following foetal scan and there seems to be no difference in outcome if the infant is delivered by caesarean section or vaginally. The aim, once the infant is delivered, is to keep the exposed bowel moist and the infant should be inserted feet first into a clear plastic sac. This method is preferred over packs soaked with saline, although these can be used in an emergency. The bag should be tied above the lesion leaving the arms free so the infant can be cannulated for IV access, as to the circulation using a long line, as TPN and a range of broad spectrum antibiotics will be required. The infant needs to be nursed supported on their side to prevent kinking the loops of bowel and transferred once stable to the surgical unit. If the infant is self-ventilating with ease and maintaining their oxygen saturations, there is no need to intubate for transfer as prolonged ventilation is damaging to newborn lungs. This infant will be intubated and ventilated for surgery and the immediate recovery period to address the requirement for suitable analgesia and for ease of nursing to ensure that the infant is kept immobile to prevent tension on the repair line.

Repairs may be primary or staged depending on the extent of the defect. If the repair is staged some sort of silo bag to contain the gut will be stitched to the abdomen. There is a variety of makes, e.g. Gore-Tex®, or the plastic from an infusion bag may be used. This silo is created to accommodate intestines and will be reduced over a period of time. This avoids creating excessive intra-abdominal pressure, allows skin to stretch and grow, and improves the cosmetic result. The bag containing the intestines needs to be supported or suspended from the incubator roof or a frame to avoid the bag containing the gut from folding over causing trauma or kinking of the bowel. A combination of the primary defect and handling the gut normally results in a paralytic ileus and these infants are usually nil by mouth for prolonged periods until peristalsis returns. The mother should be supported and strongly encouraged to

express and store her breast milk as this is the preferred feed when feeding is eventually commenced. Building up feed tolerance can be a frustrating time for the parents as by this time the defect has been repaired the wound has healed and their baby is dressed and looks 'normal'. Reverse transfers to the referring hospital may relieve some for the pressure on the family, however clear feeding re-grade plans have to be in place and suitable follow-up organised.

Exomphalos or large omphalocoele

This is another abdominal wall defect where the gut has herniated into the base of the umbilical cord. It usually looks less drastic than the gastroschisis but the prognosis can be poorer as there is quite a strong association between this and other midline defects and some of these are chromosomal in origin. Not all of these are surgically repaired as some of the smaller ones may epithelialise over.

Intussusception

This is the telescoping of one segment of intestine into the adjacent distal segment which compresses the attached associated mesentery, blood vessels and nerves as a consequence. The resulting oedema and ischaemia to the affected intestine leads to obstruction and the risk of perforation and peritonitis. Most cases affect the ileo-colic region and it is the most common cause of intestinal obstruction in children between 3 months and 6 years of age, but small abnormalities can also provide a focus for the telescoping in clinical conditions such as a Meckel's diverticulum (Milbrandt and Sigalet 2008). Intussusception is rare in infants under 3 months of age and in older children and young people. Intussusception may also be a rare postoperative complication occurring in 0.08–0.5% of laparotomies. The likely mechanism is due to a difference in activity between segments of the intestine recovering from an ileus, which produces the intussusception (Bai et al. 2009).

Signs and symptoms of intussusception

- Colicky abdominal pain.
- Vomiting, feed intolerance; the vomit may contain bile.
- Stools containing blood called 'currant jelly' stool.
- Tubular mass in the abdomen.
- Absent bowel sounds.
- Abdominal X-ray may reveal gas and or free fluid levels.

If the infant is not managed in a timely fashion with appropriate fluid resuscitation, the condition can escalate and result in shock, with the infant requiring full intensive care provision, including inotropic support.

Management of intussusception

If the infant is sufficiently well, a non-surgical intervention can be tried with the administration of either an air enema or a barium contrast enema, which will confirm the diagnosis and can also rectify the problem. The enema itself carries a risk of perforation and cannot be performed if there is a suspicion that the bowel has already perforated (Shekherdimian et al. 2009).

If the intestinal obstruction cannot be resolved by the enema, surgery is necessary to reverse the intussusception and relieve the obstruction. This can sometimes result in resection and anastomosis to remove the segment of the intestine which has become gangrenous. This procedure may be undertaken laparoscopically if there is an experienced practitioner to perform the procedure (Fraser et al. 2009).

Volvulus or malrotation

Volvulus can be defined as a twisting of a loop of intestine around its mesenteric attachment site. This twisting can occur at various sites of the GI tract, including the stomach, small intestine, caecum, transverse colon and sigmoid colon. Midgut volvulus refers to twisting of the entire midgut around the axis of the superior mesenteric artery, which can be a very serious presentation. Because of embryological maldevelopment and rotation the condition can present soon after birth or may manifest within two months of life. It can be associated with a number of other pathologies, such as duodenal atresia, Meckel's diverticulum, intussusception, small bowel atresia, prune belly syndrome, gastric volvulus, persistent cloaca, Hirschsprung disease and extrahepatic biliary anomalies.

Clinical presentation of volvulus

The acute presentation resembles an abdominal emergency and requires urgent intervention:

* Pain and tender abdomen.
* Vomiting, which is usually bilious.
* Infants or children with delayed diagnosis may present in a shocked state.

Subacute presentation, usually found in older children, is not such an urgent situation and is not usually seen in intensive care. These children may have abdominal pain which is disproportionate to abdominal distension and may have a palpable mass. Abdominal X-rays may demonstrate

small bowel obstruction with fluid–air levels, while contrast studies may demonstrate corkscrew signs.

Management of volvulus

* Management of pain.
* Gastric decompression with NGT placement and left on free drainage.
* Fluid and electrolyte replacement.
* Intravenous antibiotics.

Acute or shocked presentation necessitates early surgery to prevent the development of ischaemia and or gangrenous bowel segments. Most children will have a Ladd procedure where the appendix is removed, the mesenteric bands are divided and the small intestine is replaced to the right and the colon to the left side of the abdominal cavity.

Postoperative management

Standard postoperative care will be required. Some children with volvulus suffer with prolonged ileus postoperatively and will require parenteral nutrition as a consequence of being unable to tolerate enteral nutrition. These children will require gentle reintroduction of enteral feeding, usually determined by the surgical team. A very small number will develop acquired short bowel syndrome and will require ongoing management.

Abdominal trauma

Abdominal trauma is relatively uncommon in children and most are managed conservatively regardless of age (Gaines 2009; Tataria et al. 2007). Most abdominal trauma results from blunt force trauma. In isolation it has a low mortality but when combined with other trauma, such as neurological or thoracic, the mortality rises (Davenport and Pierro 2009). Young children's abdominal organs are vulnerable as the ribs are poorly ossified and significant injuries in the under 2 year olds should trigger 'safeguarding questions' as there may be non-accidental, welfare and supervision issues (Champion et al. 2002).

Complications of major organ lacerations

* Major haemorrhage.
* Intestinal perforation.
* Leakage of gastrointestinal secretions into the abdominal cavity.

Abdominal organs such as the liver and spleen are highly vascular and friable so they are susceptible to laceration. These injuries can be life-threatening. If suspected, the child should be urgently admitted to a PICU, as the levels of medical expertise in Emergency Departments are variable (Prentiss and Vinci 2009).The child needs circulatory access, should be fully monitored and a range of diagnostic investigations performed. There is still a role for plain abdominal X-rays, but ultrasound and a CT scan can provide a more detailed picture. As considerable amounts of blood can be lost into the abdomen with only minor increases in girth size, measuring girth is an inaccurate means of observation (Atkin and Clifford 1985) yet continues to be performed in some units. This can lead to excessive handling and increase the distress of the child. Perforation of the gut can be a complication of blunt trauma and spillage of gut contents may lead to peritonitis. This is regarded as secondary peritonitis.

The aims of medical treatment and surgical management are twofold and complementary. One focuses on the need to restore and maintain the circulatory volume and the other to locate the area(s) of damage and prevent further blood loss. If surgery is indicated, then primary repair is preferred, but when not possible excision of the affected lobe of liver or removal of the spleen may be required. The liver has an amazing capacity to regenerate but there are considerable immunity risks for the asplenic child. There is some controversy with regard to the need for prophylaxis antibiotic therapy post-splenectomy (Moffatt 2009) and practitioners should refer to their local policies in terms of treatment strategies and medications utilised.

Neonatal liver disease

In neonates, jaundice can occur as a feature unrelated to a primary liver disorder or a symptom exacerbated by coexisting diseases. It is considered here as neonates frequently get admitted to the PICU for surgery or when the neonatal unit is full. It is common among premature infants and indeed in some term babies. The speed in which jaundice occurs is significant and also the length of time the condition is present is important as these can be indicators of the general well-being of the infant. Generally, physiological jaundice appears by day 3 and with good management lasts about 2 weeks. The causes of neonatal jaundice can be split into two main groups: haemolytic, caused by increased red cell breakdown; and non-haemolytic, caused by impairment in bilirubin excretion, as in liver disease. Haemolytic hyperbilirubinaemia is usually associated with unconjugated or indirect bilirubin.

Unconjugated hyperbilirubinaemia

This accounts for most cases of jaundice. The neonatal liver is fairly immature and bilirubin is the major waste product of haemoglobin degradation, which mainly takes place in the spleen. A raised bilirubin level in the blood is called hyperbilirubinaemia. This spills out of the bloodstream into the tissues and causes the yellow discoloration associated with the condition. The main causes are listed in Table 8.6.

Management

Low-level unconjugated hyperbilirubinaemia in the neonate does not need active intervention other than to establish a means of effective enteral feeding to improve hydration and stimulate gut transit times. Blood is sampled for levels of bilirubin to be measured and plotted on a chart which indicates treatment thresholds. If the infants are very sick, these treatment thresholds may be lowered as these infants may be considered to be more vulnerable to the consequences of kernicterus. Usually, treatment is by phototherapy but extremely high levels may be managed by exchange blood transfusion.

Providing phototherapy in the PICU

Phototherapy works by using light to change bilirubin to the more water-soluble cis-form, which is easier to excrete. A range of lights, pads and blankets is now used. However, for phototherapy to be effective, the infant requires maximum skin exposure and in some cases this means being naked except for a nappy. This can cause some parents distress so attention to the environment of care using screens, turning the baby round so they are head first visible rather than bottom first, or nursing the infant at the end of the unit away from the main unit walkway.

- Maintaining maximum exposure also has implication for handling and parents keen to get to know their new baby can feel excluded.
- Sick infants can have a critically unstable temperature which exposure to phototherapy exacerbates. Central and shin temperatures should be monitored continually.
- The infant's eyes must be covered when under lights, again causing some distress to the parents, and constantly monitored to ensure the covers remain in situ. Eye care should be provided when the nappy is changed and the parents can be taught to do this.
- Skin care is important to remove acidic urine and stools, however skin creams, oils or ointment must be avoided as the heat produced by the lights may result in skin burns.

Nurses play an important part in supporting the family to come to terms with this additional complication. In the

Table 8.6 Causes of unconjugated hyperbilirubinaemia

Cause	Aetiology
Physiological jaundice	Due to excessive RBC breakdown at birth and functional immaturity of the conjugation processes in the liver. Term babies treated with phototherapy if bilirubin greater than 300 μmol/l.
Breast milk jaundice	Persistence of foetal mechanisms (e.g. beta glucuronidase) causes low-level continued jaundice in some infants. This can be exacerbated by poor feeding techniques leading to dehydration. Surveillance is required by doctor if it lasts over a month.
Systemic disease	
Rhesus and ABO incompatibility Glucose-6-phosphate dehydrogenase Sickle cell disease Thalassaemia Spherocytosis Hypothyroidism Upper-intestinal obstruction Sepsis Hypoxia/acidosis Galactosaemia Fructosaemia	All cause increased haemolysis, which is particularly problematic if encountered in the newborn period exacerbating jaundice levels because of liver immaturity.
Iatrogenic	
Trauma at birth	Bruising leading to breakdown of RBC.
Blood transfusion Administration of certain drugs	Administration process can damage RBC. Some drugs displace bilirubin from albumin so increasing the free component, e.g. diazepam, hydrocortisone, gentamicin, cefalosporins, digoxin.
Inherited disorders	
Crigler-Najjar syndrome (Types 1 and 2)	Deficiency in enzyme uridinediphosphateglucuronosyltransferase (UDPGT). Type 1 is total and needs phototherapy long term. Type 2 is partial and may ultimately be treated with enzyme inducers such as phenobarbitone.
Gilbert's syndrome	Mild, transient jaundice that needs no treatment but reassurance.

Source: Dixon et al. (2009) *Nursing the Highly Dependent Child or Infant: A Manual of Care*. Reproduced with permission from John Wiley and Sons, Ltd.

NNU phototherapy is more common and as parents see other infants having it without difficulty they are more accepting. In the PICU their infant may be the only one in a box or under a set of lamps, so the distress may be disproportional.

If exchange transfusion is considered a textbook on neonatal care should be consulted.

Conjugated hyperbilirubinaemia

This is much less common. Elevated conjugated bilirubin results from obstructive liver disease, but can be seen in many types of liver disease which affect hepatocyte func-

tion. Conjugated hyperbilirubinaemia is said to be present when >20% of the total plasma bilirubin is conjugated or when the total conjugated level is greater than 20 mmol/l. Total and conjugated bilirubin levels are measured in the laboratory and the level of unconjugated is the difference between the two. The ratios of types of bilirubin can be helpful in diagnosis of the cause. In hepatobiliary disease the total and conjugated will be raised. Total and unconjugated will be raised in hepatic disease. A split bilirubin (total and conjugated) should be performed on any baby who remains jaundiced after 2 weeks of life (3 weeks for preterm infants). If the conjugated fraction is raised as defined above, investigations for possible liver disease should be started. Liver disease in the newborn can present as:

- An ill infant with liver failure (deranged clotting unresponsive to intravenous vitamin K).
- Neonatal hepatitis syndrome.
- Biliary obstruction.

If an infant has pale stools and dark urine, this needs to be brought to the attention of the medical team urgently. These infants are going to require more investigation for their hyperbilirubinaemia, and management and treatment will be more complex as phototherapy is not indicated for this group of babies.

Biliary atresia

This is one of the most common reasons for liver transplantation in children. The cause of this remains relatively obscure and because it is rare occurring in 1/15000 (Davenport and Pierro 2009) there is little research to inform on the aetiology or epidemiology of the condition. Biliary atresia is a condition in which the normal extrahepatic biliary system is disrupted. Progressive damage of extrahepatic and intrahepatic bile ducts secondary to inflammation may occur, leading to fibrosis, biliary cirrhosis and eventual liver failure.

There are three main types of biliary atresia:

- Type I: the common bile duct is obliterated, while the proximal bile ducts are patent.
- Type II: atresia of the hepatic duct is seen, with cystic bile ducts found at the porta hepatis.
  - In type IIa, the cystic and common bile ducts are patent.
  - In type IIb, the cystic, common bile duct, and hepatic ducts are obliterated.
- Type III: discontinuity of the right and the left hepatic ducts to the level of the porta hepatis. This form of biliary atresia is common, accounting for more than 90% of cases.

The infant with biliary atresia usually appears normal at birth but develops jaundice 2–3 weeks after birth. The key symptoms are:

- Jaundice.
- Dark urine: build-up of bilirubin.
- Acholic (clay-coloured) stools.

- Hepatomegaly.
- Weight loss and irritability.

Management of biliary atresia

Surgical intervention, known as a hepatoportoenterostomy or a Kasai procedure, is the only management option for biliary atresia and is ideally undertaken before 60 days of life to limit scarring within the liver, but this is not a curative procedure and the majority of children with biliary atresia will require liver transplantation before they reach adulthood (Bassett and Murray 2008).

The Kasai procedure removes the abnormal bile ducts and a loop of intestine is mobilised and sutured to some of the smaller ducts to drain the liver. As a result, bile flows from the smaller bile ducts straight into the intestine, bypassing the need for the larger bile ducts completely. This reduces reabsorption of bile into the blood stream and ensures that digestion of enteral nutrients is supported. This corrects many of the problems of biliary atresia.

Cholangiopathies

Cholangiopathies are a wide array of congenital or acquired disorders that result in chronic cholestatic conditions which lead to liver failure (Lazaridis et al. 2004). Cholangiopathies share the common feature of primarily targeting cholangiocytes, the epithelial cells lining the intrahepatic biliary tree (Lazaridis et al. 2004). These diseases are characterised by the progressive vanishing of bile ducts (ductopenia) which results from an abnormal cholangiocyte homeostasis. It is thought that this ductopenia results from excessive cell death by apoptosis (Alvaro et al. 2007). There is a compensatory proliferative response which enlarges the liver and is one reason why these children have large swollen abdomens. Cholangiopathies are a challenge for clinicians to manage and 50% of transplants among paediatric patients are due to these disorders.

Acute liver failure (ALF)

Fulminant hepatic failure or acute liver failure (ALF) in children is a relatively rare clinical syndrome and the mortality rate is high at 60–80% in the absence of liver transplantation (Nazer 2011, Cochran and Losek 2007). The complexity of the child with hepatic failure is a challenge for the whole healthcare team. This is not the same as the transient liver dysfunction associated with critical illness which is commonly seen in PICU, however critical illness with persistent end organ ischaemia can be a contributory factor.

The three essentials for normal liver function are adequate blood flow, good oxygenation and low pressure in the biliary system. The functions of the liver are numerous but include the following:

- Carbohydrate, fat and protein metabolism.
- Removal of drugs and hormones.
- Excretion of bile and the synthesis of bile salts.
- Storage of glycogen.
- Activation of vitamin D, and synthesis of vitamins A, B_{12}, D, E and K.
- Production of apoferetin.
- Phagocytosis.

The causes of acute or fulminant liver failure are wide-ranging. The mechanisms of hepatic cellular injury which may lead to ALF are:

- Direct hepatocellular injury:
  – Herpes virus family.
  – Toxic or reactive metabolites (e.g. paracetamol).
  – Toxic metabolites of compounds – metabolic diseases.
- Immune-mediated hepatocellular injury:
  – Viral infections.
  – Drug hepatotoxicity (dihydralazine, halothane).
- Ischaemic hepatocellular injury:
  – Shock states
  – Systemic inflammatory response syndrome (SIRS).

Clinical features of ALF

Acute liver failure can develop within days or weeks depending on the underlying aetiology. The range of clinical signs will also vary; however there is a rapid onset of hepatic dysfunction with associated development of coagulopathies, metabolic derangement and the accumulation of neurotoxic by-products in the brain which cause an encephalopathic picture to emerge.

General signs of ALF

- Nausea and vomiting.
- Fatigue.
- Anorexia.
- Jaundice.
- Ascites.
- Increased bruising.

Hepatic signs of ALF

- Elevated transaminases (ALT, AST).
- Hypoglycaemia.
- Abnormally low cholesterol levels.

- Coagulopathy (not correctable with parenteral vitamin K).
- Progressively rising bilirubin.
- Elevated ammonia levels with associated encephalopathy.

Hepatic encephalopathy (HE)

HE is a gradable, reversible syndrome characterised by decreased level of consciousness, seizures or multifocal muscle twitching or coma. For HE to be diagnosed there must be an absence of other factors which could suppress cerebral function. Up to 80% of patients with HE have cerebral (cytotoxic) oedema while between 30–50% will have clinically significant raised intracranial pressure.

HE may be graded according to the neurological signs present (Table 8.7).

Management of ALF

The management of ALF is determined in part by the need to manage the complications associated with the hepatic dysfunction alongside therapies aimed at minimising ongoing hepatic cell damage and supporting the child until there is recovery of hepatic function or the child is referred for transplant (Table 8.8).

Complications arising from hepatic dysfunction include those detailed below. The most common causes of death are notated with an asterisk:

Table 8.7 Grading of hepatic encephalopathy

Grade of encephalopathy	Clinical features
Grade I (Mild)	Lethargy, disruption of day–night sleep patterns, mild motor impairment.
Grade II (Moderate)	Disorientation, confusion, inappropriate behaviours, increasing drowsiness but remaining responsive to simple commands.
Grade III (Severe)	Rousable to voice and localisation to pain, confusion, incoherent speech patterns.
Grade IV (Coma)	Unrousable, minimal response to painful stimuli, decerebrate or decorticate posturing.

Source: adapted from Arya, SheffaliGulati and Deopujari 2010; Blei and Córdoba 2001; Munoz 2008.

Table 8.8 Management strategies for ALF

Body system	Management strategies
Cardiovascular	Restoration of a euvolaemic state with judicious use of fluid and CVP monitoring. Diuresis with albumin, fluid restriction, diuretics. Support myocardial performance – use of vasoactive medications. Maintain good oxygenation to the myocardium.
Pulmonary	Intubation and mechanical ventilation may be necessary, particularly in children with grade III/–IV HE and in these children, oral intubation is indicated to prevent potential haemorrhage secondary to coagulopathy. Reduce the risk of ventilator associated pneumonia (Chapter 4).
Neurological	ICP monitoring is controversial and not proven to benefit the outcome but could be considered in children with rapidly developing signs and symptoms of raised ICP, Grade IV HE, rapidly progressing grade III HE or the presence of cerebral oedema on CT scan. Standard RICP therapy to maintain ICP <20 mmHg and CPP >50 mmHg (Chapter 7). Barbiturate coma may be used if necessary. Continuous EEG monitoring. Continuous renal replacement therapy (CRRT) such as continuous venovenous haemofiltration (CVVH) or plasmapheresis to reduce the levels of harmful nitrogenous metabolites.
Metabolic	Nil by mouth in initial stages until cause identified. Maintain serum blood glucose level above 4 mmol to minimise the possibility of hypoglycaemia and its deleterious effects. Maintain glucose intake with 15, 20, or 50% glucose as necessary. Enteral feeds/dietary intake which is low in sodium and protein (if stable – grade I–II HE). Use of PN – highest concentration of glucose tolerated if unable to maintain enteral nutrition with supplements of amino acid (trophamine) 0.5–1.0 g/kg/day and the use of lipids (20% solution) 0.5–3 g/kg/day.
Haematological	Vitamin K – 0.2 mg/kg/day (max. 10 mg) IV × 3 days, then every other day. Maintain PT at 20–25 sec (if no active bleeding). Maintain PT at <20 sec (if active bleeding). Maintain platelet count >50 000. Maintain haematocrit > 30%. Fresh frozen plasma (FFP) infusions for active bleeding. Plasmapheresis should be considered when there is severe coagulopathy and/or bleeding.
Gastrointestinal	Gastric protection to prevent ulceration and reduce the risk of gastric bleeding – H_2 receptor antagonist. Use of lactulose to reduce the transit times of ammonia containing matter through the bowel.
Renal	Conventional renal support through the use of peritoneal dialysis or CVVH may be required. Renal dysfunction with renal failure occurs in as many as 50% of patients. The kidneys are involved secondary to hepatorenal syndrome (HRS), acute tubular necrosis (ATN), drug-induced nephrotoxicity or prerenal azotaemia. *Hepatorenal syndrome* HRS is defined as functional renal failure occurring in patients with severe liver disease in the absence of any other underlying cause of renal disease. A decrease in blood flow to the kidneys has been suggested as the underlying pathophysiology (Latif and Mehmood 2010). Liver transplantation is the treatment of choice for HRS; however, some patients continue to require dialysis even following the transplant.

Source: Arya et al. 2010; Blei and Córdoba 2001; Latif and Mehmood 2010; Munoz 2008.

- Encephalopathy.
- Cerebral oedema and raised intracranial pressure.*
- Haemorrhage.
- Hypoglycaemia (profound).
- Disseminated intravascular coagulopathy.*
- Acid base derangements.
- Cardiac and circulatory instability.
- Pulmonary failure.
- Renal failure.
- MODS.*
- Sepsis.*

Bridging to transplant or recovery

Referral to a specialist centre is necessary for any child who may require liver transplantation. These centres offer a range of bridging therapies and not all children will proceed to a full transplant. Current strategies include hepatocyte transplantation or extracorporeal liver support systems. These are highly specialised therapies and practitioners should seek further information from specialist centres.

Auxiliary orthotopic liver transplantation (AOLT)

AOLT usually involves the transplanting of one or two lobes of the donor liver, although the whole liver may be used without the complete removal of the native liver. AOLT acts as a bridge to native liver recovery. If recovery occurs, then immunosuppression may be discontinued and the graft removed or allowed to atrophy to avoid long-term immunosuppression. In metabolic diseases, AOLT can provide the necessary enzymes to correct the deficiency and yet allows the patient to continue to utilise their native liver. Published studies indicate a good success rate for this therapeutic approach (Faraj et al. 2010).

Predictive outcomes of ALF

The overall survival for patients with ALF and grade III or grade IV HE has increased from 20% to 50% over the past two decades without transplant, but the best independent predictor of outcome is the aetiology of the ALF. For example, Wilson's disease has a predicted survival of <5% without liver transplant while the survival from non-ABC hepatitis is <20%.

Liver transplant

Paediatric liver transplantation is highly successful and is now an established therapeutic option (Alagille 2004). Children who have severe hepatic disease and who may require a transplant are referred via established care pathways to a paediatric liver transplant centre. There are many

Table 8.9 Indications for liver transplant

Life-threatening metabolic liver disease	Crigler–Najjar syndrome
	Urea cycle defects
	Hypercholesterolaemia
	Organic acidaemias
	Primary hyperoxaluria
Chronic liver disease	Biliary atresia
	Alpha-1-antitrypsin deficiency
	Autoimmune hepatitis
	Sclerosing cholangitis
	Caroli syndrome
	Wilson's disease
	Cystic fibrosis
	Progressive familial intrahepatic cholestasis (all types)
	Alagille syndrome
	Glycogen storage diseases types 3 and 4
	Tyrosinaemia type 1
Acute liver failure	Ingestion of toxic metabolites
Liver tumours	Unresectable hepatoblastoma (without active extrahepatic disease)
	Unresectable benign liver tumours with disabling symptoms

Source: UK Transplant 2005.

reasons why a child may need to be considered for transplant and Table 8.9 is not an exhaustive review. As children's size and age varies widely, matched grafts are unlikely to be available. This has led to the development of reduced-size graft and split liver transplantation. This has the advantage that a single donor liver can serve two or three children. Parents or adult relatives may also be screened and selected to provide a segment of their liver in living donor liver transplantation. Post-transplant management protocols usually include the use of a calcineurin inhibitor (cyclosporine or tacrolimus) and while the protocol usually depends on the surgical team's preference, tacrolimus has almost completely replaced cyclosporine in liver transplantations (Jain et al. 2002). Most centres also use steroids for some time post-transplant.

Endocrine presentations

There are a small number of endocrine presentations where the child may either in the first instance or as a secondary consequence end up in the intensive care setting.

Endocrinology is a specialised field and the general principles of management only are outlined in this section.

Diabetic ketoacidosis

Diabetes mellitus (DM) arises from inadequate insulin effects within the body. In children it almost always occurs as a result of inadequate amounts of insulin being available.

TYPES OF DM
- Type I (IDDM): the most frequent form in children.
- Type II (NIDDM): uncommon in children, however the incidence is increasing (these children are not usually prone to ketosis).

RARE TYPES OF DM
- Genetic defects of β-cell function.
- Genetic defects of insulin action.
- Diseases of the exocrine pancreas.
- Drug or chemical induced (Table 8.4).
- Uncommon forms of immune-mediated diabetes.
- Other genetic syndromes (Alberti et al. 1999).

The mechanism for the development of DM in children is not clearly understood but there are a number of possible factors which may predispose a child towards it, including genetic predisposition, following a viral infection or as part of an autoimmune process. A number of children have either defective conversion of pro-insulin to insulin or an abnormal structure of their insulin molecules which causes the development of DM.

Diabetic ketoacidosis

DKA is one of the commonest metabolic disorders seen in the paediatric population and while the majority of children will not be managed in the intensive care setting, a small number will due to their age or persistent metabolic derangement which is slower than usual to respond to treatment strategies.

Pathophysiology of diabetic ketoacidosis

DKA is characterised by severe depletion of water and electrolytes from both the intracellular (ICF) and extracellular fluid (ECF) compartments. The initial and key event in DKA is insulin deficiency, however many of physiological processes seen are mediated by increased levels of counter-regulatory hormones (glucagon, adrenaline and noradrenaline, growth hormone and/or cortisol) (Table 8.10).

As a consequence of the processes outlined in Table 8.10 the five key clinical features of DKA are hyperglycaemia, ketogenesis, hyperosmolality, dehydration and electrolyte imbalance (Figure 8.1). The key to the management of the child with DKA is thorough assessment followed by frequent reassessment of the therapies instituted. Treatment is divided into two phases: initial assessment and management on presentation; and long-term management. (For further information regarding pre-intensive care management, practitioners are advised to refer to the current British Society of Paediatric Endocrinology and Diabetes (BSPED) guidelines and local integrated care pathways.)

Management of DKA (BSPED Guidelines 2009)

Children who are likely to require high dependency or intensive care provision are identified in the following categories:

- Severe acidosis (pH <7.1) with marked hyperventilation.
- Severe dehydration (10%) with the presence of shock.
- Under 2 years of age.
- Decreased level of consciousness to the point where the airway may be compromised.

Fluids

An assessment of the degree of dehydration must be made before calculating fluid requirements. As one of the major complications of DKA is cerebral oedema, fluid management strategies must be clearly prescribed and if there is uncertainty, clarification must be sought from the prescribing practitioner. The total fluids required by the child are for maintenance and for the replacement of the calculated fluid deficit. Important formulas are identified in Figure 8.2. Caution must be taken with rehydration in:

- Young children (<2 years of age).
- Children with very high serum sodium levels or very high initial serum glucose levels.

Electrolytes

Potassium is mainly an intracellular ion and there is always a massive depletion of total body potassium even though initial serum levels may be elevated, normal or low. In a persistent acidotic state, the intracellular positively charged ions of potassium move out of the cell in exchange for the positively charged hydrogen ions (to allow access to the intracellular buffers) in an attempt to reduce the degree of acidosis. The increased serum potassium level is detected in the renal tubules and the perceived excess is excreted.

Table 8.10 Physiological changes of insulin and counter-regulatory hormones in DKA

	Physiological effects	Changes in DKA
Insulin	Helps glucose enter the cells. Stimulates glycogenesis (creation of glycogen). Stimulates glucose catabolism (breakdown). Lowers serum blood glucose level.	Decreased or absent levels mean that glucose does not enter the cells. Glycogen is not formed to store glucose and therefore the serum level of glucose rises.
Cortisol	Stimulates protein mobilisation and gluconeogenesis. Raises the serum blood glucose level.	Increased levels of proteins, which are utilised as an alternative source of energy.
Glucagon	Stimulates glycogenolysis (liberation of glycogen from the liver stores). Raises the serum blood glucose level.	Increased circulating levels of glycogen, which is metabolised to glucose but which cannot be used by the cells for energy.
Growth hormone	Decreases utilisation of carbohydrate for energy. Stimulates the liberation and catabolism of fats. Raises the serum blood glucose level.	Increased levels of fat, which is broken down into glycerol and fatty acids – neither can be accessed by cells for energy.
Adrenaline	Stimulates the liberation and catabolism of fats. Stimulates glycogenolysis (liberation of glycogen from the liver stores). Raises the serum blood glucose level.	Increased levels of fat which is broken down into glycerol and fatty acids – neither can be accessed by cells for energy. Increased circulating levels of glycogen, which is metabolised to glucose but which cannot be used by the cells for energy.

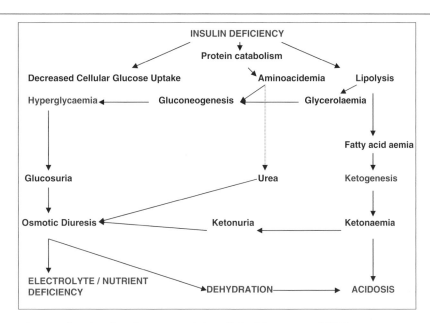

Figure 8.1 The pathways for the development of the clinical features of DKA.

Overall Fluid Requirement = Maintenance + Deficit

Deficit

% dehydration × weight (kg) × 10 = fluid deficit in ml

- To avoid excessive fluid replacement calculate total deficit as no more than 8%.

- Calculate total volume to be given over 48 hours after subtracting resuscitation fluid

  given.

- Maintenance fluid requirements are calculated according to the following guideline

  rather than the standard method usually used.

Weight (kg)	Maintenance Fluids
0 – 12.9	80mls/kg/24 hours
13 –19.9	65mls/kg/24 hours
20 – 34.9	55mls/kg/24 hours
35 – 59.9	45mls/kg/24 hours
> 60	35mls/kg/24 hours

Figure 8.2 Fluid calculations in DKA. Source: BSPED 2009.

The greater the level of acidosis, the greater the potassium exchange. Once the acidosis starts to resolve with the administration of fluids and insulin therapy however, the exchange will be reversed and hydrogen will move out of the cells while potassium moves back in. The overall next effect of this will be a total body depletion of potassium as the perceived excess lost through the kidneys will not have been replaced at this point. Although the child may present with hypokalaemia, normokalaemia or even hyperkalaemia, the recommendation is for potassium supplementation to begin immediately unless the child has elevated T-waves on the ECG or is anuric. Careful monitoring of serum electrolytes with 4-hourly sampling as a minimum is recommended.

There is always depletion of phosphate, another predominantly intracellular ion, and serum levels may be very low. There is no evidence in adults or children that replacement has any clinical benefit and phosphate administration may lead to hypocalcaemia.

The serum sodium concentration is an unreliable measure of the degree of ECF loss because the presence of glucose, essentially confined to the extracellular space, causes the osmotic movement of water into the extracel-

lular space thereby inducing dilutional hyponatraemia. There is some evidence that a drop in plasma sodium concentration during treatment may precipitate the development of cerebral oedema (Barry et al. 2010), therefore 0.9% sodium chloride is recommended as the initial fluid for the first 12 hours of treatment for the management of DKA. The child may present with hyponatraemia, hypernatraemia or normal serum values, but careful monitoring of both plasma and corrected values of the child's sodium is essential to minimise the potential risks of rebound hypo or hypernatraemia (Wolfsdorf et al. 2007).

Insulin therapy

After the child's rehydration fluids have started, blood glucose levels will start to fall. There is some evidence that cerebral oedema is more likely if insulin is started early, therefore it is now recommended that insulin infusions should not start until the intravenous fluids have been running for at least 1 hour. Continuous low-dose intravenous infusion is the preferred method for control and there is no need for an initial bolus. It is important that the insulin infusion is never discontinued while the child is receiving rehydration therapy or while they are receiving glucose in their fluids as insulin is required to switch off ketone production. Children who are already on a long-acting insulin preparation (e.g. Glargine™) often continue with this in addition to IV insulin infusion. Children who are on continuous subcutaneous insulin infusions already need to have this therapy stopped when the DKA protocol is instituted.

Anti-coagulant prophylaxis

There is a significant risk of femoral vein thrombosis in the very young and the sickest children presenting with DKA if femoral lines are used for access and fluid management, therefore low-dose anti-coagulation therapy may be required. It is also recommended that this should be considered in children who are significantly hyperosmolar, but only after discussion with senior medical staff.

Ketone monitoring

It is now recommended that near-patient ketone testing is used to confirm that ketone levels are falling adequately in response to therapy alongside the usual blood glucose monitoring (Savage et al. 2011). At initial presentation, blood ketone levels are generally >3 mmol/l and a gradual reduction in this value will indicate that the child is receiving sufficient insulin (BSPED 2009).

Complications of DKA

The most widely acknowledged complication is cerebral oedema which is unpredictable in its occurrence, affecting younger children and those with newly diagnosed diabetes more frequently. It has an associated mortality of around 25%. The pathophysiology of cerebral oedema in DKA is not clearly defined, however the following steps are recommended if it is suspected, after ensuring that hypoglycaemia is not the cause of any changes in the child's neurological status:

- Give hypertonic (2.7%) sodium chloride (5 ml/kg over 5–10 min) or mannitol 0.5–1.0 g/kg stat (2.5–5 ml/kg mannitol 20% over 20 min).
- Restrict IV fluids to half calculated maintenance and replace the deficit over 72 rather than 48 hours.
- Urgent CT scan.

Other complications include hypoglycaemia or hypokalaemia, both of which may be avoided through the careful monitoring of the child's electrolytes and serum glucose levels. A number of children initially present with abdominal pain and continuing abdominal pain is common. It may be attributed to liver swelling, gastritis, urinary retention or ileus, however, if it persists after the stabilisation of the DKA a surgical referral may be necessary to rule out any abdominal pathology (e.g. appendicitis). A raised serum amylase is also a common finding (BSPED 2009).

Adrenal insufficiency

Adrenal insufficiency is rare in children and as the presentation is nonspecific, there is often a delay in diagnosis. The most common causes are congenital adrenal hyperplasia (72% of cases), adrenoleukodystrophy (15% of cases) and autoimmune adrenalitis (13% of cases).

The adrenal gland is made up of two discrete parts: the cortex and the medulla. The cortex has three layers: the zona glomerulosa, zona fasciculata and the zona reticularis. The outer cortex is mainly stimulated by the renin angiotensin aldosterone system (RAAS) and high serum K^+ levels, which combine to regulate the release of aldosterone. The inner cortex is mainly controlled by the corticotropin-releasing hormone (CRH)–adrenocorticotrophic hormone (ACTH) system which regulates the release of cortisol in response to stress. It also produces adrenal androgens. The medulla is part of the sympathetic nervous system (SNS) and produces the endogenous catecholamines adrenaline and noradrenaline (Tortora and Derrickson 2009).The actions and effects of aldosterone and cortisol insufficiency are outlined in Table 8.11.

Adrenocortical insufficiency

Adrenocortical insufficiency may arise as a consequence of primary disease such as Addison's disease or congenital adrenal hyperplasia, secondary to an underlying disease process such as pan-hypopituitarism or as a consequence of long-term high-dose glucocorticoid therapy.

Addison's disease

Addison's disease is characterised by progressive destruction of the adrenal glands. This is usually autoimmune-based and most likely the result of cytotoxic T-lymphocytes, although 50% of patients have circulating adrenal antibodies. Clinical and biochemical insufficiency occurs once >90% of the gland is destroyed. Addison's disease affects 1–4 per 100000 people, in all age groups and both sexes. The symptoms of adrenal insufficiency usually begin gradually and the most common symptoms are chronic and worsening fatigue, muscle weakness, loss of appetite and weight loss. Hyperpigmentation or darkening of the skin can also occur. This is most visible on scars, skin folds, pressure points such as the elbows, knees and knuckles, and toes, lips and mucous membranes. Sudden, severe worsening of symptoms is called an Addisonian crisis or

Table 8.11 Actions of aldosterone and cortisol

	Actions	Effects of insufficiency
Aldosterone	Increase Na^+ and Cl^- reabsorption Increase in K^+ and H^+ secretion	Hyponatraemia Hyperkalaemia Acidosis Dehydration Azotaemia
Cortisol	Mobilises energy Increased glycogen release – induction of relative hyperglycaemia Water retention by increasing ADH (stress response)	Weakness Hypotension Shock Hypoglycaemia Eosinophilia

Source: Tortora and Derrickson 2009.

acute adrenal insufficiency. In most cases, symptoms of adrenal insufficiency become serious enough for a diagnosis to have been made and treatment instituted; however sometimes symptoms first appear during an Addisonian crisis.

Acute adrenal insufficiency or crisis

Crisis occurs when the physiological demand for these hormones exceeds the ability of adrenal glands to produce them, e.g. when the body is subjected to an intercurrent illness or stress:

- Major or minor infections.
- Injury.
- Surgery.
- Burns.
- General anaesthesia.
- Hypermetabolic states.

It should be considered when shock and vascular collapse are out of proportion to the severity of disease and degree of collapse, with unresponsiveness to volume expansion and inotropic support and or there is severe unexplained resistant hypoglycaemia. Management of acute adrenal insufficiency is focused on immediate resuscitation, volume replacement and treatment of the precipitating cause with the administration of corticosteroid therapy.

Initial resuscitation uses the ABC approach:

- High-flow O_2.
- IV/IO fluid boluses (20 ml/kg 0.9% sodium chloride).

- IV dextrose (2–5 ml/kg 10% glucose) as required according to serum blood glucose values.

Calculation and intravenous replacement of estimated dehydration:

- Usually calculated as 5% or greater and replaced over 8 hours.
- Use 5% glucose with 0.9% sodium chloride.
- Unlikely to require added potassium initially, but careful monitoring of electrolytes is essential.

Corticosteroids:

- IV hydrocortisone – 100 mg/m^2 (approximately 4 mg/kg for a child).
- IV hydrocortisone (2 mg/kg for a child) IV every 6 hours during the first 24 hours.
- Thereafter the hydrocortisone dose can usually be halved again.

If hypotension persists after initial management, additional corticosteroids may be required along with a vasoactive infusion (e.g. dopamine). Invasive monitoring (e.g. arterial and central access) may be necessary. These children rarely require intubation and invasive ventilation. Ongoing management centres on hormone replacement:

- Glucocorticoid replacement – hydrocortisone is the mainstay of treatment; the dose is divided into two-thirds in the morning and one third in the late afternoon (thus stimulating the normal diurnal adrenal rhythm).

- If there is coexistent thyroid deficiency, thyroid hormones should not be replaced before glucocorticoids, as a crisis may be precipitated.
- Mineralocorticoid replacement (fludrocortisone) – this is usually required in primary adrenal insufficiency.

Phaeochromocytoma

Phaeochromocytomas are rare tumours, with an incidence of 1–2 per million of the population. Between 10 and 20% of these tumours occur in children, however the majority appear after the age of 14 years. Approximately 6–10% of the tumours are malignant and may be associated with other syndromes such as multiple endocrinopathy (MEN) (Spoudeas 2005; Waguespack et al. 2010).

A phaeochromocytoma is a catecholamine-secreting tumour arising from chromaffin cells in the sympathetic nervous system and may be found in the adrenal medulla. Tumours located outside the adrenal glands may also be termed paragangliomas. Chromaffin cells produce the catecholamines noradrenaline and adrenaline. Noradrenaline is transformed into adrenaline by phentolamine methyltransferase. Both of these are metabolised to VMA (vanillylmandellic acid). Noradrenaline is the predominant product of this tumour in children (Barry et al. 2010), although adrenaline may also be secreted. Although there are a number of cardiovascular manifestations, the major clinical presentation is sustained or paroxysmal hypertension associated with other signs and symptoms of catecholamine excess (Prejbisz et al. 2011).

Clinical presentation

- Sustained hypertension (in around 80–90% of cases).
- Tachycardia.
- Sweating.
- Headache.
- Nausea and vomiting.
- Change in vision.
- Orthostatic hypotension.
- Abdominal pain.
- Polyuria and polydipsia.

Management of phaeochromocytoma

Before surgery to remove the tumour there needs to be a period of medical management to stabilise the child's cardiovascular status. The therapy required will depend on whether the tumour secreted both adrenaline and noradrenaline or just the latter.

Preoperative management

The key requirements of preoperative management are to restore circulating blood volume to normal and gain control of the child's cardiovascular system before surgery is planned. Effective alpha blockade should always be achieved before beta blockade is attempted to avoid precipitating congestive heart failure:

- Volume resuscitation (these tumours induce a volume-reduced circulating blood flow as a consequence of sustained hypertension).
- Hypertension control with alpha-adrenergic drugs (e.g. phentolamine and phenoxybenzamine or prazosin). For persistent hypertension after alpha blockade, consideration may be given to introducing a beta blockade using esmolol or labetalol. Beta blockade initiated without prior alpha blockade can exacerbate hypertension.

Postoperative management

The major issue postoperatively is cardiovascular instability, with intermittent hypotension being one of the primary concerns. Where possible, intravascular fluids should be used to manage this and the use of vasoactive agents avoided, however there may well be a requirement for a very low-dose noradrenaline infusion to manage hypotension. The removal of the trigger for long-standing hypertension can induce a precipitous drop in blood pressure, which may compromise cerebral perfusion. Persistent hypertension in the postoperative period may be indicative of residual tumour mass which is active.

Hypoglycaemia

Hypoglycaemia is defined as a blood glucose level of <2.5 mmol/l or 4 mmol/l in children with diabetes (Barry et al. 2010). For most healthy children glycogen stores are sufficient to maintain blood glucose levels for up to 8 hours of fasting while in infants stores are more limited and last between 4 and 6 hours. Once glycogen stores are depleted the body becomes reliant on gluconeogenesis to provide glucose for the cells. Depriving the brain of glucose produces predictable adverse consequences in terms of metabolism and growth, and may lead to permanent impairment of brain growth and function. Long-term sequelae can include profound developmental delay or retardation or recurrent seizures.

Aetiology of hypoglycaemia

The causes of hypoglycaemia include:

- Glycogen storage disease.
- Ketotic hypoglycaemia (uncommon). It is observed in children <5 years, who usually become symptomatic after an overnight or prolonged fast, especially with illness and poor oral intake. Children often present as

inexplicably lethargic or frankly comatose, having only marked hypoglycaemia with ketonuria (Cranmer 2011)

- Pan-hypopituitarism.
- Sepsis.
- Liver disease.
- Beta cell adenoma.
- Deliberate poisoning.
- Infant of a diabetic mother.
- Congenital hyperinsulinism (previously known as nesidioblastosis). This is a refractory non-ketotic hypoglycaemia caused by developmental disorganisation of the islet cells and inappropriate insulin release. There is a relative deficiency of somatostatin in this condition.

Clinical presentation of hypoglycaemia

Early symptoms are related to adrenergic activity and the autonomic response to hypoglycaemia and include sweating, palpitations and anxiety in the older child or pallor and jitteriness in the infant. Repeated or prolonged episodes of hypoglycaemia can result in the appearance of neuroglycaemic symptoms with little or no warning (termed hypoglycaemic unawareness). Symptoms include:

- Anxiety, ataxia, paraesthesia, dysarthria.
- Sweating.
- Hypothermia.
- Apnoeas and bradycardias and cyanosis in infants.
- Palpitations.
- Poor feeding.
- Seizures.
- Coma.

Management of hypoglycaemia

The management of hypoglycaemia is in part determined by the effects manifested in the infant or child.

Symptomatic

It is important where possible to collect blood for specific testing to determine the cause, while preparing a glucose infusion. A laboratory-derived blood glucose level is important (due in part to the relative inaccuracy of the some other methods of deriving blood glucose levels) and additional samples will be required to screen for metabolic disorders (e.g. markers of fatty acid metabolism). A failure to find large ketones with hypoglycaemia suggests that fat is not being metabolised from adipose tissue (hyperinsulinism) or that fat cannot be used for ketone body formation secondary to enzymatic defects in fatty acid oxidation (Cranmer 2011). Practitioners are referred to their unit's

clinical protocols for the relevant samples and the required blood volumes.

An intravenous glucose bolus dose of 10% glucose (0.5g/kg) will be required, after which a continuous glucose infusion will be needed, which provides the infant or child with 6–8mg/kg/min of glucose. The purpose of the continuous infusion is to avoid a rebound hypoglycaemia secondary to the insulin secretion triggered by the bolus dose. In the small infant the use of high glucose concentrations may be necessary to avoid a large fluid load; however, concentrations over 12.5% will require central venous access. Similarly, if the child's blood glucose level is not maintained on 10% or 12.5% glucose infusions, central access will be necessary (Barry et al. 2010).

If hypoglycaemia is refractory to glucose administration, either glucagon or hydrocortisone may be of benefit.

Hyperinsulinism

For hyperinsulinism, in addition to glucose management to maintain normoglycaemia, a glucagon infusion or the use of ocreotide may be indicated if persistent hypoglycaemia is present. When there is stability in terms of blood glucose levels, diazoxide, which acts on the potassium channel (KATP channel) to prevent insulin release, may be given orally if the cause of hyperinsulinism is not secondary to a KATP channel defect, and consideration may be given to the use of continuous enteral feeds to maintain stability.

Asymptomatic

If the infant or child is asymptomatic, appropriate oral intake or an enteral feed may be sufficient to correct the hypoglycaemia. If this is a single episode which can be attributable, then further investigation may not be merited, however if there is a repeated history, then clinical investigations must be undertaken.

Hyperammonaemia

Hyperammonaemia is a termed applied to a heterogeneous group of disorders characterised by elevated ammonia levels in the blood, resulting in altered levels of consciousness (Bosoi and Rose 2009) (Table 8.12). The incidence is rare and presentation can be in the neonatal period or later in childhood. The main causes of hyperammonaemia are organic acidaemias, fatty acid oxidation disorders (FAOD) or urea cycle disorders.

Physiology of ammonia production

Catabolism of nitrogenous compounds (endogenous and exogenous proteins) produces amino acids, which are

Table 8.12 Clinical presentation of hyperammonaemia

Neonates	Older children
Onset of features 24–72 hours after feeding (protein load) commences.	Usually present after a sudden protein load or an intercurrent infection.
Neurological manifestations	*Neurological manifestations*
• Lethargy leading to coma.	• Lethargy leading to coma.
• Hypotonia.	• Acute ataxia.
• Neonatal seizures.	• Hyperactivity.
	• Psychiatric symptoms.
Gastrointestinal manifestations	*Gastrointestinal manifestations*
• Persistent vomiting (+/– dehydration).	• Persistent vomiting (+/– dehydration).
• Poor feeding.	• Hepatomegaly.
• Hepatomegaly.	
Nonspecific	*Nonspecific*
• Hyperventilation (due to a respiratory alkalosis).	• Underlying history of recurrent episodes of above symptoms worsening is severity.
• Hypothermia.	

further metabolised to form ammonia. Ammonia is a toxic metabolite in large quantities, therefore the liver is responsible for maintaining the circulating ammonia levels at less than harmful levels.

The liver eliminates excess ammonia through two routes:

• Conversion of glutamate to glutamine.
• Conversion of ammonia to urea via the urea cycle.

Management of hyperammonaemia

Acute hyperammonaemia requires immediate intervention to prevent the harmful effects of ammonia manifesting permanently in the neurological system. The initial management will depend on whether this is the first presentation for the neonate or child. If it is, it is extremely important that blood and urine specimens required for diagnosis of an underlying metabolic disorder are taken before treatment is started. In addition, a second laboratory confirmed ammonia level should be available before treatment commences.

Management may be divided into a number of sections each with a targeted aim:

• Reduce nitrogen intake: Stop all dietary intake of protein and any intravenous amino acids (e.g. TPN).
• Reversal of the catabolic state: Deliver high-dose glucose concentration to meet metabolic demands, avoiding tissue catabolism and the breakdown of endogenous protein.

• Improve nitrogen excretion: Administration of sodium benzoate, arginine and sodium phenylbutyrate.
• Removal of toxic metabolites: Provision of continuous renal replacement therapy (CRRT); insertion of suitable vascular access and commencement of either CVVH or CVVHDF (Chapter 6).

Hyperammonaemia can cause irreversible neurotoxicity and cell death in the CNS. Acutely, the effects can conspire to cause cerebral oedema, increased intracranial pressure and ultimately death. Regardless of the aetiology, the neonate or child's prognosis depends on both the severity and duration of the ammonia level elevation. The sites of damage are not always predictable and the child will require careful neurological evaluation after the acute phase of treatment is completed (Bachmann 2003;Bosoi and Rose 2009; Summar et al. 2008).

References

Akobeng A. 2008. Assessing the validity of clinical trials. Journal of Pediatric Gastroenterology and Nutrition, 47(3): 277–82.

Alagille D. 2004. History of pediatric liver transplantation in Europe. Acta Gastroenterologica Belgica, 67(2):172–5.

Alberti K, Aschner P et al. 1999. WHO Definition, Diagnosis and Classification of Diabetes Mellitus and its Complications. www.staff.ncl.ac.uk/philip.home/who_dmc.htm #Tab3.

Alfaleh K, Anabrees J, Bassler D. 2010. Probiotics reduce the risk of necrotizing enterocolitis in preterm infants: a meta-analysis. Neonatology, 97(2):93–9.

Alvaro D, Mancino MG et al. 2007. Proliferating cholangiocytes: a neuroendocrine compartment in the diseased liver. Gastroenterology, 132:415–31.

Arnbjörnsson E, Larsson M et al. 2002.Transanastomotic feeding tube after an operation for duodenal atresia. European Journal of Pediatric Surgery, 12(3):159–62.

Arya DR, Sheffali Gulati S, Deopujari, S. 2010.Management of hepatic encephalopathy in children. Postgraduate Medical Journal (BMJ), 86:34–41.

ASERNIP-S Report. 2007. Natural Orifice Translumenal Endoscopic Surgery (NOTES)TM for Intra-abdominal Surgery. ASERNIP-S report no. 62. www.surgeons.org/AM/Template.cfm?Section=ASERNIP_S_NET_S_Database&Template=/CM/ContentDisplay.cfm&ContentFileID=24194.

Atkin R, Clifford P. 1985. Girth measurement is not a reliable investigation for the detection of intra-abdominal fluid. Annals of the Royal College of Surgeons of England, 67.

Babbitt C. 2007. Transpyloric Feeding in the pediatric intensive care unit. Journal of Pediatric Gastroenterology and Nutrition, 44(5):646–9.

Bachmann C. 2003. Outcome and survival of 88 patients with urea cycle disorders: a retrospective evaluation. European Journal of Pediatrics, 162(6):410–16.

Bai YZ, Chen H, Wang WL. 2009. A special type of postoperative intussusception: ileoileal intussusception after surgical reduction of ileocolic intussusception in infants and children. Journal of Pediatric Surgery, 44(4):755–88.

Barr J. 1998. Understanding pediatric intestinal pseudo-obstruction: implications for nurses. Gastroenterology Nursing, 21(1):11–13.

Barry P, Morris K, Ali T (Editors). 2010. Paediatric Intensive Care. Oxford UK: Oxford University Press.

Bassett MD, Murray KF. 2008. Biliary atresia: recent progress. Journal of Clinical Gastroenterology, 42(6):720–9.

Bell MJ, Ternberg JL et al. 1978. Neonatal necrotizing enterocolitis – therapeutic decisions based upon clinical staging. Annals of Surgery, 7(1):1–7.

Benifla M, Weizman Z. 2003. Acute pancreatitis in childhood: analysis of literature data. Journal of Clinical Gastroenterology, 37(2):169–72.

Blei AT, Córdoba J. 2001.Hepatic encephalopathy. American Journal of Gastroenterology, 96(7):1968–76.

Bombell S, McGuire W. 2009. Early trophic feeding for very low birth weight infants. Cochrane Database of Systematic Reviews, 3: Art. CD000504. DOI:0.1002/14651858.CD000504.pub3

Bosoi CR, Rose CF. 2009. Identifying the direct effects of ammonia on the brain. Metabolic Brain Disease, 24(1): 95–102.

Bosscha K, Nieuwenhuijs V et al. 1998. Gastrointestinal motility and gastric tube feeding in mechanically ventilated patients. Critical Care Medicine, 26(9):1510–17.

Braun F, Broering D, Faendrich F. 2007.Current concepts in clinical surgery small intestine transplantation today. Langenbeck's Archives of Surgery, 392(3):227–38.

British Society of Paediatric Endocrinology and Diabetes (BSPED). 2009. BSPED Recommended DKA Guidelines. www.bsped.org.uk/professional/guidelines/docs/DKA Guideline.pdf.

Champion M, Richards C et al. 2002. Duodenal perforation: a diagnostic pitfall in non-accidental injury. Archives of Disease in Childhood, 87(5):432–3.

Chang YJ, Chao HC et al. 2011. Acute pancreatitis in children. Acta Paediatrica, 100(5):740–4.

Cochran JB, Losek JD. 2007. Acute liver failure in children. Pediatric Emergency Care, 23(2):129–35.

Cranmer H. 2011. Neonatal Hypoglycemia Clinical Presentation. emedicine.medscape.com/article/802334-overview.

Cutler C, Davis N. 2005. Improving oral care in patients receiving mechanical ventilation. American Journal of Critical Care, 14(5):389–94.

Davenport M, Bianchi A et al. 1990. Colonic atresia: current results of treatment. Journal of the Royal College of Surgeons Edinburgh, 35(1):25–8.

Davenport M, Pierro A. 2009. Paediatric Surgery. Oxford Specialist Handbooks in Surgery. Oxford: Oxford University Press.

Davies B, Stringer D. 1997.The survivors of gastroschisis. Archives of Disease in Childhood, 77(2):258.

Dazzi A, Lauro A et al. 2007. Steroids in intestinal transplantation. Clinical Transplantation, 21(2):265–8.

Deane A, Fraser R, Chapman M. 2009. Prokinetic drugs for feed intolerance in critical illness: current and potential therapies. Critical Care Resuscitation, 11(2):132–43

Diaz LK, Akpek EA et al. 2005. Tracheoesophageal fistula and associated congenital heart disease: implications for anaesthetic management and survival. Paediatric Anaesthesia, 15(10):862–9.

Dicken BJ, Sergi C et al. 2011. Medical management of motility disorders in patients with intestinal failure: a focus on necrotizing enterocolitis, gastroschisis, and intestinal atresia. Journal of Pediatric Surgery, 46(8):1618–30.

Dinsmore JE, Maxson JT et al. 2004. Is nasogastric tube decompression necessary after major abdominal surgery in children? Journal of Pediatric Surgery, 32(7):982–5.

Dixon M, Crawford D et al. 2009. Nursing the Highly Dependent Child or Infant: A manual of care. Singapore: Wiley-Blackwell.

Donowitz L, Page M et al. 1986. Alteration of normal gastric flora in critical care patients receiving antacid and cimetidine therapy. Infection Control, 7(1):23–6.

Duro D, Kamin D, Duggan C. 2008. Overview of pediatric short bowel syndrome. Journal of Pediatric Gastroenterology and Nutrition, 47: S33–S36.

Faraj, W, Dar F et al. 2010. Auxiliary liver transplantation for acute liver failure in children. Annals of Surgery, 251(2):351–6.

Fraser JD, Aguayo P et al. 2009. Laparoscopic management of intussusception in pediatric patients. Journal of Laparoendoscopic and Advanced Surgical Techniques Part A, 19(4):563–5.

Gaines B. 2009. Intra-abdominal solid organ injury in children: diagnosis and treatment. The Journal of Trauma: Injury, Infection, and Critical Care, 67(2):S135–S139.

Grant D, Abu-Elmagd K et al. 2005. Intestine Transplant Registry. 2003 report of the Intestine Transplant Registry: a new era has dawned. Annals of Surgery, 241(4):607–13.

Heyland D, Tougas G et al. 1996.Impaired gastric emptying in mechanically ventilated, critically ill patients. Intensive Care Medicine, 22(12):1339–44.

Hirschl RB, Yardeni D et al. 2002. Gastric transposition for esophageal replacement in children: experience with 41 consecutive cases with special emphasis on esophageal atresia. Annals of Surgery, 236(4):531–41.

Jaffray B. 2005. Minimally invasive surgery. Archives of Disease in Childhood, 90(5):537–42.

Jain A, Mazariegos G et al. 2002. Reasons why some children receiving tacrolimus therapy require steroids more than 5 years post liver transplantation. Pediatric Transplant, 5(2):93–8.

Kajia T, Tanakaa H et al. 2009. Nutritional effects of the serial transverse enteroplasty procedure in experimental short bowel syndrome. Journal of Pediatric Surgery, 44(8):1552–9.

Kilby M. 2006. The incidence of gastroschisis. British Medical Journal, 332(7536):250–1.

Lacaille F, Vass N et al. 2007. Long-term outcome, growth and digestive function in children 2 to 18 years after intestinal transplantation. GUT, 57(4):455–61.

Latif N, Mehmood K. 2010.Risk factors for fulminant hepatic failure and their relation with outcome in children. Journal of Pakistan Medical Association, 60(3):175–8.

Lazaridis K, Strazzabosco M, Larusso N. 2004. The cholangiopathies: disorders of biliary epithelia. Gastroenterology, 127(5):1565–77.

Li M, Ji G et al. 2008. Living-related small bowel transplantation for three patients with short gut syndrome. Transplant Proceedings Journal, 40(10):3629–33.

Messori A, Trippoli S et al. 2000. Bleeding and pneumonia in intensive care patients given ranitidine and sucralfate for prevention of stress ulcer: meta-analysis of randomised controlled trials. British Medical Journal, 321(7269):1103.

Miedema B, Johnson J. 2003. Methods for decreasing postoperative gut dysmotility. Lancet Oncology, 4(6):365–72.

Milbrandt K, Sigalet D. 2008. Intussusception associated with a Meckel's diverticulum and a duplication cyst. Journal of Pediatric Surgery, 43(12):E21–3.

Minkes R, Mazziotti M, Langer J. 2008. Stomas of the Small and Large Intestine. emedicine.medscape.com/article/939455-overview.

Modi B, Javid P et al. 2007. First report of the International Serial Transverse Enteroplasty Data Registry: indications, efficacy, and complications. International STEP Data Registry. Journal of the American College of Surgeons, 204(3):365–71.

Moffatt S. 2009. Overwhelming postsplenectomy infection: managing patients at risk. Journal of the American Academy of Physicians Assistants. www.jaapa.com/Overwhelming-postsplenectomy-infection-Managing-patients-at-risk/article/140089.

Moore K, Persaud T. 2003. Before We Are Born: Essentials of embryology and birth defects. China: Elsevier Saunders.

Moreira T, McQuiggan M. 2009. Methods for the assessment of gastric emptying in critically ill, enterally fed adults. Nutrition in Clinical Practice, 24(2):261–73.

Moss RL, Dimmitt RA et al. 2006. Laparotomy versus peritoneal drainage for necrotizing enterocolitis and perforation. New England Journal of Medicine, 354:2225.

Munoz SJ. 2008. Hepatic encephalopathy. Medical Clinics of North America, 92:795–812.

National Institute for Health and Clinical Excellence (NICE). 2002. TA40 Guidance on the Use of Infliximab for Crohn's Disease. guidance.nice.org.uk.

National Institute for Clinical Excellence (NICE). 2007. Serial transverse enteroplasty procedure (STEP) for bowel lengthening in parenteral nutrition-dependent children. Clinical Guidance IPG232. http://guidance.nice.org.uk/IPG232.

National Institute for Health and Clinical Excellence (NICE) (2009) IPG288 Extracorporeal photopheresis for Crohn's Disease: http://guidance.nice.org.uk/IPG288.

Nazer H. 2011. Pediatric Fulminant Hepatic Failure Treatment & Management. emedicine.medscape.com/article/929028.

Nielson R, Zitsman J. 2008. Atresia, Stenosis and Other Obstructions of the Colon. emedicine.medscape.com/article/934014-overview.

Obideen K, Yakshe P, Wehbi M. 2008. Chronic pancreatitis. Emedicine Gastroenterology. emedicine.medscape.com/article/181554-overview.

Office for National Statistics. 2006. www.statistics.gov.uk/downloads/theme_health/MB3-No22/CongARVfinal.pdf.

Office for National Statistics. 2007. www.statistics.gov.uk/StatBase/Product.asp?vlnk=5799.

Park J, Del Pino A et al. 1999. Stoma complications. The Cook County Hospital experience. Journal Diseases of the Colon and Rectum, 42(12):1575–80.

Pammi M, Abrams S. 2011. Oral lactoferrin for the prevention of sepsis and necrotizing enterocolitis in preterm infants. Cochrane Database of Systematic Reviews, 10:CD007137.

Patole SK, de Klerk N. 2005. Impact of standardised feeding regimens on incidence of neonatal necrotising enterocolitis: a systematic review and meta-analysis of observational studies. Archives of Diseases in Childhood Fetal and Neonatal Ed, 90(2):F147–51.

Patel RM, Lin PW. 2010. Developmental biology of gut-probiotic interaction. Gut Microbes, 1(3):186–95.

Pierro A, Hall N. 2003. Surgical treatment of infants with necrotizing enterocolitis. Seminars in Neonatology, 8:223–32.

Pirenne J, Kawai M. 2006. Tolerogenic protocol for intestinal transplantation. Transplantation Proceedings Journal, 38(6): 1664–7.

Pittman J, Rawl S. 2009. Development of the ostomy outcome risk assessment scale and the ostomy outcome classification index. Scientific and clinical abstracts from the 41st Wound, Ostomy and Continence Nurses Annual Conference. Journal of Wound Ostomy and Continence Nursing, 36(3) (Suppl.):3.

Pobo A, Lisboa T et al. 2009. A Randomized Trial of Dental Brushing for Preventing Ventilator-Associated Pneumonia. Chest. First published online: www.chestjournal.org/content/early/2009/05/29.

Prejbisz A, Lenders JW. 2011. Cardiovascular manifestations of phaeochromocytoma. Journal of Hypertension, 29(11): 2049–60.

Royal College of Nursing (RCN). 2005. Perioperative Fasting in Adults and Children. www.rcn.org.uk/data/assets/pdf_file/0009/78678/002800.pdf.

Premji SS, Chessell L. (2007) Continuous nasogastric milk feeding versus intermittent bolus milk feeding for premature infants less than 1500 grams. Cochrane Database of Systematic Reviews, 4:Art. CD001819. DOI: 10.1002/14651858.CD001819.

Prentiss K, Vinci R. 2009. Children in emergency departments: who should provide their care? Archives of Disease in Childhood, 94(8):573–6.

Rees CM, Eaton S et al, and Members of NET Trial Group, Pierro A. 2010. Peritoneal drainage does not stabilize extremely low birth weight infants with perforated bowel: data from the NET Trial. Journal of Pediatric Surgery, 45(2):324.

Reveiz L, Guerrero-Lozano R et al. 2010. Stress ulcer, gastritis, and gastrointestinal bleeding prophylaxis in critically ill pediatric patients: a systematic review. Pediatric Critical Care Medicine, 11(1):124–32.

Richardson L, Banerjee S, Rabe H. 2006. What is the evidence on the practice of mucous fistula refeeding in neonates with short bowel syndrome? Journal of Pediatric Gastroenterology and Nutrition, 43(2):267–70.

Ruemmele F, Sauvat F et al. 2006 Seventeen years after successful small bowel transplantation: long-term graft acceptance without immune tolerance. GUT, 55(6):903–4.

Sala D, Chomto S, Hill S. 2010. Long-term outcomes of short bowel syndrome requiring long-term/home intravenous nutrition compared in children with gastroschisis and those with volvulus. Transplant Proceedings Journal, 42(1):5–8.

Savage MW, Dhatariya KK et al. for the Joint British Diabetes Societies. 2011. Joint British Diabetes Societies guideline for the management of diabetic ketoacidosis. Diabetic Medicine, 28:508–15.

Schnabl KL, Van Aerde JE et al. 2008. Necrotizing enterocolitis: a multifactorial disease with no cure. World Journal of Gastroenterology, 14(14):2142–61.

Shekherdimian S, Lee SL et al. 2009. Contrast enema for pediatric intussusception: is reflux into the terminal ileum necessary for complete reduction? Journal of Pediatric Surgery, 44(1):247–50.

Somal J, Darby J. 2006. Gingival and plaque decontamination: can we take a bite out of VAP? Critical Care, 10(4):312–13.

Stewart D, Waxman K. 2007. Management of postoperative ileus. American Journal of Therapeutics, 14(6):561–6.

Spoudeas HA (Ed). 2005. Paediatric Endocrine Tumours: A Multi-Disciplinary Consensus Statement of Best Practice from a Working Group Convened under the Auspices of the BSPED and UKCCSG (rare tumour working groups).www.bsped.org.uk.

Summar ML, Dobbelaere D et al. 2008. Diagnosis, symptoms, frequency and mortality of 260 patients with urea cycle disorders from a 21-year, multicentre study of acute hyperammonaemic episodes. Acta Paediatrica, 97(10): 1420–5.

Tataria M, Nance M et al. 2007. Pediatric blunt abdominal injury: age is irrelevant and delayed operation is not detrimental. The Journal of Trauma: Injury, Infection, and Critical Care, 63(3):608–14.

Tepas, J, Sharma R et al. 2010. Timing of surgical intervention in necrotizing enterocolitis can be determined by trajectory of metabolic derangement. Journal of Pediatric Surgery, 45(2):310.

Thomas PA, Gilardoni A et al. 2009. Colon interposition for oesophageal replacement. Multimedia Manual of Cardiothoracic Surgery. mmcts.ctsnetjournals.org/cgi/content/full/2009/0603/mmcts.2007.002956.

Tortora GJ, Derrickson BH. 2009. Principles of Anatomy and Physiology, 12th Edition. Volume 2: Maintenance and Continuity of the Human Body. Asia: John Wiley and Sons.

UK Transplants. 2005. www.uktransplant.org.uk/ukt.

Valusek P, Spilde T et al. 2007. Laparoscopic duodenal atresia repair using surgical U-clips: a novel technique. Surgical Endoscopy, 21(6):1023–5.

Van Wijck K, de Jong J et al. 2010. Prolonged antibiotic treatment does not prevent intra-abdominal abscesses in perforated appendicitis. World Journal of Surgery, 34(12): 3049–53.

Vaughan WG, Grosfeld JL et al. 1996. Avoidance of stomas and delayed anastomosis for bowel necrosis: the 'clip and drop-back' technique. Journal of Pediatric Surgery, 31(4):542–7.

Waguespack SG, Rich T et al. 2010. A current review of the etiology, diagnosis, and treatment of pediatric pheochromocytoma and paraganglioma. Journal of Clinical Endocrinology and Metabolism, 95(5):2023–37.

Walsh MC, Kliegman RM. 1986.Necrotizing enterocolitis: treatment based on staging criteria. Pediatric Clinics of North America, 33:179–201.

Weiss B, Lerner A et al. 2009.Methotrexate treatment in pediatric Crohn disease patients intolerant or resistant to purine analogues. Journal of Pediatric Gastroenterology and Nutrition, 48(5):526–30.

Werlin SL. 2003.Pancreatitis in children. Journal of Pediatric Gastroenterology and Nutrition, 37:591–5.

Wikin K. 2002. A critical analysis of the philosophy, knowledge and theory underpinning mouth care practice for the intensive care unit patient. Intensive Critical Care Nursing, 18(3):181–8.

Williams TA, Leslie GD. 2004. A review of the nursing care of enteral feeding tubes in critically ill adults: part I. Intensive Critical Care Nursing, 20(6):330–43.

Wolfsdorf J, Craig ME et al. 2007. Diabetic ketoacidosis. Pediatric Diabetes, 8:28–42.

Zhang Y, Ortega G et al. 2011. Necrotizing enterocolitis requiring surgery: outcomes by intestinal location of disease in 4371 infants. Journal of Pediatric Surgery, 46(8): 1475–81.

Resources and further reading

History of Pediatric Liver Transplantation. emedicine.medscape.com/article/1012447-overview.

Biliary Atresia. Health Development Advice. www.hda-online.org.uk/digestive-diseases/atresia/index.html.

X-ray and Imaging.www.learningradiology.com/notes/ginotes/livertraumapage.htm

Stoma appliances.

www.convatec.co.uk/engb/cvtuk-lopostmsuk/cvt-portallev1/0/detail/0/1183/2134/little-ones-paediatric-stoma-care-systems.html.

www.coloplast.co.uk/ecompany/gbmed/homepage.nsf/0/cbbdc6ea0c88f73880256ed3003ee357/$FILE/Charter29Article.pdf.

Chapter 9
CARE OF A CHILD WITH MUSCULOSKELETAL INJURY

Mark Fores[1] and Doreen Crawford[2]

[1] Clinical Skills Unit, Leicester Royal Hospital, University Hospitals of Leicester NHS Trust, Leicester, UK
[2] School of Nursing and Midwifery, Faculty of Health and Life Sciences, De Montfort University, Leicester, UK

Introduction

This chapter first considers the developmental anatomy and physiology of the musculoskeletal system, bone injury and healing, then focuses on the management of some of the types of trauma encountered on the PICU.

Because children are different

Children are smaller and have different proportions from adults so there are different implications for the care and management of the injured child. Trauma has greater significance as the forces are focused on a smaller surface area. A smaller muscle mass and a thinner fat layer mean the child's skeleton has less protection. In addition, the child's skeleton and surrounding tissues have greater flexibility which means that the child's skeleton affords less protective capacity than the adult skeleton, so impacting forces are transported more readily to the internal structures. The implication this has for assessment is that the absence of a serious external injury may not exclude damage to internal structures and organs.

Other factors in relation to an immature skeleton need to be taken into account when dealing with a child's musculoskeletal injury. These include an increased resilience to stress, a thicker periosteum, an increased potential to remodel, shorter healing times and the presence of a physis. The bone density and healing time of children with pre-existing pathogenic bone conditions need to be taken into account as these will be compromised by their underlying condition.

Developmental anatomy and physiology

The musculoskeletal structure provides the bony framework of the body and with the musculature, tendons and ligaments provides the support and mobility associated with survival. During growth and development every bone undergoes a series of changes and total skeletal mass increases to a maximum in the third decade of life, after which there is gradual diminution.

The adult human skeleton consists of 206 bones, most of which are paired. By contrast, children are born with more than 300 bones and cartilaginous structures, as during early child development and growth, parts of the skeleton fuse together to form single bones, eventually culminating in the formation of the adult skeleton. The embryonic skeleton is composed of fibrous membrane and hyaline cartilage. During week 4 of gestation, embryonic connective tissue in the region of the future skeleton shows signs of differentiation (MacGregor 2008). At about week 8, bone tissue begins to develop and eventually replaces most of the existing fibrous or cartilage structures. Ossification and osteogenesis are synonyms meaning the process of bone formation. In embryos this process leads to the formation of the bony skeleton. Most bony nuclei of long bones and round bones ossify after birth.

Two types of bone formation occur: intramembranous ossification and endochondral ossification.

Intramembranous ossification

This is bone formation within loose fibrous connective tissue and most bones formed by this process are flat, for example the bones of the skull and the clavicles. Several events take place in intramembranous bone formation:

- Increased vascularity of tissue.
- Active proliferation of mesenchymal cells. The mesenchymal cells give rise to osteogenic cells, which develop into osteoblasts.
- Osteoblasts begin to lay down osteoid. Osteoid is the organic part of bone without the inorganic constituent.
- Osteoblasts either retreat or become entrapped as osteocytes in the osteoid.
- The osteoid calcifies to form spicules of spongy bone. The spicules unite to form trabeculae. The inorganic salts carried in the blood vessels supposedly bring about calcification. The salts are deposited in an orderly fashion as fine crystals (hydroxyapatite crystals) intimately associated with the collagenous fibres. These crystals are only visible with the electron microscope.
- Bone remodelling occurs and periosteum and compact bone are formed.

Endochondral ossification

This is bone which forms within the hyaline cartilage. Essentially, and with the exception of the clavicles, all bones below the base of the skull form by endochondral ossification.

This type of ossification involves the replacement of a cartilaginous model by bone and is best observed in long bones, such as the humerus or femur. Events of endochondral ossification include:

- Primary ossification centre. The first change indicative of the beginning of ossification takes place about the centre of the future bone shaft. Here the cartilage cells hypertrophy and the cartilage matrix becomes calcified. Subsequently, part of the calcified matrix disintegrates, opening cavities that communicate with the connective tissue and vessels at the surface.
- The bone collar forms simultaneously with the primary ossification centre. Cells of the perichondrium begin to form bone. The bone collar holds together the shaft, which has been weakened by the disintegration of the cartilage. The connective tissue about the bone collar, previously a perichondrium, is now called periosteum.
- Periosteal buds are connective tissue buds or 'sprouts' containing mesenchymal cells (which give rise to osteogenic cells) and blood vessels, which grow from the periosteum to reach the primary ossification centre. Osteoblasts attach to spicules of calcified cartilage in the primary ossification centre and begin to produce osteoid. Thus, bone is formed and the process continues towards both epiphyses. While this is occurring, the cartilage outside the primary ossification centre increases in size by interstitial and appositional growth.

About the time of birth, a secondary ossification centre appears in each end (epiphysis) of long bones. Periosteal buds carry mesenchyme and blood vessels in, and the process is similar to that occurring in a primary ossification centre. The cartilage between the primary and secondary ossification centres is called the epiphyseal plate, and it continues to form new cartilage, which is replaced by bone, a process that results in an increase in length of the bone. Growth continues until the individual is about 21 years old or until the cartilage in the plate is replaced by bone. The point of union of the primary and secondary ossification centre is called the epiphyseal line.

In relation to postnatal bone growth, during infancy and childhood, long bones lengthen entirely by interstitial growth of the epiphyseal plate cartilage and its replacement by bone, and all bones grow in thickness by appositional growth.

This ongoing skeletal development is summarised in Table 9.1.

Essentially the skeleton is composed of two frameworks: the axial skeleton and the appendicular skeleton.

The axial skeleton consists of the ribs, sternum, vertebral column and skull. The skull and vertebral column house and protect complex vulnerable structures such as the spinal cord but permit exit and origins of the spinal nerves (see Figure 9.1). The appendicular skeleton consists of the bones that make up the upper and lower limbs and the bones referred to as girdles (the pectoral and pelvic girdles) which attach the limbs to the axial skeleton.

Fracture classification and bone healing following injury

Despite the remarkable strength and indeed plasticity in young children, their bones are susceptible to fracture. Currey and Butler (1975) found immature bone to be

Table 9.1   Summary of skeletal development

Age	Anatomical development
Upper limbs	
Weeks 4–6	Limb buds develop, upper extremities with pronated forearms appear and begin to rotate externally.
Week 7	Ten upper digit rays appear and continue to differentiate until weeks 12–13, when the hands appear.
Week 12	Formation of the body's solid framework begins; systematically each cartilage model becomes solid bone. Primary centres of ossification appear in the diaphysis of most bones. Secondary centres for ossification do not present until birth.
Vertebrae	
Weeks 3–5	Formation of vertebrae, segmentation and chondrification.
Weeks 6–8	Two halves of the neural arch fuse, and further fusion to centrum.
First year to 3–6 years	The anterior arch of the first cervical vertebra begins to ossify and approximately 30% of children are completely ossified by 3 months and over 80% by 1 year. Complete closure of the synchondroses is completed in all children by 3 years.
11–13 years	Final height of vertebral column is reached in girls.
14–16 years	Final height of vertebral column is reached in boys.
25 years	Ossification complete.
Pelvis	
Week 8	Ilium appears.
Week 12	Ischium appears.
Week 16	Pubis appears.
7 years	Ischial and pubic rami fuse.
15 years	'Y'-shaped cartilaginous physis of the three bones fuse soon after puberty.
Femur	
Week 8 week	Appearance of the centre of the shaft.
Week 40 (term)	Appearance of the centre of the lower end of the femoral shaft.
1 year	Centre appears in the femoral head.
3 years	Centre appears in the greater trochanter.
12 years	Centre appears in the lesser trochanter.
18 years	Centres fuse with the femoral shaft.
Patella	
3 years	Centre appears at the patella.
Puberty	Ossification is complete soon after puberty.
Tibia	
Week 8	Primary centre of the tibial shaft appears.
9 months	Upper epiphysis appears.
2 years to puberty	Distal epiphysis ossifies, secondary centre of tibial tuberosity appears.
18 years	Distal epiphysis joins the shaft.
20 years	Upper epiphysis joins the shaft.
Fibula	
Week 8	Primary centre appears.
2 years	Centre of lower end of the fibula ossifies.
4 years	Centre of the proximal end of the tibia ossifies.
18 years	Lower end of the fibula fuses with the tibial shaft.
20 years	Proximal end of the fibula fuses with shaft.

Table 9.1 (*Continued*)

Age	Anatomical development
Foot	
Week 26	Ossification of calcaneus.
Week 30	Ossification of talus.
Week 40	Ossification of cuboid.
1st year	Bones of tarsus are ossified.
3rd year	Lateral ossification of the cuneiforms.
4th year	Medial ossification of the cuneiforms.
5 years	Intermediate ossification of the cuneiforms. Navicular ossifies.
18 years	Metatarsal epiphyses (feet) ossify. Metatarsals fuse.
Clavicle	
Week 5	The first bone in the skeleton with two centres that rapidly fuse.
Adolescence	Elongation of the sternal end, cartilaginous epiphysis appears and fuses several years later. Clavicle last bone to complete growth.
Scapula	
Weeks 6–8	Scapula forms by chondrification of the mesenchyme followed by bony centres appearing in the glenoid angle.
10 years to puberty	Appearance of the base of the coracoid appears and fuses with the glenoid at puberty.
Puberty to 25 years	Secondary centres appear at puberty in acromion, medial border, inferior angle and coracoid, fusing by the age of 25.
Humerus	
Weeks 6–8	At week 6 the humerus is cartilaginous, primary centre of ossification appears at week 8.
Radius	
Weeks 6–8	At week 6 appears in cartilage, primary centre of ossification appears during week 8.
2 years	Secondary centre appears.
4 years	Radial head appears.
18 years	Radial head fuses with shaft.
Ulna	
Weeks 6–8	At week 6 cartilaginous framework appears, primary centres appear in shaft at week 8.
6 years	
8–18 years	Head ulna ossifies.
20 years	Olecranon epiphysis appears, fusion does not involve articular surfaces. Head fuses with shaft.
Hand	
In utero	Shafts of metacarpals and phalanges ossify.
Year 1	Each carpal bone ossifies from one centre, the largest. Carpal ossifies in the first year of life.
Year 2	Ossification of hamate.
Year 3	Ossification of triquetal.
Year 4	Ossification of lunate.
Year 5	Ossification of trapezium.
Year 6	Ossification of scaphoid.
Year 7	Ossification of trapezoid.
Year 10	Ossification of pisiform.

Source: modified from Chamley et al. 2005.

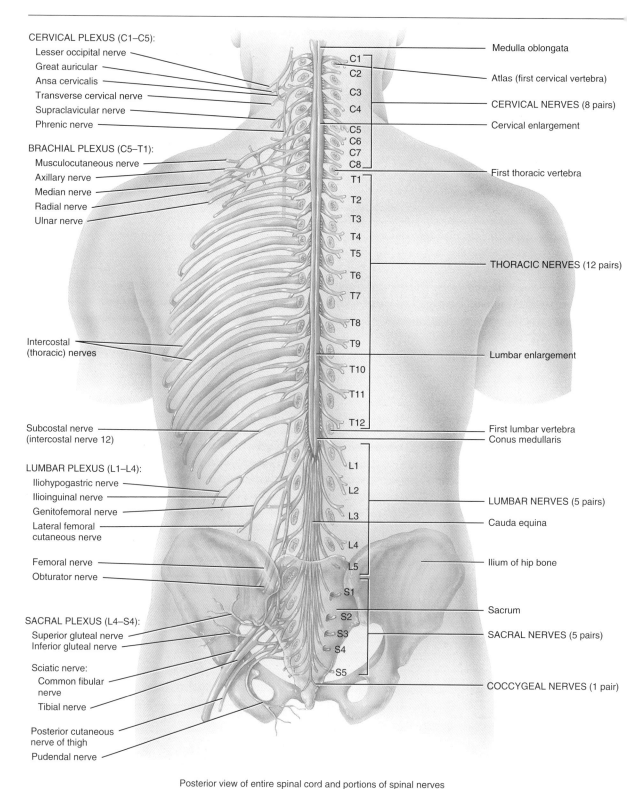

CERVICAL PLEXUS (C1–C5):
Lesser occipital nerve
Great auricular
Ansa cervicalis
Transverse cervical nerve
Supraclavicular nerve
Phrenic nerve

BRACHIAL PLEXUS (C5–T1):
Musculocutaneous nerve
Axillary nerve
Median nerve
Radial nerve
Ulnar nerve

Intercostal
(thoracic) nerves

Subcostal nerve
(intercostal nerve 12)

LUMBAR PLEXUS (L1–L4):
Iliohypogastric nerve
Ilioinguinal nerve
Genitofemoral nerve
Lateral femoral
cutaneous nerve

Femoral nerve
Obturator nerve

SACRAL PLEXUS (L4–S4):
Superior gluteal nerve
Inferior gluteal nerve

Sciatic nerve:
Common fibular
nerve
Tibial nerve

Posterior cutaneous
nerve of thigh
Pudendal nerve

C1
C2
C3
C4
C5
C6
C7
C8
T1
T2
T3
T4
T5
T6
T7
T8
T9
T10
T11
T12
L1
L2
L3
L4
L5
S1
S2
S3
S4
S5

Medulla oblongata

Atlas (first cervical vertebra)

CERVICAL NERVES (8 pairs)

Cervical enlargement

First thoracic vertebra

THORACIC NERVES (12 pairs)

Lumbar enlargement

First lumbar vertebra
Conus medullaris

LUMBAR NERVES (5 pairs)

Cauda equina

Ilium of hip bone

Sacrum

SACRAL NERVES (5 pairs)

COCCYGEAL NERVES (1 pair)

Posterior view of entire spinal cord and portions of spinal nerves

Figure 9.1 The spinal cord and the spinal nerves. From Tortora, G.J. and Derrickson, B.H. (2009) *Principles of Anatomy and Physiology*, 12th edn. Reproduced with permission from John Wiley and Sons, Inc.

weaker in bending strength but able to absorb more energy prior to fracture. During childhood most fractures result from trauma that twists or smashes the bones (e.g. sports injuries, road traffic accidents, falls and non-accidental injuries).

Fractures can be classified initially as:

- Position of the bone ends after fracture, i.e. non-displaced or displaced fracture.
- Completeness of the break, i.e. incomplete or complete.
- Orientation of the break relative to the long axis of the bone, i.e. linear or transverse.
- Whether or not the bone penetrates the skin resulting in an open fracture (Marieb and Hoehn 2010).

Fractures can also be described in terms of location of the fractures and the type of break, for example, fragmented, spiral, compression, depressed, greenstick or epiphyseal.

In simple terms a fracture is usually treated by reduction, realignment and immobilisation. Healing times are usually about 6–8 weeks in adolescence but may be quicker in younger children. Immobilisation following closed reduction usually involves application of a cast to maintain the corrected position, non-weight-bearing activities for lower limb injuries, or open reduction whereby the bone ends are surgically reduced with pins, wires or application of an external fixator.

Bone healing stages

Haematoma formation

When a bone breaks, blood vessels in the bone and periosteum and perhaps in the surrounding tissues are torn and haemorrhage. As a result, a haematoma forms at the fracture site. Soon bones cells deprived of nutrition die and tissue at the site becomes swollen, painful and inflamed.

Fibrocartilaginous callus formation

Within a few days a soft callus forms. Capillaries grow into the haematoma and phagocytic cells invade the area and begin cleaning up the debris. Meanwhile fibroblasts and osteoblasts invade the fracture site. The fibroblast begins by producing collagen fibres which span the break and connect the broken bone ends, some differentiate into chondroblasts which secrete cartilage matrix. Osteoblasts then begin forming spongy bone. This results in the formation of a fibrocartilaginous callus that splints the bone.

Bony callus formation

Within a week new bone trabeculae begin to appear in the fibrocartilaginous callus and gradually converts it to a bony (hard) callus of spongy bone. Bony callus formation continues until a firm union is formed about 2 months later.

Bone remodelling

This begins during bony callus formation and continues for several months after the bony callus is remodelled. Excess material is removed and compact bone is laid down to construct the shaft walls. The final structure resembles that of the original unbroken bony regions because it responds to the same mechanical stressors.

Musculoskeletal trauma

Reasons for trauma depend on age, mobility and risk-taking. Trauma is the leading cause of death in children >1 year of age in the developed world and unintentional injury ranks as the leading cause of death between 1 and 34 years. Fatality rates are higher for children when compared with adults who have similar injuries. Motor vehicle collisions and falls account for the majority of multiple trauma (Barry et al. 2010) and most paediatric trauma is regarded as blunt trauma (Leonard et al. 2011).

Birthing injuries, such as shoulder dystocia and fractures, are rare, however they will need to be suspected and considered if there is deformity, impaired movement or if the infant seems in pain following birth. The under 5 year olds are at greater risk of non-accidental injury (NAI) and falls, and health protection campaigns have been launched to warn parents of small children of the dangers of open windows.

Injuries in pre-teenage years and adolescents result from more risk-taking behaviours. Road traffic accidents (RTA) cause the more serious injuries, but general activities such as sports, trampolines and falls are the most common.

Initial assessment when a child has traumatic injury

The paediatric approach to trauma is to prioritise and treat life-threatening events. This will involve undertaking a primary survey to identify and treat these injuries. This will initially take place at the scene of the incident and will be undertaken again once the child arrives in the Emergency Department.

Primary survey

A: Airway with cervical spine stabilisation.

B: Breathing with oxygen.

C: Circulation with haemorrhage control and IV access.

D: Disability neurological assessment (Glasgow Coma Score).

E: Exposure completes the assessment of the child.

Secondary survey

Once the primary survey is complete and the child is stable, the secondary survey will be performed to inform ongoing management. On occasion, due to the severity of the child's injuries, this may be performed in the intensive care environment. A good, clear history is vital, for example, the mechanism of injury, preceding events and AMPLE may be used to clarify events:

A: Allergies.
M: Medications.
P: Past medical history
L: Time of the child's last meal.
E: Events preceding the accident.

Investigations required

Laboratory studies (full blood count, urea and electrolytes, blood glucose, coagulation, blood type cross-match) and radiological studies (cervical spine, chest, pelvis) that were not undertaken during the initial resuscitation should now be performed and a definitive management plan made. The identification and treatment of musculoskeletal injury at this time is already in progress; indeed, the first part of the initial assessment is airway with C-spine immobilisation. The secondary survey is a top to toe, front to back assessment where recognition of the severity of the injury may be identified and appropriate interventions undertaken. It is at this point that the value of positioning, splinting of injuries and pain management comes into play.

On arrival on intensive care it is vital that a correct, relevant and accurate history of events and interventions is documented and communicated effectively to the medical and nursing staff. Handover of the patient is a vital link in this chain of planning and providing care in the intensive care environment. Thorough, clear documentation and checklists may aid this communication. More recently, simulated events within the relevant clinical environment have been used to improve this process. For example, the simulated event of an admission from A&E to the PICU may be used. Many different specialities are involved in the immediate care of a paediatric trauma casualty: Emergency Department staff, paediatricians, surgical teams, orthopaedic teams and radiology.

The number of specialities involved could in itself result in a breakdown of communication and information transfer. These events are quite rare and teams need to work well together. By simulating this event the teams can get to know each other and appreciate each other's strengths. Areas for improvement can be identified, not just in the performance of individuals but in the organisational system's performance; this will result in enhanced care, procedures and policy development to improve clinical practice.

Because fractures in themselves are rarely life-threatening, when dealing with children who have multiple systems injuries the splinting of obvious fractures will generally be sufficient as the initial orthopaedic management, while the child's general condition is stabilised. Loder (1987) reported that in 78 children who had multiple injuries, the early operative stabilisation of fractures within the first 2 or 3 days after injury led to a shorter hospital stay, a shorter stay in the ICU and a shorter time on ventilator assistance. In addition, there were fewer complications in those who underwent surgical treatment of the fractures less than 72 hours after injury.

When reviewing the top-to-toe evidence on the assessment and management of spinal musculoskeletal injuries it is important to acknowledge that some of the evidence and recommendations for management of certain injuries are based on adult findings and data. Until child-based evidence is available, adaptation of adult studies has been utilised.

Spinal cord injury (Table 9.2)

Spinal cord injuries (SCI) can be classified as complete or incomplete transection. A complete lesion is irreversible and will result in a loss of sensory, motor and autonomic functioning. The sensory, motor and autonomic functioning damage from incomplete lesions varies. Werndle and colleagues (2012) found variability in the management of adults with SCI. Although there are fewer spinal cord injury centres for children, given that many are nursed, initially at least, on general PICUs, the same lack of standardisation is likely to apply. This chapter focuses on conservative management. Although Singhal and colleagues (2008) found that the neurological outcome in surgically treated patients was comparable to that of conservatively treated patients and that the advantage of surgical management in closed cervical spine injuries (better alignment, easier manual handling and early mobilisation) was traded for poorer neurological outcome in adults, there are as yet no comparable studies for children.

Spinal cord injuries (SCI) in children are relatively rare. In Europe the incidence of non-fatal SCI is 0.09–2.12 per 100 000 children per year (Barry et al. 2010). They are hard to diagnose because of the problem of obtaining a clear history due to developmental age (McCall et al. 2006) and the difficulty of imaging an immature spine. In addition, children usually regress developmentally in times of stress and injury, making communication challenging.

Table 9.2 Spinal cord injuries in infants, children and young people

Location of injury	Injury characteristics
Cervical spine	Site of approximately 60% of spinal injuries in children from birth to 10 years. An injury at C3 and above is usually fatal as these cause respiratory arrest. Survivors will require long-term ventilation. Injury from C5 will not affect diaphragmatic function. If the injury is at C6–7 children will retain some function in the upper limbs although this may be limited. With C-spine injuries there will be loss of sensation and sphincter control, leading to continence problems.
Types and cause of cervical spine injury	Occipitoatlantal dislocation – a rare injury, which usually occurs in RTAs and is associated with a high mortality. The mechanism of injury can be caused by hyperextension–rotation, combined with a distraction force. Care must be taken not to increase the dislocation. This requires immediate stabilisation and a halo applied before operation facilitates reduction and allows posterior occipitoatlantal fusion to be performed under optimum conditions. Atlas fracture– fracture of the ring of C1, caused by an axial compressive force applied to the head which results in direct compression of the ring of C1 by the occipital condyles. Traumatic atlantoaxial instability– in the older child (as in adults) this is most often a result of injury to the transverse ligament and the alar ligaments, resulting in an increased distance between the atlas and the dens of axis. Odontoid fractures – these account for approximately 10% of all C-spine fractures and dislocations in children. The injury in the child occurs at the synchondrosis at the base of the dens and displaces anteriorly. The mechanism of injury is usually associated with falls from a height or RTAs, however in children <4 years the mode of injury (MOI) could be relatively minor such as a fall from a cot or bed. Pedicle fractures of C2 – the MOI is usually extension and axial loading, with a high incidence of injuries to the face and head. The mechanism of injury is usually associated with falls from a height or RTAs. Fractures and dislocations of the subaxial spine – these are relatively rare in young children but may be seen in children >8 years and may include fracture dislocations, burst fractures, compression fractures, posterior ligamentous injuries, facet fractures and facet dislocations.
Thoracic spine	Account for approximately 20% of spinal injury usually between 8 and 14 years. Children may retain control of upper limbs but have poor trunk balance. Injuries above T6 can result in autonomic dysreflexia, which can be a medical emergency, so recognising and treating the earliest signs and symptoms efficiently can avoid the dangerous complication of hypertension.
Thoracic/lumbar spine	Retain control of muscles in abdomen and upper back. Children with injuries in this region retain trunk balance.
Lumbar spine	Injuries from L2 to L4 may occur because of poorly placed lap seat belts. Children who have injuries below L3 may retain the functioning of upper leg muscles but lose foot and ankle control.

Source: adapted from Ball and Bindler 2008.

The patterns of injury in children >10 years are similar to those of adults, with a greater incidence of subaxial injuries than in younger children. In younger children spinal injuries are more commonly seen in the atlas, axis and upper cervical vertebrae owing to the relatively large size of the head, the immature skeleton and the immature supporting muscle and tissue structures which results in the fulcrum of injury being above C3. It is also important to remember that SCI may have occurred with the absence of abnormality on plain X-rays; SCIWORA (spinal cord injury without radiological abnormality). The clinical features may range from tingling and numbness to paralysis. Thoracic SCIWORA should also be considered in accidents involving high-speed direct impact, distraction from lap seat belts and crush injury by a slow-moving vehicle.

The mechanism of injury generally relates to the age of the child. At birth C-spine injury is not clearly defined, however breech and forceps deliveries are associated with SCI (Ruggieri et al. 1999).

SCI in infants and small children may be associated with NAI, therefore very careful consideration and care should be taken in relation to assessment and treatment. As stated, under 5 year olds are also at risk from falls and during pre-teens and adolescence RTA injuries predominate.

Cervical spine injury (C-spine injury)

C-spine injury should be suspected in any child who has sustained a significant head injury, has suffered blunt trauma to or above the clavicles, has a history of an RTA (as a pedestrian or car passenger), fall from a height, diving into shallow water, associated sporting injury (e.g. a scrum collapse in rugby, horse riding injury, etc.), hangings, NAI with suggested shaking injury or the unconscious child brought into A&E. This list is by no means exhaustive but if the mechanism of injury suggests potential spinal injury, care should be taken to stabilise the head and C-spine. One of the most common presenting complaints when a C-spine injury is present in an alert child is the presence of torticollis (limited neck motion) in which the child will hold the head to one side with the chin pointing to the opposite side.

Spinal protection

A conscious, frightened child with an actual or suspected SCI is very difficult to immobilise completely and attempts at immobilising are inconsistent (Skettet et al. 2002), although excessive movement and instability need to be limited. In order to try to prevent the extension of the injury, management must be tailored to the patient's age, neurological status, type and level of injury (Duhem et al. 2008). Initial attempts to protect the spinal cord can involve

using a range of devices (cervical collar, spinal board, scoop stretcher, vacuum mattress), sedation and taking appropriate measures when rolling or moving the patient (log rolling).

If there is any concern in relation to C-spine injury the C-spine should be immobilised, usually by using an appropriate-sized hard collar and sand-bags (or equivalent medical device and tape). However, if the child becomes uncooperative or combatant, then they should simply have a hard collar applied (if they will tolerate it). When immobilisation of the head is too rigid there may be an increase in the leverage on the neck as the child struggles, therefore this should be avoided. It is important that the child is treated in a calm atmosphere and communicated with appropriately for their age and level of development so that anxiety and stress are minimised. Parents should ideally remain at the bedside to help facilitate this.

In relation to positioning, Herzenberg and colleagues (1989) reported on 10 children under 7 years of age with unstable C-spine injuries who were found to have an anterior angulation or translation on the lateral radiograph when the patient was positioned on the traditional backboard. They recommend using a bed or a backboard with a posterior recess for the head to drop posteriorly and prevent angulation of the neck.

Log-rolling

Spinal cord instability should be assumed in all patients with significant trauma injuries until such an injury is excluded. These patients should be log-rolled during the initial assessment and the entire spine should be inspected and palpated for ecchymoses, soft tissue swellings, step-offs and tenderness. Every patient with a suspected spinal injury also needs a thorough and careful neurological examination.

Physical examination

The physical examination should be undertaken by an experienced clinician and the neck palpated for tenderness, muscle guarding or the presence of a gap in the spinous process that would indicate a posterior ligamentous injury.

Radiography

Radiographic evaluation should be performed along with other C-spine imaging according to local protocols. A complete radiographic examination should include a lateral view, anterior-posterior (AP), and odontoid (open mouth) view, but omit if a CT scan of the head is also required as then a CT of the upper C-spine should be done instead. Oblique views if the lower C-spine is inadequately visualised on the lateral view (this is rarely needed in children) can be notoriously difficult to obtain in young children. The use of the CT scanner has increased in recent years and when CT scanning the head-injured patients bound for intensive care, it seems logical to scan the neck at the same time. A CT scan of the neck reduces the risk of missing an injury of the C-spine (Morris et al. 2004). An MRI scan may be required if there are features of neurological deficit.

Thoracic and lumbar spinal injuries

In children these are less common than C-spine injuries; children under 10 years are more likely to sustain upper thoracic injuries (T4–T10) as a result of a fall or motor vehicle/ pedestrian collision. Between the ages of 10 and 20 years they are more likely to sustain injuries at the thoracolumbar junction (T12–L1), again predominantly as a result of motor vehicle injuries or recreational pursuits.

Some key concepts need to be considered in relation to thoracic and lumbar injuries. First, the ligaments are more elastic and forgiving, second, there is a higher ratio of cartilage to bone, and third, the facets are more horizontal allowing greater motion. The three column spine also requires understanding a concept introduced by Denis (1983). Denis realised that complete rupture of the posterior ligamentous structures did not produce instability. Rather, instability in flexion requires not only rupture of the posterior ligaments but also disruption of the 'middle column' – the posterior longitudinal ligament, the posterior annulus fibrosus and the posterior wall of the vertebral body. The anterior column consists of the anterior longitudinal ligament, the anterior annulus fibrosus and the anterior vertebral body. The posterior column is made up of the posterior arch and posterior ligamentous complex. Injuries to the thoracic and lumbar spine are usually the result of high energy forces. They can also be difficult to diagnose as these patients may frequently have associated injuries and an altered state of consciousness. The force that produces the injury is more commonly flexion, which may be combined with compression, distraction or shear forces.

Acute spinal cord injury in context

An injury to the spinal cord potentially exposes the child to the systemic factors which can be related to injury such as inflammation and infection. Also interruption to the central control of the sympathetic outflow and lack of 'back-up' spinal reflexes supporting this, particularly in the weeks immediately following an SCI, means that cardiovascular control, compensation for postural change and the effect of gravity are functionally absent below the level of the lesion.

Management in intensive care

When planning the management and care of these injuries the focus will depend on the site of injury/fracture and its severity. Whether it is a C-spine, thoracic or lumber a spinal injury care should be taken when moving these patients. In the initial phases, if there is concern about the C-spine, then it should be immobilised with the 'Holy Trinity' of sandbags, collar and tape. The next level of intervention may depend on whether or not surgery, such as halo traction, is required to stabilise the injury.

If the injury does not require immediate surgery, the child will be maintained in an intensive care environment for conservative continuation of care as the general consensus seems to be that the next stage is a waiting game; initially it may be impossible to determine the extent of the injury until the child is awake and a more detailed neurological examination can take place. The primary insult has occurred at the time of the initial injury, therefore the general principle is to prevent a secondary insult by taking care and immobilising the injury. Time is something that the child has, but this uncertainty can be a frustrating and anxious time for the family as they wait to find out the full extent of the injury. This frustration can be shared by the intensive care team as prediction under this degree of uncertainty is unwise.

Steroid use

A number of pharmacological agents have been used in an attempt to improve recovery after SCI. The aims of using these agents are to reduce swelling and oedema and prevent ischaemic injury. A number of drugs have been tried, but only methylprednisolone has received widespread clinical attention. There is some controversy in the use of steroids in terms of balancing the benefits and outcomes of a high dose against the increased incidence of pneumonia and a potentially longer ICU stay, but no change in mortality and a decrease in rehabilitation periods have been identified (Gerndt et al. 1997). Despite this, many units administer methylprednisolone to patients with SCI within 3 hours of injury and maintain them on this treatment regime for 48 hours.

Spinal neurological shock

Continuous monitoring should be undertaken in all critically injured patients and the intensive care nurse should observe the patient for signs of shock caused by neurological injury. Signs include a fall in blood pressure and a drop in heart rate (in hypovolaemia one would usually observe a fall in blood pressure with an accompanying tachycardia).

Moving and handling

Spinal immobilisation should be continued in the intensive care environment. The difficulty in relation to paediatric intensive care patients is that they may often be ventilated and sedated/muscle relaxed and may also have other associated injuries. The simple rule is that all of these patients should be assumed to have spinal column instability until the injury can be excluded. This creates quite a challenge in paediatric intensive care.

In relation to C-spine immobilisation one of the disadvantages of the rigid collar is that it gets soiled and may result in pressure sores if used long term. An alternative is an Aspen collar. This is a two-part collar with the front detaching to give access the patient. It also has interchangeable foam inserts which can be changed when performing cares.

When undertaking nursing procedures, the care of the child's C-spine requires two people and clear communication must be maintained throughout. This is particularly important in any procedure where a collar and any anchoring tapes have to be temporarily removed to assess skin integrity or maintain hygiene. One person should manually stabilise the head and neck while the other removes the tapes and sandbags, etc., and then undertakes the procedure.

When changing sheets or the position of the patient the child should be moved by log-rolling. The main issue with this manoeuvre is how many people are required as this will have a demand on the nursing staff. PICUs operate on a 1:1 nurse–patient ratio. If a unit has six patients and one of these patients is an adolescent with a spinal injury, then it may take four people to roll and one person to undertake the nursing care –five in all. This is where a multidisciplinary approach is vital as medical staff and physiotherapists should be co-opted to assist. Therefore, all staff should be trained in log-rolling and handling techniques to care for a patient with a spinal injury. As an alternative, the patient may be nursed on a spinal bed such as a Stryker frame which permits turning in various planes without the movement of individual parts. This is not suitable for small children or for young people who demonstrate loss of physiological stability when turned prone (see autonomic dysreflexia).

If the patient needs to be moved for further imaging investigations such as CT or MRI, this creates another set of obstacles to be overcome. The use of vacuum mattress-type devices has been introduced into paediatric intensive care mainly to transport critically ill children. The value of this should not be underestimated for intra-hospital transfers either. Mattresses could be utilised in taking the patient to CT as many of these devices are now CT-compatible and will allow the safe transfer of patient from bed to CT scanner and back again. Before taking a child for an MRI the compatibility of vacuum mattress needs to be confirmed.

Special considerations with high spinal injury

Children with high spinal lesions need to be handled with care to avoid autonomic dysreflexia which is a medical emergency, so it is important to recognise and treat the earliest signs and symptoms:

- Headache.
- Cutis anserina (goose bumps).
- Red, blotchy and sweaty above the level of injury.
- Slower than usual pulse, hypertension.
- Nausea.
- Cold, clammy skin below level of spinal injury.

Autonomic dysreflexia can be caused by any stimuli such as irritants, pressure and pain to the body below the level of spinal injury. Things to consider include an overstretched bladder, UTI or bowel over-distension due not only to constipation or impaction, but also tight clothing or uncomfortable bedding.

On-going management

The care of the patient with an SCI can be both challenging and rewarding for the intensive care team. It produces a unique set of challenges due to the site and severity of the injury sustained and the consequences. This will vary from individual to individual but this group of patients will generally be initially immobilised, on bed rest, may be sedated and ventilated and will potentially be at risk of developing pneumonia, sepsis, pressure sore injury and DVT, and will need complete supportive management.

Respiratory care

Initial respiratory care will focus on appropriate ventilatory care and prevention of nosocomial infection. This group of patients may be at risk of developing pneumonia or sepsis. Therefore, it is important that careful attention is paid to providing good respiratory care Chapter 4.

In terms of the patient with an SCI, attention should considered for long-term management. The level, innervation and severity of the injury will dictate long-term management. C3, C4 and C5 innervate the diaphragm. Therefore spinal cord injury at this level will dictate whether the patient will be ventilator-dependent and may also require a tracheostomy in the long term. In the immediate environment of intensive care this is generally viewed as routine care management, but to family and the patient this is a life-changing event and the psychological impact should not be underestimated. This will put an immense strain on any family. For example, as a result of a major RTA, the infant who sustains a C3 fracture will be ventilator-dependent for life. If this is the case, support mechanisms should be put in place as soon as possible, utilising all the skills of the multidisciplinary team to facilitate care, including the community respiratory care teams. Once the patient is stable and recovering, plans should be put in place for the continuation of care. This is where the importance of a good high dependency facility is so important and access to one of these can allow for transfer. Some contact should also be made with units that specialise in the intermediate and long-term care of patients with an SCI as they can have a lot to offer.

Specialist feeding

As with any intensive care patient calorific requirements are vital to recovery. Nasogastric or naso-jejunal feeds should be commenced in line with unit policy. Dietetic involvement and a nutritional management plan are a necessity in care provision (Chapter 12).

Elimination

The patient will be catheterised with the appropriate urinary catheter for the age of the child. Attention should be paid to accurate fluid balance monitoring in relation to input and output. Urine output should ideally be 1 ml/kg/hr. Catheter care should be undertaken as part of hygiene management but the risk remains that the patient could develop a urinary tract infection, therefore careful monitoring of the character and composition of urine should be undertaken when measuring output. The PIC nurse needs to be aware of the signs of underlying infection (raised temperature, tachycardia, offensive smelling urine, protein in the urine, etc.) as the consequences will depend on the site and severity of injury. The spinal nerves that relate to bladder and bowel function innervate at lumbar level, therefore as with respiratory care, long-term planning is vital.

As a result of the injury the child may have to use intermittent catheterisation in the long term and need appropriate bowel management. This is where early communication with specialist services such as a urology nurse specialist is vital in planning and coordinating immediate and future care.

Pain

As with any musculoskeletal injury, pain management is vital. Initially, the child may be sedated and ventilated, depending on the severity of the injury and any coexisting injuries such as a head injury. There may be cases, however, when the child has sustained an injury that may not require sedation or ventilation (e.g. a thoracic SCI). In these circumstances, pain assessment scores and appropriate analgesic intervention will be required. A pain score should be utilised that is appropriate for the child's age and development, and analgesia administered as prescribed. Opiates should be avoided when dealing with non-ventilated tetraplegia or high paraplegia as they can cause respiratory depression. Diclofenac tends to be the drug of choice for these patients although most other general analgesics can be used (Chapter 13).

Bone loss, contractures and scoliosis

Although the mechanism of future bone loss in these children is not fully understood, it is likely to be a complex interplay between hormones, drug therapy, gender and genetic predisposition. The loss of mechanical stimuli of bone has a major impact on bone integrity, and in individuals with SCI, bone loss begins immediately after injury (Dionyssiotis 2011). This makes these children more prone to subsequent bone injury below the spinal cord injury, so effective and efficient management of movement and positioning learned from the start of rehabilitation may prevent later fractures and complications. Associated muscular atrophy and spasticity can complicate rehabilitation, and positioning supports, splints, footboards, boots and braces all have a role in preventing contractures and optimising residual function. Scoliosis can complicate positioning and respiratory function if the injury was sustained before the skeleton was mature.

Psychosocial concerns

Adverse psychological and social effects are part of the process of an enforced hospital stay and an admission to intensive care, accompanied by the fact that damage from a SCI may be permanent and the consequences life-changing. Helping the child and family accept the situation is not solely the role of the intensive care nurse as the child will be transferred to rehabilitation and ongoing care units. However the children's nurse working in the PICU can provide a solid platform by being honest and transparent and never providing false hope or colluding with denial.

Even during the early stages the family can benefit from counselling and the idea introduced that the child will need long-term psychological support and not just physical care. While the child is in PIC the children's nurse role stops short of motivational coaching, but allowing the family to sink into deep despair is not in anyone's interests. There are some remarkable role models who have overcome disability and achieved incredible results in every sphere of life.

Ruling out C-spine injury and providing clearance
Ruling out C-spine injury is notoriously difficult in the 0–3 years age range (Anderson et al. 2010) and in the unconscious ventilated patient as generally requirements such as no radiological abnormality, no pain, paraesthesia or paralysis, normal neuro-muscular status observed and can communicate these findings effectively, will be impossible to determine. There are no guidelines to assist the decision-making process. The decision should be taken by an orthopaedic surgeon or neurosurgeon and until the spinal injury is considered clear, then the standard nursing management in relation to care of the spinal injury (i.e. immobilisation and log-rolling, etc.) will apply.

Pelvic injury
Pelvic ring stability is provided by an intact ring of bones and by strong connecting ligaments, therefore pelvic stability is as much about the state of the ligaments which make the connections as the skeletal framework. These are:

- Iliolumbar ligaments.
- Dorsal sacroiliac ligaments.
- Sacrotuberous ligaments.
- Ventral sacroiliac ligaments.
- Sacrospinous ligaments.
- Posterosuperior interosseous ligaments.

Fractures to the pelvis are rare in children. Motor vehicle accidents account for about 60% in adults (Frakes and Evans 2004) and about 75–90% of all pelvic fractures in children. Whereas adults are likely to have been drivers or passengers in an RTA, children are more likely to have been a pedestrian who has been struck by a vehicle. The high energy that produces these injuries may also result in visceral and vascular injury, which can be fatal. Mortality associated with pelvic fractures in children is lower than that of adults at about 5% (Ismail et al. 1996). The likelihood of associated injuries is higher in those with multiple fractures of the pelvic ring and those with unstable fractures are more likely to have greater resuscitation requirements. Resuscitation takes priority. In the past, pelvic injuries were managed non-operatively, using compression devices, plaster casts and bed rest. Over time, outcome studies have demonstrated that post-traumatic anatomic deformities and pelvic instability correlated with persistent pain and functional limitation (McCormack et al. 2010).

Classification of pelvic injury
There are several types of pelvic injury classification (Table 9.3). Torode and Zieg (1985) used a four-part classification based on radiological findings:

Type I: Avulsion fractures.
Type II: Iliac wing fractures.
Type III: Simple pelvic fracture.
Type IV: Unstable ring disruption fractures.

Complications of pelvic fracture
The most common associated injuries involve the genitourinary system and lower abdominal organs. These may include bladder rupture or damage to the urethral vessels, contusions or laceration of the spleen, liver, kidneys, mesenteric injuries or injuries to the large or small intestine. Due to the MOI of pelvic fractures, head injury is the most common associated neurological injury and associated musculoskeletal injuries such as fractured femur (25% of cases) may be present. Associated vascular injuries are often due to venous bleeding leading to retroperitoneal haematoma, which can potentially lead to a very unstable child at risk of hypovolaemic shock. These children will require immediate stabilisation and volume replacement, initially this may be with 0.9% sodium chloride, however these patients will generally also require whole blood or packed cells. Major arterial bleeds are much rarer.

A more interventional approach to the management of the fractured pelvis may lead to fewer long-term effects such as limb length discrepancies, growth disturbance of the acetabulum, resulting in acetabular dysplasia, hip subluxation or hip joint incongruity (Holden et al. 2007). Osteonecrosis of the femoral head may develop after acetabular fractures and is associated with hip dislocation. Other complications include myositis ossificans and neurologic deficits secondary to sciatic, femoral, and/or lumbosacral plexus nerve injuries (Holden et al. 2007).

Clinical examination
MOI should alert the clinician to suspecting pelvic injury. As children may also have associated head injury they may be confused, making communication and clinical examination difficult and as a result the pelvic injury may be difficult to diagnose. A child's pelvic X-ray can be difficult

Table 9.3 Pelvic fractures

Type of injury	Possible cause and possible management
Type I: Avulsion fractures	Usually caused by athletic injuries with boys more affected than girls. A typical history is of someone who has performed a strenuous activity such as kicking a ball and feels a sudden, sharp pain. The powerful contraction of the muscle results in avulsion of the bone. Conservative treatment is usually successful: rested on crutches and non-weight-bearing. It is unlikely that this injury on its own will be seen in the intensive care environment.
Type II: Iliac wing fractures	Account for about 15% (2261) of fractures in children (this is higher than adults) often as a result of being struck by a motor vehicle The MOI is usually an external force on the iliac wing which results in a disruption of the iliac apophysis or a lateral compression-type wing fracture wing. These injuries can result in significant blood loss. Treatment usually consists of assessment of haemodynamic status and intervention if required. Unstable pelvic fractures may be stabilised by using external or internal fixation. These are painful fractures so should be managed accordingly. A paralytic ileus may develop after a wing fracture which will require evaluation by a paediatric general surgeon and treatment of the ileus (bowel rest/ placement of NG tube), bed rest.
Type III: Simple pelvic ring fractures	This is the most common fracture type in children, accounting for up to 55% of all pelvic fractures in children (2261). This injury includes fractures of the two ipsilateral pubic rami, disruptions of the pubic symphysis, fracture or separation of the sacroiliac joints, or displaced fractures in which no clinical instability can be detected. Children can have a fracture in a single aspect of the pelvic ring, possibly due to the elasticity of the sacroiliac joints and pubic symphysis, unlike adults in whom a pelvic fracture in one part of the ring must be associated with a fracture in another part. Treatment is usually conservative with symptomatic pain management and patients usually do very well with a short period of bed rest followed by progressive weight-bearing rehabilitation. Type III fractures are also associated with a higher incidence of musculoskeletal injuries.
Type IV: Pelvic ring disruption fractures	These include bilateral pubic rami fractures (so-called straddle fractures), double ring fractures or disruptions and fractures of the anterior structures and acetabular portion of the pelvic ring. These fractures have the highest incidence of associated genitourinary, musculoskeletal, neurological and intra-abdominal injuries. If the orthopaedic management of these involves external fixation such as Hoffmann A frame or a Ganz pelvic clamp, diligent care of the insert point will be required to prevent ascending infection. Internal fixation is by a range of plates, screws, bars and wires.

Source: Garvin et al. 1990; Nieto-Lucio, Camacho-González and Reinoso-Pérez 2010; Tile 1988; Torode and Zieg 1985.

to interpret. The physical examination should ideally be undertaken by an experienced orthopaedic surgeon and should be thorough and organised, starting with an examination of the entire body, inspecting for bruising, lacerations and deformity. The inspection should include the perineal area, the external urethral meatus should be inspected for blood, followed by an assessment of pelvic stability pressing over the iliac crests for tenderness and for abnormal mobility this should only be done once to minimise the risk of dislodging clots and re-starting bleeding.

Radiological examination

An initial AP pelvic radiograph should be obtained as soon as possible in the A&E Department. Other views may be required, including inlet and outlet views. MRI scans are very helpful in assessing the nature of the injuries and the extent of the damage; however the handling involved can destabilise the critically ill child.

Care of the child with a pelvic injury

Initially, if it is suspected that a child has sustained a pelvic injury then, as with an SCI, great care should be taken when moving and handling the child. Children with pelvic fractures can be haemodynamically unstable so care initially will focus on stabilising the child's haemodynamic status by administering fluid (in trauma initial fluid bolus 10 ml/kg sodium chloride 0.9%). These children often require blood products early in their management. Splinting may help stabilise the child. In adults pelvic splints are available but one may have to improvise for a child, using a sheet and fluid bags. In the authors' experience this has proved invaluable. Splinting injuries is a relatively simple technique and generally helps reduce blood loss and aids with pain relief. The child with a pelvic injury or a suspected pelvic injury should have their urine tested for blood.

Children with pelvic fractures are lifted not log-rolled for care, as log-rolling could potentially cause further injury.

Fractures to the limbs – extremity injury

In the event of a trauma admission to the PICU the child may have sustained extremity injuries or fractures. Initial observation of the extremities should be undertaken in the secondary survey and the patient should be clinically examined and observed for bruising, swelling and deformity, and palpated for tenderness. Crepitus and abnormal movement may be found but should not be elicited as these are painful. The pattern and degree of tenderness alone will identify the need for X-ray. Assess peripheral circulation, including pulses and capillary return. Although it is important to assess the peripheral sensation for sensitivity to touch, the pin-prick test should not be used in a frightened child. Further investigations may include MRI scans and angiograms. Management of the extremity injury is important and children may fixate on 'it hurts here'. However, it is vital that the extremity injury does not distract from the main focus of the primary assessment and interventions required to treat life-threatening events.

Upper limb injuries and fractures

Clavicle

Clavicle fractures are common in childhood and are generally not serious. Most result from a fall onto the shoulder. Clavicle fractures may also occur during birth and may present acutely as a pseudoparalysis (normal hand and forearm movement without movement of the arm) from birth or a few weeks after the delivery.

In the PICU, a fractured clavicle may complicate other shoulder injuries and will contribute to the pain and deformity of these. With a displacement the child should

be observed for vascular injury presenting as pulse abnormalities. Enlarging and discoloured swelling may suggest laceration or compression of the subclavian blood vessels. Diagnosis of fracture is confirmed on AP X-ray. Most clavicle injuries heal well and reduction is rarely required. In children a sling or shoulder strap will provide immobilisation and pain relief. In the PICU, careful handling of the limb should be undertaken. Infants are also managed conservatively and require analgesia and gentle handling of the limb.

Shoulder

Shoulder dislocations are rare in children and if seen in PICU will complicate other trauma. Anterior dislocations are more common than posterior. On presentation there will be pain and deformity compared with the opposite shoulder. AP and true scapular lateral or transaxillary radiographs are diagnostic. Reduction will be required and this is accomplished with traction–counter-traction, scapular manipulation or external rotation techniques after adequate sedation and analgesia.

Humerus

A fractured humerus will complicate the primary reason for admission to PICU, such as a head injury following a fall from a jungle gym. Children's fractures which involve the growth plates can be identified according to the Salter–Harris classification (Table 9.4). It is important to be aware of this as the growth of the bone may be affected if they are not managed well.

A Salter–Harris Type 1 fracture of the proximal humerus is most common between the age of 5 and 11 years of age.

A Salter–Harris Type 2 is most common between the age of 11 and 15 years and most are not displaced. If the fracture is displaced most orthopaedic surgeons currently rec-

Table 9.4   Salter–Harris classification

Classification	Description
1	Fracture along the growth plate resembling a slipped epiphysis.
2	Fracture through the epiphyseal plate with triangle of bone shaft attached.
3	Fracture through the epiphysis extending into epiphyseal plate.
4	Fracture of epiphysis and shaft crossing the epiphyseal plate.
5	Damage to epiphyseal plate.

ommend reduction and pinning (Omid et al. 2008) to enhance the prospect of full functional recovery.

In most cases, analgesia, sling and immobilisation are adequate means of management, however internal fixation may be required if the proximal epiphysis is significantly displaced. Humeral shaft fractures may be the result of a direct blow and NAI should be considered in injuries which are found in a child <3 years of age, especially with a spiral humerus fracture.

Elbow

Elbow fractures account for 5–10% of all fractures in children. It is often helpful to address elbow fractures from an anatomical perspective, as each fracture poses unique challenges in diagnosis and treatment. The elbow joint is a complex articulation of three bones (humerus, radius and ulna) which allows motion in all three planes (Hart et al. 2011). Diagnosis of elbow injuries is by radiography. This can be difficult and is usually complicated by the presence of numerous epiphyses and ossification centres. These injuries are usually the result of a fall onto an outstretched arm. Types of injury that occur are supracondylar humerus fractures, fracture of the medial and lateral condyle, medial epicondylar injuries, fracture separation of the distal humerus physis, elbow dislocations and radial head subluxation. Generally, these require reduction and may need surgical fixation depending on the severity of the injury. Orthopaedic consultation is warranted immediately to determine treatment interventions. As with all extremity injuries the limb should be closely observed for neurovascular complications. Findings such as pallor, cyanosis of the fingers, prolonged capillary refill, altered sensation and absence of radial pulse should be acted on immediately.

Radius and ulna

Fractures to the radius and ulna are very common during childhood, heal well and are unlikely to cause long-term problems. They should be suspected if there is any type of deformity about the elbow, forearm or wrist. For children in PICU there may be other priorities, but management is generally a closed reduction and a cast. There is increasing evidence that children are best managed with semi-rigid casts for simple fractures (Taranu et al. 2011).

Hand and wrist

Anatomically, the hand and wrist are a complex structure of bones, muscles, ligaments and tendons, which enable the child to perform complex functions with considerable dexterity. For children admitted to PICU, minor injuries to the hand and wrist are not likely to be considered impor-

tant, however the hand has a rich blood supply from the radial and ulna arteries. Children with hand and wrist injuries must have their vascular status assessed and regularly monitored. Where there is consciousness and cooperation the tip of each digit for should be examined for sensation. A cold hand with absent or reduced pulses accompanied with intense pain might indicate ischaemia, compartment syndrome and/or embolus (Larson 2002). Orthopaedic review should be undertaken once the patient is stable and, if required, the injury should be reduced and immobilised. Some injuries may require surgical intervention (internal or external fixation). This will be dictated by the type and severity of injury and orthopaedic opinion. Major hand trauma (e.g. crush injury) can have considerable implications for the future of the child and a referral to a specialist hand consultant is required. The primary focus of any treatment is to achieve optimal restoration of function (Larson 2002).

If hand fractures are suspected, they should be X-rayed, any rings removed, any bleeding stopped and wounds covered with an appropriate dressing. Where possible the child's arm should be elevated to reduce the risk of swelling. Whenever possible, IV lines should not be sited over or near areas of skeletal trauma.

Lower limb injuries and fractures

Femur

Femoral shaft fractures represent approximately 1.6% of all bony injuries in children (Kasser and Beaty 2006). The first peak of these injuries occurs in early childhood and the second in adolescence. Although femoral shaft fractures are dramatic and disabling, most unite rapidly without significant complications or sequelae. In the past, traction and casting were the standard treatments, however a variety of treatments now maybe considered including external fixation, compression or submuscular plating and flexible or locked intramedullary nailing. This means that the child may be in for a shorter hospital stay than in the past, decreasing impairment, increasing convenience and decreasing cost of care (Kasser and Beaty 2006).

The aetiology of femoral fractures varies with age. In children younger than walking age up to 80% of femoral fractures may be caused by abuse (Beals and Tufts 1983). Older children are unlikely to have femoral fractures caused by abuse as their bone is sufficiently strong to withstand forceful blows and can survive torque without fracture. In older children, femoral fractures are most likely to be caused by high energy impacts such as RTAs, which account for over 90% of fractures in this age group (Hedlund and Lindgren 1986). Therefore, the child's

Table 9.5 Treatment options for femoral shaft fractures in children and adolescents

Age	Treatment
Birth–24 months	Pavlik Harness (newborn to 6 months).
	Immediate spica cast.
	Traction, then spica cast.
2–5 years	Immediate spica cast.
	Traction, then spica cast.
	External fixation (rare).
	Flexible intramedullary rod (rare).
6–11 years	Traction, then spica cast.
	Flexible intramedullary rod.
	Compression plate.
	External fixation.
12 years–maturity	Flexible intramedullary rod.
	Compression plate.
	Locked intramedullary rod.
	External fixation.

Source: modified from Kasser and Beaty 2006.

admission to intensive care is likely to be due to other injuries sustained (e.g. in a multiple trauma event) and that the femoral shaft fracture is an associated injury.

The fractures may be classified as transverse, spiral or oblique; fragmented or non-fragmented; and open or closed

Treatment depends generally on age and size and whether it is an isolated injury or a result of polytrauma (Table 9.5).

Enthusiasm for treatments that decreases hospital stay (an important consideration in intensive care management) has led to the use of external fixation and flexible intramedullary nails in children 6 years of age and older. Also, skeletal fixation is frequently used in children with multiple trauma, head injury, vascular compromise, floating knee injuries or multiple fractures.

Ward et al. (1992) reported the use of compression plates for the treatment of femoral shaft fractures in 25 children 6–16 years of age, 22 of whom had associated fractures or multisystem injuries. According to these investigations, plate fixators offer the advantages of anatomic reduction, ease of insertion, simplified nursing care, rapid mobilisation without casting and applicability to any size femoral shaft. Disadvantages include the long incision necessary and risks of plate breakage and stress fracture after plate removal.

Knee injuries

Fractures involving the physis about the knee are particularly prone to complications and associated injuries and must be approached with care.

There is quite a significant risk of permanent injury to the physis, which may lead to growth disturbance and requires follow-up after fracture healing. As with all extremity trauma the injury should be acknowledged but should not detract from emergency care management of the multiple-injured patient. In addition, associated injuries to nerves, vascular structures, ligaments and the possibility of compartment syndrome require significant attention to detail and nursing care in the evaluation and management of these injuries. A series of 63 distal femoral physeal fractures in children aged 2–11 years were almost invariably caused by severe trauma, however those occurring in older children were usually secondary to less extensive trauma, most often sports injuries (Riseborough et al. 1983). The Salter–Harris classification is useful for description and treatment planning.

The mechanism of injury for fractures of the proximal tibial epiphysis is usually due to motor vehicle trauma. The proximal tibial physis has intrinsic anatomic stability and is reasonably well protected. For this reason separation of the proximal tibial epiphysis is quite rare.

Management depends on classification of injuries and other relevant factors, such as the child with multiple injuries. Management may involve manipulation, reduction and immobilisation or closed reduction and fixation, or open reduction.

Fractures of the patella in children usually are the result of a direct blow and are much less common than in adults. The diagnosis of patella fractures in children is prone to delay (Belman and Neviaser 1973). Primary osseous fractures of the patella in children are treated similarly to adults, with internal fixation of displaced fractures.

Tibia and fibula

Tibia and fibula are common paediatric long bone injuries (Shannak 1988). The average age of occurrence is 8 years and 70% of paediatric tibial fractures are isolated injuries and unlikely to be seen in PICU.

Non-displaced tibial metaphyseal fractures are stabilised with a long leg cast, whereas displaced tibial fractures require closed reduction with a general anaesthetic. Uncomplicated shaft fractures can be treated by manipulation and casting, and displaced fractures can be reduced under sedation and then immobilised. In general, operative treatment is rarely needed and the indications for this are open fractures, fractures with an associated compartment syndrome, fractures in children with spasticity (head injury or cerebral palsy), fractures in which open treatment facilitates nursing care (floating knee, multiple long bone fractures, multiple system injuries) and unstable fractures that fail closed manipulation and casting (Bartlett et al. 1997). Common methods of fixation include percutaneous metallic pins, bio-absorbable pins, external fixation and plates with screws.

The use of flexible intramedullary nails or intramedullary Steinman pins is increasing common.

A fractured fibula in very young children on its own without associated injury to the tibia is uncommon as the fibula is well covered by soft tissue except at the lateral malleolus. As children get older and become involved in sports, fibula fracture is more common and occurs in association with rolled/twisted ankle injury, particularly with significant weight-bearing forces. It can also occur as a result of high impact and awkward landings from a jump or an agility task such as landing from a vault or a balance beam. Contact sports (e.g. karate) and a direct blow to the outer lower leg or ankle may cause a fibula fracture, as may sports that involve a change of direction at speed (e.g. football, rugby, hockey, netball) so the injury is seen in adolescents and young adults. It would not be seen in isolation in intensive care or high dependency units and although treatment involves the need for anatomical reduction to realign the bone by manipulation under anaesthetic followed by a means to stabilise the fracture, possibly with plates and screws. The child may need a protective boot and crutches for a number of weeks. However, such a fracture is not usually a high priority in the intensive care environment.

Foot and ankle

Ankle injuries account for approximately 5% of the workload in an Emergency Department (Wardrope and English 1998). Most patients will have a simple ankle sprain. However, in the intensive care environment they may have sustained an ankle or foot injury as part of a multi-system trauma event.

These injuries, although important, should not detract from the primary survey to identify and treat life-threatening events. As with all musculoskeletal injuries, history-taking and understanding the mechanism of injury are important, with the primary focus of any treatment being to achieve optimal restoration of function (Larson 2002). The examination should be structured, and symptoms such as bruising, swelling, pain and obvious deformity should be taken into account. Deformity may require immediate intervention. A fractured or dislocated ankle can disrupt normal neurovascular supply to the foot, therefore foot pulses and sensation should be assessed (where possible) during the assessment of injury and following the reduction (Holt and Dolan 2000). Once reduced, the limb should be immobilised in a plaster of Paris or splint prior to X-ray. To prevent oedema the limb should be elevated and to help reduce swelling ice packs may be used.

Growth plate injuries

Physeal injuries can be sustained in many ways but the most frequent mechanism is fracture. Most commonly the fracture injury is direct, with the fracture pattern involving the physis itself. However, it can also be the result of and associated with a fracture elsewhere in the limb segment.

In general, fractures in children heal more rapidly than in adults and physeal injuries should be managed methodically, including general assessment and stabilisation of the poly-traumatised patient, evaluation of the neurovascular and soft tissue status of the traumatised limb, and the reduction and stabilisation of the fracture. Except for the possibility of subsequent growth disturbance, the potential complications of physeal injuries are no different from other traumatic musculoskeletal injuries (see Table 9.4, Salter–Harris classification).

Open fracture

Most serious open fractures result from high-velocity blunt injury involving vehicles. Penetrating injuries are much less common in children than in adults.

In children with multiple injuries approximately 10% of the fractures are open (Schalamon et al. 2003). When open fractures are present 25–50% of patients have additional injuries involving head, chest, abdomen and other extremities (Kay and Skaggs 2006).

Wound classification can be used to describe the injuries to the tissue adjacent to the open fracture:

- Type I fractures usually result from a spike of bone puncturing the skin. The wound is less than 1 cm in size and there is minimal soft tissue damage or contamination.
- Type II wound is generally larger than 1 cm and is typically associated with a transverse or oblique fracture with minimal comminution. There is adjacent soft tissue injury, including skin flaps or skin avulsion, and a moderate crushing components of adjacent soft tissue is usually present. Skin grafts of flaps should not be needed.
- Type III. These are the most severe open fractures and are associated with extensive soft tissue injury, large open wound and significant contamination

- IIIA: There is soft tissue coverage of the bone which is often a segmental fracture.
- IIIB: Bone is exposed at the fracture site, with treatment typically requiring skin and or muscle flap coverage of the bone.
- IIIC: Fractures are defined as those with an injury to a major artery in that segment of the extremity. These injuries are often associated with extensive soft tissue loss and contamination.

(Gustillo et al. 1984).

The treatment of open fractures in children is similar to management in adults. Primary goals are to prevent infection of the wound and fracture site, while allowing soft tissue healing, fracture union and a return to optimal function.

Initial primary care may include application of a sterile betadine dressing and preliminary alignment and splinting of the fracture. If profuse bleeding is present, a compression dressing is applied. The second stage is primary surgical intervention, including initial debridement of tissue until the wound appears viable. The fracture is reduced and stabilised at this time. The third and final stage is the bony reconstruction as required and ultimately rehabilitation.

Wound care is a vital aspect of the continued management to promote healing and avoid infection. Initially the child may require serial irrigation and debridement every 2–3 days until the wound is clean and appears viable (Chapter 14).

Antibiotic therapy decreases the risk of infection in open fractures. Wilkins and Patzakis (1991) reported a 13.9% infection rate in 79 patients who received no antibiotics whereas there was a 5% infection rate in 815 patients with similar injuries who had antibiotic prophylaxis. Antibiotic therapy is usually limited to 48–72 hours after surgical treatment of the open fracture.

Internal and external fixators

The type of operative stabilisation depends on the nature and type of injury and also the training and experience and personal preference of the orthopaedic surgeon. For stabilisation of closed long bone fractures the most common methods are usually intramedullary rod fixation, external fixation and AO compression plating, although Kirschner wires or Steinman pins may be used in conjunction with casts. The most common indications for the use of external fixation in a child with multiple injuries have been for open fractures with significant soft tissue injury, fractures in association with a head injury and coma, and so-called floating knee fractures of the femur and tibia. If an external fixator is used, pins sites should be closely monitored for early detection of pin tract infection.

Amputation

In severe injury the general principle is to preserve all extremities, however in extreme injury where the limb is beyond salvage an amputation may be required. If amputation is necessary, then as much length as possible should be preserved. If an amputation is the only option then once the child is recovering they will require immense input in terms of physical rehabilitation and psychological and emotional support.

Compartment syndrome

Compartment syndrome is a potential complication of musculoskeletal trauma. Early identification is vital as if it is left untreated it may result in limb loss or death.

Muscles, nerves, blood vessels and bones are surrounded by a tough inelastic tissue called fascia. Each group of tissues enveloped by fascia forms a compartment. As the fascia is inelastic it will not tolerate any movement and therefore will not accept any increase in volume or pressure in that particular compartment. It occurs when the injury induces increased pressure within a confined space. Because the early signs of compartment syndrome are often subtle it may be difficult to make an early diagnosis in the intensive care patient as they may be obtunded or sedated and ventilated.

Compartment syndrome is generally described as resulting from high pressure in the muscle compartment in the closed fascial space (Maher et al. 1994) which results in cellular anoxia, muscle ischaemia and death (Olson and Glasgow 2005). In children it can be seen following fractures of the supracondyle humerus or tibia, however the actual incidence in children is unknown. The increase in compartmental pressure occurs as a direct result of the injury to the muscle and tissues, which causes haemorrhage and swelling. In conjunction ischaemia produces anoxia in muscles, which in turn causes release of histamine-like substances which increase capillary permeability and lead to intra-muscular oedema. The increasing intramuscular oedema produces a progressive increase in the intrinsic tissue pressure of the muscles. The taut fascial envelope creates venous compression which further increases the intramuscular intrinsic pressure (Eaton and Green 1975).

Both mechanisms increase compartmental pressure, causing vascular obstruction and nerve impairment. If left untreated muscle necrosis may result, potentially requiring amputation. If still not treated, renal failure can occur and may result in death (Newton 2007). Once in progress the recognised treatment for this potentially devastating cycle is prompt wide surgical decompression of the fascial compartment. The surgical techniques for a fasciotomy depend on the anatomical location and it is vital that all of the relating compartments associated with the injury are released.

Monitoring the pressure

Normal compartmental pressure is 0–8 mmHg (compartment syndrome is said to be present when the pressure is elevated above this) (Mubarak et al. 1978). Measuring this pressure involves inserting a needle or catheter into the compartment and attaching it to a transducer or manometer apparatus. There is some debate about when surgical interventions should be performed in relation to pressure readings (Elliott and Johnstone 2003). Mubarak and colleagues (1978) recommended 30 mmHg, Matsen et al. (1980) and Gibson and colleagues (1986) suggested 45 mmHg. Others, such as McQueen and Court-Brown (1996), used differential pressures and advised surgical decompression between 10 and 30 mmHg. Willis and Rorabeck (1990) provide an overview of compartment syndrome management in children.

Non-invasive methods of diagnosis have also been tried recently. Wiemann and colleagues (2006) used pulsed phased-locked loop ultrasound and Joseph and colleagues (2006) used a measurement of tissue hardness to diagnose compartment syndrome in children.

Once compartment syndrome has been diagnosed surgical intervention in the form of a fasciotomy will be required. Long surgical cuts are made in the fascia to relieve the pressure. The wounds are generally left open (covered with a sterile dressing) and closed during a second surgery, usually 48–72 hours later. Skin grafts may be required to close the wound (Chapter 14).

In relation to circumferential plaster casts, bandages or back-slabs, if they are causing the problem, they should be loosened or cut down to relieve the pressure. With prompt diagnosis and treatment, the outlook is excellent for recovery of the muscles and nerves inside the compartment. However, the overall prognosis will be determined by the injury leading to the syndrome.

Elevating limbs

Given that compartment syndrome is difficult to diagnose in children and the difficulty is compounded in sedated children the best treatment is avoidance. It is important to remember that the only early sign may be pain, particularly pain on passive stretching. Pallor, pulselessness, paralysis

and paraesthesia are unreliable and may be late signs and often only present after permanent damage has occurred (Bea et al. 2001). Therefore, continued close monitoring of the injured limb is vital in early diagnosis and will be a prominent nursing role due to their unique position in caring for the patient.

Wright (2007) describes a neurovascular assessment and the clinical signs and symptoms of compartment syndrome (Table 9.6). Observations for neurovascular impairment should be carried out hourly in children at risk or more frequently if there is a clinical concern. Wright (2007) considered a validated assessment tool and stressors, the importance of good documentation and effective communication of concerns to the multidisciplinary team. It needs to be acknowledged, though, that whichever assessment tool is used it may still be difficult to conduct neurovascular assessment in young children due to their immature development and communication skills.

General care of plaster of Paris and casts

The presence, position and sometimes weight of a cast can have impact on the range of mobility and movement (for pressure area care, see Chapter 14). Splinting and stabilising using casts on children's fractures take a lower priority in PICU than some of the other coexisting features of their trauma. However, the application of these is performed for ease of nursing and for ongoing care. The PICU nurse may not see many simple casts, so for ease of memory some main points related to these are reproduced below.

Casts take time to dry; a fibreglass takes about 30 minutes, a plaster of Paris (POP) about 48 hours. If POP is used, care should be taken in handling and positioning the child during this time as indents on a soft POP can result in loss of alignment and a potential area of pressure below. To help reduce swelling following application of a cast the limb should be elevated and the fingers and toes observed to monitor the blood circulation to the periphery.

Fingers and toes should remain pink and warm and the pulses palpable. If not, a medical review is required. In some cases where swelling is expected a back-slab may be used which allows for some swelling and following 48–72 hours the back-slab can be converted to full POP. Back-slabs are very useful as in an emergency they can be removed using scissors to cut though the bandage. The basis of the back-slab can be retained and crepe or gauze bandage can be used to re-splint.

If the cast cracks, it is ineffective and needs to be reviewed. If the edges are rough, the rough edge can be

Table 9.6 Signs, symptoms and observations

Signs and symptoms	Nursing observation
Increasing pain, out of proportion to the injury or surgical intervention is the first most reliable sign (Wright and Bogoch 1992)	Regular pain assessments using an age-appropriate pain tool. Give all prescribed analgesia.
Pallor	Observe perfusion of digits on the affected limb. Assess to see if capillary refill time is less than 1 second.
Paraesthesia	Ask if the child can feel pins and needles in the digits. Lightly touch all digits, asking the child to confirm that they can feel the touch and that the feeling is normal or the same as the non-affected hand.
Paralysis	Ask the child to move the affected digits. The child may be reluctant because of pain, but should be able to do so.
Pulselessness, the last sign. If pulselessness occurs, then the compartment syndrome is well established and amputation is likely	Record the pulse distal to the site of injury. It may be necessary to make a hole in the plaster to access the pulse.
Coldness	Feel the digits for warmth and compare with the other limb.

Source: Wright 2007.

covered by pink plaster or zinc oxide plaster strips (check that the child is not allergic to these types of plaster). If the skin becomes sore, the plaster will need to be trimmed and the sore skin treated as pressure areas (Chapter 14).

POPs must be kept dry and this has implications for maintaining hygiene and toileting depending on the location of the cast. If the cast encases a wound and there is breakthrough bleeding the cast will be soggy and ineffective. A window over a wound is the preferred option.

When a full POP is used and needs to be removed a plaster saw has to be employed. Children may need to be sedated or have ear muffs to reduce the noise and potential distress of this process.

Conclusion

This chapter has reviewed some of the essential elements to consider when caring for a child who has suffered extensive trauma. It should be noted that orthopaedic children's nursing is in itself an advanced speciality and as soon as the child is sufficiently stable to attain maximum function and rehabilitation the child should be transferred to receive this specialist care.

References

Anderson R, Kan PM et al. 2010. Utility of a cervical spine clearance protocol after trauma in children between 0 and 3 years of age. Journal of Neurosurgery Pediatrics, 5(3):292–6.

Ball W, Bindler C. 2008. Pediatric Nursing. Hemel Hempstead: Prentice Hall.

Barry P, Morris K, Ali T. 2010. Paediatric Intensive Care. Oxford Specialist Handbooks. Oxford: Oxford University Press.

Bartlett C, Weiner L, Yang E. 1997. Treatment of type II and type III open tibia fractures in children. Journal of Orthopaedic Trauma, 11(5):357–62.

Bea D, Kadiyala K, Walters P. 2001. Acute compartment syndrome in children: contemporary diagnosis, treatment, and outcome. Journal of Pediatric Orthopaedics, 21(5): 680–8.

Beals R, Tufts E. 1983. Fractured femur in infancy: the role of child abuse. Journal of Pediatric Orthopaedics, 3(5):583–6.

Belman D, Neviaser R. 1973.Transverse fracture of the patella in a child. Journal of Trauma, 13(10):917–18.

Chamley C, Carson P et al. 2005. Developmental Anatomy and Physiology of Children: a practical approach. Oxford: Churchill Livingstone.

Currey J, Butler G. 1975. The mechanical properties of bone tissue in children. Journal of Bone and Joint Surgery, 57(6):810–14.

Denis F. 1983. Spinal instability as defined by the three-column spine concept in acute spinal trauma. Clinical Orthopaedics and Related Research Medicine. missouri.edu/ortho/secure/docs/s-spine/Denis%201983.pdf.

Dionyssiotis Y. 2011. Spinal cord injury-related bone impairment and fractures: an update on epidemiology and physiopathological mechanisms. Journal of Musculoskeletal and Neuronal Interactions, 11(3):257–65.

Duhem R, Tonnelle V et al. 2008. Unstable upper pediatric cervical spine injuries: report of 28 cases and review of the literature. Childs Nervous System, 24(3):343–8.

Eaton R, Green W. 1975. Volkmann's ischemia: a volar compartment syndrome of the forearm. Clinical Orthopaedics and Related Research, 113:58–64.

Elliott K, Johnstone A. 2003. Diagnosing acute compartment syndrome. Journal of Bone and Joint Surgery, 85(5): 625–32.

Frakes M, Evans T. 2004. Major pelvic fractures. Critical Care Nurse, 24(2):18–30.

Garvin KL, McCarthy RE et al. 1990.Pediatric pelvic ring fractures. Journal of Pediatric Orthopaedics, 10:577–82.

Gerndt S, Rodriguez J et al. 1997. Consequences of high-dose steroid therapy for acute spinal cord injury. Journal of Trauma – Injury, Infection and Critical Care, 42(2):279–84.

Gibson MJ, Barnes MR et al. 1986. Weakness of foot dorsiflexion and changes in compartment pressures after tibial osteotomy. Journal of Bone and Joint Surgery, 68-B: 471–5.

Gustillo R, Mendoza R, Williams D. 1984. Problems in the management of type III (severe) open fractures: a new classification of type III open fractures. Journal of Trauma, 24(8):742–6.

Hart E, Turner A et al. 2011. Common pediatric elbow fractures. Orthopaedic Nursing, 30(1):11–17.

Hedlund R, Lindgren U. 1986. The incidence of femoral shaft fractures in children and adolescents. Journal of Pediatric Orthopedics, 6(1):47–50.

Herzenberg J, Hensinger R et al. 1989. Emergency transport and positioning of young children who have an injury of the cervical spine. The standard backboard may be hazardous. Journal of Bone and Joint Surgery, 71(1):15–22.

Holden C, Holman J, Herman M. 2007. Pediatric pelvic fractures. Journal of the American Academy of Orthopaedic Surgeons, 15(3):172–7.

Holt L, Dolan B. 2000. Accident and Emergency Theory into Practice. Oxford: Baillière Tindall.

Ismail N, Bellemare J et al. 1996. Death from pelvic fracture: children are different. Journal of Pediatric Surgery, 31(1): 82–5.

Kasser J, Beaty J (Eds). 2006. Supracondylar fractures of the distal humerus. In Rockwood and Wilkins' Fractures in Children (6th edition, pp. 543–89). Philadelphia: Lippincott Williams & Wilkins.

Kay R, Skaggs D. 2006. Pediatric polytrauma management. Journal of Pediatric Orthopaedics, 26(2):268–77.

Joseph B, Varghese R et al. 2006. Measurement of tissue hardness: can this be a method of diagnosing compartment syndrome non-invasively in children? Journal of Paediatric Orthopaedics, 15(6):443–8.

Larson D. 2002. Assessment and management of hand and wrist fractures. Nursing Standard, 16(36):45–53.

Leonard JC, Kuppermann N et al. 2011. Factors associated with cervical spine injury in children after blunt trauma. Annals of Emergency Medicine, 58(2):145–55.

Loder R. 1987. Pediatric polytrauma: orthopaedic care and hospital course. Journal of Orthopaedic Trauma, 1(1): 48–54.

MacGregor J. 2008. Introduction to the Anatomy and Physiology of Children. New York: Routledge.

Maher AB, Salmond SW, Pellino TA. 1994. Orthopaedic Nursing. Philadelphia: WB Saunders.

Marieb E, Hoehn K. 2010. Human Anatomy and Physiology. Harlow: Pearson Education.

Matsen F, Winquist R, Krugmire R. 1980. Diagnosis and management of compartment syndromes. Journal of Bone and Joint Surgery, 62:286–91.

McCall T, Fassett D, Brockmeyer D. 2006. Cervical spine trauma in children: a review. Neurosurgical Focus, 20(2). thejns.org/doi/pdf/10.3171/foc.2006.20.2.6.

McCormack R, Strauss E et al. 2010. Diagnosis and management of pelvic fractures. Bulletin of the NYU Hospital for Joint Diseases, 68(4):281–91.

McQueen M, Court-Brown C. 1996. Compartment monitoring in tibial fractures: the pressure threshold for decompression. Journal of Bone and Joint Surgery, 78(1):99–104.

Morris C, McCoy E, Lavery G. 2004.Spinal stabilisation for unconscious patients with multiple injuries. British Medical Journal, 329(7464):495–9.

Mubarak SJ, Owen CA et al. 1978. Acute compartment syndromes: diagnosis and treatment with the aid of the wick catheter. Journal of Bone and Joint Surgery of America, 60(8):1091–5.

Newton E. 2007. Acute complications of extremity trauma. Emergency Clinics of North America, 25:751–61.

Nieto-Lucio L, Camacho-González S, Reinoso-Pérez J. 2010. Surgical treatment of type IV unstable pelvic fractures in pediatric patients using the Torode and Zieg classification. Acta Ortopédica Mexicana, 24(5):337–42.

Olson S, Glasgow R. 2005. Acute compartment syndrome in lower extremity musculoskeletal trauma. American Academy of Orthopaedic Surgeons, 13(7):436–44.

Omid R, Choi P, Skaggs D. 2008. Supracondylar humerus fractures in children. Journal of Bone and Joint Surgery, 19(5):485–94.

Riseborough EJ, Barrett IR, Shapiro F. 1983. Growth disturbances following distal femoral physeal fracture-separations. Journal of Bone and Joint Surgery, 7(65):885–93.

Ruggieri M, Smárason A, Pike M. 1999. Spinal cord insults in the prenatal, perinatal, and neonatal periods. Developmental Medicine and Child Neurology, 41(5):311–17.

Schalamon J, Bismarck S et al. 2003. Multiple trauma in pediatric patients. Pediatric Surgery International, 19(6):417–23.

Shannak AO. 1988. Tibial fractures in children: follow-up study. Journal of Pediatric Orthopedics, 8(3):306–10.

Skettet S, Tibby S et al. 2002. Immobilisation of the cervical spine in children. British Medical Journal, 324(7337): 591–3.

Singhal B, Mohammed A et al. 2008. Neurological outcome in surgically treated patients with incomplete closed traumatic cervical spinal cord injury. Spinal Cord, 46(9): 603–7.

Taranu R, Webb J et al. 2011. Using semi-rigid casts in the management of buckle fractures. Paediatric Nurse, 20(2): 25–8.

Tile M. 1988. Pelvic ring fractures: Should they be fixed? Journal of Bone and Joint Surgery, 70B:1–12.

Torode I, Zieg D. 1985. Pelvic fractures in children. Journal of Pediatric Orthopedics, 5(1):76–84.

Tortora GJ, Derrickson BH. 2009. Principles of Anatomy and Physiology, 12th Edition. Volume 2: Maintenance and Continuity of the Human Body. Asia: John Wiley and Sons.

Ward W, Levy J, Kaye A. 1992. Compression plating for child and adolescent femur fractures. Journal of Pediatric Orthopedics, 12(5):626–32.

Wardrope J, English B. 1998. Musculo-Skeletal Problems in Emergency Medicine. Oxford: Oxford University Press.

Werndle MC, Zoumprouli A et al. 2012. Variability in the treatment of acute spinal cord injury in the United Kingdom: results of a national survey. Journal of Neurotrauma, 29(5):880–8.

Wiemann J, Toshiaki U et al. 2006. Non-invasive measurements of intramuscular pressure using pulsed phased-locked loop ultrasound for detecting compartment syndromes: a preliminary report. Journal of Orthopaedic Trauma, 20(7): 458–63.

Wilkins J, Patzakis M. 1991. Choice and duration of antibiotics in open fractures. Orthopedic Clinics of North America, 22(3):433–7.

Willis RB, Rorabeck CH. 1990. Treatment of compartment syndrome in children. Orthopedic Clinics of North America, 21(2):401–12.

Wright E. 2007. Evaluating a paediatric neurovascular assessment tool. Journal of Orthopaedic Nursing, 11(1): 20–9.

Wright J, Bogoch E. 1992. Compartment syndrome: a diagnostic dilemma. Journal of the American Academy of Physician Assistants, 5(2):94–8.

Resource

Pelvic Ring Fractures. emedicine.medscape.com/article/394515-overview#a01.

Chapter 10
CARE OF THE INFANT OR CHILD WITH THERMAL INJURY

Jane Leaver[1] and Clare Thomas[2]

[1] School of Nursing and Midwifery, Faculty of Health, Birmingham City University, Birmingham, UK
[2] Burns Centre, Birmingham Children's Hospital, Birmingham, UK

Introduction

A major burn can have a huge impact on the child and family as it will cause disfigurement, disability and psychological trauma. This means that the involvement of an experienced team that can meet all of the needs of a burnt child is essential. This chapter focuses on the care and management required for a child with a burn in PICU.

Causes of burns

Burns to the skin can be caused by several different mechanisms: fire (e.g. house fires, barbecues, bonfires), hot fluids (e.g. baths, hot drinks, cooking fat), contact with hot objects (e.g. hair straighteners, irons, electrical fires, radiators), electrical burns (e.g. low-voltage domestic electrical appliances, high-voltage high-tension cables), chemicals (e.g. acids, alkali), or radiation (e.g. sunburn).

Scalds are more common than flame burns in paediatrics, especially in the pre-school age group (Hankins et al. 2006). However, it is the large scalds and flame burns that are more likely to require admission to PICU and those burns where patients have sustained an inhalation injury.

Most burn injuries in paediatrics are accidental, although it must be remembered that there may be child protection issues such as neglect and non-accidental injury (Chester et al. 2006). This needs to be taken into consideration when caring for the child and family and if necessary appropriate safe-guarding referrals made (Chapter 18).

Burn physiology

The skin is the largest organ of the body and consists of two layers: the epidermis and dermis. The epidermis consists of 4–5 cell layers with the lower basal cell layer repeatedly dividing and regenerating. As the cells mature and die they move up to the corneum stratum, which is a layer of dead cells that are constantly being shed. It is this layer that helps to provide a constant skin pH. The dermis contains the hair follicles, sweat and oil glands, nerves, blood vessels and sensory receptors. It is the dermis that gives the skin its elasticity and strength; however, unlike the epidermis it cannot regenerate.

The skin has a number of functions, including protection of underlying organs, maintenance of body temperature, first line of protection against infection, waterproofing, excretion of waste products, sensation of pain and touch, and formation of vitamin D. Therefore, if damage or loss of the skin occurs, as in a burn, these functions will be impaired and treatment needs to take this into account.

Damage to the skin has both local and systemic effects. Locally, the skin is destroyed to varying depths, depending on the temperature and duration of contact with the

Paediatric Intensive Care Nursing, First Edition. Edited by Michaela Dixon and Doreen Crawford.
© 2012 John Wiley & Sons, Ltd. Published 2012 by John Wiley & Sons, Ltd.

causative agent. The higher the temperature and the longer the contact time the deeper the burn. Also, children have much thinner skin than adults and so are more likely to suffer deep burns (Williams 2009).

Jackson (1953) first described the burn wound as having three zones. The zone of coagulation at the point of contact at the centre of the burn is where protein in the cells is destroyed, causing tissue death. Surrounding this area of necrosis there is less damage but the circulation is compromised; this is the zone of stasis and it has the potential to recover, but if there are further insults, such as infection, oedema or continued hypovolaemia, then it will become necrotic, causing the burn wound to become deeper and larger. The outermost zone, the zone of hyperaemia, in a large burn can involve the rest of the body. This zone has an increased tissue perfusion due to inflammatory mediators and will usually recover. However burn wounds are dynamic and heterogeneous so can change, particularly in the first few days (Australia and New Zealand Burn Association 2006), so caution should be used when estimating the depth and informing the family.

When the local tissue is destroyed this sets off an inflammatory response releasing cytokines and other chemical mediators. This release in a burn of greater than 30% of total body surface area (TBSA) will have a systemic effect on the whole body (Hettiaratchy and Dziewulski 2004) causing cardiovascular, respiratory, renal, metabolic and immunological changes. The systemic response can be more of a threat to the child than the actual wound.

The release of histamine, bradykinin, prostaglandins and other chemical mediators from the wound cause capillary permeability, which in turn leads to oedema from the plasma leak and hypovolaemia (Kramer et al. 2007). The plasma leak is usually at its greatest in the first 8–12 hours, then gradually decreases over the next 48–72 hours (Ahrns 2004). The release of inflammatory mediators due to the tissue trauma and hypovolaemia can affect cardiac function, causing an increase in pulmonary and systemic vascular resistance (SVR) and myocardial depression and thus a reduced cardiac output. A reduced cardiac output can occur even after adequate fluid therapy (Kramer et al. 2007). The increased SVR is also partly due to increased blood viscosity from the loss of plasma in the blood, which leads to an increased haemoconcentration (Cook 2002). The hypovolaemia and reduction in cardiac output can lead to a decrease in tissue perfusion and hypoxia, which in turn leads to ischaemia of the gastrointestinal tract and kidneys if not corrected. It can also cause anaerobic metabolism and acidosis. Acidosis can also be a result of pulmonary oedema from the effect of the inflammatory mediators on the lungs and hypoproteinaemia (Herndon 2007). It is also thought that the systemic inflammatory response resulting from a large burn can cause respiratory distress syndrome. Cerebral oedema in children with large burns can also occur (Kramer et al. 2007).

The cardiovascular effects in a severe burn can lead to a hypermetabolic response. This severe increase in the metabolic rate is characterised by a raised core temperature, greater oxygen and glucose consumption, and the accelerated breakdown of proteins, sugars and fats, which is revealed as an increase in urine urea and creatinine levels (Norbury and Herndon 2007). This hypermetabolic state can also have a detrimental effect on the body's immune system and wound healing. It can persist for a couple of years after the burn has healed (O'Ceallaigh and Shah 2008; see also Chapter 14).

Electrical burns have some differences in pathophysiology. Initially, an electrical burn may look quite small. However, if the electricity was of a high voltage (>1000 volts) the electrical current will enter at the point of contact and travel to the exit point at earth. As the current passes through the tissues damage will occur from the heat generated (Australia and New Zealand Burn Association 2006). This can cause more damage than first seen, as internal damage may have occurred to the tissue, muscles, nerves, blood vessels and even bone. This makes it harder to assess the extent of the burn. There may also be other trauma present, such as factures and dysrhythmias due to muscle tetany and electrical activity.

Burn assessment

Size

To calculate the size of a burn, a Lund and Browder chart (Figure 10.1) should be used. The areas of burn injury are transcribed onto the chart with as much accuracy as possible and the percentage is calculated for each area, then added up to give the total body surface area (TBSA) burnt. It is important to take into consideration the age of the child when performing this calculation as the ratio of head size to the rest of the body surface area changes with age. Small areas of burnt or unburnt skin can be calculated using the child's hand size (palm and fingers) which equates to approximately 1% TBSA (Barret and Dziewulski 2006; Hettiaratchy and Papini 2004).

Depth

The depth of the burn is defined by the depth of skin tissue damaged. This can be classified as superficial, partial thickness or full thickness (Cook 2002); or alternatively as epidermal, superficial dermal, deep dermal and full thickness (Hettiaratchy and Papini 2004) (Table 10.1).

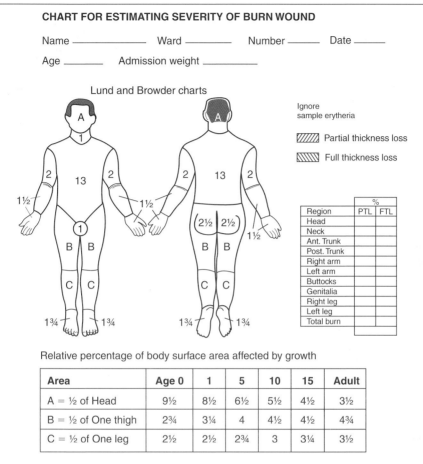

CHART FOR ESTIMATING SEVERITY OF BURN WOUND

Name —————— Ward ———— Number ——— Date ———

Age ——— Admission weight ——————

Lund and Browder charts

Ignore
sample erytheria

///// Partial thickness loss

\\\\\ Full thickness loss

Region	PTL	FTL
Head		
Neck		
Ant. Trunk		
Post. Trunk		
Right arm		
Left arm		
Buttocks		
Genitalia		
Right leg		
Left leg		
Total burn		

Relative percentage of body surface area affected by growth

Area	Age 0	1	5	10	15	Adult
A = ½ of Head	9½	8½	6½	5½	4½	3½
B = ½ of One thigh	2¾	3¼	4	4½	4½	4¾
C = ½ of One leg	2½	2½	2¾	3	3¼	3½

Figure 10.1 Lund and Browder chart. From Dixon, M., Crawford, D., Teasdale, D. & Murphy, J. (eds) (2009) *Nursing the Highly Dependent Child or Infant: A Manual of Care*, p. 225. Reproduced with permission from John Wiley & Sons, Ltd.

The assessment of burn depth is multifactorial and involves visual observation, clinical assessment of sensation, bleeding and blanching, the history of the thermal source, contact time and any first aid given.

The deeper the burn the less sensation – a superficial burn is very painful, whereas a full thickness burn has no sensation as all the nerve endings have been destroyed. Similarly, bleeding on a pin prick is brisk in a superficial burn but is delayed in a deep dermal burn and nonexistent in a full thickness burn. However, these can be difficult to assess and a more accurate, non-invasive method is to assess the capillary return on blanching of the burn wound with pressure. In a superficial burn the capillary return is brisk. This becomes slower as the deeper the burn until there is no blanching in deep dermal and full thickness burns.

Laser Doppler imaging can also be used to aid burn depth assessment alongside the clinical assessment (Sainsbury 2008). This uses a red laser to scan the burn wound and then produces a diagrammatic colour image of the blood flow in the wound. This can be helpful in determining borderline deep dermal/full thickness depths and whether surgery is indicated.

Management of burns

Primary and secondary survey

A primary survey is required, using the ABCDE approach as for any child following trauma, but additional consideration needs to be given to particular areas specifically related to the burn injury.

Airway

The history of the injury will give vital clues as to the risk of airway involvement, for example if they were in an enclosed environment, smoke present, burns to the face, singeing of nasal hair and/or eyebrows, hoarseness,

Table 10.1 Burn depth

Epidermal or superficial burn	Only part of the epidermis is destroyed. The area looks red and is very painful. There is brisk capillary refill and the burn usually heals within a week.
Superficial dermal or superficial partial thickness burn	The epidermis is fully destroyed as is part of the papillary dermis. The area may have blisters and looks red and wet on examination. Brisk capillary refill and sensate. Usually heals within 2 weeks.
Deep dermal or deep partial thickness burn	All the epidermis, papillary dermis and part of the reticular dermis are destroyed. The area is paler and may be mottled in colour and often drier in appearance. Sluggish capillary refill. Sensation is reduced. Usually heals within 3 weeks, although grafting may be considered depending on size and area.
Full thickness burn	Both the epidermis and dermis are destroyed and sometimes underlying tissues. The area will be charred, leathery-looking or waxy white in colour and thus can be sometimes be mistaken for unburnt skin. Insensate and no capillary refill. All but very small full thickness burns usually need excision and grafting as they will take longer than 3 weeks to heal with potential complications.

Source: Herndon 2007.

breathing difficulties and change of conscious level, this would give a high index of suspicion of airway involvement.

Anaesthetic assessment should be sought for any burns to the face and neck if there is a possibility of smoke inhalation injury or any respiratory impairment. It is recommended that if there is a threat to the airway, intubation occurs earlier rather than later due to the risk of swelling (Australia and New Zealand Burn Association 2006). An uncut ET tube should be used as the face is likely to swell considerably. Cotton tapes rather than adhesive tape should be used to secure the ET tube as these can be adjusted as required.

As with any other trauma injury the cervical spine should be protected until clinically cleared (Chapter 9).

Breathing

A full respiratory assessment is required, including arterial blood gas and carbon monoxide (CO) levels. Oxygen is required to maximise tissue oxygenation and perfusion and to combat any CO intoxication.

An escharotomy (an excision through the burnt eschar to viable tissue to relieve constriction allowing for chest expansion) may be required for circumferential full thickness burns to the chest in order to facilitate adequate ventilation.

Circulation

The child's peripheral and central circulation needs to be assessed and any bleeding stopped. This is an important part of the initial assessment, especially if there has been

a delay in treatment as there is a risk of hypovolaemia due to fluid being lost from the burn. It is also important to assess the peripheral circulation in case there are circumferential deep burns that are causing inadequate tissue perfusion which can lead to compartment syndrome and may need an escharotomy to release the pressure. Any jewellery should be removed due to risk of impairment to tissue perfusion from swelling. Good, reliable venous access (ideally in unburnt skin) should be obtained, bloods taken for urea and electrolytes, full blood count cross-match, CO levels and fluids commenced as per burn fluid regimen and any additional boluses to stabilise the child (ATLS 2008).

Disability

Assessing the child's neurological level is required using the AVPU (alert, voice, pain, unconscious) score initially and then an age-appropriate tool. Hypoxia from smoke inhalation and/or CO intoxication will cause reduced consciousness levels. These need to be ruled out before consideration is given to other causes of altered neurological status, such as head injury or alcohol intoxication.

Exposure

Once the life-threatening issues have been assessed it is important to do a thorough examination to assess the extent of the burn and look for any other injuries. The child should be kept warm and exposure kept to a minimum.

The secondary survey

This includes an AMPLE (allergies, medicines, past medical history, last meal, event) history and relevant

X-rays should be undertaken in line with the trauma guidelines (Australia and New Zealand Burn Association 2006). The child should be reassessed regularly to ensure any change in their condition is not missed.

Airway management and inhalation injury

The majority of children admitted to the PICU with a thermal injury have been intubated and require assistance with their respiratory system. This is due to the extent of the injury or the suspicion that the child has had an inhalation injury (Chapter 4).

The most common signs and symptoms associated with an inhalation injury are discussed in the primary survey section and, as stated, it is better to intubate earlier rather than later as the intubation will be more difficult if facial, tongue and upper airway swelling has occurred. Bronchoscopy is often used to confirm an inhalation injury along with clinical signs and symptoms.

Classification of inhalation injury can be divided into upper airway and lower airway injury, where the tissue is damaged by heat and inhaled chemicals, and systemic toxicity which occurs when the absorption of toxic substances occurs through the alveoli (Australia and New Zealand Burn Association 2006). Studies have shown that the addition of an inhalation injury along with a thermal injury increases mortality risk (Lafferty 2010).

Most inhalation injuries are caused if the child has been involved in a house fire or in an enclosed space where they have inhaled heat and toxic smoke particles and fumes causing irritation, which can lead to airway and gas-exchange complications. Many household materials produce toxic gases when ignited (Traber et al. 2007), including CO and hydrogen cyanide. Inhalation injury can also be caused by steam, which tends to stay hotter for longer and thus causes a lower airway thermal injury.

CO poisoning occurs because of its higher affinity than oxygen to haemoglobin, forming carboxyhaemoglobin. It is important to realise that CO poisoning can give a false high pulse oximetry reading. Treatment is the administration of 100% oxygen until the CO levels are <10%.

The treatment for smoke inhalation includes toileting of the bronchial tree with regular lavage and suction until the particles are no longer visible, regular chest physiotherapy and regular repositioning of the patient with the aim to remove any foreign particles as quickly as possible to reduce complications. In recent years there has been much debate on the use of drug adjuncts to treat an inhalation injury. This includes the use of nebulised heparin, acetylcysteine, salbutamol (Palmieri 2009) or sodium bicarbonate (Prior et al. 2009).

The ventilation of the child follows the same principles as for all ventilation, using the least possible level of oxygen and pressure to get an acceptable level of gas exchange (O'Ceallaigh and Shah 2008). It is beyond the scope of this chapter to cover the many strategies for pulmonary ventilation in children with burns with or without inhalation injuries. However, the principles of lung protective ventilation strategies are now widely used and include high-frequency flow ventilation, positive end expiratory pressure and low tidal volumes. There have been some reported cases of using extracorporeal membrane oxygenation (ECMO) on patients with smoke inhalation injury (Niederbichler et al. 2009). However, performing surgery on children with a large cutaneous burn while on ECMO would put them at risk.

Securing the endotracheal tube can be difficult in children who have burns to the face. Whatever method is used, the nurse must ensure it is secure, checked regularly, the area kept clean and that the mechanics of ventilation do not cause more damage to the face by the action of pressure.

In some cases a child requires a prolonged period of ventilation and a tracheostomy may be performed. Although there are complications with tracheostomies some studies support this early intervention (O'Ceallaigh and Shah 2008). Consequently, in many cases if the patient has had a deep thermal injury to the face and neck, the neck area where the tracheostomy will be sited will be grafted as a priority to allow the site to heal and stabilise prior to cannulation.

Fluid resuscitation and patient monitoring

Children with burns >10% TBSA will need fluid resuscitation to ensure adequate tissue perfusion due to the amount of fluid lost through capillary permeability from the circulation. This is particularly relevant in the first 8 hours following burn injury, but in the more severely burnt child may be prolonged.

There are many burn fluid resuscitation formulas and all take into consideration the size of burn and weight of the child. In the United Kingdom, the Parkland formula (Table 10.2) is commonly used (Baker et al. 2007), as it is a relatively simple and easy to use crystalloid-based regime. The Cochrane Review (Schierhout and Roberts 1998) on the use and risks of albumin in fluid resuscitation caused considerable debate about whether it should be used. More recently it has been suggested that the advantage of using crystalloids is that they have smaller molecules than albumin so do not get trapped in the extravascular space when capillary permeability is reduced, leading to third spacing. However, crystalloids are more easily lost from the circulation, leading to oedema, whereas the larger molecules of albumin stay in the circulation longer (Duncan

Table 10.2   The Parkland formula

Requirement	
Resuscitation fluid	
The amount of fluid to be given in the first 24 hours from the time of injury	4 ml Hartmann solution × Wt (kg) × TBSA Half of the calculated volume is given in the first 8 hours post injury and the remaining half of the volume given over the following 16 hours
Maintenance fluid	
Maintenance fluid should take into account any oral or enteral feeds. This maintenance fluid should not be hypotonic as this increases the risk of hyponatraemia (National Patient Safety Agency 2005)	100 ml/kg/24 hour up to 10 kg of body weight plus 50 ml/kg/24 hour between 10–20 kg of body weight plus 20 ml/kg/24 hour for each kg over 20 kg of body weight

Adapted from Australia and New Zealand Burn Association (2006).

and Dunn 2008). Albumin is also more expensive and carries a great risk of an adverse reaction, which has caused Perel and Roberts (2007) to question the use of colloids. Their review showed no evidence that the use of colloids compared to crystalloids in resuscitation reduced mortality. Some burn services, although using crystalloids initially, will introduce albumin after about 8 hours when the capillary permeability leak begins to decline. This is more to replace the oncotic protein loss than increase the circulatory volume (Hettiaratchy and Papini 2004). Further research is currently being undertaken in burn fluid management using other types of fluid, such as starches.

Children have a greater requirement of fluid than adults, especially if they have an inhalation injury (Traber et al. 2007) which is why resuscitation fluid is given in addition to maintenance fluid. Maintenance fluid should take into account any oral or enteral feeds and should not be hypotonic as this increases the risk of hyponatraemia (National Patient Safety Agency 2007), but it should contain glucose to prevent hypoglycaemia as children have lower glycogen reserves than adults (Duncan and Dunn 2008; Lee and Herndon 2007).

The fluid required is calculated from the time of the burn not the time the child arrives in the Emergency Department, so extra fluid may need to be given on admission to the PICU to catch up with the regime.

Replacement of fluid is not a precise procedure and the formulas are only a guide. Care needs to be taken to avoid complications due to too little fluid resuscitation such as organ under-perfusion and too much fluid resuscitation which could lead to excess oedema, cerebral oedema and cellular hypoxia (Duncan and Dunn 2008).

Monitoring the child's fluid status is important to detect any deviations from their norm. In the PICU setting this can be achieved through pulse, arterial blood pressure, blood for a blood count, urea and electrolytes, blood gas for pH, base excess and lactate, the difference between peripheral and central temperatures, oesophageal Doppler for cardiac output and capillary refill. Central venous pressure can also be used in conjunction with other clinical measures, but as an isolated reading it can be inaccurate in burn patients (Duncan and Dunn 2008).

Urine output is another important measure that needs to be considered when monitoring the child's fluid resuscitation status. Therefore, a child in PICU would need to be catheterised as approximately 1 ml/kg/hr of urine is required. If their urine output is <0.5 ml/kg/hr, consideration should be given to increasing the amount of resuscitation fluid; conversely, if it is >2 ml/kg/hr, consideration needs to be given to decreasing the amount of resuscitation fluid. An exception is when rhabdomyolysis (the breakdown and destruction of muscle) occurs. Then, the urine output needs to be increased to flush debris through the renal tubules to prevent renal failure. Should renal failure occur haemofiltration (and sometimes dialysis) is required. Haemofiltration may also be considered if the child becomes septic and hyperpyrexic.

In patients with a large thermal injury the use of inotropes may be necessary to maintain an adequate blood pressure if the problem is not due to insufficient fluids. As the cutaneous blood flow will be compromised there is risk that the burn will deepen, therefore it is important that the inotropic support be stopped as soon as possible.

Wound management

Wound management is a vital part of burn care. On arrival at the PICU the wounds will probably be covered with cling film. Once the child has been stabilised the burns surgeon can reassess the wound and ensure that the correct TBSA and depth has been calculated. This will influence both the fluid and wound management.

The main aims of wound management are prevention of infection, excision of dead tissue and wound closure, taking into account the need to preserve function and the aesthetic result. Early excision and wound coverage have been shown to reduce mortality and minimise blood loss (Papini 2004) and also to remove potential harmful bacteria, reduce pain, hasten recovery and shorten the hospital stay (Janzekovic 1977).

Most full thickness burn wounds will need to be excised and grafted to achieve early wound coverage and minimise infection and scarring. The gold standard for wound coverage is the patient's own skin (autograft), but there are times when there is insufficient autograft to cover the wound so a skin substitute needs to be sourced. These come in various forms:

- Temporary skin replacements such as allograft (skin from another human) or Biobrane™ (a nylon mesh containing silicone and porcine collagen). These skin substitutes are temporary dressings and although they initially cause closure of the burn wound, reducing pain and fluid loss, and encouraging migration of epithelial cells, they will lift off after a week or so when epithelisation has occurred. However, caution needs to be used if devitalised tissue or colonisation is present due to risk of infection.
- Bioengineered products that act as a permanent dermal substitute, for example Integra™ (a dermal matrix containing bovine collagen and glycosaminoglycan with a silicone top layer).
- Cultured autologous skin cells, which can be applied in the form of a spray or sheets. However, for these cells to be grown, a skin biopsy needs to be taken at an early stage.

These skin substitutes are expensive and should be applied to a clean, well-prepared wound bed, by experienced staff.

The ideal dressing for a burn is one that protects against infection, promotes moist wound healing, absorbs the large amount of wound exudate produced and is comfortable. As with any wound, the wound appearance and the aim of treatment need to be taken into consideration when deciding on a dressing; for example, is the aim protection, debridement or treating infection? There are many dressings that can be used on burns (Wasiak et al. 2008). In paediatric major burn care many of the dressings used are anti-microbial with a silver, iodine or chlorhexidine base (e.g. Acticoat™, Urgotul silver, betadine soaks and bactigra). However, care needs to be taken that they are appropriate for the child's age due to the risk of toxicity.

Frequent dressing changes will occur and, depending on condition of the child, may be performed in theatre or the cubicle. Cleaning the burn wounds is an important aspect of wound management. There are differing opinions regarding this (Watret and Armitage 2002). Some advocate not cleansing wounds as it will interfere with the healing process. They are generally talking about clean, healthy, granulating wounds, whereas a burn wound is at greater risk of infection which may cause systemic sepsis so needs aggressive cleaning, which may include showering and the use of antiseptic agents (e.g. iodine, chlorhexidine, cetrimide).

Certain areas of the body (e.g. the face) require specific consideration especially as there is a greater risk of contamination from secretions. The face is very vascular and has good healing potential, but it is not easy to dress well. Therefore, the treatment of choice for the face is regular cleaning to remove exudate, followed by the application of white paraffin or Polyfax or a dressing (e.g. aqualcel Ag®) or allograft to prevent bacterial contamination. If the wound extends under the hairline, the hair may need to be shaved to facilitate accurate assessment, wound care and to prevent a matted mess that encourages bacterial growth. If the ears are burnt, care needs to be taken that any exposed cartilage does not dry out and die. Any burns around the eye area should have an ophthalmic assessment as corneal damage may have occurred.

Once the burn wound has healed there is a high probability of scarring. Although it is not possible to avoid scarring some management techniques can improve the appearance of the scar. The most common are moisturising, pressure and silicone (Gollop 2002).

Pain

Burns can be excruciatingly painful whatever the depth. Although the nerve endings in full thickness burns have been destroyed, in the surrounding area the nerve endings may be intact or only partially affected and thus will cause pain. The inflammatory response which releases chemical mediators will also activate the pain-sensing nerves (nociceptors) causing pain (Latarjet 2002). Prolonged burn pain can cause hyperalgesia and lead to chronic pain (Summer et al. 2007). Therefore an important aspect in the care of a child admitted to PICU with a thermal injury is pain management. This is complex and multifaceted as it will involve the control of background pain (from the burn and

ET tube), breakthrough pain, postoperative pain and procedural pain, such as with dressing changes and therapy. A combination of various types of analgesic may be needed to address the different types of pain (nociceptive and neuropathic) and anxiety.

It is important to provide adequate analgesia from the outset and many burn services have their own guidelines for pain management, all of them including pharmacological intervention. Intravenous opioid analgesia is usually the first choice; it should be titrated to the needs of the child. These children may require larger doses than expected over a period of time due to low pain tolerance (Meyer et al. 2007; Patterson and Sharar 2001). The use of regular paracetamol alongside the opiate can be very effective for controlling background pain. Non-steroidal anti-inflammatory drugs should be used with caution in the acute phase.

Sedation may also be required when the child is ventilated and/or having dressing changes as anxiety can have detrimental effect and increase pain levels. Gabapentin has also been shown to be effective in combating neuropathic pain from burn injuries in children (Mendham 2004) and should be considered with amitriptyline and clonidine.

Along with the child's clinical status, the use of an appropriate pain scale to score the amount of pain is advantageous in assessing the child's pain management and aiding the adjustment of the analgesia (see Chapter 13 for further information on pain assessment and management). In the event that the child is conscious, distraction therapy can be an effective way to reduce their distress and pain level. Other non-pharmacological interventions have been shown to be effective in reducing anxiety and pain (e.g. music therapy, massage and hypnotherapy).

Nutritional requirements

Nutrition is an important aspect of burn care. A large wound has been created so there is an increased requirement for proteins, carbohydrates, vitamins and minerals to facilitate good wound healing. Albumin is lost through the burn wound exudate so extra protein is required to compensate and there is an increased hypermetabolic response due to the stress from the trauma and the nature of the burn wound which requires an increased calorie intake.

It is important that a proper nutritional assessment is carried out by a dietician and the appropriate nutritional requirements calculated on a regular basis. In addition, it is important to monitor the adequacy of nutrition through the estimation of the body's nitrogen balance from 24-hour urine collections and a weekly weight and blood results.

It is recommended that the serum level of trace elements is monitored, as trace elements, in particular zinc, copper and selenium, have an important role to play in growth and repair, metabolism, immunity and as antioxidants. Voruganti (2005) noted that these trace elements are reduced in burns and thus it is advocated that high doses of trace elements are given IV to children with major burns (Berger et al. 1998).

In the PICU children will not usually be able to eat and drink, however they would not be able to achieve their increased nutritional requirement even if awake, thus supplementary feeding is essential. Ideally, the enteral feed should be administered via a naso-jejunal tube so their feeding regime is not interrupted as much from frequent theatre visits as there is evidence to suggest that jejunal feeding can safely continue during surgery (Jenkins et al. 1994). Feeding should commence within 24 hours of injury if possible to help prevent paralytic ileus, reduce bacterial translocation and maintain the integrity of the gut (Norman et al. 2002). There are many formulas used to estimate the calories the child requires following a burn injury. This changes depending on the physical state of the child (e.g. pyrexia, wound coverage, level of pain and stress) (Saffle and Graves 2007).

The burnt child is prone to a Curling ulcer (stress ulcer) due to the stress response to the burn injury, and appropriate medication, such as an H_2 receptor blocker, should be given prophylactically for prevention (Beierle and Chung 2007).

In recent years the focus has been on trying to reduce catabolism and weight loss in the burn patient. This has been attempted with some documented success by using drugs such as oxandrolone (Demling and Orgill 2000), growth hormone and propranolol (Jeschke et al. 2008).

Toxic shock syndrome

Toxic shock syndrome is a systemic illness which occurs mainly when *Staphylococcus aureus* exotoxins or, less commonly, streptococcus exotoxins enter the blood stream. It has a reported incidence in children with burns and is thought to be due to the fact that the child has not yet developed the appropriate antibodies (White et al. 2005). If a child with a burn injury becomes unwell with a pyrexia and other symptoms such as rash, vomiting, irritability, lethargy and low white blood cell counts, then toxic shock should be considered.

Toxic shock can develop very rapidly from observation of the first signs and symptoms to multi-organ failure and death, so early recognition and prompt treatment are required. This may include admission to a PICU for organ support. Specific treatment is the administration of fresh frozen plasma or IV immunoglobulin concentrate which contain the antibodies required. Intravenous antibiotics (e.g. flucloxacillin) should also be given to prevent further growth of the staphylococcus aureus.

Environmental and continuing care considerations

The environment in which these patients are nursed is an important part of their care. Due to the high risk of infection in burn patients protective isolation is required, which includes a high standard of hand hygiene, the wearing of protective clothing and the restriction of the number of visitors.

A thermo-regulated cubicle is required as the child has sustained skin loss and requires an environment that can help keep them warm (especially as their core temperature is raised due to the hypermetabolic response), prevent fluid loss due to evaporation, help reduce hypermetabolism and reduce the risk of infection. This cubicle should ideally be regulated between 28°C and 33°C (Barrow and Herndon 2007). It is worth noting that is important to keep visitors and nursing staff hydrated as they are also in a room with a high temperature.

These patients require the same fundamental nursing care as all patients in PICU, including oral care, catheter care, maintenance of invasive lines and ventilation equipment, normal hygiene needs and play activities. Children with perineal and buttock burns present their own difficulties due to risk of infection. Flamazine® is used in the nappy of younger children, whereas sometimes in the older child it is feasible to use a bowel management system to keep the area free from faecal contamination. Occasionally, an elective bowel stoma may be required.

The child will require pressure area management with specialised pressure-relieving equipment. The position these patients are nursed in is also important, as this may affect their long-term outcome. Children with neck burns should be nursed without a pillow to encourage neck extension. Depending on where the burns are, their head or limbs may need to be elevated. Splints to stop contractures and prevent complications due to immobility of some areas (e.g. hands, feet and axillas) will be required and the appropriate care of these adjuncts is essential. Physiotherapists and occupational therapists have an important role to play in the care of these children.

Due to the inflammatory response following a major burn, patients can become hypercoagulable and be at risk of thrombosis (Barret and Dziewulski 2006), therefore the need for prophylactic anticoagulation therapy should be considered.

Psychosocial needs

Due to both the burn injury and admission to PICU this is an extremely stressful time for the child and their family. In some circumstances due to the nature of the incident there may be more than one family member injured, which has an increased impact on the family. The family may have had to travel to the treatment centre and may need accommodation. The involvement of a family support worker and social worker can be of great benefit.

The family will need explanations about the treatment and plan of care for their child, and may need psychological help in order to cope with their child's altered appearance. The psychological trauma is not just at the time of the accident or the PICU admission; consequently the patient and family may require involvement of the psychologist and family support over a long period, especially after discharge, in order to come to terms with an altered body image and any consequences of the accident. This may include rehousing, claiming financial benefits, help returning to school and reintegrating with their peers. There are various support groups nationwide that can be of benefit, such as Changing Faces (www.changingfaces. org.uk) and the Children's Fire and Burn Trust (www. childrensfireandburntrust.org.uk).

It is also worth remembering that the staff involved in caring for these patients may also need support.

Conclusion

The multidisciplinary teamwork of assessing, planning and providing the total care required for these complex patients is essential to ensure a successful discharge from PICU so that the child and their family can continue their progress and rehabilitation. This team support will continue beyond admission and discharge in order that the child gets back to their pre-hospital life as far as possible.

References

Advanced Trauma Life Support (ATLS). 2008. Student Manual (8th edition). Chicago: American College of Surgeons.

Ahrns K. 2004. Trends in burn resuscitation: shifting the focus from fluids to adequate endpoint monitoring, edema control and adjuvant therapies. Critical Care Nursing Clinics of North America, 16(1):75–98.

Australia and New Zealand Burn Association. 2006. *Emergency Management of Severe Burns*. Hobart, Australia.

Baker R, Akhavani MA, Jallali N. 2007. Resuscitation of thermal injuries in the United Kingdom and Ireland. Journal of Plastic Reconstructive Aesthetic Surgery, 60:682–5.

Barret J, Dziewulski P. 2006. Complications of the hypercoagulable status in burn injury. Burns, 32:1005–8.

Barrow R, Herndon D. 2007. History of treatment of burns. In D Herndon (Ed). Total Burn Care (3rd edition, chapter 1). Philadelphia: Saunders Elsevier.

Beierle E, Chung D. 2007. Surgical management of complications of burn injury. In D Herndon (Ed). Total Burn Care (3rd edition, chapter 38). Philadelphia: Saunders Elsevier.

Berger M, Spertini F et al. 1998. Trace element supplementation modulates pulmonary infection rates after major burns: a double blind, placebo-controled trial. American Journal of Clinical Nutrition, 68(21):365–71.

Chester D, Jose R et al. 2006. Non-accidental burns in children – are we neglecting neglect? Burns, 32:222–8.

Cook D. 2002. Pathophysiology of burns. In C Bosworth Bousfield (Ed). Burn Trauma (2nd edition, chapter 1). Management and Nursing Care. London: Whurr.

Demling R, Orgill D. 2000. The anticatabolic and wound healing effects of the testosterone analog oxandrolone after severe burn injury. Journal of Critical Care, 15(1):12–17.

Duncan R, Dunn K. 2008. Physiological responses to burn injury and resuscitation protocols for adult major burns. In C Stone (Ed). The Evidence for Plastic Surgery (chapter 6). Shrewsbury: tfm Publishing.

Gollop R. 2002. Burns aftercare and scar management. In C Bosworth Bousfield (Ed). Burn Trauma. Management and Nursing Care (2nd edition, chapter 13). London: Whurr.

Hankins C, Tang X, Philips A. 2006. Hot beverage burns: an 11-year experience of the Yorkshire regional burns centre. Burns, 32(1):87–91.

Herndon D (Ed). 2007. Total Burn Care, 3rd edition. Philadelphia: Saunders Elsevier.

Hettiaratchy S, Dziewulski P. 2004. ABC of burns: pathophysiology and types of burns. British Medical Journal, 328:1427–9.

Hettiaratchy S, Papini R. 2004. ABC of burns: initial management of a major burn; II – assessment and resuscitation. British Medical Journal, 329:101–3.

Jackson D. 1953. The diagnosis of the depth of burning. British Journal of Surgery, 40(164):588–96.

Janzekovic Z. 1977. The treatment of burns. Burns, 4:61–6.

Jenkins K, Gottschlich M et al. 1994. Enteral feeding during operative procedures. Journal of Burn Care and Rehabilitation, 15:199–205.

Jeschke M, Finnerty C et al. 2008. Combination of recombinant human growth hormone and propranolol decreases hypermetabolism and inflammation in severely burn children. Pediatric Critical Care Medicine, 9(2):209–16.

Kramer C, Lund T, Beckum O. 2007. Pathophysiology of burn shock and burn edema. In D Herndon (Ed). 2007. Total Burn Care (3rd edition, chapter 8). Philadelphia: Saunders Elsevier.

Lafferty KA. 2010. Smoke Inhalation. emedicine.medscape.com/article/771194-overview.

Latarjet J. 2002. The management of pain associated with dressing changes in patients with burns. World Wide Wounds. European Wound Management Association Journal, 2(2):5–9.

Lee J, Herndon D. 2007. The pediatric burn patient. In D Herndon (Ed). Total Burn Care (3rd edition, chapter 36). Philadelphia: Saunders Elsevier.

Mendham J. 2004. Gabapentin for treating itching produced by burns and wound healing in children: a pilot study. Burns, 30(8):851–3.

Meyer W, Patterson D et al. 2007. Management of pain and other discomforts in burned patients. In D Herndon (Ed). Total Burn Care (3rd edition, chapter 64). Philadelphia: Saunders Elsevier.

National Patient Safety Agency, 2007. Reducing the Risk of Hyponatraemia When Administering Intravenous Infusions to Children. Patient Safety Alert. 2007-03-28 -V1.

Niederbichler A, Jokuszies A et al. 2009. Extracorporeal life support devices (ECMO, ILA) in severely burned patients: Bridging the gap? Burns, 35:S45–S45.

Norbury WB, Herndon D. 2007. Modulation of the hypermetabolic response after burn injury. In D Herndon (Ed). Total Burn Care (3rd edition, chapter 31). Philadelphia: Saunders Elsevier.

Norman L, Anderton D, Hubbard S. 2002. Nutritional care for an individual following burn trauma. In C Bosworth Bousfield (Ed). Burn Trauma. Management and Nursing Care (2nd edition, chapter 10). London: Whurr.

O'Ceallaigh S, Shah M. 2008. Improving outcome in paediatric burns. In C Stone. (Ed). The Evidence for Plastic Surgery (chapter 7). Shrewsbury: tfm Publishing.

Palmieri TL. 2009. Use of β-agonists in inhalation injury. Journal of Burn Care and Research, 30(1):156–9.

Papini R. 2004. ABC of burns: management of burn injuries of various depths. British Medical Journal, 329:158–60.

Patterson D, Sharar S. 2001. Burn pain. In J Loeser (Ed). Bonica's Management of Pain (3rd edition, chapter 42). Philadelphia: Lippincott, Williams and Wilkins.

Perel P, Roberts I. 2007. Colloids versus crystalloids for fluid resuscitation in critically ill patients. Cochrane Database Systemic Reviews, 17(4):CD000567.

Prior K, Nordmann G et al. 2009. Management of inhalational injuries in UK burns centres – a questionnaire survey. Journal of the Intensive Care Society, 10(2):141–4.

Saffle J, Graves C. 2007. Nutritional support of the burn patient. In D Herndon (Ed). Total Burn Care (3rd edition, chapter 30). Philadelphia: Saunders Elsevier.

Sainsbury D. 2008. Critical evaluation of the clinimetrics of laser Doppler imaging in burn assessment. Journal of Wound Care, 17(5):193–200.

Schierhout G, Roberts I. 1998. Fluid resuscitation and colloid or crystalloid solutions in critically ill patients: a systematic review of randomised trials. British Medical Journal, 316(7136):961–4.

Summer GJ, Puntillo KA et al. 2007. Burn injury pain: the continuing challenge. Journal of Pain, 8(7):533–48.

Traber D, Herndon D et al. 2007. The pathophysiology of inhalation injury. In D Herndon (Ed). Total Burn Care (3rd edition, chapter 18). Philadelphia: Saunders Elsevier.

Voruganti V, Klien G et al. 2005. Impaired zinc and copper status in children with burn injuries. Burns, 31(6):711–16.

Wasiak J, Cleland H, Campbell F. 2008. Dressings for superficial and partial thickness burns. Cochrane Database of Systematic Reviews, 4:Art. CD002106. DOI: 10.1002/14651858.CD002106.pub3.

Watret L, Armitage M. 2002. Making sense of wound cleaning. Journal of Community Nursing. 16(4):27–34.

White M, Thornton K, Young A. 2005. Early diagnosis and treatment toxic shock syndrome in paediatric burns. Burns, 31(2):193–7.

Williams C. 2009. Successful assessment and management of burn injuries. Nursing Standard, 23(32):53–62.

Chapter 11
CARE OF THE CHILD WITH CANCER

Karen Selwood, Caroline Langford and Michelle Wright

Oncology Services, Alder Hey Children's Hospital, Royal Liverpool Children's NHS Trust, Liverpool, UK

Introduction

Caring for a child with cancer in an ICU requires an understanding of their underlying diagnosis and treatment, which in turn requires knowledge of associated symptoms, their effects on quality of life and recovery, and causes and implications of symptoms in order to meet the multidimensional needs of the patient (Kaplow 2001).

Children and young people with cancer may require treatment on an ICU at different times in their treatment journey. Paediatric cancer survival rates have increased dramatically over recent years, with 7 out of 10 children now being cured (CCLG 2007). Much of the success of paediatric oncology treatments is related to clinical trials and the development of protocol-driven, randomised controlled trails (CCLG 2007). Treatment protocols have dramatically increased survival rates; however, treatment often involves intensive chemotherapy and stem cell or bone marrow transplants, with children having a greater susceptibility to infection and septicaemia and a greater requirement of intensive care support (Keengwe et al. 1999). However, while advances in oncological care and supportive care have led to improved survival, they may lead to admissions to ICU for postoperative, acute concurrent illness (de Boer et al. 2005) and more commonly in paediatric patients, complications related to cancer therapy

or a diagnosis of cancer itself with its related diagnosis-specific complications. Oncology emergencies can be defined as haematological, structural, metabolic or complications relating to cancer treatment (Higdon and Higdon 2006).

The aim of this chapter is to look at those children admitted to ICU with oncology-related problems. The chapter is divided into sections, with an introduction including an overview of oncological treatments, differences in looking after children with cancer and related issues. Specific problems in which children are admitted to ICU will then be discussed, divided into groups of disease-related complications, treatment-related comorbidities and transplant issues. A brief introduction regarding general side-effects of chemotherapy will also be provided.

Leukaemia remains the most common cancer in children, followed by brain tumours. Table 11.1 describes the majority of paediatric oncology conditions with treatment options and prognosis.

Treatment

Treatment for children with malignancies includes chemotherapy, radiotherapy, surgery, stem cell/bone marrow rescue and transplantation, and novel therapies such as gene

Paediatric Intensive Care Nursing, First Edition. Edited by Michaela Dixon and Doreen Crawford.
© 2012 John Wiley & Sons, Ltd. Published 2012 by John Wiley & Sons, Ltd.

Table 11.1 Paediatric oncology conditions with treatment options and prognosis

Condition	Definition	Treatment	Prognosis
Wilms' tumour	Malignant tumour of the kidney	Combination of chemotherapy, surgery and occasionally radiotherapy (dependent on staging)	Overall survival around 90% depending on staging of disease
Non-Hogkin's lymphoma	Malignancy of lymphoid cells. There are four categories: Burkitt's – 40% Large B-cell – 20% Anaplastic large cell – 10% Lymphoblastic – 30%	Combination of chemotherapy, surgery and occasionally radiotherapy (dependent on staging)	Dependent on type of disease, but all non-Hodgkin's lymphoma survival rates have increased dramatically
Hodgkin's	Malignancy of lymphatic system	Chemotherapy and/or radiotherapy	95–100% cure rate at 5 years
Leukaemia	Malignancy of the blood forming or haematopoietic tissues. There are three categories: Acute lymphoblastic (ALL) Acute myeloid leukaemia Chronic leukaemia	Chemotherapy (ALL) Chemotherapy +/– bone marrow/stem cell transplant (AML) Chemotherapy +/– transplant (relapse ALL) Radiotherapy for leukaemia with central nervous system involvement and conditioning for transplant	ALL 80% event-free survival AML 60% event-free survival
Neuroblastoma	Malignancy derived from nerve cells in the adrenal glands and usually spreading rapidly within the abdomen and body (60% of children have stage 4 disease)	Stage 4 disease includes chemotherapy, radiotherapy, surgery and high-dose chemotherapy with stem cell transplant rescue	Stage 4 disease is associated with significant mortality
Sarcomas	Ewing's sarcoma – sarcoma which can develop in bone and soft tissue (fat or muscle) Osteosarcoma – sarcoma which can develop in any skeletal bone	Chemotherapy, reconstructive limb-salvage surgery or amputation and usually radiotherapy	Prognosis is very much dependent on the presence of metastatic disease, the size of the tumour and histological findings when the tumour has been removed
Central nervous system tumours	Represent 20% of paediatric cancers. Common types include astrocytoma and medulloblastoma, named after type of cell or area they develop in	Surgery, chemotherapy, radiotherapy, or a combination	Dependent on type of tumour. Brain tumours are associated with significant morbidity and mortality
Retinoblastoma	A malignant tumour of the retina	Dependent on size and location, may include enucleation, chemotherapy, laser therapy, cryotherapy, thermotherapy or radiotherapy	Very favourable prognosis

(Continued)

Table 11.1 (*Continued*)

Condition	Definition	Treatment	Prognosis
Soft tissue sarcomas	A group of malignancies including tumours of contractile, connective and supportive tissues Include: rhabdomyosarcoma, non-rhabdomyosarcoma	Chemotherapy, radiotherapy, surgery, usually a combination	Prognosis dependent on site and extent of disease
Hepatoblastoma	Malignant tumour of the liver; of embryological origin	Surgery, chemotherapy and in some cases radiotherapy	80% survival rate for children with a complete surgical resection at diagnosis and adjuvant chemotherapy
Germ cell tumours	Develop from cells that produce sperm or eggs, most common places to develop include the bottom of the spine and brain	Chemotherapy and/or surgery	Dependent on staging

Source: Cancerbacup 2008, 2009; Carli et al. 2004; Colby-Graham and Chordas 2003; Flamant et al. 1998; Hargrave et al. 2004; Kushner and Cheung 2005; Lymphoma Information Network 2007; McDowell, Messahel and Oberlin 2004; Melamud, Palekar, and Singh 2006; Metzger and Dome 2005; Patte 2004; Pearson and Pinkerton 2004; Selwood, Wright and Crawford 2009; Shafford and Pritchard 2004; Smith and Hann 2004; Whelan and Morland 2004.

therapy. Children may receive one or a combination of these treatments dependent on their underlying diagnosis.

Chemotherapy

Chemotherapy is the most common treatment for paediatric malignancies. Cancer is a disease of uncontrolled cell growth. Chemotherapy is a drug which has anti-cancer or cytotoxic (cell-killing) properties and can be given intravenously or orally dependent on the diagnosis and treatment protocol. Chemotherapy kills or damages cells at different stages in the cell cycle, with different chemotherapy effective at different stages. In order to fully understand chemotherapy it is essential to have an understanding of the cell cycle, cell replication and division of the healthy cell and readers are advised to refer to an anatomy and physiology textbook of their choice (Selwood et al. 2009). The side-effects (which may be fatal) are related to the inability of chemotherapy to distinguish between healthy cells and malignant cells, therefore having a systemic effect on the whole body, with damaging effects on all cells in the bone marrow (platelets, red blood cells and white cells).

Radiotherapy

Radiotherapy is often used as a treatment for paediatric malignancies, and can be used individually or with chemotherapy or surgery, dependent on the child's diagnosis and treatment protocol (Hopkins 2008). Radiotherapy is commonly used in the treatment of Ewing's sarcoma, rhabdomyosarcoma, Hodgkin's disease, neuroblastoma, Wilms' tumour and leukaemia with central nervous system involvement (see Table 11.1); however it can also be used for children receiving palliative care to control the symptoms of progressive disease (Hopkins 2008). Radiotherapy works using high-energy rays which kill malignant cells by causing internal damage to the cells' components or molecules (Cancer Research UK 2007). The side-effects are dependent on the area of the body receiving radiotherapy and can be divided into long-term and short-term side-effects. Healthy tissues react differently to radiotherapy dependent on the proliferation rate of the tissue, for example skin, bone marrow and hair follicles proliferate quickly and therefore effects can be seen quickly; organs such as the brain and kidneys proliferate at a slower pace, therefore cellular damage occurs at a later stage (Hopkins and Scott 2008).

Surgery

Surgical treatment of malignancy has changed over the years in paediatric oncology from often being an isolated treatment to now playing an integral part of the overall management of a child with cancer alongside other modes of treatment such as chemotherapy and/or radiotherapy (Hollis et al. 2008). Surgery is commonly used in conjunction with other treatments for osteosarcoma, neuroblastoma, Ewing's sarcoma, hepatoblastoma, Wilms tumour and brain tumours. Children with malignant brain tumours often require surgery initially when they are diagnosed; however other solid tumours such as osteosarcoma and Ewing's sarcoma receive initial chemotherapy in an attempt to reduce the tumour prior to surgery. This also allows assessment to the response of chemotherapy from the histology of the removed tumour (Selwood et al. 2009). Children requiring surgery are usually cared for on a general surgical ward, have a planned intensive care bed and in unusual cases may require an emergency intensive care bed due to the complications of surgery. As a general rule children having surgery are in relatively good condition as bone marrow recovery is often essential prior to surgery, therefore children require the skills of general surgical and intensive care nurses as opposed to the skills of an oncology nurse.

Novel therapies

Novel therapies are emerging in the treatment of paediatric malignancies. These include molecular-targeted therapies, gene therapy and tumour vaccines. Molecular-targeted therapies are the therapy which really seems to be increasing within paediatric oncology and works by inhibiting growth of malignant cells without damaging surrounding healthy cells, which is very encouraging (Selwood et al. 2009).

Bone marrow and stem cell transplantation

Bone marrow and stem cell transplantation is associated with high levels of morbidity for many reasons. Bone marrow or stem cell transplantation involves bone marrow or stem cells from a donor being transplanted by intravenous infusion. Before the recipient receives the transplanted cells they are given high doses of chemotherapy with or without total body irradiation in an attempt to wipe out the immune system and associated disease completely (Selwood et al. 2009). An allogeneic transplant involves receiving a transplant from another source, either a relative or an unrelated donor, dependent on the suitability of the match (Bennett-Rees and Hopkins 2008a; Selwood et al. 2009), and usually occurs in children with high-risk leukaemia, relapsed leukaemia or children with particular haematological conditions (Selwood 2008a).

Autologous transplantation involves cells being harvested from the patient and then reinfused following high doses of myeloablative chemotherapy (Bennett-Rees and Hopkins 2008a). This procedure is often referred to as a stem cell/bone marrow rescue and is predominantly used for children with solid tumours, commonly children with stage 4 neuroblastoma (Selwood 2008a).

The side-effects of a bone marrow/stem cell transplant are severe and life-threatening, due to the nature of high-dose chemotherapy and the prolonged period of neutropenia (Selwood 2008a). Nursing care focuses on prevention of infection, through barrier nursing, mouth care, dietary restrictions, skin care and infection screening (Bennett-Rees and Hopkins 2008c). Stem cell transplantation is associated with high mortality rates, with multiple infectious and non-infectious causes, often requiring support of an ICU (Pene et al. 2006). Children are at high risk of infection due to the prolonged period of neutropenia, veno-occlusive disease as a result of conditioning chemotherapy and other side-effects related to oncological treatments mentioned in this chapter. An allogeneic transplant is often further complicated by the presence of graft-versus-host disease (GVHD) (Pene et al. 2006). GVHD involves the donor's T-cells attacking the recipient's tissues and can be fatal. GVHD can be acute or chronic and can involve many systems in the body including skin, gastrointestinal tract and liver (Bennett-Rees and Hopkins 2008b). GVHD can have a positive effect due to its ability to recognise and eliminate any malignant cells seen; this is known as graft versus leukaemia (Bennett-Rees and Hopkins 2008b). GVHD is common during transplantation and may require further immunosuppressive therapy such as steroids, which in turn increase the risk of mortality (Pene et al. 2006). Although mortality remains high for patients following a bone marrow/stem cell transplant, improvements in supportive care in the ICU have significantly improved the survival of haemato-oncology patients (Naeem et al. 2006).

So, the question remains, are oncology children different from other children who are looked after in the ICU? Immunosuppression is often the most significant difference. Children with cancer who are admitted to the ICU, with the exception of children who have had planned surgery, are often neutropenic and severely immunocompromised following chemotherapy or bone marrow/stem cell harvest. It is important, however, to be aware that although children post-surgery may not be neutropenic at that time, if they have had fairly recent chemotherapy they may still have a degree of immunosuppression.

It is important to remember when looking after a child who is receiving or who has received chemotherapy that as well as the immune system being damaged, the physiological response to infection is not as effective and the physical barriers may be damaged. This damage (e.g. to the skin, gastrointestinal tract, etc.) is often due to side-effects of chemotherapy such as mucositis. The normal responses to infection are not always present as a result of chemotherapy and/or steroids, for example a child may have a serious life-threatening infection without a fever.

Historically, patients with cancer admitted to the ICU were associated with a very high mortality rate. Over recent years, however, there is limited evidence to support such a statement (Farquhar-Smith and Wigmore 2008), particularly in the paediatric population. It has been suggested that the cancer diagnosis itself is not the risk factor in survival, but the acute disturbance in the physiological processes that has a detrimental effect on overall outcome (Farquhar-Smith and Wigmore 2008). Differing risk factors are suggested as being risk factors in oncology patients on the ICU, one of which is mechanical ventilation, which is strongly linked with mortality (Soares et al. 2005). It has been suggested that there is a link between survival of oncology children on the ICU and the use of inotropes, with the amount of inotropes having a negative effect on overall survival (Keengwe et al. 1999). It has also been documented that gram-negative infections, in particular *Pseudomonas* and *Klebsiella*, are linked with high levels of ICU admission and death (Adamski et al. 2008). The major differences in caring for children with a malignancy on the ICU are often related to the treatment the child has received in the past or are currently receiving and the potential side-effects. Side-effects, such as prolonged neutropenia and severe weight loss, have a huge impact on the body's ability to recover from illness and side-effects. Gaining an understanding of chemotherapy and its side-effects will enable the reader to have an awareness of the anticipated problems and predicted side-effects of children with a malignancy.

Literature also suggests that the earlier children are admitted to an ICU the better the survival outcome in critically ill cancer patients (Thiery et al. 2005). Children with a malignancy are looked after in specialised paediatric oncology units, from where children are often moved to ICU late on, due to the specialist care they receive on the oncology unit and as it is often a risk to move such chil-

dren, particular children post-bone marrow or stem cell transplant, being nursed in strict isolation.

It is important to consider that the care of the oncology patient within an ICU environment has the added dimension of the complex ethical issues faced by medical and nursing staff (Collins and Mozdzierz 1996). Nursing staff may struggle with often divergent views and different clinical perspectives, particularly relating to perception of treatment effectiveness and prognosis between intensivists, oncologists and occasionally other specialists (Kaplow 2001).

Conditions related to the disease process

In this section we discuss conditions specifically related to the disease process, at diagnosis, relating to disease progression or as a direct result of initial treatment.

Superior vena cava syndrome

The superior vena cava is a major blood vessel, which drains venous blood from the head, neck, upper extremities and upper thorax, back to the heart (Kallab 2005). Superior vena cava syndrome is an obstruction of venous blood flow though the SVC (Selwood et al. 2009). The majority of cases of SVC syndrome are seen in patients with a malignant disease; in fact up to 90% of cases involve patients with a malignancy (Creel et al. 2008). The frequency of SVC syndrome in the paediatric population is unknown due to the lack of published data; however it is known that cases of the syndrome are caused by central venous catheter thrombosis and more commonly as a direct result of a tumour compressing the SVC (Creel et al. 2008). Tumour compression of the SVC can occur at diagnosis or relapse/disease progression and can be caused by many tumours including T-cell leukaemia (Hon et al. 2005), non-Hodgkin's lymphoma, Hodgkin's lymphoma, chest tumours and any malignant process causing a mediastinal mass (Selwood et al. 2009).

Signs and symptoms are directly related to the increased venous pressure in the upper part of the body (Wilson et al. 2007), resulting in oedema in the upper extremities and face, engorgement of the face, subconjunctival haemorrhage and protruding eyes (Beeson 2007). Oedema leads to compromise of the pharynx or larynx, resulting in a cough, dyspnoea, stridor and dysphagia, with cerebral oedema leading to confusion, headaches and, in some cases, coma (Wilson et al. 2007). Haemodynamic compromise can also occur due to decreased venous return (Wilson et al. 2007). Onset can be insidious but can happen very quickly leading to acute respiratory distress (Selwood et al. 2009), with the most common symptom development being over a two-week period (Wilson et al. 2007).

Diagnosis

Diagnosis can be established through imaging such as chest X-ray or CT scan, however a diagnosis is often established through clinical examination and an accurate history-taking (Haut 2005; Kallab 2005).

Management

Management of SVC syndrome has a two-pronged approach, involving treatment of the malignant condition and managing and relieving the symptoms of the obstruction itself (Wilson et al. 2007). Diagnosing the underlying aetiology of the tumour is essential to ensure appropriate treatment is commenced as quickly as possible (Kennebeck 2005). Adjunctive therapy such as steroids and diuretics are commonly used in relieving the symptoms (Beeson 2007). Steroids are also very effective in reducing tumour burden in patients with non-Hodgkin's lymphoma, and thereby reducing the obstruction (Wilson et al. 2007). The nursing care of a child with SVC syndrome is a challenge (Hon et al. 2005), with children often requiring immediate intubation and ventilation when the syndrome is suspected (Haut 2005). Psychological care is essential in caring for children with SVC syndrome, as the child and family are dealing with an acute, life-threatening episode and trying to deal with the prospect of ongoing cancer treatment, with limited knowledge (Selwood et al. 2009).

Spinal cord compression

Spinal cord compression in children is a medical emergency and a serious complication of a malignant process (Haas 2003). Children with spinal cord compression may be looked after in the intensive care environment and are associated with considerable mortality and morbidity (Joseph and Tayar 2005; Osowski 2002). Spinal cord compression in the paediatric population is usually associated with a variety of malignant diseases at diagnosis, including lymphoma, Ewing's sarcoma, osteosarcoma, leukaemia, neuroblastoma, posterior fossa brain tumours and with metastatic disease (Haut 2005; Selwood 2008b). However, it can also cause problems in the palliative stage of a malignant disease.

Spinal cord compression is a compression of the intrathecal sac caused by a mass in the epidural space (Quinn and DeAngelis 2000). Malignant invasion of the spinal cord can occur at any point along the 26 vertebrae (Flounders and Ott 2003) and can cause irreversible neurological damage if not treated promptly (Selwood 2008b), therefore

imaging is crucial in order to diagnose the condition and ensure speedy and appropriate treatment.

Signs and symptoms

Signs and symptoms are related to the location of tumour and the extent of spinal cord compression (Marrs 2006). Back and neck pain is an early complaint (Slocombe and Boynes 2005), and pain may progress from a discomfort into weakness in limbs, autonomic dysfunction, loss of sensation and occasionally paralysis (Osowski 2002; Selwood 2008b).

Diagnosis

Diagnosis of spinal cord compression involves a thorough physical examination, including a neurological examination, an accurate history and an MRI scan (Kwok et al. 2006).

Management

Options for the treatment of children with spinal cord compression include decompression surgery, radiotherapy and chemotherapy. Dexamethasone is commonly used to reduce swelling and inflammation and therefore giving temporary pressure relief (Haas 2003). Spinal cord compression is one of the few situations in which chemotherapy is administered as an emergency (Selwood 2008b). Radiotherapy is commonly given for spinal cord compression in the palliative stages of care.

As with superior vena cava syndrome it is important when nursing these children to give consideration to psychological care and education, as these children and their families may have to deal with an acute oncological event, as well as the prospect of further treatment and the possibility of long-term neurological problems (Selwood 2008b). Nursing management focuses on assessing ongoing neurological function and pain relief (Flounders and Ott 2003), as well as preventing and treating associated complications such as sensory-motor deficits and immobility (Wilkes 1999).

Tumour lysis syndrome

Children who are most at risk of tumour lysis syndrome (TLS) usually have bulky disease with a large tumour burden (e.g. B-cell or T-cell lymphomas) or have a high white cell count leukaemia. It is sometimes seen in children with solid tumours. TLS can occur before treatment is commenced but is most common 12–72 hours after the initiation of treatment (Rheingold and Lange 2006). TLS consists of several metabolic abnormalities that results from the rapid death of tumour cells and can be fatal. There is a resulting increase in the breakdown products of uric acid, phosphate and potassium, and the symptoms will relate to these changes.

Prevention and early recognition of any problems are vital. An awareness of the children likely to encounter this problem is important with relevant medical personnel involved fully aware of the situation. Aggressive hydration, without added potassium, at $3 \, l/m^2$ of the body surface area should be started before treatment is commenced and during initial chemotherapy. A renal ultrasound performed before treatment is commenced will also establish whether there are any abnormalities that may compromise renal function. Frequent observation of the renal function should be undertaken for early recognition of abnormalities followed by prompt treatment, which may be needed 4–6 hourly. An accurate fluid balance, twice daily weights and 4-hourly blood pressures also help assess and highlight any potential problems promptly. Although rare, leukapheresis has been performed to reduce really high white cell counts before treatment is commenced (Porcu et al. 2000).

There are two medications that are used to help promote the breakdown of uric acid: allopurinol and recombinant urate oxidase. Allopurinol is administered orally and works by inhibiting the enzyme xanthine oxidase which is necessary for the production of uric acid. It does not reduce any uric acid that is already present (Jeha 2001). Recombinant urate oxidase is administered intravenously and works by catalysing the conversion of uric acid into allatonin, which is more easily excreted in the urine with less potential for precipitation (Jeha 2001). Any blood samples of children who are on recombinant urate oxidase need to be put on ice immediately because if they are transported at room temperature the uric acid in the sample degrades and the results will give a false low (Lim et al. 2003). Allopurinol is used routinely in all children who have a risk of TLS, whereas recombinant urate acid tends to be used in children who present with a large tumour burden or high white cell count or with a uric acid that is increasing throughout treatment.

Even if these steps are taken, some children will end up with metabolic abnormalities that will need treatment. Some will develop renal failure that will require haemodialysis to help reduce the plasma uric acid, high levels of potassium and high phosphate. Hyperkalaemia will need to be corrected by decreasing potassium intake, facilitating the shift of extracellular potassium and excretion. Correction of the hyperphosphataemia should increase the low calcium that occurs when phosphate is high. Successful management of the child with TLS relates to recognition of those at risk, prevention and early recognition of any

abnormalities. Most of these children will be diagnosed and treated in the oncology unit, but some may present straight to intensive care for management.

Other issues where children who require specialist input may present in ITU

There are many malignancies which may present in an ICU, in particular malignancies that present with a mediastinal mass, such as lymphoma. Often such children require intubation and ventilation and may require procedures such as chest drains. Treatment is a two-way approach: treating the current symptoms and establishing a diagnosis so effective treatment of the malignancy can commence.

Side-effects of chemotherapy

Chemotherapy affects the malignant cells but can also damage any rapidly dividing cells in the body. This can lead to significant side-effects which can range from mild to life-threatening. Some of the side-effects that may be seen in the intensive care environment are discussed here. It should be noted that these children can have multiple side-effects and this should be considered when nursing them.

Bone marrow suppression

The majority of chemotherapy agents cause some form of bone marrow suppression leading to three main problems seen in the oncology patient: anaemia, thrombocytopenia and neutropenia. These are commonly seen 7–14 days post-chemotherapy.

Anaemia

This is a deficiency of red blood cells or haemoglobin (Hb) leading to a decrease in the oxygen-carrying capacity of the blood (Hastings et al. 2006). It can lead to breathlessness, pallor, headaches, loss of appetite, dizziness, fatigue and irritability. Transfusion is usually performed when the child is symptomatic of anaemia or may be considered when the Hb falls below 7–8 g/dl. However, there is no consensus on the level that the Hb can fall to before transfusion is indicated; this will depend on local practice.

Thrombocytopenia

This is a result of a fall in the circulating platelets resulting in bleeding, purpura or petechiae (Selwood 2008a). Often the management of thrombocytopenia is conservative, although this will vary with local practice. Platelets are usually transfused when a patient is symptomatic or about to undergo an invasive procedure although they may be given if the platelet count is less than 10×10^9l. Pre-procedure (e.g. a lumbar puncture), platelets may be transfused to ensure there are enough platelets circulating. If a child has a fever, infection or enlarged liver, their effectiveness may be decreased and more platelet transfusions may be required (British Committee for Standards in Haematology 2003).

There is a risk with administering blood products, including adverse reactions and the potential for infection, and these will need to be considered as with any patients. Cytomegalovirus (CMV) carries a significant risk of morbidity and mortality in the immunocompromised patient. This has been reduced since the induction of leukodepleted blood products although most oncology patients will still receive CMV-negative blood products. Irradiated blood products are required for patients immediately pre- and post-stem cell transplantation, patients with Hodgkin's disease and patients who have received treatment with a purine analogue (e.g. fludarabine). Irradiation destroys the ability of transfused lymphocytes to respond to host foreign antigens thereby preventing graft versus host disease in these patients (BCSH Blood Transfusion Task Force 1996).

Neutropenia

The definition of neutropenia differs between hospitals but is commonly referred to as an absolute neutrophil count of $<0.5 \times 10^9$l (normal $2.5–7.5 \times 10^9$l). This is a common complication of cytotoxic chemotherapy and can occur 7–10 days post-treatment and usually recovers by 21 days. There is a significant risk of morbidity and mortality associated with the risk of life-threatening infections and it also leads to delays in chemotherapy. Children should attend for assessment if they have a temperature of 38.5°C or two recordings of 38°C 1 hour apart as temperatures are often the only symptom that there is an infective process taking place. All other inflammatory processes are altered in the immunocompromised child and may not show any signs of infection. On arrival the child should be treated as an oncological emergency and should commence broad spectrum antibiotics within 30–60 minutes once a full assessment has taken place otherwise there is an increased risk of mortality or morbidity (Pizzo 1999).

Immunocompromised children are at risk from both gram-negative and gram-positive sepsis. Gram-negative sepsis (*Escherichia coli*, *Pseudomonas aeruginosa* and *Klebsiella*) used to be the most common organisms seen. Now gram-positive sepsis is more common, mainly caused by the endogenous flora of the patient (e.g. coagulase-negative staphylococci and streptococci) (Oren et al. 2001).

There is a risk of fungal infections in the immunocompromised child and this can also be life-threatening. Children with prolonged neutropenia are at greater risk of invasive fungal infections (Lehrnbecher et al. 1999) and breaches of mucosa which coexist with neutropenia allow a portal for infection into the body. Prolonged use of antibiotics and steroids is an additional risk factor. Antifungal treatment is often given to children who are recognised to be at risk at prophylactic doses. These are then increased to treatment dose as the child presents with an infection.

The majority of these children are managed successfully within the oncology unit; however when the patient has systemic sepsis with evidence of circulatory insufficiency and inadequate tissue perfusion leading to shock, intensive care will be required (Tan 2002). These children can present to the oncology unit in a collapsed state or deteriorate within the unit. There should be some consideration as to where these children are nursed within the intensive care environment; ideally, a single room should be available although the most important aspect of preventing pathogens is washing of hands.

The use of granulocyte colony-stimulating factor (GCSF) is not used routinely to decrease the incidence of febrile neutropenia. Some of the more intensive protocols recommend its use; otherwise it is used when patients have prolonged neutropenia or are unwell.

Gastrointestinal problems

As chemotherapy affects all the rapidly dividing cells, many gastrointestinal problems can occur, most commonly 7–10 days post-chemotherapy and last until the neutrophil count recovers, usually about day 21. Increased risk is due to opportunistic infections that may involve the gastrointestinal tract.

Mucositis

The endothelial cells of the mouth, oropharynx and gut as a whole can be affected by chemotherapy. This can lead to a sore, inflamed mouth and as the mucosa becomes broken there is a risk of infection translocating into the blood stream, leading to a systemic infection (Brown and Wingard 2004).

Signs and symptoms of mucositis

- Pain.
- Inflammation.
- Ulceration.
- Dry mouth.
- Dry, cracked lips.
- Bleeding.

Management

Prevention is the ideal, but is not always possible. Children and families are educated to clean their teeth with a soft toothbrush and fluoride toothpaste at least twice a day (Glenny 2006). This should continue if the child is hospitalised, however if the mouth is painful, adequate analgesia will be required before it can be achieved. Analgesia can be a combination of topical and systemic relief depending on the severity of pain and the age of the child. Often the hospitalised child will require intravenous opioid infusions to achieve adequate pain control and subsequently allow them to clean the oral cavity and maintain some form of nutrition. The oral cavity should be assessed at least daily. Gibson and Nelson (2000) adapted a guide developed by Eilers et al. (1988) for use in children with an algorithm of care; ideally a national tool and algorithm would be beneficial.

Nausea and vomiting

Nausea and vomiting are distressing side-effects of chemotherapy. Some chemotherapy drugs are more emetic than others. It can occur at any time but is more common during treatment, although some children may experience prolonged vomiting. This may be exacerbated by aversions to food or smells and contribute to poor nutrition. The symptoms can generally be controlled with antiemetic drugs which should be commenced prior to treatment and continued throughout the chemotherapy and for several days post-treatment. The drugs administered generally depend on the emetic potential of the treatment and most units will have some form of algorithm to follow. As well as considering drugs to control nausea and vomiting, non-pharmacological methods may be required (Dibble et al. 2007).

Diarrhoea

Diarrhoea is an abnormal increase in stool liquidity caused by impairment of absorption, secretion and rapid movement through the gut (Hogan 1998). It may be due to anxiety, altered diet, the use of nutritional supplements, medication, infection and chemotherapy and can lead to dehydration, electrolyte imbalances and general debility (Hogan 1998). It is important to try to establish the primary cause and treat this if possible. Once infective causes have been eliminated one of the opioid-receptor agonists (e.g. loperamide) may be used to reduce peristalsis of the gut (Wadler et al. 1998). Regular observation of the anal area is vital to recognise excoriation and inflammation and ensure prompt treatment.

Constipation

Constipation is a decrease in the frequency of or passing hard stools. It can occur in the immunocompromised child due to chemotherapy, opioid analgesia, intestinal obstruction and poor diet (Smith 2001). Prevention should be the main aim with adequate fluids and diet, although these children may not often feel like eating. Regular assessment of bowel action is vital and if the child has not opened their bowels, action should be taken, usually in the form of stool softeners or laxatives. Occasionally, suppositories and enemas are required but these should be used with caution as there is risk of trauma to the anal area leading to infection, bleeding and anal fissures.

Nutrition

Weight loss is common in immunocompromised children and can occur at any time. Poor nutrition has a poor prognostic effect, as children who are well nourished are better able to resist infection and tolerate treatment (Den Broeder et al. 2000). There are a number of contributory factors, including nausea and vomiting, taste changes, mucositis, diarrhoea and constipation. It is important to assess nutrition; however there is not an established tool available for this at present. Weight is important and should be performed on each admission to look at the trend. Nutritional advice should include recommendations of good diet and appropriate nutritional supplements. This can be difficult and may turn into a battle between the child and parents.

If extra nutrition is required, then enteral feeding (via a nasogastric tube or PEG tube) should be considered initially if the child has a functioning gut as this is often successful (Den Broeder et al. 2000). If the gut is not functioning or there is ongoing weight loss, then parenteral nutrition should be considered (Lowis et al. 2004).

Neutropenic enterocolitis

Neutropenic enterocolitis (typhlitis) is a transmural inflammation with variable degrees of necrosis and infection of the colon, especially the caecum (Haut 2005). The organisms commonly involved are anaerobes and gram-negative bacilli (Walsh et al. 2006). Bacterial flora, neutropenia and chemotherapy contribute, causing multifactorial disruption of the mucosal barrier. Infection may lead to ischaemia, progressing to necrosis and perforation of the bowel wall. These conditions are associated with a high mortality rate (50–100%) (Shamberger et al. 1986).

Signs and symptoms

Signs and symptoms include fever, acute abdominal pain (usually in the right lower abdominal quadrant) and abdominal distension. The child may also experience diarrhoea. In more severe cases the bowel may perforate, which may manifest as hypovolaemia or septic shock (Haut 2008).

Diagnosis

Diagnosis is usually by radiological examination. A CT scan is preferred, although ultrasound scans are often easier to obtain. They both identify ileal and caecal colonic wall-thickening and inflammatory changes (Haut 2008).

Management

Management is usually conservative and includes resting the bowel, broad spectrum antibiotics, including an antibiotic against anaerobes (e.g. metronidazole), analgesia and nutritional support in the form of total parenteral nutrition. Surgical intervention usually occurs if the bowel perforates or there is general deterioration of the child (Jain et al. 2000). GCSF may be used to help stimulate recovery of the neutrophils to aid recovery as survival of these patients has been attributed to neutrophil recovery (Wade et al. 1992).

Potential surgical problems – bowel obstruction

The commonest complaints among patients with cancer are related to the gastrointestinal system, with 40% of patients complaining of abdominal pain (Ilgen and Marr 2009). Presentations of abdominal pain vary and can stem from the underlying malignancy and/or treatment, to the full range of pathologies seen in the healthy population (Ilgen and Marr 2009). It is estimated that 30% of infectious complications arise from the gastrointestinal tract, with subsequent abdominal complications requiring surgical intervention (Koretz and Neifeld 1985). Appendicitis and neutropenic colitis are the most common surgical complications noted in children with leukaemia (Sherman et al. 1973). Right lower quadrant intra-abdominal pathological processes are of particular concern, and the differential diagnosis of abdominal pain in the paediatric patient with cancer includes acute appendicitis, typhlitis, intussusception and obstructive ileus (Schlatter et al. 2002).

Tumours of the gastrointestinal tract are extremely rare in paediatric patients, estimated at <5% of all neoplasms (Ladd and Grosfeld 2006). The most common malignancy of the gastrointestinal tract in children is non-Hodgkin's lymphoma. Clinical presentation can vary from an abdominal mass to more urgent signs of intestinal obstruction with bilious vomiting or abdominal pain from perforation (Bethel et al. 1997; Skinner et al. 1994). Children with Burkitt's lymphoma may present with intussusception.

These patients tend to be older than general paediatric patients with this condition. Intestinal obstruction may result from either direct compression of the lumen by an expanding mass or by the intraluminal projection of a small tumour mass (Magrath 1997). The malnourished state of many of these patients has been associated with poor outcomes and perforations (Rivera-Luna et al. 1987).

It is recognised that presentation and clinical findings may be altered in a child with abdominal pain and an underlying haematological malignancy. Neutropenia and multiple medications can cause an altered inflammatory response, meaning infectious complications often present atypically posing a diagnostic challenge for clinicians (Sternberg 1999). Chemotherapeutic agents, particularly corticosteroids, frequently mask blunt signs and symptoms such as abdominal tenderness and peritoneal irritation (Exelby et al. 1975). It may be difficult for the clinician to differentiate between an acute abdominal condition and the physiological alterations brought about by neutropenia and chemotherapy toxicity. Misdiagnosis has serious implications in terms of treatment where the adverse effects of chemotherapy should be managed medically as opposed to an acute abdominal condition, which may require surgical intervention. In addition, early diagnosis in the paediatric oncology patient is paramount to avoid systemic infectious complications that result from delayed diagnosis (Hobson et al. 2005). A documented mortality rate approaching 40% is associated with undiagnosed intra-abdominal pathology leading to gram-negative sepsis (Singer 1977).

Improvement in outcome is multifactorial and can be attributed to improved supportive care such as antibiotics, availability of blood products and enhanced anaesthetic and critical care (Chirletti et al. 1993).

Chemotherapy-induced intestinal perforation after treatment is a recognised complication. However, differentiating the symptoms of pain owing to perforation and pain secondary to chemotherapy-induced mucositis can be challenging. Not surprisingly, bowel perforations in paediatric oncology patients are associated with high mortality rates likely resulting from spillage of gastric contents in an immunocompromised patient (Baildam et al. 1989).

Children with cancer who suffer intestinal necrosis or perforation often require surgery. There may be reluctance to perform an intestinal anastomosis due to the risk of leakage or sepsis. Intestinal stoma may prove the best option. Surgery in these patients is associated with considerable morbidity and mortality (Rokhsar et al. 1999). Because immunosuppressed patients have abnormalities in the number or function of circulating neutrophils, platelets and coagulation factors, they are susceptible to wound

Table 11.2 GI complications – causative factors

Gastric haemorrhage	Steroids
Typhlitis	Neutropenia
Perirectal abscess	Prolonged neutropenia
Pancreatitis	Asparaginase

infections and bleeding after abdominal surgery. If, following a gastrointestinal complication, an intestinal stoma is required, it is likely an immunocompromised child will require the stoma for a longer duration than a typical paediatric patient with a stoma. Stoma closure is normally delayed until completion of chemotherapy due to increased infection risks and poorer healing conditions.

Other complications and likely causative factors are illustrated in Table 11.2.

A multidisciplinary approach among surgeons, oncologists and intensivists is fundamental in developing individualised treatment plans that address the many complex challenges.

Neurological insult

Paediatric oncology patients are prone to central nervous system (CNS) complications due to many factors including the disease itself, or metastases, deranged blood counts, toxicity from treatment or dysfunction from failure of other organ systems.

These patients usually present with acute or subacute neurological symptoms of differing severity, ranging from mild neurological deficit to seizure or coma. Many of these neurological complications are exclusive to children with malignant conditions.

Brain tumours are one of the most common solid tumours in children, with an incidence of approximately 1–5/100 000 (Walker et al. 1985). In the United Kingdom, approximately 350 cases are diagnosed annually in 0–15 year olds (Pizer and May 1997). Presentation is usually with signs and symptoms of raised intracranial pressure with or without evidence of cranial nerve dysfunction (Pizer and May 1997). When epilepsy is associated with brain tumours, the cause may be tumour-related or treatment-related. However, seizures are an uncommon presentation of brain tumours in children, occurring in approximately 10% of cases.

Mental status changes, from somnolence or delirium to coma, are second only to headache as the most frequent reason for a neurological consultation in children with cancer (Antunes and De Angelis 1999). The potential seri-

ousness of the underlying cause and the difficulty in defining the origin in these severely ill children explain the high number of neurological consultations. It can be difficult to differentiate a structural from a toxic origin in patients prone to developing intracranial mass lesions but who are also treated with drugs causing decreased alertness or metabolic imbalances.

The main causes of cerebrovascular accidents (CVA) are intracranial bleeding resulting from thrombocytopenia and cerebral infarction, often secondary to infection, commonly aspergillosis. Management is similar to that of patients without a malignancy. Importance should be placed on the correction of any thrombocytopenia or coagulopathy, and infectious sources should be ruled out or treated. Mortality following the development of CVA in bone marrow recipients has been shown to be approximately 69%, irrespective of age, diagnosis, type of transplant and time of presentation (Coplin et al. 2001).

Newly diagnosed oncology patients may also need intensive care treatment due to neurological symptoms secondary to hyperleucocytosis. This can occur when the patient's total white cell count exceeds 100 000 mm³, leading to increased blood viscosity and emboli in the circulation, causing intracranial haemorrhage or thrombosis. Treatment will include intensive support while correcting blood abnormalities via blood products and cytotoxic agents.

Thrombosis is a significant problem in patients with cancer. Use of new agents and aggressive therapy for cancer is associated with an increase in their occurrence (Bick 2003).

Haemorrhagic stroke accounts for approximately half of strokes in childhood. With an incidence of 2–3/100 000 children, stroke is among the top 10 causes of death in childhood (Lynch et al. 2002) and is as common as brain tumours in children.

Haematological abnormalities are reported to be the major risk factor in 10–30% of haemorrhagic stroke (Blom et al. 2003). Therefore, paediatric oncology patients fall into this at-risk group, as the treatment they receive will undoubtedly cause haematological abnormalities.

Cytotoxic treatment within paediatric oncology protocols can cause neurological side-effects. Asparaginase, used to treat acute leukaemia, has a known risk for CVAs. It causes deficiencies in plasma haemostatic proteins and fibrinogen factors (Priest et al. 1982), leading to thrombosis (Feinberg and Swenson 1988). Hypertensive encephalopathy is another side-effect experienced in children receiving steroids or ciclosporin A for their condition (Schwartz et al. 1995). Methotrexate, an antifolate cytotoxic agent, is widely used to treat various forms of childhood cancer. Neurotoxicity is a well-recognised complication of the therapy (Bleyer et al. 1973). Maytal and colleagues (1995) reported a significant risk of acute symptomatic seizures in patients with leukaemia which are most frequently related to side-effects of intrathecal methotrexate or L-asparaginase treatment.

Cranial irradiation is known to cause neurological damage. With the use of higher doses of irradiation, plus combined treatment with chemotherapy, the survival from childhood cancers has improved, however toxicity to normal brain tissue has also increased.

Lumbar puncture for analysis and treatment of cerebrospinal fluid (CSF) is a frequent procedure in the management of paediatric oncology patients. Prophylactic platelet and/or fresh frozen plasma (FFP) transfusions may be given beforehand if required as these patients will commonly have coagulopathy. Despite this, extradural haematoma can occasionally occur as a complication after a lumbar puncture.

Infectious complications are one of the most significant causes of morbidity and death in the paediatric cancer patient (Brown 1984). Infection of the brain sometimes occurs from a pulmonary focus or direct extension through the walls of the paranasal sinuses to involve the brain (Epstein et al. 1991). Brain abscesses in paediatric patients are uncommon with the exception of children with cancer, who are particularly susceptible because of the underlying malignancy and the immunosuppressive effect of treatment. Fungi are the major causative organisms of brain abscesses in immunosuppressed cancer patients.

Viral pathogens account for the greatest portion of infections in children in remission (Kosmidis et al. 1980). Varicella zoster virus, cytomegalovirus, herpes simplex virus and measles virus are the most frequently encountered viral pathogens.

Kuskonmaz and colleagues (2006) looked at neurological complications in paediatric acute lymphoblastic leukaemia patients (excluding leukaemic infiltration) and found that the most common complication was meningitis, which developed in 25% of episodes, generally caused by iatrogenic infection. About 20% of the children with leukaemia have been reported to develop treatment-related abnormalities detectable by MRI (Lo Nigro et al. 2000). The differential diagnosis of the neurological complications related to chemotherapy and other neurological complications of cancer is often difficult and it may be impossible to identify precisely which of the chemotherapeutic agents is responsible for the adverse neurotoxicity (Ray et al. 2002).

To conclude, paediatric oncology patients are prone to neurological complications which can require intensive care and support. Such patients should be treated with a high index of clinical suspicion when they present with even subtle acute neurological symptoms.

Liver

Sinusoidal obstructive syndrome

Sinusoidal obstructive syndrome (SOS) (also known as veno-occlusive disease) is characterised by obstruction of small intrahepatic venules (Miano et al. 2008). The incidence is reported at 27–40% and is most common following haematopoietic stem cell transplant but can occur in other patients, especially those who have had actinomycin or 6-thioguanine chemotherapy. The more severe cases are associated with a significant morbidity and mortality.

Signs and symptoms
- Enlarged liver.
- Ascites.
- Jaundice.
- Right upper quadrant pain.
- Weight gain with fluid retention (Rheingold and Lange 2006).

It may also be associated with multi-organ failure.

Diagnosis

Diagnosis is usually made clinically. The serum bilirubin is elevated, as are the enzymes ALT and AST. They may also have refractory thrombocytopenia, low albumin and clotting abnormalities. A Doppler ultrasound of the liver may show occlusion of the blood vessels and reversal of blood flow, but the findings are not always consistent (Veys and Rao 2004).

Management

Prevention is the ideal. The use of oral ursodeoxycholic acid, which is thought to work by making endogenous bile acids more hydrophilic thereby decreasing proinflammatory cytokine production, is often used, although it is only available as an oral preparation which may make compliance difficult, especially if the child has nausea or a sore mouth (Eisenberg 2008).

IV defibrotide can also be used prophylactically but is also used to treat SOS. It has an antithrombolytic, anti-ischemic and anti-inflammatory action but does not have an immediate effect, therefore supportive care is vital. This includes restricting fluids to prevent third spacing and maximise renal perfusion and administration of diuretics to relieve ascites (Bennett-Rees and Hopkins 2008b).

Occasionally, abdominal paracentesis may be required to relieve any respiratory distress. From a nursing perspective an accurate fluid balance and twice daily weights are an important aspect of care of these children as they can influence daily management.

Cardiac

The anthracycline chemotherapy drugs can cause cardiac problems and it is usually dose-related, however some children develop problems after very little treatment. These can be immediate, with acute arrhythmias, conduction abnormalities and decreased left ventricular function, however most are long-term and commence after treatment has been completed. Regular echocardiograms detect any abnormalities with the ejection fraction, although the child may also present with symptoms of cardiac failure.

Renal

Renal function can be affected by chemotherapy drugs, especially cisplatin, methotrexate and ifosfamide. Observation of renal function is vital, including assessment of glomerular filtration rate (GFR), and subsequent chemotherapy doses may need to be reduced if abnormal. This will also impact on the doses of other renal toxic medication (e.g. gentamicin).

Respiratory

Respiratory problems can be related to chemotherapy regimens, including bleomycin, methotrexate, cyclophosphamide and lomustine, although bleomycin is the most common cause, especially if given with radiotherapy (Limper 2004). They can lead to fibrosis of the lungs. A child that has received bleomycin and radiotherapy may also have problems with anaesthetics.

Pneumocystis carinii is a fungal infection that can become an opportunistic infection in the immunocompromised child. Prevention is the aim, with the use of prophylactic co-trimoxazole. Children present with this infection in a subtle manner with pyrexia, dyspnoea and a nonproductive cough. The chest X-ray has a typical ground glass appearance (Bastow 2000).

Management

This is initially high-dose co-trimoxazole and high-dose steroids. Often other antibiotics or antifungals are administered until a definite diagnosis is obtained. These children may deteriorate quickly and require respiratory support in the ICU environment.

Skin

The child may have problems with the skin following chemotherapy, especially high-dose cytarabine. This can cause rashes which can lead to irritation and blistering. Ensuring the skin is kept well moisturised is important and that any changes are acted upon. It is also important to assess the integrity of the skin when the child is in with a neutropenic episode as a broken area may be a portal for infection and should be monitored.

Hearing

Children receiving cisplatin and carboplatin are at risk of hearing loss. This can be severe and irreversible (Bertolini et al. 2004). Antibiotics (e.g. gentamicin) can also be ototoxic and should be used with caution.

Viral infections

Viral infections can be fatal to the immunocompromised child.

Varicella

This can be a problem as it can disseminate to the lungs, brain, liver and skin (Rogers 1995). Any child that has been exposed to varicella and does not have antibodies against it should receive prophylactic oral acyclovir or receive passive immunisation with varicella zoster immune globulin (VZIG). If the child develops chickenpox, they should be treated with IV acyclovir and nursed in isolation.

Measles

Measles in the immunocompromised child can lead to pneumonia and encephalitis. If a child has had contact with measles then they should receive passive immunisation with human immunoglobulin (HIG) and if given within 72 hours the virus can be prevented from infecting the patient (Stalkup 2002).

References

Adamski J, Steggall M et al. 2008. Outcome of gram negative infection in immunocompromised children. Pediatric Blood and Cancer, 51(4):499–503.

Antunes NL, De Angelis LM. 1999. Neurologic consultations in children with systemic cancer. Cited in NL Antunes. 2002. Mental status changes in children with systemic cancer. Pediatric Neurology, 27:39–42.

Baildam AD, Williams GT et al. 1989. Abdominal lymphoma – the place for surgery. Cited in SR Goldberg, K Godder, DA Lanning. 2007. Successful treatment of a bowel perforation after chemotherapy for Burkitt lymphoma. Journal of Pediatric Surgery, 42:E1–E3.

Bastow V. 2000. Identifying and treating PCP. Nursing Times, 96(37):19–20.

BCSH Blood Transfusion Task Force. 1996. Guidelines on gamma irradiation of blood components for the prevention of transfusion-associated graft-versus-host disease. BCSH Blood Transfusion Task Force, 6(3):261–71.

Beeson MS. 2007. Superior Vena Cava Syndrome. www.emedicine.com/emerg/topic651.htm.

Bennett-Rees N, Hopkins S. 2008a. Background to the haematopoietic stem cell transplantation. In F Gibson, L Soanes (Eds). Cancer in Children and Young People (pp. 97–106). London: John Wiley & Sons.

Bennett-Rees N, Hopkins S. 2008b. Complications of stem cell transplantation. In F Gibson, L Soanes (Eds). Cancer in Children and Young People (pp. 143–62). London: John Wiley & Sons.

Bennett-Rees N, Hopkins S. 2008c. Protective isolation. Nursing issues. In F Gibson, L Soanes (Eds). Cancer in Children and Young People (pp. 135–42). London: John Wiley & Sons.

Bertolini P, Lassalle M et al. 2004. Platinum compound-related ototoxicity in children: long-term follow-up reveals continuous worsening of hearing loss. Journal of Pediatric Hematology/Oncology, 26(10):649–55.

Bethel CAI, Bhattacharyya N, et al. 1997. Alimentary tract malignancies in children. Cited in AP Ladd, JL Grosfeld. 2006. Gastrointestinal tumors in children and adolescents. Seminars in Pediatric Surgery, 15:37–47.

Bick RL. 2003. Cancer-associated thrombosis. Cited in JT Wiernikowski, UH Athale. 2006. Thromboembolic complications in children with cancer. Thrombosis Research, 118: 137–52.

Bleyer WA, Drake JC, Chabner BA. 1973. Neurotoxicity and elevated cerebrospinal-fluid methotrexate concentration in meningeal leukaemia. Cited in WCW Chu, V Lee et al. 2003. Imaging findings of paediatric oncology patients presenting with acute neurological symptoms. Clinical Radiology, 58:589–603.

Blom I, De Schryver EL et al. 2003. Prognosis of haemorrhagic stroke in childhood: a long-term follow-up study. Cited in LC Jordan, AE Hillis. 2007. Hemorrhagic stroke in children. Pediatric Neurology, 36:73–80.

British Committee for Standards in Haematology. 2003. Guidelines for the use of platelet transfusion. British Journal of Haematology, 122(1):10–23.

Brown AE 1984. Neutropenia, fever and infection. Cited in WC Chu, V Lee et al. 2003. Imaging findings of paediatric oncology patients presenting with acute neurological symptoms. Clinical Radiology, 58:589–603.

Brown CG, Wingard J. 2004. Clinical consequences of oral mucositis. Seminars in Oncology Nursing, 20(1):16–21.

Cancerbacup. 2008. Ewing's Sarcoma in Children. www.cclg.org.uk/search/index.php?zoom_sort=0&zoom_query=bone+tumours&zoom_per_page=10&zoom_and=1&zoom_cat%5B%5D=-1.

Cancerbacup. 2009. Germ Cell Tumours in Children. www.cancerbackup.org.uk/Cancertype/Childrenscancers/Typesofchildrenscancers/Germcelltumours

Cancer Research UK. 2007. info.cancerresearchuk.org/cancerandresearch/learnaboutcancer/treatment/radiotherapy.

Carli M, Cecchetto G, et al. 2004. Soft tissue sarcomas. In R Pinkerton, PN Plowman, R Pieter. Paediatric Oncology (3rd edition, pp. 339–71). London: Arnold.

CCLG (Children's Cancer and Leukaemia Group). 2007. www.cclg.org.uk.

Chirletti P, Barillani P, et al. 1993. The surgical choice in neutropenic patients with haematological disorders and acute abdominal complications. Cited in MJ Hobson, DE Carney et al. 2005. Appendicitis in childhood hematologic malignancies: analysis and comparison with typhlitis. Journal of Pediatric Surgery, 40:214–20.

Colby-Graham MF, Chordas C. 2003. The childhood leukemias. Journal of Pediatric Nursing, 18(2):87–95.

Collins E, Mozdzierz G. 1996. Ethical considerations in treating oncology patients in the intensive care unit. Critical Care Nursing Quarterly, 18(4):44–53.

Coplin WM, Cochran MS et al. 2001. Stroke after bone marrow transplantation: frequency, aetiology and outcome. Cited in H Pawson, A Jayaweera, T Wigmore. 2008. Intensive care management of patients following haematopoietic stem cell transplantation. Current Anaesthesia and Critical Care, 19:80–90.

Creel AM, Crawford D, Prabhakaran P. 2008. Anaphylaxis and superior vena cava thrombus in a pediatric patient with acute lymphoblastic leukemia. Pediatric Emergency Care, 24(11):771–3.

De Boer S, de Keizer NF, de Jonge E. 2005. Performance of prognostic models in critically ill cancer patients – a review. Critical Care, 9:458–63.

Den Broeder E, Lippins RJJ et al. 2000. Association between the change in nutritional status in response to tube feeding and the occurrence of infections in children with solid tumour. Pediatric Hematology Oncology, 17(7):567–75.

Dibble SL, Luce J et al. 2007. Acupressure for chemotherapy-induced nausea and vomiting: a randomized clinical trial. Oncology Nurses Forum, 34(4):813–20.

Eilers J, Berger AM, Petersen MC.1988. Development, testing, and application of the oral assessment guide. Oncology Nursing Forum, 15(3):325–30.

Eisenberg S. 2008. Hepatic sinusoidal obstruction syndrome in patients undergoing haematopoietic stem cell transplant. Oncology Nursing Forum, 35(3):385–97.

Epstein NE, Hollingsworth R et al. 1991. Fungal brain abscesses: aspergillosis/Mucormycosis in two immunosuppressed patients. Cited in WCW Chu, V Lee et al. 2003. Imaging findings of paediatric oncology patients presenting with acute neurological symptoms. Clinical Radiology, 58:589–603.

Exelby PR, Ghandchi A et al. 1975. Management of the acute abdomen in children with leukaemia. Cited in MJ Hobson,

DE Carney et al. 2005. Appendicitis in childhood hematologic malignancies: analysis and comparison with typhlitis. Journal of Pediatric Surgery, 40:214–20.

Farquhar-Smith WP, Wigmore T. 2008. Outcomes for cancer patients in critical care. Current Anaesthesia and Critical Care, 19:91–5.

Feinberg WM, Swenson MR.1988. Cerebrovascular complications of L-asparaginase therapy. Cited in WCW Chu, V Lee et al. 2003. Imaging findings of paediatric oncology patients presenting with acute neurological symptoms. Clinical Radiology, 58:589–603.

Flamant F, Rodary C. et al. 1998. Treatment of non-metastatic rhabdomyosarcomas in childhood and adolescence. Results of the second study of the International Society of Paediatric Oncology: MMT84. European Journal of Cancer, 34(7): 1050–62.

Flounders JA, Ott BB. 2003. Oncology emergency modules: spinal cord compression. Oncology Nursing Forum, 30(1). C:DOCUME~1\PKarmaz\LOCALS~1\Temp\K1DGK7R3. htm.

Gibson F, Nelson W. 2000. Mouth care for children with cancer. Paediatric Nursing, 12(1):18–22.

Glenny A. 2006. *Mouth Care for Children and Young People with Cancer: Evidence-based Guidelines*. UKCCSG-PONF Mouth Care Group.

Haas F. 2003. Management of malignant spinal cord compression. Nursing Times, 99(15):32–4.

Hargrave DR, Messahel B, Plowman PN. 2004. Tumours of the central nervous system. In R Pinkerton, PN Plowman, R Pieters. Paediatric Oncology (3rd edition, pp. 287–322). London: Arnold.

Hastings CA, Lubin BH, Feusner J. 2006. Hematologic supportive care for children with cancer. In PA Pizzo, DG Poplack (Eds). Principles and Practice of Pediatric Oncology (5th edition, pp. 1231–68). Philadelphia: Lippincott, Williams & Wilkins.

Haut C. 2005. Oncological emergencies in the pediatric intensive care unit. AACN Clinical Issues, 16(2):232–45.

Haut C. 2008. Typhlitis in the pediatric patient. Journal of Infusion Nursing, 31(5):270–7.

Higdon ML, Higdon JA. 2006. Treatment of oncologic emergencies. American Family Physician, 74(11):1873–80.

Hobson MJ, Carney DE et al. 2005. Appendicitis in childhood hematologic malignancies: analysis and comparison with typhlitis. Journal of Pediatric Surgery, 40:214–20.

Hogan CM. 1998. The nurse's role in diarrhoea management. Oncology Nursing Forum, 25(5):879–86.

Hollis R, Denton S, Chapman G. 2008. General surgery. In F Gibson, LM Soanes. Cancer in Children and Young People (pp. 187–217). Chichester: John Wiley & Sons.

Hon KE, Leung A et al. 2005. Critical airway obstruction, superior vena cava syndrome, and spontaneous cardiac arrest in a child with acute leukemia. Pediatric Emergency Care, 21(12):844–6.

Hopkins M. 2008. Administration of radiotherapy. In F Gibson, LM Soanes. Cancer in Children and Young People (pp. 289–309). Chichester: John Wiley & Sons.

Hopkins M, Scott C. 2008. Acute and sub-acute side-effects of radiotherapy. In F Gibson, LM Soanes. Cancer in Children and Young People (pp. 321–41). Chichester: John Wiley & Sons.

Ilgen JS, Marr AL. 2009. Cancer emergencies: the acute abdomen. Emergency Medicine Clinics of North America, 27(3):381–99.

Jain Y, Arya LS, Kataria R. 2000. Neutropenic enterocolitis in children with acute lymphoblastic leukaemia. Pediatric Hematology and Oncology, 17(1):99–103.

Jeha S. 2001. Tumour lysis syndrome. Seminars in Haematology, 38(4, supplement 10):4–8.

Joseph M, Tayar R. 2005. Spinal cord compression requires early detection. European Journal of Palliative Care, 12(4): 141–3.

Kallab AM. 2005. Superior Vena Cava Syndrome. Emedicine. www.emedicine.com/me/topic2208.htm.

Kaplow R. 2001. Special nursing considerations. Critical Care Clinics, 17(3):769–89.

Keengwe IN, Stansfield F et al. 1999. Paediatric oncology and intensive care treatments: changing trends. Archives of Disease in Childhood 80: 553–555.

Kennebeck SS. 2005. Tumors of the mediastinum. Clinical Pediatric Emergency Medicine, 6:156–64.

Koretz MJ, Neifeld JP. 1985. Emergency surgical treatment for patients with acute leukemia. Cited in MJ Hobson, DE Carney et al. 2005. Appendicitis in childhood hematologic malignancies: analysis and comparison with typhlitis. Journal of Pediatric Surgery, 40:214–20.

Kosmidis HV, Lusher JM et al. 1980. Infections in leukemic children: a prospective analysis. Cited in WCW Chu, V Lee et al. 2003. Imaging findings of paediatric oncology patients presenting with acute neurological symptoms. Clinical Radiology, 58:589–603.

Kushner BH, Cheung NV. 2005. Neuroblastoma – from genetic profiles to clinical challenge. New England Journal of Medicine, 353(21):2215–17.

Kuskonmaz B, Unal S, et al. 2006. The neurologic complications in pediatric acute lymphoblastic leukemia patients excluding leukemic infiltration. Leukemia Research, 30:537–41.

Kwok Y, Tibbs PA, Patchell RA. 2006. Clinical approach to metastasis epidural spinal cord compression. Hematology/Oncology Clinics of North America, 20:1297–305.

Ladd AP, Grosfeld JL. 2006. Gastrointestinal tumors in children and adolescents. Seminars in Pediatric Surgery, 15:37–47.

Lehrnbecher T, Groll AH, Chanock SJ. 1999. Treatment of fungal infections in neutropenic children. Current Opinions in Pediatrics. 10:47–55.

Lim E, Bennett P, Beilby J. 2003. Sample preparation in patients receiving uric acid oxidase rasburicase therapy. Clinical Chemistry, 49(8):1417.

Limper AH. 2004. Chemotherapy-induced lung disease. Clinics in Chest Medicine, 25(1):53–64.

Lo Nigro L, Di Cataldo A, Schiliro G. 2000. Acute neurotoxicity in children with B-lineage acute lymphoblastic leukemia B-ALL treated with intermediate risk protocols. Cited in B Kuskonmaz, S Unal et al. 2006. The neurologic complications in pediatric acute lymphoblastic leukemia patients excluding leukemic infiltration. Leukemia Research, 30:537–41.

Lowis SP, Goulden N, Oakhill. A. 2004. Acute complications. In R Pinketon, PN Plowman, R Pieters (Eds). Paediatric Oncology (3rd edition). London: Arnold.

Lymphoma Information Network. 2007. www.lymphomainfo.net/childhood/hodgkins.html.

Lynch JK, Hirtz DG et al. 2002. Report of the National Institute of Neurological Disorders and Stroke workshop on perinatal and childhood stroke. Cited in LC Jordan, AE Hillis. 2007. Hemorrhagic stroke in children. Pediatric Neurology, 36:73–80.

Magrath IT. 1997. Malignant non-Hodgkin's lymphoma in children. In PA Pizzo, DG Poplack (Eds). Principle and Practice of Pediatric Oncology (pp. 661–96). Philadelphia: Lippincott, Williams and Wilkins.

Marrs JA. 2006. Nurse, my back hurts: understanding malignant spinal cord compression. Oncology Nursing, 10(1): 114–18.

Maytal J, Grossman R et al. 1995. Prognosis and treatment of seizures in children with acute lymphoblastic leukaemia. Cited in M Moleski 2000. Neuropsychological, neuroanatomical, and neurophysiological consequences of CNS chemotherapy for acute lymphoblastic leukemia. Archives of Clinical Neuropsychology, 15(7):603–30.

McDowell HM, Messahel B, Oberlin O. 2004. Hodgkins disease. In R Pinkerton, PN Ploughman, R Pieters. Paediatric Oncology (3rd edition, pp. 267–86). London: Arnold.

Melamud M, Palekar R, Singh, A. 2006. Retinoblastoma. American Family Physician, 73(6):1039–44.

Metzger ML, Dome JS. 2005. Current therapy for Wilm's tumor. Oncologist, 10(10):815–26.

Miano M, Faraci M et al. 2008. Early complications following haematopoetic SCT in children. Bone Marrow Transplantation, 41:S39–S42.

Naeem N, Reed MD et al. 2006. Transfer of the haematopoietic stem cell transplant patient to the intensive care unit: does it really matter? Bone Marrow Transplantation, 37:119–33.

Oren I, Haddad N et al. 2001. Invasive pulmonary aspergillosis in neutropenic patients during hospital construction: before and after chemoprophylaxis and institution of HEPA filters. American Journal of Hematology, 66(4):257–62.

Osowski M. 2002. Spinal cord compression: an obstructive oncological emergency. Topics in Advanced Practice Nursing. eJournal2(4).www.medscape.com/viewarticle/442735.

Patte C. 2004. Non-Hodgkin's lymphoma. In R Pinkerton, PN Ploughman, R Pieters. Paediatric Oncology (3rd edition, pp. 254–66). London: Arnold.

Pearson ADJ, Pinkerton R. 2004. Neuroblastoma. In R Pinkerton, PN Ploughman, R Pieters. Paediatric Oncology (3rd edition, pp. 386–415). London: Arnold.

Pene F, Aubron C et al. 2006. Outcome of critically ill allogeneic haematopoietic stem-cell transplantation recipients: a reappraisal of indications for organ failure supports. Journal of Clinical Oncology, 24(4):643–8.

Pizer B, May P. 1997. Paediatric surgical oncology. 8: Central nervous system tumours in children. Cited in K Ibrahim, R Appleton. 2004. Seizures as the presenting symptom of brain tumours in children. Seizure, 13:108–12.

Pizzo PA. 1999. Current concepts: fever in immunocompromised patients. New England Journal of Medicine, 341(12):893–900.

Porcu P, Cripe LD et al. 2000. Hyperleukocytic leukemias and leukostasis: a review of pathophysiology, clinical presentation and management. Leukaemia and Lymphoma, 39(1–2):1–18.

Priest JR, Ramsay NK et al. 1982. The effect of L-asparaginase on antithrombin, plasminogen, and plasma coagulation during therapy for acute lymphoblastic leukaemia. Cited in WCW Chu, V Lee et al. 2003. Imaging findings of paediatric oncology patients presenting with acute neurological symptoms. Clinical Radiology, 58:589–603.

Quinn J, DeAngelis L. 2000. Neurological emergencies in the cancer patient. Seminars in Oncology, 27:311–21.

Ray M, Marwaha RK, Trehan A. 2002. Chemotherapy related fatal neurotoxicity during induction in acute lymphoblastic leukemia. Cited in B Kuskonmaz, S Unal et al. 2006. The neurologic complications in pediatric acute lymphoblastic leukemia patients excluding leukemic infiltration. Leukemia Research, 30:537–41.

Rheingold SR, Lange BL. 2006. Pediatric Oncology (5th edition, pp. 1202–30). Philadelphia: Lipincott Williams & Wilkins.

Rivera-Luna R, Martinez-Guerra G et al. 1987. Treatment of non-Hodgkin's lymphoma in Mexican children. The effectiveness of chemotherapy during malnutrition. American Journal of Pediatric Hematology and Oncology, 4:356–66. Cited in SR Goldberg, K Godder, DA Lanning. 2007. Successful treatment of a bowel perforation after chemotherapy for Burkitt lymphoma. Journal of Pediatric Surgery, 42:E1–E3.

Rogers TR. 1995. Infectious complications of treatment. Baillière's Clinical Paediatrics 3(4):683–98.

Rokhsar S, Harrison EA et al. 1999. Intestinal stoma complications in immunocompromised children. Journal of Pediatric Surgery, 34(12):1757–61.

Schlatter M, Snyder K, Freyer D. 2002. Successful nonoperative management of typhlitis in pediatric oncology patients. Cited in MJ Hobson, DE Carney et al. 2005. Appendicitis in childhood hematologic malignancies: analysis and comparison with typhlitis. Journal of Pediatric Surgery. 40:214–20.

Schwartz RB, Bravo SM et al. 1995. Cyclosporine neurotoxicity and its relationship to hypertensive encephalophathy: CT and MR findings in 16 cases. Cited in WCW Chu, V Lee et al. 2003. Imaging findings of paediatric oncology patients presenting with acute neurological symptoms. Clinical Radiology, 58:589–603.

Selwood K. 2008a. Side-effects of chemotherapy. In F Gibson, F, L Soanes (Eds). Cancer in Children and Young People (pp. 33–71). London: John Wiley & Sons.

Selwood K. 2008b. Oncological Emergencies. In F Gibson, L Soanes (Eds). Cancer in Children and Young People (pp. 73–84). London: John Wiley & Sons.

Selwood K, Wright M, Crawford D. 2009. Care of the child with haematological and oncological conditions. In M Dixon, D Crawford et al. (Eds). Nursing the Highly Dependent Child or Infant. A manual of care (pp. 250–68). Chichester: Wiley-Blackwell.

Shafford EA, Pritchard J. 2004. Liver tumours. In R Pinkerton, PN Ploughman, R Pieters. Paediatric Oncology (3rd edition, pp. 449–68). London: Arnold.

Shamberger RC, Weinstein HJ, et al. 1986. The medical and surgical management of typhlitis in children with acute nonlymphocytic myelogenous leukaemia. Cited in MD van de Wetering, HN Caron et al. 2004. Severity of enterocolitis is predicted by IL-8 in paediatric oncology patients. European Journal of Cancer, 40:571–8.

Sherman NJ, Williams K, Woolley MM. 1973. The surgical complications in patients with leukaemia. Cited in MJ Hobson, DE Carney et al. 2005. Appendicitis in childhood hematologic malignancies: analysis and comparison with typhlitis. Journal of Pediatric Surgery, 40:214–20.

Singer C. 1977. Bacteremia and fungemia complicating neoplastic disease. Cited in MJ Hobson, DE Carney et al. 2005. Appendicitis in childhood hematologic malignancies: analysis and comparison with typhlitis. Journal of Pediatric Surgery, 40:214–20.

Skinner MA, Plumley DA et al. 1994. Gastrointestinal tumors in children: an analysis of 39 cases. Cited in AP Ladd, JL Grosfeld. 2006. Gastrointestinal tumors in children and adolescents. Seminars in Pediatric Surgery, 15:37–47.

Slocombe A, Boynes S. 2005. Malignant spinal cord compression. Radiology, 11:293–8.

Smith S. 2001. Evidence based management of constipation in the oncology patient. European Journal of Oncology Nursing, 5(1):18–25.

Smith OP, Hann I. 2004. Pathology of leukaemia. In R Pinkerton, PN Ploughman, R Pieters. Paediatric Oncology (3rd edition, pp. 83–100). London: Arnold.

Soares M, Jorge IF et al. 2005. Characteristics and outcomes of cancer patients requiring mechanical ventilator support for >24 hrs. Critical Care Medicine, 33(3):520–6.

Stalkup JR. 2002. A review of the measles virus. Dermatologic Clinics, 20(2):209–15.

Sternberg R. 1999. A plea for incidental appendectomy in pediatric patients with malignancy. Cited in MJ Hobson, DE Carney et al. 2005. Appendicitis in childhood hematologic malignancies: analysis and comparison with typhlitis. Journal of Pediatric Surgery, 40:214–20.

Tan SJ. 2002. Recognition and treatment of oncologic emergencies. Journal of Infusion Nursing, 25(3):182–8.

Thiery G, Azoulay E et al. 2005. Outcome of cancer patients considered for intensive care unit admission: a hospital-wide prospective study. Journal of Clinical Oncology, 23:4406–13.

Veys, P, Rao, K. 2004. Advances in therapy: megatherapy allogenic stem cell transplantation. In R Pinkerton, PN Plowman, R Pieters (Eds). Paediatric Oncology (3rd edition). London: Chapman & Hall.

Wade DS, Nava HR, Douglass HO Jr. 1992. Neutropenic enterocolitis. Clinical diagnosis and treatment. Cited in DB Wilson, A Rao et al. 2004. Neutropenic enterocolitis as a presenting complication of acute lymphoblastic leukemia: an unusual case marked by delayed perforation of the descending colon. Journal of Pediatric Surgery, 39(7): e18–e20.

Wadler S, Benson III et al. 1998. Recommended guidelines for the treatment of chemotherapy-induced diarrhoea. Journal of Clinical Oncology, 16(9):3169–78.

Walker AE, Robins M, Weinfeld F. 1985. Epidemiology of brain tumours: the national survey of intracranial neoplasms. Cited in K Ibrahim, R Appleton. 2004. Seizures as the presenting symptom of brain tumours in children. Seizure, 13:108–12.

Walsh TJ, Rolidies E. et al. 2006. Infectious complications in pediatric cancer patients. In PA Pizzo, DG Poplack (Eds). Principles and Practice of Pediatric Oncology (5th edition, pp. 1269–1329). Philadelphia: Lippincott, Williams & Wilkins.

Whelan J, Morland B. 2004. Bone tumours. In R Pinkerton, PN Ploughman, R Pieters. Paediatric Oncology (3rd edition, pp. 83–100). London: Arnold.

Wilkes G. 1999. Neurological disturbances. In C Yarbro, M Frogge, Goodman. Cancer Symptom Management (2nd edition, pp. 344–81). Boston: Jones and Barlett.

Wilson LD, Detterbeck FC, Yahalom J. 2007. Superior vena cava syndrome with malignant causes. The New England Journal of Medicine, 356(18):1862–9.

Section 3
ESSENTIAL CARE

Chapter 12
NUTRITION AND FLUID MANAGEMENT

Doreen Crawford

School of Nursing and Midwifery, Faculty of Health and Life Sciences, De Montfort University, Leicester, UK

Introduction

This chapter provides an overview of the physiology of fluid and electrolytes within the child's body then considers problems that can be encountered when there are deviations from these. The chapter briefly turns to metabolism and reviews strategies to improve or sustain a child's nutritional status. This is important as all children have a daily fluid and calorie requirement, which varies with age and condition, and in the intensive care environment it may not be possible to administer these by the enteral route. The standard fluid allowance for neonates, infants and children is calculated in terms of volume of oral feed required to meet the calorific needs of the healthy growing child over a 24-hour period. Table 12.1 illustrates normal fluid requirements according to age.

This apparently disproportionate fluid requirement reflects the fluid composition of the body and the need to sustain that. Total body water (TBW) varies with gender, weight and age. Infants and young children have a greater water concentration than adults, with TBW approximating 75–80% of body weight in the full-term infant and an even greater proportion in the premature infant. In older children and young people the range is 40–60%. The infant also has a greater water turnover due to their higher metabolic rate, larger surface area in relation to body mass and the infant's inability to concentrate urine due to immature

kidneys. Table 12.2 illustrates the differences in the proportion of the body which is fluid related to age.

The distribution and movement of body fluids

The water content of the body is contained within various compartments. Intracellular fluid (ICF) is water contained within the cells; extracellular fluid (ECF) is water outside of the cells. ECF fluid is further divided into intravascular fluid (plasma), interstitial fluid (fluid surrounding tissue cells) and transcellular fluid (cerebral spinal fluid, synovial fluid, pleural fluid and peritoneal fluid). ECF contains large amounts of sodium and chloride, moderate amounts of bicarbonate and small amounts of potassium, magnesium, calcium and phosphate. This is very different from the content of ICF, which has hardly any calcium, small amounts of sodium, chloride, bicarbonate and phosphate, moderate amounts of magnesium and large amounts of potassium.

There are several factors which influence the movement of fluid in and out of the vascular space; these are osmotic, oncotic and hydrostatic pressure, together with changes in capillary permeability. Table 12.3 reviews the physiology of these.

In addition to these mechanisms of body fluid distribution, fluid balance is influenced by changes in both the osmolality and volume of the plasma (Pearson 2002). Water is lost from the body by insensible loss (skin and

Paediatric Intensive Care Nursing, First Edition. Edited by Michaela Dixon and Doreen Crawford.
© 2012 John Wiley & Sons, Ltd. Published 2012 by John Wiley & Sons, Ltd.

Table 12.1 Fluid requirements

Daily fluid requirements	Hourly fluid requirements
Preterm infants: 200 ml/kg/day	1–10 kg: 4 ml/kg/hr
Term infants 150 ml/kg/day	11–20 kg: 2 ml/kg/hr
Children/adolescents: 2–3 l/day	>20 kg: 1 ml/kg/hr

Source: adapted from APLS Guidelines 2005; Dixon et al. 2009.

Table 12.2 Body water content and blood volume

Age group	Approximate water content in body	Approximate blood volume
Premature infant	90%	85–90 ml/kg
Newborn infant	70–80%	80–90 ml/kg
12–24 months	64%	75–80 ml/kg
Adult	60%	65–70 ml/kg

respiration) and sensible mechanisms (kidneys and urine production).

The normal regulation of water balance

Water is taken into the body by the oral intake of fluid and food. The water from fluids and solid foods is absorbed from the gastrointestinal tract. A small amount of water is generated from the body's metabolic processes. Regardless of age, all healthy persons require approximately 100 ml of water per 100 calories metabolised for dissolving and eliminating metabolic wastes. It should be remembered that the metabolic rate will increase with fever and where there is a need to repair tissue and recover from damage. Water loss is mainly through the kidneys, although it is also lost through the skin, lungs and gastrointestinal tract.

There are two main physiological mechanisms which synergistically regulate body water. These are manifest by the child's drive to seek fluid which is regulated by thirst, and the antidiuretic hormone (ADH) which conserves water. Thirst is controlled by the thirst centre in the hypothalamus. This centre is stimulated by two stimuli: cellular dehydration caused by an increase in extracellular osmo-

Table 12.3 The distribution and movement of body fluids

Pressure or mechanism	Contributing factors
Osmotic pressure	This is directly related to the number of particles that are dissolved in a fluid. The number of dissolved particles per litre of fluid is known as osmolality. These particles are mainly electrolytes and proteins. Sodium is the main electrolyte determining intravascular osmotic pressure. The osmotic pressure of intravascular, interstitial and intracellular fluids will be equal, however if there is an acute fall in osmotic pressure of the intravascular compartment, then fluid will move out into the tissues with potentially disastrous results.
Oncotic pressure	This is mainly determined by the plasma proteins. A normal level of plasma protein will keep fluid within the intravascular space. A significant loss of plasma proteins will result in water moving from the intravascular space into the tissues, causing tissue oedema and hypovolaemia.
Hydrostatic pressure	This can be described as the pressure of water in the blood vessels or tissues. The force of the heart pumping the blood through the blood vessels causes a hydrostatic pressure that is slightly higher than that in the tissues. This is counteracted by the oncotic pressure so that there is no net loss of fluid into the tissue spaces.
Capillary permeability	In health the capillary pores are too small to allow the passage of plasma proteins. However, if the capillary permeability increases, the plasma proteins have the potential to leave the capillaries and this drags water with them into the interstitial space leading to hypovolaemia. The permeability of the capillary wall changes in inflammatory disease states.

Source: Dixon et al. 2009.

lality and detected by osmoreceptors situated near the thirst centre; and by a decrease in blood volume. Stretch receptors, known as baroreceptors, which are situated in the carotid sinus and aorta, are sensitive to changes in arterial blood pressure together with low pressure baroreceptors, which are located in the left atrium and major thoracic veins.

A third important stimulus for thirst is angiotensin 2. Its secretion increases in response to low blood volume and low blood pressure. ADH is responsible for the reabsorption of water by the kidneys. ADH is also known as vasopressin. If too little ADH is secreted, the kidneys' ability to reabsorb water diminishes, resulting in excessive urine output (polyuria). The levels of circulating ADH are controlled by extracellular volume and osmolality.

In the critically ill infant and child there is a propensity for fluid to be retained because of the increased production of ADH and aldosterone. The factors that may cause this to occur include hypotension, pain, stress, positive pressure ventilation and severe pulmonary hypertension. The increased production of ADH results in an increase of intravascular volume and a reduction in intravascular osmolality, while the increased secretion of aldosterone results in increased sodium and water reabsorption. It is essential that the children's nurse is able to accurately assess the fluid balance status of the child. This can be done by maintaining and documenting an accurate fluid balance with an hourly measurement of input and output and by continual clinical assessment of the child. This includes the monitoring of the vital signs, such as measuring the pulse volume and BP.

The child's physical appearance is a great indicator of wellbeing: the texture and turgor of the skin, the moistness of the tongue and the tension of the fontanels when they are present. The central venous pressure (CVP) provides a measurement of the pressure in the right atrium of the heart. The CVP recording is an indication of the fluid homeostasis of the body. However, they are not without risk and should only be used in areas where the doctors and nurses are used to caring for them.

Clinical considerations

Dehydration

Infants under the age of 2 years are more at risk of becoming dehydrated due to their physiology. However, dehydration can occur at any age and sick children are at greater risk. Children may be admitted to CICU because of dehydration induced by vomiting, poor absorption, diarrhoea, diabetes, not replacing gastric or intestinal aspirate, thermal injury, fever and the use of diuretics. Dehydration can result from either inadequate fluid intake or excessive fluid loss. In addition to dehydration it is likely that the child will have abnormal levels of electrolytes. Dehydration is usually classified according to its level of severity (mild, moderate or severe) and also according to the serum sodium and osmolality levels:

- Isotonic.
- Hypotonic (hyponatraemic).
- Hypertonic (hypernatraemic).

Isotonic dehydration occurs when the loss of water and sodium are proportional. Serum sodium remains normal and as a result there is equal distribution of fluid loss between the interstitial and intravascular spaces.

Hypotonic dehydration results if a greater proportion of sodium is lost than that of water. Serum sodium falls resulting in decreased serum osmolality and shifting of fluid from intravascular to interstitial and cellular spaces. Hypotonic dehydration is likely quickly to show signs and symptoms of low intravascular volume.

Hypertonic dehydration occurs when water is lost in greater proportion to sodium. Serum sodium increases, which shifts fluid from the cellular and interstitial spaces to the intravascular space. This will help maintain intravascular volume so signs of dehydration may not be evident until fluid loss is substantial. Classification and signs and symptoms of dehydration can be seen in Table 12.4. When assessing children for signs dehydration it is essential that a complete history is taken and that the child's age and type of dehydration is taken into account as signs and symptoms may vary.

Treatment of dehydration

Dehydration in children can be assessed by the use of tools and scales (Bailey et al. 2010). Unless treated, moderate to severe dehydration will lead to a compromise of cardiac output and systemic perfusion. If this occurs, the body uses compensatory mechanisms to try to maintain systemic and essential organ perfusion, which in turn may lead to metabolic acidosis, multi-system failure and ultimately death. These systems are interdependent (see Chapters 5 and 6).

Whether the dehydration is isotonic, hypotonic or hypertonic in origin the aim of treatment is restoration and maintenance of intravascular volume and systemic perfusion, together with correction of any electrolyte balance. In mild dehydration and, depending on cause and age of child, rehydration may be achieved through oral therapy. However, very sick children will need the insertion of one, and preferably two, wide-bore intravenous cannula. If IV

Table 12.4 Classification and signs and symptoms of dehydration

Clinical presentation	Mild dehydration	Moderate dehydration	Severe dehydration
Body weight loss	Infant 5% (50 ml/kg) Child 3% (30 ml/kg)	10% (100 ml/kg) 6% (60 ml/kg)	15% (150 ml/kg) 9% (90 ml/kg)
Heart rate	Mild tachycardia	Moderate tachycardia	Extreme tachycardia
Blood pressure	Normal	Normal	Hypotensive
Peripheral pulses	Normal	Weakened	Very weak or absent
Skin perfusion	Normal/warm	Pale/cool	Mottled/grey/cold
Skin texture and turgor	Texture dry, skin fold springy, return slightly reduced	Texture very dry, moderately reduced skin fold visible for <2 seconds	May be flaky and scaly, severely reduced skin fold visible for >2 seconds
Mucous membrane and tongue	Dry	Very dry	Extremely dry
Capillary refill time	Normal to slightly prolonged	Slightly/moderately prolonged	Severely prolonged
Urine output	Slightly reduced	Mild oliguria	Severe oliguria or anuria
Neurological	Normal/irritable	Irritable/lethargic	Unresponsive
Anterior fontanels	Flat or depressed	Moderately depressed	Significantly depressed
Ocular tension (resistance of the eye to deformation when estimated digitally)	Normal, highly resistant	Eye can be slightly depressed	Very depressed, eyes sunken

Source: adapted from Dixon et al. 2009.

access is difficult to obtain, an intraosseous needle should be considered while preparation is made for a cutdown into a vein. When access to the circulation is established, the insertions of a central venous pressure monitor should be considered.

The dehydrated child must be assessed for signs of shock. This is ascertained by clinical and biochemical examination. The cause of the dehydration also needs to be established and an effective treatment regime to allow for rehydration and correction of abnormalities in electrolyte balance over a 24–48-hour period (APLS 2005). The acid base balance also needs to be considered and treated accordingly.

The fluid resuscitation of a child in hypovolaemic shock secondary to fluid loss is the rapid administration of crystalloid. The starting volume is 20 ml/kg. This can be repeated if there is inadequate clinical response with no evidence of intravascular overload. The type of fluid used should approximate in electrolyte concentration to that of serum. Commonly used fluids are 0.9% saline or Hartmann's solution. The presence of hyper- or hyponatraemia does not affect the choice of fluids during this stage of resuscitation (APLS 2005).

Over-hydration and fluid overload

The child requiring intensive care is susceptible to fluid overload and oedema. Fluid overload is a problem as it results in more circulatory volume than the heart can effectively cope with. This may eventually result in heart failure, which typically manifests as pulmonary oedema and peripheral oedema. There should be hourly calculation of fluid input and output, continuous monitoring supplemented by continual clinical reassessment.

There are four main factors which can cause oedema (Table 12.5).

Signs and symptoms of fluid overload include:

• Oedema.
• Tachycardia.
• Hypertension.
• Respiratory distress.
• Decrease in saturations.
• Enlarged liver.
• Raised central venous pressure.
• Weight gain.
• Signs of alveolar flooding or fluid streaks on chest X-ray.
• Frothy pink secretions if intubated.

Table 12.5 Factors contributing to oedema

Increased capillary pressure	A result of increased vascular volume caused by heart failure, kidney disease, thermal injury.
	A result of venous obstruction caused by acute pulmonary oedema, liver disease with portal vein congestion.
	A result of decreased arteriolar resistance caused by drugs blocking the calcium channels.
Decreased colloidal osmotic pressure	A loss of plasma proteins caused by kidney disease such as nephrotic syndrome, extensive burns.
	A decrease in the production of plasma proteins results in liver disease, starvation and malnutrition.
Increased capillary permeability	Result of extensive tissue injury or thermal injury, allergic reactions or inflammation.
Obstruction of lymphatic flow	Result of malignant obstruction or obliteration of lymphatic structures.

Source: adapted from Porth and Matfin 2004.

Table 12.6 Normal values of electrolytes

Electrolyte	Premature infant	Term infant	Child	Daily requirements
Potassium	4.5–7.2 mmol/l	3.6–6.4 mmol/l	3.5–5 mmol/l	1–2 mmol/kg
Sodium	135–45 mmol/l	135–45 mmol/l	135–45 mmol/l	2–4 mmol/kg
Calcium	2.1–2.7 mmol/l	2.1–2.7 mmol/l	2.1–2.7 mmol/l	0.3 mmol/kg
Magnesium	0.6–1 mmol/l	0.6–1 mmol/l	0.6–1 mmol/l	0.07–0.2 mmol/kg
Phosphate	1–2.6 mmol/l	1–1.8 mmol/l	1–1.8 mmol/l	0.04–1.5 mmol/kg

Source: adapted from Pearson 2002, in Dixon et al. 2009.

Treatment of fluid overload will be determined by the cause, for example, if the primary cause of fluid overload is due to cardiac failure, then the use of inotropic and/or diuretic therapy may be indicated in order to increase cardiac output. However, if the fluid overload is due to over-hydration and intravascular overload, then the patient is likely to need fluid restriction and the administration of diuretics.

Electrolytes

Electrolytes are ions with the ability to conduct a charge and they account for approximately 95% of the solute molecules in body water, the other 5% being non-electrolytes such as glucose, urea and creatinine (McCance and Huether 2002). The main electrolytes are sodium, potassium, calcium, magnesium, chloride, bicarbonate and phosphate. The main intracellular electrolyte is potassium, while the main extracellular electrolyte is sodium. Normal values (Table 12.6) and daily requirements differ according to age and laboratories have slightly different reference ranges. Refer to the local policy and seek advice if unsure about a value for a particular child.

Electrolyte action

Having an excess or deficiency of an electrolyte can potentially be very dangerous for any child and even more so for the child who needs intensive care.

Sodium (Na^+)

As the main electrolyte in the ECF compartment Na^+ has a major effect on osmosis and osmolality. Hyponatraemia is classified as a Na level <135 mmol/l. Deficits of Na alter the ability of cells to depolarise and repolarise normally.

Signs and symptoms of hyponatraemia include lethargy, headaches, seizures and coma. If hyponatraemia is accompanied by a loss of ECF, then signs of hypovolaemia may be displayed, including tachycardia, hypotension and diminished urine output. In other situations hyponatraemia may be due to water retention and detected by weight gain and oedema (McCance and Huether 2002). Treatment will depend on the cause, biochemical results and clinical manifestation. Rapid falls in sodium can be corrected quickly but these situations are unusual. Sodium levels usually fall gradually and correction should also be so. Natural corrected with fluid restriction is possible.

Hypernatraemia is a sodium level >145 mmol/l. It can be caused by excessive water loss, decreased water intake or excessive sodium intake. Signs and symptoms may include thirst, oliguria/anuria, high specific gravity of urine and increased serum osmolality. If decreased intravascular volume occurs, then tachycardia, hypotension and peripheral shutdown may also present. Neurological symptoms resulting from the movement of water out of brain cells may include headache, seizures and coma. Identification of the cause by history, clinical examination and biochemical investigations will define treatment. The cause needs to be treated but will also include rehydration.

Potassium (K+)

Potassium is the most common intracellular ion, with an intracellular concentration of 140–150 mmol/l. The extracellular levels are much lower. K^+ is regulated by two main mechanisms: through the kidney, which either conserves or eliminates K^+, and through the transcellular shifts between the intracellular and extracellular compartments, which allows K^+ to enter body cells when plasma levels are high and move out when the plasma levels are low (Porth and Matfin 2004). The control of K^+ within normal range is essential as only a slight derangement from normal levels can result in life-threatening cardiac dysrhythmias.

K^+ is essential for many body functions, including growth, conduction of nerve impulses, acid base balance and the use of carbohydrates for energy. Hypokalaemia is a plasma potassium level <3.5 mmol/l. Causes of hypokalaemia include inadequate intake, excessive loss usually through gastro-intestine, skin and kidneys and redistribution of K+ between the ICF and ECF compartments.

Signs and symptoms include polyuria, vomiting, muscle cramps, confusion, metabolic alkalosis and cardiac arrhythmias. Treatment consists of treating the cause and, if necessary, administering potassium supplements either by orally or if necessary intravenously.

K^+ is a powerful electrolyte. Children with abnormal K^+ levels ought to be electrocardiographically monitored. Hypokalaemia can cause ECG changes, including prolonged PR interval, depression of ST segment and the flattening of the T-wave. IV K^+ must be administered by a nurse or doctor who is appropriately trained and skilled in its administration. It needs to be given slowly at an infusion rate >0.4 mmol/kg/hr. K^+ should only be administered

through a good vascular access. The child should be ECG-monitored.

Hyperkalaemia is an increase in plasma potassium level >5 mmol/l. It is that is very rarely seen in the well child but can occur in the highly dependent patient. The main causes are excessive rapid administration of potassium, decreased renal excretion as in acute renal failure and from the movement of potassium between the ICF and ECF compartments. The signs and symptoms include nausea and diarrhoea, dizziness and muscle cramps. The main risk of hyperkalaemia is cardiac dysrhythmia, which can lead to cardiac arrest. The child should be ECG-monitored. Treatment options include decreasing or stopping intake, increasing renal excretion and increasing cellular uptake (Porth and Matfin 2004).

Calcium (Ca+), phosphate (PO4−) and magnesium (Mg)

Ca and Mg are closely linked to PO_4 levels (Pearson 2002). They are obtained from the diet and absorbed from the intestines, with any excess eliminated in the urine. The majority of the body's calcium and phosphate is found in bones and approximately 50 percent of magnesium is found within bones. The majority of the remaining amounts of each electrolyte is found intracellularly. Only a very small amount of calcium, magnesium and phosphate is present within the extracellular fluid and are regulated by vitamin D, parathyroid hormone and calcitonin production.

Calcium

The main source of calcium is milk and milk products. The calcium content of the bone provides strength and stability to the skeletal system. It is also used to maintain extracellular levels. The small amount of extracellular calcium is either a protein-bound complex or is ionised. It is only the ionised form that is free to leave the vascular compartment and participate in cellular function. The function of ionised calcium includes participation in enzyme reaction, an effect on membrane potential, neuronal excitability, contraction in skeletal, cardiac and smooth muscle, influences cardiac contractility and automaticity and is essential for blood clotting (Porth and Matfin 2004).

Children who are critically ill or highly dependent need are at risk of hypocalcaemia as they may have an impaired ability to gain calcium from bone stores, may have high losses from the kidney or more may bind with protein and then be unavailable. Hypocalcaemia may be acute or chronic. In the acute stage it can cause jitteriness, convulsions, ECG abnormalities, arrhythmias and heart failure. Treatment will be to identify and treat cause and by administration of calcium infusion according to local treatment regime and policy. Hypercalcaemia is rare but may occur because of excessive bone resorption as a result of cancer with bone metastases, leukaemia, lymphoma and multiple myeloma. It may occur as a result of prolonged and extensive immobilisation and in paraplegics and quadriplegics. Other causes include endocrine diseases, recovery phase of acute renal failure and Williams' syndrome. Signs and symptoms include seizures, muscle flaccidity and tachyarrhythmias. Many patients with hypercalcaemia will be volume-depleted and will respond to fluid resuscitation followed by diuretic therapy. Other forms of treatment include renal replacement therapy (Pearson 2002).

Hypocalcaemia

Measurement of calcium can be done as total calcium or ionised calcium. The value range differs. It is important to know which one has been measured and requested.

- Total: 2–2.7 mmol/l.
- Ionised: 1.2–1.3 mmol/l.

Clinical manifestations of hypocalcaemia are due to disturbances in cellular membrane potential, resulting in neuromuscular irritability. Muscle cramps involving the back and legs are common. Insidious hypocalcaemia may produce symptoms of encephalopathy. Papilloedema occasionally occurs, and cataracts may develop after prolonged hypocalcaemia. Severe hypocalcaemia with plasma Ca <1.75 mmol/l may cause tetany, laryngospasm and generalised seizures.

Phosphate (HPO₄) – negative electrolyte

Phosphate is essential to many bodily functions. It helps bone formation, is essential for certain metabolic processes, including the formation of ATP and the enzymes necessary for metabolism of glucose, fat and protein, it serves as an acid base buffer in ECF and in the renal excretion of hydrogen ions (Porth and Matfin 2004). Like calcium, only a small amount of phosphate is located in the ECF compartment. Causes of hypophosphataemia include decreased intestinal absorption, for example, by severe and prolonged diarrhoea, lack of vitamin D, increased renal losses and malnutrition. The treatment is by replacement therapy and treatment of the cause. The most common causes are impaired renal function and tumour lysis syndrome. If hyperphosphataemia is present, symptoms similar to hypocalcaemia will be seen.

Hyperphosphataemia

Skeletal fractures or disease, kidney failure, hypoparathyroidism, haemodialysis, diabetic ketoacidosis, acromegaly, systemic infection and intestinal obstruction can all cause phosphate retention and build-up in the blood. The disorder occurs concurrently with hypocalcaemia. Individuals with mild hyperphosphataemia are typically asymptomatic, but signs of severe hyperphosphataemia include paraesthesia, tingling in hands and fingers, muscle spasms and cramps, convulsions and cardiac arrest.

Hypophosphataemia

Low serum phosphate levels may be caused by hypomagnesaemia and hypokalaemia. Severe burns, diabetic ketoacidosis, kidney disease, hyperparathyroidism, hypothyroidism, Cushing's syndrome, malnutrition, haemodialysis, vitamin D deficiency and prolonged diuretic therapy can also diminish blood phosphate levels. There are typically few physical signs of mild phosphate depletion. Symptoms of severe hypophosphataemia include muscle weakness, weight loss and bone deformities (osteomalacia).

Magnesium

This is a very important electrolyte. Its function includes the following: it is essential to all reactions that require ATP; and essential for replication and transcription of DNA and for the translocation of messenger RNA. It is required for cellular energy metabolism, functioning of the sodium–potassium membrane pump, nerve conduction and calcium channel activity (Porth and Matfin 2004). Magnesium is found in green vegetables, meat, nuts and seafood and body levels are mainly regulated by the kidney.

Hypomagnesaemia can be caused by impaired intake or absorption as in starvation and malabsorption. It can also be caused by increased losses as in diuretic therapy and diabetic ketoacidosis. Signs and symptoms include tetany, cardiac arrhythmias and nystagmus. Treatment is by magnesium replacement but caution is required if the intravenous route is used.

Hypermagnesaemia is rare and is mainly caused by renal failure. Signs and symptoms include lethargy, confusion, hypotension and cardiac arrhythmias. Treatment should include stopping any administration and the administration of calcium, which is an antagonist of magnesium.

Nutritional needs of the child

Children in the intensive care environment are uniquely vulnerable. Their nutritional care plan must match the total metabolic needs of the body and allow for repair and growth (Table 12.7). Energy input is obtained from three main classifications of food groups: carbohydrates, fats

Table 12.7   Terms that are associated with metabolism include the following

Homeostasis	The maintenance of a stable environment.
Anabolism	The building of large molecules from smaller ones, requiring energy, for example, making fat from fatty acids and glycerol.
Catabolism	The breakdown of large complex molecules into smaller ones releasing energy, for example, releasing amino acids from a peptide chain.
Adenosine tri-phosphate (ATP)	Energy generated and used by the cells.
Glycolysis	A stage in glucose metabolism where glucose is broken down resulting in the production of ATP.

Table 12.8   Effects of insulin on carbohydrate, fat and protein metabolism

Carbohydrate metabolism	Insulin is important for the transport of glucose into the adipose cells, providing the glycerol portion of the fat molecule for the depositing fat in these cells.
Fat metabolism	Insulin decreases the utilisation of fat as a source of energy. It inhibits the action of lipase. In the absence of insulin increased breakdown and utilisation of fat for energy occurs, which leads to excessive amounts of acetoacetic acid being formed which cannot be metabolised by the body and leads to a systemic build-up of acid.
Protein metabolism	Little is understood about the effects of insulin on protein synthesis and storage other than that insulin causes active transport of amino acids into the cells. Insulin has a direct effect on ribosomes by increasing the translation messenger RNA, so forming new proteins, and insulin inhibits the catabolism of proteins decreasing the rate of amino acid release from cells.

and proteins. Energy is derived from the oxidation of carbon and hydrogen from dietary molecules.

Carbohydrate metabolism

Carbohydrates are absorbed from the digestive tract. During digestion large carbohydrate molecules, such as starch and lactose, are broken down to simple sugars, such as glucose, fructose and galactose. These are then absorbed into the bloodstream and transported to the liver by the hepatic portal vein. From the liver they are then transported systemically. Any excesses are stored as glycogen in the liver and skeletal muscle. Glycogen can be readily broken down into glucose when required. The importance of this mechanism is that some cells (e.g. brain cells) rely almost exclusively on glucose as their source of energy for ATP production.

Fat metabolism

Fat molecules are absorbed from the digestive system in small clusters known as chylomicrons. Chylomicrons tend not to enter the blood stream directly but are absorbed by the lymphatic system. This means they are transported directly to the heart and the rest of the body. Fat consists of glycerol and fatty acids and both can be used to produce energy. Glycerol is a carbohydrate and the liver uses it to synthesise glucose. Fatty acids are fed into the Krebs cycle in the mitochondria leading to further production of ATP. Fat contains more energy per gram than carbohydrate.

Protein metabolism

Proteins consist of chains of amino acids. These chains are broken down by enzymes in the digestive system releasing amino acids, which are then absorbed into the blood stream. Amino acids are first transported to the liver and then to the rest of the body. Amino acids are not usually used as a source of fuel, their primary function being for growth and development. However, if other sources of energy are not available, they are utilised as a source of energy. The breakdown of amino acids results in the production of ammonia, which is then converted to urea by the liver before being excreted by the kidney.

In order for the cells to be able to utilise the products of metabolism two hormones, insulin and glucagon are needed; these are secreted by the pancreas.

Insulin

Insulin is secreted by the β cells in the pancreas from the islets of Langerhans. It is a very large polypeptide and its main role is the maintenance of blood glucose by binding with large protein receptors in the cell wall. Table 12.8

reviews the action of insulin on the product of carbohydrate, fat and protein metabolism.

Glucagon

Glucagon is secreted by the α cells of the islets of Langerhans in the pancreas. It has the opposite action to insulin. The effects of glucagon include the increased breakdown of glycogen stores to form glucose, the increased breakdown of fats and glucose synthesis.

Growth of the infant and child

Growth only occurs when more nutrition is provided than is required to meet basic metabolic needs and have a balanced intake of both macro- and micronutrients. Macronutrients include carbohydrates, lipids and proteins. Micronutrients include minerals such as calcium, magnesium, phosphate, iron, zinc and copper, water-soluble vitamins B and C and fat-soluble vitamins A, D, E and K.

It is expected that normal growth pattern would see an infant doubling its birth weight by age 6 months, trebling birth weight by 12 months and quadrupling birth weight by 24 months. Sixty per cent of children's energy needs are utilised by their major organs in order to maintain normal function. Basal metabolic rate reaches its maximum around the age of 2 years, then decreases with age.

Nutritional assessment

The assessment of the child's nutritional state when first admitted to an ICU might not be one of the highest priorities, but this can contribute to the prevalence of malnutrition among critically ill patients, especially those with a protracted clinical course (Mehta and Compher 2009). Both over- and underfeeding are common. In part this is owing to the difficulties in calculating requirement as metabolic response to stress, injury, surgery or inflammation cannot be accurately predicted and the metabolic alterations may change during the course of illness (Mehta et al. 2009). Weighing patients may be difficult if they are attached to machinery and the weight recorded may not be true indication of nutritional status if they are oedematous. Calorimetry is possible but not common; illness may alter or mask biochemical results. There is a range of equations designed to calculate requirement, but none is deemed the gold standard, leading to a need for clinical creativity. Much more research is required in this area (Frankenfield and Ashcraft 2011). Enteral feeding in the highly dependent child needs to be commenced as soon as possible, interrupted and disturbed as little as possible and reviewed frequently.

Types and methods of feeding

Children require more calories per kg body weight than adults due to their higher metabolic rate and any child who has an illness or disease will need additional calorific intake (Singh 1997). Consideration of nutrition, including type, volume and administration of feed, needs to be made as early as possible to prevent harmful physiological effects (Alexander 1999). Enteral feeding is the method best suited to achieving maximal nutritional status in the child with high dependency needs. There are obvious advantages: it is efficient and economical, readily available and the majority of nurses have the skill and expertise needed to administer enteral feeds safely enterally. Enteral feeding maintains the gut barrier structure and function. It is an important stimulus to mature the gut of a premature infant, maximises the immunological properties of the gut and minimises the risk of bacterial translocation. However, for a number of reasons it may not be possible for the child to receive their nutritional requirement in this way. These include recent gut surgery, short gut syndrome, paralytic ileus, non-absorption of feeds, severe breathlessness and respiratory distress.

Another consideration of method and frequency of feeding is the age of the child. The volume capacity of the stomach alters with age (Table 12.9) and this, together with the condition of the child, needs to be taken into account.

Whenever possible intermittent oral feeding is the preferred method, and for the infant breast milk is at least the basis of the preferred feed. However, there are many situations where oral feeding may not be an option or indeed intermittent feeding may not be appropriate, for example, where there is endotracheal intubation, absent or impaired

Table 12.9 Stomach capacity by age

Age	Capacity
Newborn	10–20 ml
1 week	30–90 ml
2–3 weeks	75–100 ml
1 month	90–150 ml
3 months	150–200 ml
1 year	210–360 ml
2 years	500 ml
10 years	750–900 ml
16 Years	1500 ml
Adulthood	2000–3000 ml

Source: Moules and Ramsey 1998.

swallowing reflexes, coma or severe breathlessness. In these situations enteral feeding can be administered by the use of naso- or orogastric tubes, nasoduodenal or nasojejunal tubes or in the situation where long-term tube feeding is anticipated, a gastrostomy or jejunostomy may be performed. Frequency of feeding can be adapted from intermittent to continuous in order to meet the individual needs and condition of the child.

Bolus or continuous enteral feeding, gastric or transpyloric feeding

There is controversy over commencing infants and young children on bolus or continuous feeding. Bolus is physiologically more appropriate and in the neonatal unit currently the administration of a slow bolus seems to be preferred. This style of management reflects what is done in most neonatal units, although the clinical benefits and risks of continuous versus intermittent nasogastric tube milk feeding cannot be reliably discerned from the limited information available from randomised trials (Premji and Chessell 2007). Arguments for intermittent bolus gavage include the fact that this is physiologically normal and promotes the cyclical surge of gut hormones which are normally seen in healthy term infants and gastrointestinal hormones such as gastrin, gastric inhibitory peptide and enteroglucagon require the presence of intraluminal nutrients to stimulate secretion. Continuous tube feeding has been cited as being better tolerated in some ITU patients (Rhoney et al. 2002). Continuous transpyloric (TP) feeding has been suggested as a means to manage feed intolerance (Sánchez et al. 2007) and TP enteral nutrition is a useful and simple feeding method that enables a high calorie feed to be delivered to children who are receiving high-dose sedatives and muscle relaxants (Sánchez et al. 2007). Continuous TP feeding has been cited as causing prolonged diarrhoea but is effective in maintaining nutrition and has the advantage of not contributing to gastric pooling. TP feeding permits feeding to be stopped for shorter periods prior to attempts at extubation (Babett 2007).

In the absence of evidence, from a patient safety perspective a nurse administering a bolus has to be physically present and attentive during its administration, whereas continuous feeds continue to be administered regardless of the presence of the nurse. In lightly sedated children weaning off ventilation the irritation of an NGT taped to their face may result in restlessness and partial removal. Where bolus feeding is practised this would be quickly noticed and the NGT re-passed; where continuous feeds are used it could be some time before displacement becomes apparent. The mechanism to assess the location

of the tube and strategies for enteral tube management (NPSA 2011) is well documented and universally adopted and will not be considered here.

Types of enteral feeds

Breast milk is universally advocated as the feed of choice for infants. Current recommendations are for exclusive breast milk feeds for the first 6 months and as a dietary supplement for up to 2 years (WHO 2002). Not surprisingly it is well tolerated even in seriously compromised guts. Approximately 50% of energy in breast milk is provided by fats, whereas in infant formulas it is approximately 25%. Breast milk has protective properties (e.g. immunoglobulin A – IgA) and has antibodies which are active against a wide range of bacterial, viral, fungal and parasitic antigens. Lactoferrin binds with free iron in milk and is thought to inhibit the growth of *E. coli* and lysosome which attacks bacteria membranes.

Growth factors in breast milk may have a role in maintaining the protective nature of the intact gastrointestinal mucosa as breast milk promotes the growth of normal gut flora. Breast-fed infants are less likely to experience infections compared to formula-fed infants, particularly where there are risks of unhygienic preparation and storage of the feed. For the infants of mothers who were unable to express breast milk or who are unable to express sufficient milk to feed their infant, donor milk is becoming more readily available.

Most infant feeding formulas are based on cow's milk which has been modified to resemble the nutritional composition of mature breast milk. Modified cow's milk feeds can be divided into three groups (Table 12.10):

• Whey-dominant – whey:casein ratio similar to breast milk, e.g. Aptamil First™, Cow & Gate Premium™, Farley's First Milk™, SMA Gold™.

Table 12.10 Types of formula feed

Age	Type of formula feed
Preterm <2 kg	Nutriprem SMA low birth weight
Preterm >2 kg	Nutriprem 2, Premcare
Full term and under 1 year	EBM, SMA Gold, C&G Premium or Plus, Aptimil, Farley's First
1–6 years (8–20 kg)	Nutrini, Nutrini-fibre, Nutrini-energy Multifibre
7–12 (21–45 kg)	Tentrini Multifibre, Tentrini energy with fibre
13 years+	Nutrison Multifibre

- Casein-dominant – whey:casein ratio similar to cow's milk, there is no scientific evidence to support the claim that a casein-dominant feed will help to satisfy a hungry infant.
- Follow-on formula for infants over 6 months of age has a higher iron content.

The best enteral feed for the child

Consideration of the type of enteral feed used should include patient condition, availability of feed and parental choice. Dieticians should be involved in ensuring that high dependency patients are receiving the appropriate feed, including any additional supplements, in order to meet the growth and metabolic needs of the child. Types of enteral feed available are listed in Tables 12.11 and a strategy by which the enteral feed can be commenced and built up is considered in Figure 12.1.

Where bolus feeding is practised the question as to the administering of a flush at the end of a feed arises. Feeding tubes are prone to clog for a variety of reasons. One is accumulation of formula sediment in the lower segment of the tube, especially during the slow administration of calorically dense formulas or those containing fibre (Bankhead et al. 2009). Clogging is also more likely in small diameter tubes. Another common cause is the administration of medications via the tube. Bankhead and colleagues (2009) recommended flushing feeding tubes in neonatal and paediatric patients should be performed using the lowest volume of sterile water necessary to clear the tube.

A further consideration in continuous enteral feeding concerns the time the formula should hang before removal. Bankhead and colleagues (2009) recommend that decanted formulas or reconstituted formulas hang for no more than 4 hours and the giving set changed every 8 hours to prevent contamination. Reconstituted formula has demonstrated some instability of the fat and carbohydrate fractions (Galt and Josephson, 1982), however the 4-hour recommendation is well within any risk. Sterile formula in a closed system can be left for up to 24 hours (Bankhead et al. 2009).

The length of time a NGT should be in place is controversial as their use is not without complications. Generally, only the smaller diameter, soft silicone NGTs are appropriate for long-term feeding, to avoid irritation, pressure area damage and erosion of the nasal mucosa in the nasal cavity. Other complications include nose bleeds, sinusitis, sore throats and ear infections.

Some of these tubes have guide wires to facilitate insertion and these have been implicated in a number of adverse incidents, among them oesophageal perforation, pulmonary aspiration, pneumothorax and intracranial placement of the tube. There are strict mechanisms to assess the location of the tube and strategies for enteral tube management. The recommendations of the National Patient Safety Agency (2011) are well documented and universally adopted and will not be considered further here. The future might include enzyme testing paper to confirm placement which will reduce the need for X-ray confirmation of a tube placement when the nurse is confronted with ambiguous pH readings.

Long-term enteral tube feeding

Long-term feeding devices should be considered when the need for enteral feeding is 4 weeks or longer (Bankhead et al. 2009). Following the placement of a PEG tube, feeding can commence after 6 hours (Brown et al. 1995; Choudhry et al. 1996). PEG tubes should be considered as the feeding tubes of choice if the child requires maxillary facial surgery or has a base of skull fracture. They can be placed in the CICU under local anaesthetic, reducing the

Table 12.11 Types of enteral feed

Oral supplements	Not complete diets but used to supply more energy.
Polymeric diets	For children with normal/near-normal gut function. Contains protein, long-chain fatty acids, complex carbohydrates, vitamins and minerals (e.g. Pediasure and Ensure).
Pre-digested diets	For children with severely impaired gastrointestinal function. Contains free amino acids, di- and tripeptides, short carbohydrate polymers and fat, as well as vitamins, minerals and essential fatty acids (e.g. Pregestimil).
Elemental diets	For patients with severe gastrointestinal dysfunction.
Disease-specific diets	Diets formulated for specific conditions such as renal failure, hepatic encephalopathy, chylothorax.
Modular diets	Individual components of a feed can be adjusted to achieve optimum diet.

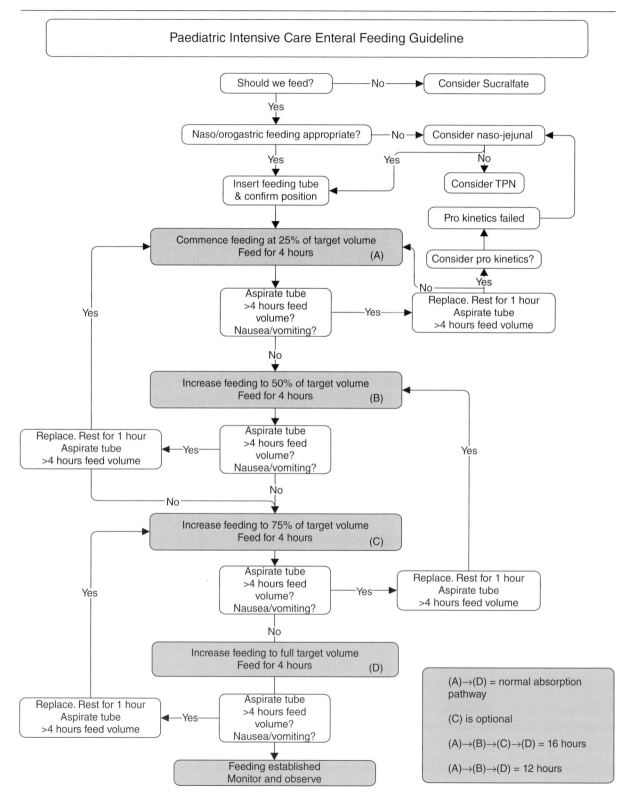

Figure 12.1   Progressing feeds. From Martin and Cox 2000.

risk of transferring the child to theatre. They are better tolerated than NGTs and result in less gastro-oesophageal reflux and a reduction in aspiration pneumonia. They are associated with a low incidence of complications and are a cost-effective alternative when considering long survival and transfer back to the community (Avitsland et al. 2006).

Parenteral nutrition (PN)

Parenteral means administered by any means other than the mouth. Giving nutrition directly into the blood stream is a common feature in children who require intensive care to replace or to supplement what can be administered into the gut. The infusion consists of a sterile prescription of water, amino acids, glucose, minerals and vitamins. Emulsified fats can also be administered. PN is hyperosmolar and must be infused slowly into a large vessel where there is a good circulating volume to dilute and buffer the infusion. The subclavian or jugular veins are frequently used. These are major blood vessels and to avoid ascending infection or loss of patency the line needs to be handled aseptically and kept flushed even when nutrition is not being administered. This is particularly important if the child is mobile and should be emphasised to the parents who have children on long-term PN and are being taught to administer this at home. If the requirement is going to be a long-term one a Hickman or Broviac line may be surgically inserted.

The solution usually needs to be protected from light to prevent the formation of free radicals and should be stored in a refrigerator until preparation is being made for it to be infused. It is usually taken out of the refrigerator approximately 2–4 hours before use, depending on bag size, to bring the solution up to room temperature.

There are a number of standard PN 'recipes' commercially available, but many pharmacies augment these according to the individual child's requirements. Different feeding regimes are advocated; some try to replicate the normal peaks and troughs that would be experienced if the child was on a normal bolus diet; others try and maintain a status quo.

There is a range of sophisticated infusion devices and filters available for use with PN and these detect air emboli to prevent these from entering the child's circulation. For children who are ambulant, small battery-powered packs available.

There are a number of reasons why PN might be necessary:

- The child is severely undernourished.
- As support following extensive surgery, radiotherapy or chemotherapy.

- The child is in a hypercatabolic state following severe burns.
- The child cannot absorb nutrients or suffers from chronic diarrhoea and vomiting;
- The gut is too immature or insufficient.
- The gut is paralysed (e.g. after major surgery).
- The child is unconscious and enteral feeding is not possible.

The decision to commence PN is not taken lightly as there are a considerable number of complications though many of these are preventable:

- Emboli and thrombosis.
- Infection.
- Fluctuations in blood sugar.
- Phlebitis.
- Cholestasis.

The reason for some of these is that catheter remains in place for a relatively long time and the body has the capacity to recognise foreign materials and acts defensively with fibrin deposits or blood clots that can obscure the line. As these lines can be critical to survival these are serious complications (Chwals 2006; Kakzanov et al. 2008).

Children with long lines and who are having TPN have a higher risk of sepsis (Beghetto et al. 2005), especially those who are already immunocompromised. Children who have prolonged exposure to PN are at risk of PN-associated cholestasis and intestinal failure-associated liver disease (IFALD), and this has a high mortality and morbidity (Willis et al. 2010). In part this is because it may have progressed to a fairly advanced stage by the time it becomes evident via laboratory or physical signs. Woodward and colleagues (2009) recommend MRI scanning of the liver to pick up early indicators of damage. (For consideration of infection of the long line and septic shock, see Chapter 8.)

Managing swings in blood sugar

Insulin may sometimes be added to the PN but more commonly it is administered by a separate infusion. Sometimes a change in the way the PN is administered can be effective. Sometimes the recipe might need to be changed. The children's nurse needs to remain aware that an unstable blood sugar can be an indication of sepsis as well as poor tolerance of the PN prescription.

Phlebitis

This is inflammation of the vein and is usually associated with blood clots but with PN it can be the lining of the vein's reaction to the chemical stimulus of the solution. The signs and symptoms are often nonspecific; there may be redness along the track of the vein if a large peripheral vessel was used; or there may be a burning pain or a low-grade fever. This is a serious complication.

Cholestasis

Bile is a secretary function of the liver. Cholestasis means that bile does not flow from the gallbladder into the intestine. This may be a result of lack of intestinal stimulus to trigger its release. The metabolic complications of this are considered in Chapter 7.

Management of TPN at home

Unstable children are not nursed at home; however an increasing number of technology-dependent but otherwise stable children who used to occupy ITU cots can be transferred to the community with help and support. Many will require PN. The aim of domiciliary PN is to keep children alive and well and able to enjoy as normal a life as possible. They should, where possible, be independent and mobile between infusions. Success depends on the commitment of the family and a stable and secure home. The parents need to have a reasonable understanding of the rationale behind asepsis and they need good communication skills to act as advocates for their child when needed. As setting up infusions can be fiddly they will need considerable manual dexterity. Even given favourable circumstances, with excellent support and care most children are readmitted to hospital because of some complication such as an infection, or displacement or blockage of the catheter.

Future options

There is a range of surgical options in conserving or increasing the surface area of the intestine for absorption. Specific strategies include the STEP procedure (see Chapter 8).

Acknowledgements

The editors would like to thank Jan Murphy and Jill Cochrane, co-authors of a previous chapter on high dependency nursing, on which this chapter is based. A full acknowledgement is given to the staff at Birmingham Children's Hospital for sharing aspects of their good practice with us, and to Martin and Cox who constructed the original flow chart to progress feeding.

References

Advanced Paediatric Life Support Group (APLS). 2005. Advanced Paediatric Life Support: the practical approach (4th edition). London: BMJ Publishing Group.

Alexander JW. 1999. Is early enteral feeding of benefit? Intensive Care Medicine, 25:129–30.

Avitsland TL, Kristensen C et al. 2006. Percutaneous endoscopic gastrostomy in children: a safe technique with major symptom relief and high parental satisfaction. Journal of Pediatric Gastroenterology and Nutrition, 43(5):624–8.

Babett C. 2007. Transpyloric feeding in the pediatric intensive care unit. Journal of Pediatric Gastroenterology and Nutrition, 44(5):646–9.

Bailey B, Gravel J et al. 2010. External validation of the clinical dehydration scale for children with acute gastroenteritis. Academic Emergency Medicine, 17(6):583–8.

Bankhead R, Boullata J et al. 2009. ASPEN enteral nutrition practice recommendations. Journal of Parenteral and Enteral Nutrition, 33(2):122–67.

Beghetto M, Victorino J et al. 2005. Parenteral nutrition as a risk factor for central venous catheter–related infection. Journal of Parenteral and Enteral Nutrition, 29(5):367–73.

Brown D, Miedema B et al. 1995. Safety of early feeding after percutaneous endoscopic gastrostomy. Journal of Clinical Gastroenterology, 21:330–1.

Choudhry U, Barde C et al. 1996. Percutaneous endoscopic gastrostomy: a randomized prospective comparison of early and delayed feeding. Gastrointestinal Endoscopy, 44:164–7.

Chwals W. 2006. Vascular access for home intravenous therapy in children. Journal of Parenteral Enteral Nutrition, 30(1):65–9.

Dixon M, Crawford D et al. 2009. Nursing the Highly Dependent Child or Infant: A manual of care. Singapore: Wiley-Blackwell.

Frankenfield D, Ashcraft C. 2011. Estimating energy needs in nutrition support patients. Journal of Parenteral and Enteral Nutrition, 35(5):563–70.

Galt L, Josephson R. 1982. Stability and osmolality of a nutritional food supplement during simulated nasogastric administration. American Journal of Hospital Pharmacy, 39:1009–12.

Kakzanov V, Monagle P, Chan C. 2008. Thromboembolism in infants and children with gastrointestinal failure receiving long-term parenteral nutrition. Journal of Parenteral and Enteral Nutrition, 32(1):88–93.

Martin L, Cox C. 2000. Enteral feeding practice guidelines. Paediatric Nursing, 12(1):28–33.

McCance K, Huether, S. 2002. Pathophysiology: the biologic basis for disease in adults and children (4th edition). Missouri: Mosby.

Mehta N, Bechard L et al. 2009. Cumulative energy imbalance in the pediatric intensive care unit: role of targeted indirect calorimetry. Journal of Parenteral and Enteral Nutrition, 33(3):336–44.

Mehta N, Compher C. 2009. ASPEN clinical guidelines: nutrition support of the critically ill child. Journal of Parenteral and Enteral Nutrition, 33(3):260–75.

Moules T, Ramsey J. 1998. Textbook of Children's Nursing. London: Stanley Thornes.

National Patient Safety Agency (NPSA)/ NHS. 2011. Reducing the harm caused by misplaced nasogastric feeding tubes in adults, children and infants. http://www.nrls.npsa.nhs.uk/alerts/?entryid45=129640

Pearson, G. 2002. Handbook of Paediatric Intensive Care. London: WB Saunders.

Porth C, Matfin G. 2004. Essentials of Pathophysiology: Concepts of altered health states. Philadelphia: Lippincott, Williams & Wilkins.

Premji S, Chessell L. 2007. Continuous nasogastric milk feeding versus intermittent bolus milk feeding for premature infants less than 1 500 grams (review). The Cochrane Library. Onlinelibrary.wiley.com/doi/10.1002/14651858. CD001819/pdf/standard.

Rhoney D, Parker D et al. 2002. Tolerability of bolus versus continuous gastric feeding in brain-injured patients. Neurological Research, 24(6):613–20.

Sánchez C, Lopez-Herce J et al. 2007. Early transpyloric enteral nutrition in critically ill children. Nutrition, 23(1):16–22.

Singh NC. 1997. Manual of Pediatric Critical Care. Philadelphia: WB Saunders.

Willis T, Carter B et al. 2010. High rates of mortality and morbidity occur in infants with parenteral nutrition-associated cholestasis. Journal of Parenteral and Enteral Nutrition, 34(1):32–7.

Woodward J, Priest A et al. 2009. Clinical application of magnetic resonance spectroscopy of the liver in patients receiving long-term parenteral nutrition. Journal of Parenteral and Enteral Nutrition, 33(6):669–76.

World Health Organisation (WHO). 2002. Infant and Young Child Nutrition: Global strategy on infant and young child feeding. Apps.who.int/gb/archive/pdf_files/WHA55/ea5515.pdf.

Further reading

Lissauer T, Clayden, G. 2011. Illustrated Textbook of Paediatrics (4th edition). London: Elsevier.

Chapter 13
MANAGEMENT OF PAIN AND SEDATION IN INTENSIVE CARE

Doreen Crawford[1] and Michaela Dixon[2]

[1] School of Nursing and Midwifery, Faculty of Health and Life Sciences, De Montfort University, Leicester, UK
[2] Paediatric Intensive Care Unit, Bristol Royal Hospital for Children, University Hospitals Bristol NHS Foundation Trust, Bristol, UK

Introduction

This chapter focuses infants, children and young people who need management of their pain and who may be sedated in order to facilitate aspects of their care. Nurses are reminded of the need to practise within the code of professional conduct (NMC 2008) and adhere to both local frameworks and the standards for medicines administration (NMC 2007) although it should be noted that these standards are generic and not paediatric-specific.

The care of infants and children needs to be holistic, they may be in hospital for the duration of their illness or they may have shared care packages involving community specialists and come into hospital for varying lengths of time, for specific interventions or during crises. They may have intricate treatment protocols or infusions of complex pharmacology running as part of their care requirements, but they are first and foremost children and require all the special psychosocial considerations appropriate for their age.

The neurophysiological framework by which infants and children feel pain is considered. This may be anatomically similar to adults' but the interpretation and the meaning of the event is unique to the child. There are many definitions of pain. An acceptance that pain is what the person says it is (McCaffery 1980) is a useful definition for the children's nurse when dealing with communicative children in the ward or in high dependency areas as it makes allowance for the fact that the pain experience need not be proportional to the degree of observable injury or disease to cause distress. This definition has limitations when dealing with children in intensive care or when dealing with younger less articulate individuals and infants.

There are also the more biological definitions and there is increasing understanding of how pain is processed. Pain as a perceptive experience differs between children and young people and there are further difficulties in managing the pain of the preverbal and questionably cognitive patient.

Quite possibly pain, distress and discomfort should always be assumed in the children's intensive care unit (ICU), unless the patient indicates otherwise. Certainly, until evidenced otherwise it might be good practice to assume that any admission to a strange, noisy environment such as the CICU is likely to increase the pain and distress and plan care accordingly. However, severe, unremitting and unbearable pain in a highly dependent child or critically sick child is not exclusive to the ICU areas and pain and distress can affect children in many areas, including at home.

Pain as a vital sign

Pain can be regarded as a special sensory response (it is the end product of a sense). It can be regarded as a normal function and a normal reaction to wholly abnormal circumstances. Acute pain has a role in the body's protection, maintenance and defence. A normal response and reaction to a stimulus which causes acute pain is spontaneous withdrawal and this is learned from infancy. Sociocultural, developmental and psychological factors influence how the individual responds. Pain can impede recovery as distressed states use calories and create a hormonal imbalance. At its most primitive, the response to pain is reflexive. Finer interpretation of the stimulus, its localisation and identification requires the functioning of a remarkable and imperfectly understood structure – the nervous system.

Development of the nervous system

Potentially the most complex system, development of the nervous system is summarised in Table 13.1 (see also Chapter 7).

The biology behind the nervous system

The nervous system is responsible for an individual's ability to react to their environment as well as respond to internal triggers. It is a network of complex structures which can receive, emit and transmit electrochemical signals between tissues, organs and systems. The nervous system functions as a unified whole but for convenience is divided into the central nervous system (CNS) and peripheral nervous system (PNS).

The CNS comprises the brain and the spinal cord encased and protected by the skull and spine. The PNS consists of nerve tissue outside the brain and spinal cord. These are nerve bodies/ganglia not entirely encased in the skull and spine and include the 12 pairs of cranial nerves and the 31 pairs of spinal nerves. Some of the cranial nerves are highly specialised and critical to the function of the senses of taste, sight, hearing and smell. The PNS is differentiated into afferent and efferent pathways.

Neural transduction and transmission is complex, but put simply means that ascending nerves carry information impulses to the brain and the descending nerves carry information and impulses from the brain to muscle tissue and glands and so effect the nervous system's response. Affecters and effecters are specialist neurones and the reader is advised to refer to an anatomy and physiology text such as those listed in the reference section to further augment their understanding.

The nervous system is divided into branches representative of their function, each complementary and working synergistically with the CNS and PNS. The autonomic nervous system is also subdivided into sections; the nerves of the sympathetic and parasympathetic have a primary role in regulating the individual's internal homeostasis.

The autonomic nervous system exerts control mainly by involuntary action, which in health does not impact on the conscious awareness of the individual.

Components of the nervous system

The nervous system comprises two basic types of cell: the neurones (Figure 13.1) and the supporting cells such as the neuroglial cells. Neurones vary in size from micrometres to about a 1 metre (i.e. the length of the spine in a young adult) and their shape and complexity differ with function and location. Generally speaking, the neurones do not have direct access to good capillary networks and receive nutrients such as glucose more indirectly. Neurone axons may be covered in a fatty sheath which acts as an insulator. Gaps in this covering allow ions to flow at these intermittent junctions rather than along its full length. This is thought to increase velocity.

The covering of the axons take place according to a developmental timetable and may be incomplete at birth. The interpretation of this knowledge led to some postulating that infants could not feel pain as their nervous system was immature. It is now accepted that the absence of a myelin sheath does not impede the transmission of stimuli, which will then be perceived and experienced as pain. Foetuses and preterm infants from 24 weeks of gestation have a fully functional nociceptor system (Lee et al. 2005; Wolf 1999).

Neurones are categorised according to the number of branches they have. Unipolar have one process, bipolar two and multipolar several. Generally, sensory neurones transmitting information to the CNS are unipolar and motor neurones transmitting information away from the CNS are multipolar.

Developmental aspects of the central nervous system

Neurones in the CNS do not regenerate. More neurones than are required are initially formed and some continue to divide following birth, with clear implications for

Table 13.1 Embryological and foetal development of the central nervous system and spinal cord

Gestational age	Tissue and structure development
Embryonic period, gastrulation Days 15–17	Gastrulation refers to the trilaminar period. The formation of the primitive streak is one of the signs. Cells along this streak migrate towards the interior (ingression), which results in the formation of three layers: the endoderm, mesoderm and ectoderm. A thickening of the ectoderm forms the neural plate.
Neurulation Days 18–26	A cluster of cells central to the neural plate become columnar, giving the appearance of a groove and linear crests, rather like guttering. These crests progressively fold towards each other and when the edges come into contact, fuse to form the neural tube. This eventually becomes the brain and the spinal cord. Complete closure of the neural tube takes about 4–6 days. During the early part of the neurulation stage the neural tube is fused except for a small posterior neuropore and a larger anterior neuropore. The anterior neuropore will eventually subdivide into three vesicles representing the forebrain, midbrain and hindbrain. The anterior neuropore closes by day 24. The posterior neuropore closes by day 26. Ectodermal cells from the margins of the neural tube detach to form dorsal clusters of cells called neural crest cells. These migrate peripherally to become sensory ganglia cranial and spinal nerves, etc.
Early brain development Weeks 4–6	The complex nature and shape of the human brain is determined during embryogenesis by flexures that result from bursts of rapid cell proliferation within the confines of the cranial vault. During the three-vesicle stage, representing the forebrain (prosencephalon) midbrain (mesencephalon) and hindbrain (rhombencephalon), the three-part brain is C-shaped. By week 5 the forebrain gives rise to the paired telencephalic vesicles which will eventually become the cerebral hemispheres and the diencephalon from which develop the optic vesicles. The midbrain remains tubular and undivided. The rhombencephalon (hindbrain) subdivides into the metencephalon and a more caudal myelencephalon. By week 6, the cellular growth in a restricted area has resulted in the formation of the cephalic flexure, the pontine flexure and the cervical flexure. The metencephalon will form the pons and the myelencephalon will eventually form the medulla oblongata By weeks 5 and 6 all the cranial nerves (except the optic and the olfactory) are recognisable.
Week 8	A period of rapid differentiation and neuroblast multiplication of the brain and spinal cord. By week 8 a cross-section of the cord would reveal the characteristic butterfly shape of grey matter. A primitive spinal reflex arc is present. The lateral walls of the spinal cord thicken leaving a longitudinal groove which extends the full length of the spinal cord and into the midbrain. The divided grey matter forms dorsal and ventral plates. These plates signal the location of sensory and motor neurones and will eventually result in the sophisticated network of afferent and efferent neurones which will receive, transmit and respond to stimuli. The ventricular system is established early from the division of the telencephalon.
Weeks 12–20	Rapid vascularisation occurs. The ventricles are well-defined, C-shaped structures. A rich capillary network develops on the roof of the midbrain and hindbrain which will become the choroid plexus and will secrete the cerebral spinal fluid which will bathe the CNS. Rapid growth in restricted space forces the developing cerebral hemispheres to shroud and cover the midbrain. Initially, the cerebral cortex is smooth. Neurones start to myelinate. After 18 weeks neurones no longer divide. Surface area landmarks of the brain are increasingly identifiable. Neurones for nociception located in dorsal root ganglion.

Table 13.1 (*Continued*)

Gestational age	Tissue and structure development
Weeks 21–24	Density of cortical plate synapses increases. Rapid growth of cerebral hemispheres causes convolution of the cortex and form sulci and gyri increasing the surface area. Rapid increase in neurone cytoplasm gives rise to increase in cell size.
Borderline viability–term	As gestation progresses cortical plate matures into the six layers of cerebral cortex. Pain experience elicits typical facial expression. Rapid myelination occurs and will continue into the postnatal period.

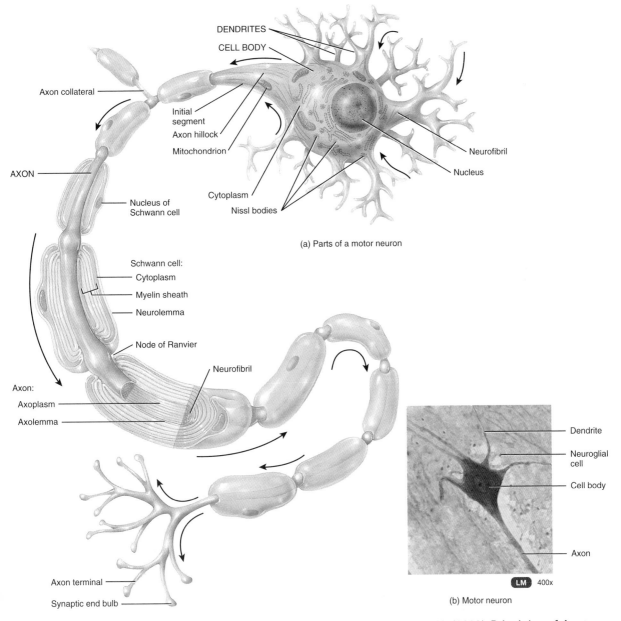

(a) Parts of a motor neuron

(b) Motor neuron

Figure 13.1 Structure of a neurone. From Tortora, G. J. and Derrickson, B. H. (2009) *Principles of Anatomy and Physiology*, 12th edn. Reproduced with permission from John Wiley and Sons, Inc.

early oxygenation and nutrition. If these neurones are not used and become part of a functional system they will die and this has possible implications for neonatal and infant experiences. Axons have limited capacity to repair, but successful function following injury depends on the type of injury and location of lesion. The formation of scar tissue, which is an end product of repair, can impede transmission. The olfactory neurones in the nose are unique in that they continue to divide and are replaced throughout life.

How nervous tissue works

Neurones are not passive; they generate and respond to electrochemical impulses by selectively changing the electrical charge over their membranes. All body cells are polarised, with the inside of the cell more negatively charged than the outside. This difference is due to the composition of the intracellular fluid compared to the composition of the extracellular fluid. There is more potassium inside the cells than outside and more sodium outside the cells; this difference is maintained by active transport on the surface of the cell membrane. Understanding this at its most basic level means that when this equilibrium is disturbed above a threshold the neurone depolarises and the signal transmitted along the axon. Most sensory nerve fibres are unimodal in that they respond to one type of stimulus (e.g. sound waves or light intensity). The afferent nerve fibres of the PNS are different in several respects; they are polymodal and have the ability to respond to mechanical, chemical or thermal reception stimuli. Once this information is transported to the CNS at the level of the spinal cord it means a variety of stimuli can be responded to and there is some ability to discern between degrees of intensity as they have complex multi-transduction channels which can distinguish between different forms of stimulation and between intensities (McCance and Huether 2006). The spinal cord is a long, thin, tubular bundle of nerve tissue and support cells which extends from the medulla oblongata to the lumbar vertebrae. It is the pathway for information connecting the brain to the peripheral nervous system. In cross-section the cord consists of white matter tracts containing sensory and motor neurons and a grey, butterfly-shaped central region made up of nerve cell bodies. The spinal cord is bathed in cerebrospinal fluid.

Δ (delta) and C fibres are regarded as first-order neurones for the detection of acute pain. The transmission of stimuli from these fibres can be transmitted up the spinothalamic tract for interpretation by the third- and higher-order neurones in the cerebral cortex, reticular and limbic areas of the brain, a little like a hierarchy of people passing on important messages to the management team. Understanding the essentials of this puts into perspective the value of the gate theory of pain first proposed by Melzack and Wall (1965).

Once neurones have fired there is a period of readjustment, called the refractory period, during which the neurone cannot fire again. In some cases (e.g. following an inflammatory response) cells can be regarded as hypopolarised and be more excitable than normal, as it takes less to trigger a signal. This hyperalgesia state has direct implications for the transmissions of signals which go on to be perceived as pain and for the management of it, as this state can prove to be very resistant to treatment.

Neurones do not physically connect, although they are in close proximity. The gaps between them are called synapses, with impulses being transmitted across the gaps by electrochemical messengers (Figure 13.2). Transmission occurs by chemical neurotransmitters, which are synthesised and stored by the neurones and released on instruction into the synaptic cleft. These chemicals pass across the synapse to reach a postsynaptic membrane and, depending on the level of excitation, have the potential to transmit the signal onwards.

Neurotransmitters

Substances which function as neurotransmitters continue to be identified. Some are chains of amino acids, some are recognised as hormones, and it is apparent that some have several roles, which vary according to location. For example, norepinephrine can be both excitatory and inhibitory. Some have direct pain implications such as the neuropeptides, the endorphins and the encephalins, which are widely distributed throughout the CNS and the PNS. The increasing understanding of what happens in the synapse will potentially result in more selective analgesics which will be capable of targeting and blocking the passage of stimuli. This will result in suppressing aversive sensations without impeding function; for example, in a limb, pain will be removed but the reception of other information such as the position and temperature of the limb will remain.

The importance of the biochemistry of the synapse is apparent every day in theatre and in ICU as this is the site of action which allows neuromuscular blockade; this permits a state of relaxation to allow intubation and ventilation, overcoming the normal body defence mechanism of cough and gag.

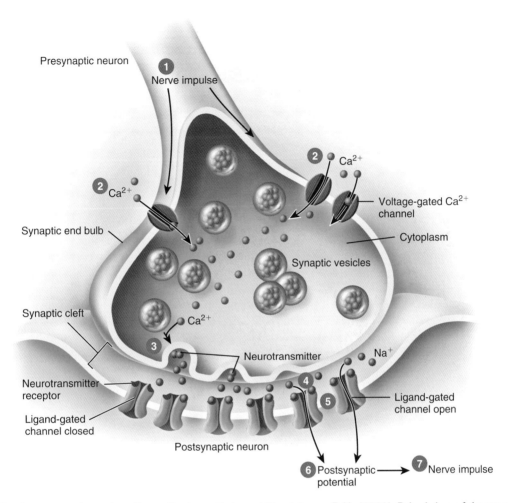

Figure 13.2 A synapse in action. From Tortora, G.J. and Derrickson, B.H. (2009) *Principles of Anatomy and Physiology*, 12th edn. Reproduced with permission from John Wiley and Sons, Inc.

Chemically-induced paralysis takes place at the neuromuscular junction, which is the point where the motor neurones extending from the spinal cord make contact with the muscle fibres. Present, at that point, are the potential transmitters which, if triggered, will result in a muscle contraction. Neuromuscular blocking drugs (Table 13.2) target this action and prevent the transmission of electrical impulses in a number of ways. They can bind with the receptor sites of the neurotransmitters so blocking the normal pathway, or they can compete with the neurotransmitters and bind with the site while not causing a muscle contraction.

The use of paralysing agents in the intensive care environment is vital to maintain an airway, prohibit the normal cough and gag response an endotracheal tube would stimulate and ensure the child will tolerate the tube and not try to breathe against the ventilator. Unfortunately, they make the child very vulnerable and dependent on good nursing care and management. These children need one-to-one nursing and all ventilator pressure alarms set in case of accidental disconnection. In addition, all monitors which record the child's vital signs need to be set within age-appropriate parameters in case of accidental extubation.

Table 13.2 Muscle relaxants used in ITU

Drug	Examples	Actions
Non-depolarising neuromuscular blocking drugs	Aminosteroid group: pancuronium rocuronium vecuronium Benzylisoquinolinium group: atracurium cisatracurium mivacurium.	Non-depolarising neuromuscular blocking drugs have a slow onset and can be classified by the length of time they maintain their action. There is a caveat of dosage. Short-acting: 15–30 minutes. Intermediate-acting: 30–40 minutes. Long-acting: 60–120 minutes. Although the child may be still and apparently sleeping the children's nurse needs to remember that non-depolarising neuromuscular blocking drugs have no sedative or analgesic effects. These are powerful drugs and have complex side-effects. If used, the nurse should refer to the BNF for Children for guidance.
Depolarising neuromuscular blocking drugs	Suxamethonium	This has the fastest onset of action of any of the neuromuscular blocking drugs. Its effect is brief so it is ideal for rapid-sequence induction for tracheal intubation. Most intubation policies give additional agents such as analgesia and atropine before an agent such as suxamethonium.

NB: When muscle relaxants are used in an ICU setting it is good practice to discontinue them every 24 hours so that the level of sedation and analgesic can be assessed.
Source: BNF for Children 2011–12.

Biology of pain and sedation

The understanding of pain is incomplete and research continues to build on current knowledge. At present there is a consensus that there are two types of acute pain: fast and slow. The perception of fast pain occurs almost instantly. It is precisely located, unique in character and identified by sudden sharp, pricking sensations. In contrast, slow pain is of later onset, perhaps a second or so after the initial stimulus. The unpleasant situation builds and escalates in intensity, becoming burning, aching and/or throbbing. It is less easy to localise and in some cases may be referred (Jenkins et al. 2006). Relating the biology to the perception of pain is called nociception and depends on the intact functioning of the nervous system. The biology may be clear-cut but the individual's experience of pain is less so. To counter pain experience and manage the clinical situation, pharmacological, cognitive strategies and holistic strategies should be employed in a multimodal approach.

The stimulus of acute pain is transmitted in two pathways: via a three-neurone system to the cerebral hemisphere on the opposite side of brain from the pain location and by a two-neurone system transmitting the stimulus to the cerebral hemisphere on the same side of the brain to

the sensation (Waugh and Grant 2006). For pain to be experienced the following sequence has to take place:

- There has to be an event, a stimulus and a trigger strong enough to fire a receptor neurone. This stimulus will travel by neurone 1 to the spinal cord by the posterior route.
- Once in the spinal cord decussation takes place; this can be compared to a circuit, with some messages being transported via one route and other messages by another. At this level it can be seen why some impulses generate a crude reflex withdrawal and others are conveyed for more precise interpretation.
- These impulses are transmitted via the anteriorolateral spinothalamic tract to the thalamus and neurone 3, where processing at the perceptual level can begin (Marieb 2004).

Pain processing

Neurone 3 conducts the stimulus to the higher brain centres of the limbic system and the cerebral cortex. Areas of the cerebral cortex correspond to parts of the body and these

Table 13.3 Linking biology to the clinical interpretation of a child's pain

Aspect of pain	Implication for the child
Pain threshold	The level at which the stimulus will exceed sensory tolerance and be perceived as pain. This seems not to vary much among individuals or in the same person over time.
Perceptual dominance	The phenomenon which seeks to explain why an individual with several sites of pain focuses on the most extreme pain experience.
Pain tolerance	The duration of time in which an individual will tolerate pain until prompted to seek relief. This varies considerably among individuals and within an individual over time.
Radicular pain	The pain which arises from a major nerve and is felt along the distribution of the nerve.
Referred pain	The pain perceived in an area removed from its point of origin. The point of origin is mainly visceral and is thought to occur as a result of the internal organs having few sensory nerves.
Incidence pain	Occurs when pain is provoked or intensified by movement or activity.

areas are probably responsible for the interpretation of what is perceived as pain. In an instant this is matched with previous experiences – the stored memories of pain. The pain stimulus is, in essence, made sense of and placed in context. There is also an understanding of what the individual's pain experience might mean to an outside observer and further lightning-quick networking influences decision-making about how the individual should react. This is conscious processing and is complex. (For greater understanding refer to texts in anatomy and physiology.) For children, there are fewer memories and less experience on which to draw, resulting in fewer learned clues on how to react. These factors account for the wide variety of pain responses and behaviours seen in children.

For the preterm and young infant there may be no previous experience and stored data on which to draw. There is significant debate as to the reception and perception of pain in the foetus (Fitzgerald 1995; Glover and Fisk 1996; Harrison 1996; James 1998; Lee et al. 2005). This debate could be extrapolated to include the extremely preterm infant (Slater et al. 2006). What can be accepted is that preterm and neonatal pain is physiologically disruptive and impacts on physiological stability as it occurs at a time when the infant is developmentally unprepared for the stimulus. Exposure to stimuli resulting in pain may promote a heightened peripheral sensitivity or dampen down the normal expected behavioural responses to pain indicative of altered development (Anand and Hall 2006). Neonatal nursing textbooks cover the topic extensively but it is astounding that, in some textbooks of neonatal medicine, pain is not found in the index. From a children's nurse perspective, an additional worry is the fact that children vary in their ability to develop the concept of

time and infants have no concept of time; accordingly, they do not have the ability to understand that the experience they are suffering is usually temporary and time-limited. Table 13.3 demonstrates the links between biology and practice.

Pain classifications

The terms nociceptive pain and non-nociceptive pain are an attempt to classify pain using biology as a basis and create a taxonomy aimed at understanding the condition usually from a mechanical perspective.

Nociceptive pain or non-nociceptive pain

Nociceptive pain originates from cell damage, resulting in the release of inflammatory mediators; these bathe and sensitise the nociceptors which activate the pain cascade (Butcher 2004). Nociceptive pain can be superficial, from the skin, subcutaneous tissue or mucous membranes and can be characterised by a well-localised, sharp, pricking and throbbing experience (Butcher 2004) or may be somatic, from the deeper tissues such as muscle tendons and joints. This is less well localised and is characterised by aching, gnawing and constant pain. Visceral pain results from affected organs, causing sensations of deep, dull, dragging spasms or squeezing, colicky pain and is frequently associated with vomiting and alterations in vital signs (Butcher 2004).

Non-nociceptive pain, such as neuropathic pain, can vary in nature and severity. This pain is often caused by over-sensitisation of the nerves and is frequently associated with numbness or paraesthesia (Butcher 2004). The symptoms of which the patient complains reflect the nerve fibre affected. Burning and itching indicate that the C fibres are the causative nerves, whereas colour and temperature changes are a result of activity of the B fibres (Butcher 2004).

Acute or chronic pain

Pain is further divided into chronic and acute pain in an attempt to define it according to a time frame. Chronic pain is usually defined as pain which persists for 3 months beyond the usual course of an acute disease or reasonable time for an injury to heal or is associated with a chronological pathological process which causes continuous pain, or pain which recurs at intervals for months or years. Prolonged pain is disabling and can interfere with physical functioning (Shaw 2006).

From a clinical perspective there can be problems with all the information summarised in previous sections. Nurses seek to interpret what information is elicited from the assessment of an individual but this is complicated when the child is cognitively impaired (Dowling 2004), pre-verbal or sedated. Signs, symptoms and a history of the event will assist, but the most effective pain assessment requires qualitative as well as quantitative analysis.

Signs and symptoms of pain

- Pain behaviour (may be socioculturally variable).
- Anxiety, vocal distress and facial expression.
- Tachycardia – elevated heart rate/pulse greater than developmental norm.
- Tachypnoea – elevated respiratory rate greater than developmental norm.
- Fixed body posture and muscle tension.
- Potential for alternation in blood gas.
- Hypertension.
- Diaphoresis – evidence of sweating (e.g. beads of perspiration on upper lip).
- Elevated temperature.
- Elevated metabolic rate.
- Hyperglycaemia.
- Gastrointestinal disturbance.

In chronic pain many of the signs and symptoms of pain maybe unaltered, making assessment more complex. The administration of an analgesic may not be sufficient to control the sensation or make the experience manageable. In these cases there may be a need to use a joint approach with careful use of sedation.

Assessing a child's need for sedation

There are many validated tools for assessing an infant's or child's pain. There are fewer to assess the level of sedation

(Bennett 2003). Sedation may be understood as a substance which works by producing a depression of the CNS; the greater the degree of depression the deeper the sedation. Sedation is required in the ICU as part of a strategy to prevent ICU syndrome (Baker 2004). Arguably the distress caused by childhood exposure to 'healthcare' can adversely affect an individual for the remainder of their life (Young 2000). There is some overlap between distress and pain and this has led to the development of joint sedation and pain tools such as the Nottingham Score (Bennett 2003a).

Crying and facial expression are universal indicators of distress in infants and very young children and some pain tools have utilised these very effectively, for example, the use of neonatal facial coding system (NFCS) developed by Grunau and Craig (1990) used a range of facial expressions based on recognised responses to pain: open mouth, lip stretch, taut tongue, eye squeeze and brow furrow. However, in some clinical conditions facial expression is impaired. This is also the case if the child is effectively sedated and would complicate assessment if a muscle relaxant had been used. Extrapolating from this, facial expression is not always a reliable indicator of comfort in the care of HD children. The appearance of a sleep state may give the erroneous assumption of comfort. In these circumstances the multidisciplinary team has little alternative but to focus on the physiological indications of pain and distress.

Sedation and analgesics are provided according to unit protocol and emerging clinical standards and the child continually monitored for any indication of breakthrough distress or pain. There is some evidence that there is scope for improvement in the way sedation is practised in children's hospitals (Babl et al. 2006). Sedatives are powerful drugs and can be an extremely useful mechanism for ensuring a child's cooperation and are used in many areas of a hospital if a temporary quiet state is required for the duration of a procedure (Ruddle 2003).

However, the use of sedation is not without risk. It should be remembered that when these agents are employed children need continuous monitoring and supervision and should be regarded as high dependency children. Vital signs can be used to monitor physiological stability and may provide an indication of improvement or recovery. Continual monitoring can provide the nurse with information on the health status of the child but a further, less quantifiable indicator is developed through experience and involves a level of informed intuition. This is what Benner (1984) alluded to and it does not sound very scientific but the multidisciplinary care team can take some confidence in their combined years of clinical experience and an awareness that they are all calling on different assessment skills for the comfort of the child. At the same time, the team needs to be mindful that the physiological indicators (e.g. heart rate and blood pressure) can vary for a myriad of reasons and that a child experiencing unrelieved distress and pain cannot stay in a heightened state of arousal indefinitely, as their body systems will seek to achieve a balance and compensate. This biologically compensated status might result in the impression that the child is distress and pain free.

The child who requires invasive modes of respiratory support will also require infusions of muscle relaxants, sedation and analgesics. There is significant interest in the development and validation of a universal sedation scoring system (Table 13.4) and this will need to be used in combination or adjacent to a pain tool. Sedation assessments like pain tools seek to measure a patient's status but like the pain tool, measurement is not without difficulty as the data harvested cannot be quantified as interval or ratio. Assessment and measurement are complicated by the fact that there is significant subjectivity between assessors and this can be influenced by a nurse's and doctor's attitude to pain and distress and what they are inclined to do about it (Grap et al. 2006; de Lima et al. 1996; Melhuish and Payne 2006; Razmus and Wilson 2006).

The higher the score the less well sedated the child is, but low scores are not necessarily indicative of good sedation. The child must be assessed against their entire clinical picture and every other detriment to a child's comfort taken into account, such as the risk of urine retention through

Table 13.4 Example of a simple sedation scoring chart

Situation	Score
Unresponsive/hypotonic on handling	1
Moving or reacting to suctioning or major handling procedures	2
Moving and reacting to handling but poorly coordinated	3
Moving spontaneously with some coordination; can be roused by voice	4
Moving spontaneously with good coordination will respond to directions	5
Awake but settled and relaxed	6
Irritable	7
Unmanageable	8

immobility and pain (Steggal 2007) or a full postoperative bladder (Cropper 2003) and the need to facilitate optimum positioning (Griffiths and Gallimore 2005).

Pharmacological means of managing a child's distress

As a general principle medicines should only be given to children when necessary and the benefits should be calculated against the risks and side-effects of the medicine. It is good practice to discuss treatment options carefully with the child and family, seek consent and provide choice when possible. However, these elements of good practice are sometimes limited in the ITU.

Many of the more powerful medications prescribed to children in pain and requiring sedation are subject to the Misuse of Drugs Regulations (2001), particularly preparations which are classified under schedules 2 and 3. In hospital, special principles apply to the administration of these medications. Safe storage and rigorous guidelines protect both staff and patients, in addition the supply and continuity of the agents are ensured. In the community, the situation has to be more flexible to allow for travel and holidays, and parents may need to be reminded about safe storage, protocols for keeping adequate supplies and the legal requirements, particularly if travelling abroad.

The pharmacology
Chloral hydrate and triclofos

These are popular hypnotics for use in hospital. They induce sedation and can be used for procedures or to maintain quiescent equilibrium for a short period. Their effects are cumulative and so should be avoided in conditions complicated by renal and hepatic impairment. Children may build up tolerance and dependence and abrupt withdrawal ought to be avoided. They have an unpleasant taste and are gastric irritants. A gastric irritant effect can result in vomiting which leaves the quantity of drug available to sedate the child open to speculation and an alternative plan may need to be in place for vital investigations to take place and avoid the need to cancel scheduled CT and MRI scans (Gray 2002).

In neonates, chloral hydrate is used where sedation is required without analgesia for example, to facilitate a 12-lead ECG or cardiac echo. It should be used with caution in preterm infants as there have been a high number of adverse cardiorespiratory side-effects (Anand and Hall 2006).

Trimeprazine, chlorphenamine and promethazine

These are sedating antihistamines with a relatively short action (promethazine may be active for up to 12 hours).

They are useful for occasional use such as insomnia in hospital or to promote a drowsy, sedated state, but should be used with caution in conditions complicated by renal or hepatic impairment. They have a range of side-effects and in some cases have a paradoxical reaction. Older children may complain of a 'hangover' during the next day.

The benzodiazepines

Benzodiazepines (diazepam, lorazepam and midazolam) are indicated for short-term use (2–4 weeks) as there is a risk of habituation. Like the other sedatives they need to be used with caution in conditions complicated by renal and hepatic impairment. They can cause respiratory depression and drowsiness, which can persist for several hours after the initial administration. They are useful in that they can induce amnesia which is helpful in getting the child to readjust from their stay in HD areas. Lorazepam has a sedative action of 8–12 hours and has a potent anticonvulsant action where first-line medications fail. Midazolam has been the subject of frequent studies and is no longer recommended for sedation in neonates as its use is associated with changes in the cerebral blood flow and haemodynamic instability (Anand and Hall 2006).

Barbituates

Barbiturates such as phenobarbital have no analgesic properties. They are useful either in isolation or in conjunction with other therapies for conditions where there is excess sensitivity and excitability, such as the abstinence syndromes. They have a long history of use in neonates and there is some prescribing confidence but, because of the potential serious side-effects such as hypotension and respiratory depression, infants need close supervision (Anand and Hall 2006).

Nitrous oxide (Entonox)

This is a sweet-smelling, colourless gas associated with anaesthetics but can be used in 50% combination with oxygen to induce procedural analgesic and cooperation without loss of consciousness (Bruce and Franck 2000). It must not be used if a pneumothorax is suspected as it expands in a closed space and would further compromise ventilation. It is increasingly popular for instant and short duration use and is becoming popular with children who need frequent interventions (Williams et al. 2006). Examples of where children would benefit from the use of Entonox include drain removal, clip/suture removal, urethral catheterisation and application of traction, complex dressings and packing of wounds.

Ketamine

In older children this drug has been extensively studied and provides analgesia, sedation and amnesia (Anand and Hall 2006). Ketamine is still occasionally used to induce sub-anaesthetic sedation. The main disadvantage is the risk of hallucinations and nightmares, although children under 16 years are regarded as less at risk. Recovery is relatively slow (BNF for Children 2008). In infants ketamine can cause a slight increase in blood pressure, slight tachycardia and bronchodilation. Further studies are required. Anand and Hall (2006) recommend its use mainly when under approved research protocols.

Pain management

Use of tools for assessment

Because pain is private and subjective, it can only be measured indirectly either by self-report or by observing behaviours which are regarded as universal indicators of pain (Mathews et al. 1993) (the latter are learned behaviours and can be culturally associated and socially influenced). There is now a range of pain tools which can be used to observe infants and children and identify those in pain. These use a variety of assessment methods which are designed to be applied to the different ages and cognitive abilities. These ranges from the preverbal tool FLACC (face, legs, activity, cry, if consolable) (Merkel et al. 1997) and NIPs to the well-known Wong and Barker-type faces scale. The idea has now been adapted and refined following a number of studies (Beyer and Wells 1989; Beiri et al. 1990; Hicks et al. 2001). A useful resource for the nurse studying infants and children's pain assessment tools can be found in the RCN's guidelines (2009).

Many assessment tools require cooperation and are inappropriate for the fully supported child who cannot do this. The ICU scales are more focused on a combination of vital sign recordings and subjective assessment of comfort. They are only as good as the nurses who use them and there are frequently discrepancies between the individual assessors. Each patient should be independently assessed at various points during the day and, although there is some evidence to suggest that nurses with different experiences assesses children differently (Hall, 2002; Twycross 1997), there is little point in taking an assessment and not doing anything about it. There needs to be a plan of action designed to manage the child and this should be discussed from a multidisciplinary perspective in consultation with the parents and then implemented (Garland and Kenny 2006).

Despite the plethora of pain tools and the management of a child's pain having a high profile in the National

Service Framework (NSF, Standard 7, 4.28–4.33), there is evidence that children's pain is still not well addressed. Coles and colleagues (2007) measured compliance in one Strategic Health Authority and if their results are indicative, the national picture is not good. Although all Trusts audited claimed to have and use pain tools, there remained too few paediatric-specific pain teams in practice and the Health Care Commission Report (2007) confirmed that children's pain is still being ignored.

The use of pharmacology

Analgesics are more effective in preventing pain than relieving established pain. Situations which are likely to cause pain and distress to children can often be anticipated and therapy planned and implemented in advance.

Analgesics – first-level therapy

The non-opioid analgesics such as paracetamol and some non-steroidal anti-inflammatory drugs (NSAIDs) do have a role in ICU. If used regularly and prescribed to therapeutic levels, they can be quite effective in the control of pain and discomfort. Individually tailored use of these can often avoid the need for stronger preparations. Paracetamol (acetaminophen) is a useful therapeutic agent and can be administered in a variety of ways avoiding the use of the enteral route where necessary. Paracetamol has rapid action once absorbed, an anti-pyretic effect and does not depress the respiratory drive. Paracetamol has relatively few side-effects and reported adverse effects are rare, but the drug is extremely dangerous in over-dosage and strict adherence to the recommended dose is stressed. A disadvantage is that it has no discernible anti-inflammatory action and so is often used in combination with other agents where this is thought to be beneficial. Many NSAIDs have analgesic action but can also be helpful in other ways as they can reduce inflammation. The pain-relieving properties of these drugs should take effect soon after administration but the anti-inflammatory mode of action may take time to build to its most effective level. Ibuprofen also has an anti-pyretic action which, when given for this, may also improve the overall comfort of the child.

Drugs classified as an NSAID have a similar mode of action: they reduce the metabolism of arachidonic acid to prostaglandins. Arachidonic acid is normally present in cell membranes; it is released when tissues are disturbed by disease process, trauma or irritation. Although prostaglandins do not cause pain in themselves, they sensitise the nerve endings to such an extent that ordinary, non-pain-producing stimulation can result in the perception of pain.

NSAIDs are particularly useful in skeletal conditions – bone, joint and muscle pain. They form the cornerstone of management for rheumatic and arthritic conditions but may also be used for headache, dysmenorrhoea and dental pain.

Side-effects of NSAIDs are numerous and include gastrointestinal disturbances, hypersensitivity and bronchospasm. In general, children seem to tolerate these drugs better than adults and as there are many, if one is not tolerated, another can be tried. Children vary in their individual ability to tolerate and metabolise these agents. If NSAIDs were employed with the therapeutic aim of reducing the pressure caused by swelling or the discomfort from the inflammatory process and seem to be non-effective, a short course of steroids might be tried. The decision to use corticosteroids in children is not taken lightly as there are many serious side-effects and it should be remembered that these agents do not have direct analgesic action, so if anti-inflammatory agents were being used in part for this purpose, the child's painkilling strategy may have to be revised.

Second- and third-level therapy

The moderate and strong analgesic agents codeine and morphine are opioid agonists and these drugs can build up dependence as an unwanted side-effect, but this is not a reason to withhold them from children. There used to be a general reluctance to prescribe opioids to infants because of these risks but MacGregor and colleagues (1998) indicated that there were no differences between children who received morphine and a group that did not. Other studies have suggested that not providing analgesia affects later behaviour and responses to pain (Johnston and Stevens 1996).

Opioids cause respiratory depression, impaired cognitive function, hypotension and gastrointestinal disturbance. Often these side-effects necessitate the use of other agents to treat and manage them, and this can result in a whole host of further potential interactions. When this occurs, child medication becomes complicated.

Opioids have been the subject of extensive research and there is much more to be uncovered. The effect of 'poppy juice' has been known for centuries. For therapeutic and legal reasons the drugs synthesised from the plant have been classified and reclassified as greater understanding occurs. Different synthesised analogues of opium have different actions and this depends on the extent to which they mimic agonist or antagonist action.

Fundamental to the understanding of pharmacology is the appreciation of the difference between agonists and antagonists:

- A neurotransmitter is considered to have agonist activity and initiates a pharmacological effect.
- An agent that is capable of blocking the action of a neurotransmitter is an antagonist.

Both have pharmaceutical roles. However, it does not follow that opioid agents are all agonists and the antidote naloxone hydrochloride is an antagonist. The biochemistry is more complex and there are many receptor types and subtypes. As a consequence, many of the narcotic agents are both receptor agonists and antagonists. This accounts for the varying degrees of action and the differing side-effects of the natural opioids and the synthetic morphine substances. A mixed agonist/antagonist can offer the child analgesia without depressing the respiratory drive and is thought to have less potential for creating dependency.

As opioid-type substances have a relatively short duration of action they are best administered either frequently or continuously in high dependency children. There are a few preparations that are considered to be long-acting such as MST, the sustained-release version of morphine salts. These modified-release preparations are most used in palliative care. Essentially, the total morphine requirements for 24 hours are given in two doses 12 hours apart but plans must be in place for the management of breakthrough pain (British National Formulary for Children 2008).

In general, the more common and minor analgesics should be tried first and their impact assessed before moving on to the stronger drugs, which are more likely to have serious side-effects. Analgesic drugs can be used singularly, in combination with each other or in combination with anti-inflammatory agents or sedation to keep a child comfortable. This progression through the levels of potency can be considered almost as a stepladder, with the common and minor drugs situated on the lower rungs of the ladder and the stronger opioids at the top. In all cases the nurse should employ the most appropriate means of administration.

Many children hate needles and the intramuscular route is usually the last resort. Needle phobia can develop but can be effectively managed (Thurgate and Heppell 2005). Arguably, part of the phobia is the exposure to strangers who have less time to prepare the child or may be perceived as less sympathetic; this makes a good case for nurses to extend their role safely and learn to cannulate (Collins et al. 2006).

The rectal route can be a useful means for administrating medication and the fully sedated child will not be as embarrassed as the conscious child, however the family may need careful preparation. This mode of administration is more common in continental Europe. The principles are the same as any other administration method and this route can be extremely useful where oral administration is not possible and there is limited IV access. Where possible the parents' wishes need to be respected and whenever possible the consent of the child or the family should be obtained and real choices offered (Watt 2003).

One area where medical technology has advanced to the benefit of the patient is in the way medication can be delivered. Intravenous access and infusions have become so common that their use is almost taken for granted. However, the insertion of these can be a source of pain in itself. A topical application of local anaesthetic cream is recommended (Arrowsmith and Campbell 2000) but some of these mixtures have side-effects; the location of application ought to be considered with care and the directions for use should be closely followed (Proudfoot and Gamble 2006). In addition, there are potentially serious side-effects to such access devices (Hamilton 2006a, 2006b) so nurses need to be vigilant and observe the sites closely. It would be ironic that a cannula sited to give pain relief ended up causing pain and distress.

Delivery systems for IV infusion

A simple infusion system can be used for infants and for children who are unable to use a patient-controlled analgesic device (PCA) (Table 13.5). The nurse should titrate to the level of analgesia required with a loading dose, maintain this above minimum effective analgesic concentration (MEAC) with the infusion, aiming to keep side-effects to a minimum, that is, below minimum toxic concentration (MTC). Beware particularly of increasing sedation without undertaking a holistic review of the child. Lower doses are required in young infants due to pharmacodynamic and kinetic differences.

Patient-controlled analgesia (PCA)

PCA is fundamentally different from other means of administration in that patients can exercise control. It represents a paradigm shift in the way a patient's pain is

Table 13.5 Continuous infusion using morphine as an example

Age	Loading doses	Maximum infusion
0–1 month	25 mcg/kg	5 mcg/kg/hr
1–3 months	50 mcg/kg	10 mcg/kg/hr
>3 months	100–150 mcg/kg	40 mcg/kg/hr

Morphine: 1 mg/kg in 50 ml normal saline gives a concentration of 20 mcg/kg/ml.

managed. As technology has become more reliable and the pharmacological solutions more stable, the PCA means of managing pain has become popular and safe. PCA enables the child to control their pain by keeping the analgesic above the MEAC, without waiting for a nurse to administer the analgesic, but also balance this against any side-effects. PCA can be administered intravenously, subcutaneously or by the epidural route, although epidural PCA use is uncommon in children (Llewellyn and Moriarty 2007).

PCA is frequently used in paediatric practice for both postoperative pain control and acute episodes, such as sickle cell crisis and mucositis associated with neutropenia induced by chemotherapy. The technique can be used to augment background analgesia and the child is in control of the bolus on demand as part of postoperative management or anticipated painful procedures. Alternatively, PCA may be used as a means of weaning the child down from stronger continuous infusions, for example in step-down care from ITU. As the analgesic requirement reduces, the device can be used when working the child towards oral maintenance. Weaning is not usually problematic. Local experience suggests that children naturally wean themselves off and frequently request removal of the devices as they become more mobile. However, it does require a clear explanation and reinforcement to the child and family and encourage pre-emptive use. A variety of pumps are available, but essentially they all have the same features: a patient-activated button, a microprocessor-controlled pump that deliver a bolus dose with a timed lockout, and total dose limit given in a fixed period, as a background infusion is usually required in children. There is good evidence of improved efficacy without the increased side-effects. When initiating treatment, adequate analgesia must be established by titrating with an intravenous dose of morphine (Table 13.6).

Patients from the age of 5 years can use the devices safely, but all children will need individual assessment and preparation. Ideally, this will be done by a specialist pain nurse. The preparation of the child is important and the technique is best used with an agreed pain assessment tool. Such cooperation is indicative of the unique trust and sensitivity that can be established between children and their carers.

Nurse-controlled analgesia

NCA is basically a morphine infusion using a PCA pump. It allows the nursing staff to give recorded bolus doses quickly and simply and is used in infants and young children (Table 13.7).

Continuous subcutaneous infusion

CSI can be used to provide an anti-emetic for the effective management of nausea and vomiting (Thompson 2004) or sedation. This can be particularly useful as a short-term procedure when the number of venous sites is limited or inaccessible. The technique, known as hypodermoclysis, was first described in the early 1900s but fell out of favour during the 1960s principally owing to misuse and the increasing safety of intravenous fluid and drug administration (Baura and Bhowmick 2005; Khan and Younger 2007). However, in selected cases for specific substances and with proper preparation the technique could emerge once again to the benefit and ease of management in children and young people who need flexibility in the administration of therapy.

Side-effects of opioids and reversal

All opioids have a similar range of side-effects if given at equal-analgesic doses, though there is marked inter-patient variability. Side-effects include respiratory depression,

Table 13.6 Example of a PCA programme

Patient-controlled analgesia (PCA) morphine

If the pump programme is not within the guidelines, ensure that the reason is documented in the clinical notes and on the audit form.

Morphine 1 mg/kg in 50 ml normal saline gives a concentration of 20 mcg/kg/ml

	<50 kg	>50 kg	Complex pain
Background	6 mcg/kg/hr (i.e. 0.3 ml/hr) on 1st–2nd postoperative day	6 mcg/kg/hour (0.3 ml/hr) on 1st–2nd postoperative day	
Bolus	1 ml (20 mcg/kg) over 1 minute	1 ml (20 mcg/kg) over 1 minute	
Lockout	5 minutes	5 minutes	5 minutes
2 hour maximum	200 mcg/kg/2 hr	12 ml	12 ml

Table 13.7   Example of an NCA programme

Nurse-controlled analgesia (morphine)
Morphine 1 mg/kg in 50 ml normal saline
Gives a concentration of 20 mcg/kg/ml

	Term–1 month (neonate)	1–3 months	>3months
Background	5 mcg/kg/hr	10 mcg/kg/hr	10–20 mcg/kg/hr
Bolus	5 mcg/kg	10–20 mcg/kg	10–20 mcg/kg
Lockout	20 minutes	20 minutes	20 minutes
2 hours maximum	25 mcg/kg/2 hr	50 mcg/kg/2 hr	200 mcg/kg/2 hr

Table 13.8   Common local anaesthetic drugs

Drug	Action
Lidocaine	Short-acting, mainly used in Dental and Accident Departments and for topical analgesia on mucosal surface (e.g. the urethra and oropharynx). Maximum dose 3 mg/kg.
Bupivacaine	This is a long-acting mainstay for local and regional blocks. Maximum dose 2.5 mg/kg. However, there are serious concerns about CNS and cardiac toxicity as most blocks are established in anaesthetised children when signs of impending catastrophe are masked. Neonates are particularly susceptible due to their high cardiac output and low drug-binding capacity, resulting in high peak levels. Unpredictable accumulation due to reduced hepatic metabolism also occurs, so epidural infusions should be limited to 48 hours and at lower rates than for older children.
L-bupivacaine and ropivacaine	Single L/S enantiomers of bupivacaine and propivacaine respectively. They offer a wider therapeutic index than racemic mixtures having less CNS and cardiac toxicity in animal and human models.

sedation, dysphoria, nausea and vomiting, constipation, urinary retention and pruritus. Small infants occasionally become twitchy/jerky on morphine infusions; this may be a sign of excessive dosing and usually responds to stopping the infusion for an hour and restarting at a lower rate.

Naloxone is a specific opioid antagonist at the μ receptor. This can be used to antagonise the opioid side-effects, especially respiratory depression or excessive sedation. The dose (10 mcg/kg repeated every 2–3 minutes) should be titrated to effect to avoid rebound pain, hypertension, cardiac dysrhythmias and (rarely) pulmonary oedema. Smaller doses (0.5mcg/kg) can be used to treat urinary retention and pruritus. An infusion of 0.25–1 mcg/kg/hr reduces recurrent pruritus and resistant nausea without reversing the analgesia.

Antiemetic intravenous agents (e.g. $5HT_3$ antagonists, ondansetron 0.1 mg/kg 8–12 hr, antihistamines, cyclizine 0.1 mg/kg/8 hr, or dexamethasone up to 0.5 mg/kg, maximum 8mg) are often required when opioids are prescribed, especially in adolescent girls and post-strabismus or middle ear surgery. Pruritus is alternatively often treated with the antihistamine chlorpheniramine 0.1 mg/kg/8 hr.

Local anaesthesia

Local anaesthetic techniques are extensively used in paediatric practice (e.g. to prevent needle phobia) by preemptive use of topical local anaesthesia prior to intravenous cannulation and intraoperatively to provide excellent postoperative pain relief (Table 13.8). The use of epidural analgesia has revolutionised postoperative management. It

Table 13.9 Loading dose for epidural 0.5 ml/kg of 0.25% plain bupivacaine

	Epidural solution	Infusion rate	Maximum bupivacaine infusion rate
Neonate	0.1% bupivacaine No adjuvants	0.1–0.25 ml/kg/hr	0.25 mg/kg/hr
Child and adolescent	0.1% bupivacaine	0.1–0.5 ml/kg/hr	0.5 mg/kg/hr
	0.1% bupivacaine with 2 mcg/ml fentanyl	0.1–0.5 ml/kg/hr	maximum of 15 ml/hr
	0.1% bupivacaine with 2 mcg/ml clonidine	0.1–0.5 ml/kg/hr	

is highly effective in controlling acute pain in the lower limbs, pelvis, abdomen and chest (Weetman and Allison 2006). Most epidurals are administered without incident (1:2000) (Llewellyn and Moriarty 2007) but there is a risk of life-threatening complications and safe administration requires an informed, skilled, multi-disciplinary approach (Royal College of Anaesthetists 2004). The general surgical children's wards in district general hospitals sometimes do not have adequate staff levels to observe epidural infusions and this has led to otherwise conscious and stable children being cared for in ICU environments. This will have unfortunate results in the way these children can rest and recover. Sleep and rest are complex phenomena and there is increasing evidence to implicate deprivation in altered healing (Bennett 2003b). The ICU unit is not a tranquil area in which to spend postoperative time and may contribute to a child's emotional distress.

Local blocks

Specific nerve blocks performed during anaesthesia (e.g. penile, ilio-inguinal/ilio-hypogastric, and axillary) for postoperative analgesia lasting 4–24 hours or sometimes in Accident Departments (e.g. femoral, digital to give analgesia for fracture reduction or suturing). A variety of techniques is used to locate nerves, including anatomical landmarks, nerve stimulators or ultrasound imaging. Peripheral blocks are associated with less morbidity and possibly mortality.

Regional

Spinal

Used as a sole technique for high-risk preterm babies undergoing herniotomy or muscle biopsy or as a supplement to general anaesthesia for high-risk neonatal cardiac surgery where it reduces the stress response to surgery better than high-dose opioids.

Epidural

The caudal route is a common single-shot access point for postoperative analgesia during sub-umbilical surgery in children. Dose is 0.5–1.0 ml/kg 0.25% bupivacaine depending on the height of the block required. The duration of the block can be increased by adding preservative-free clonidine (1–2 mcg/kg), ketamine (0.5 mg/kg) or morphine (50 mcg/kg) (Table 13.9).

Postoperative epidural infusions of local anaesthetic, usually with an adjuvant, provides analgesia for 3–4 days after major surgery. An epidural catheter is inserted after induction of general anaesthesia, the level of insertion governed by the site of the surgery, though in young infants some units prefer to use the caudal route and advance the catheter to the appropriate level.

Insertion of a catheter into the epidural space of a child and especially an infant needs a skilled experienced operator. The depth of the space in the newborn is <1 cm (as a general rule 1 mm per kg weight is a useful guide). An 18 G Tuohy needle is most frequently used though a 19 G is required for infants <5 kg. However, this smaller needle comes with a smaller, thin-walled, single end-holed catheter that is liable to kink and leak. The space is identified with a loss of resistance to saline technique (LOR with air has been associated with significant morbidity and deaths). The catheter is usually inserted at the level corresponding to the dermatomal level needed to be blocked. The spinal cord is more caudal at L3 in the infant, so most epidurals other than caudals are inserted at a level where there is a potential for spinal cord damage.

Advantages of regional analgesia

It affords superior analgesia for major surgery compared to opioids, associated with improved respiratory function, less atelectasis, better cough, with a reduction in the requirement for sedation, ventilation and earlier step down from ITU and discharge from hospital.

Contraindications and complications of regional analgesia

These include a lack of patient or parental consent, local infection or untreated systemic sepsis, bleeding or clotting abnormalities, raised intracranial pressure and spinal abnormalities:.

- Bloody tap – potential for epidural haematoma, dural tap +/– post-dural puncture headache, accidental total spinal anaesthesia, direct damage to the spinal cord or nerve roots, infection (including meningitis and epidural abscess), catheter problems, premature loss, kinking, blockage, leaks (very common especially in small infants) and delivery system problems, including drug errors and mistakes in the programming of pumps.
- Profound motor block with analgesia has led to pressure ulcers, profound analgesia may cause delay in compartment syndrome, retention of urine in approximately 20% of children so pre-emptive catheterisation is usually performed intraoperatively. Hypotension is unusual in children <8 years because of reduced peripheral venous volume, reduced sympathetic innervation to legs and less cardiac deceleration compared to adolescents and adults. A reversible Horner's block is not infrequent in a high thoracic epidural but rarely associated with significant respiratory complication.
- Toxic effects of local anaesthetics: Seizures and cardiovascular collapse have been described, especially in infants given excessive initial doses, prolonged infusions or who have received an accidental intravenous injection of local anaesthetic.
- Pharmacological effects of adjuvant drugs: Epidural opioids, clonidine and ketamine may all cause systemic side-effects, though the principal reason for using the epidural route is to use much lower total dose of drug and thereby reduce the incidence of this problem.

The role of the paediatric acute pain team

The use of complex analgesic techniques, including epidural infusions, morphine infusions and PCAs, cannot be achieved safely without the investment of a huge amount of professional time and some capital expense. The development of a multi-professional acute pain team to support these innovations is fundamental to their success. Guidelines on the indication, the prescription of simple analgesic and infusions, the equipment used and especially the level of monitoring should be developed for each institution's needs and facilities. The pain specialist provides education for nursing and medical staff and sees children and their families on a daily basis to review and audit efficacy.

Long-term implications of pain

There is some controversy over the possible or likely long-term effects of pain and distress on survivors of the neonatal unit and the CICU/PICU/HDU. The long-term sequelae of pain events are not fully understood (Taddio and Katz 2005). So in conjunction to analgesics and pain management is the need to be aware that some counselling, behavioural follow-up or psychodynamic therapy may be useful in chronic or unresolved problems, which may follow from the original pain state or as a result of the child's management.

Appendix 13.1 Drugs used for pain management

Drug	Paracetamol	Ibuprofen	Diclofenac	Codeine	Morphine
Dose	Consult BNF Example dose: 1–5 years 20–90 mg/kg in divided doses 6–12 years as above but not to exceed 4 g daily or for longer than 48 hours	Consult BNF Example dose Infant up to 3 months 5 mg/kg 3–4 times daily after feed	Consult BNF Example dose Child 6–18 years Rectal 0.5–1 mg/kg (max 75 mg) 2 times daily up to 4 days	Refer to BNF Example dose Child 1 month–12 years 0.5–1 mg/kg every 4–6 hours max 240 mg daily	Consult BNF Example dose Infant 1–6 months Bolus IV 100–200 mcg/kg Infusion 20–30 mcg/kg/hr
Mode	Oral – tablets, melts or suspensions. Intravenous Rectal	Oral – tablets and suspensions	Oral – tablets and dispersible tablets Rectal	Oral – tablets and syrup Rectal Injection – SC, IM and IV	Oral – tablets and liquid Injection – SC, IM and IV
Physiological effects	Inhibits cyclo-oxygenase in CNS but not in periphery Analgesic but not anti-inflammatory effect	Inhibits cyclo-oxygenase in the periphery gives analgesic and anti-inflammatory effects	Inhibits cyclo-oxygenase in the periphery gives analgesic and anti-inflammatory effects	Acts on opioid receptors in the CNS and the periphery to block pain transmission	Acts on opioid receptors in the CNS and the periphery to block pain transmission
Contraindication/ caution	Hepatic failure	Cardiac failure, Liver disease. Renal impairment. Peptic ulceration. CAUTION: Risk of bronchospasm	Cardiac failure, Liver disease. Renal impairment. Peptic ulceration. CAUTION: Risk of bronchospasm	Hepatic impairment Renal impairment Respiratory conditions and impairment	Raised intracranial pressure Hepatic impairment Renal impairment Respiratory conditions and impairment
Side-effects	Rare occasional rashes. Hepatic failure in very high doses	Gastrointestinal upset nausea hypersensitivity reaction	Gastrointestinal upset nausea hypersensitivity reaction	Respiratory depression Constipation Drowsiness Nausea	Respiratory depression Constipation Drowsiness Difficulty in micturition Nausea and vomiting Flushes and rash

References

Anand K, Hall R. 2006. Pharmacological therapy for analgesia and sedation in the newborn. Archives of Disease in Childhood, 91(6):448–53.

Arrowsmith J, Campbell C. 2000. A comparison of local anaesthetics for venepuncture. Archives of Disease in Childhood, 82(4):309–10.

Babl F, Munro J et al. 2006. Scope for improvement hospital wide sedation practice at a children's hospital. Archives of Disease in Childhood, 91(8):716–17.

Baker C. 2004. Preventing ICU syndrome in children. Paediatric Nurse, 16(10):32–5.

Baura P, Bhowmick B. 2005. Hypodermoclysis; a victim of historical prejudice. Age and Aging, 34(3):215–17.

Beiri D, Reeve R et al. 1990. The faces pain scale for the self-assessment of the severity of pain experienced by children: development, initial validation and preliminary investigation for ratio scale properties. Pain, 41(2):139–45.

Benner P. 1984. From Novice to Expert: Excellence and power in clinical nursing practice. Menlo Park: Addison-Wesley.

Bennett M. 2003a. Guidelines for sedation of the critically ill child. Paediatric Nurse, 15(9):14–18.

Bennett M. 2003b. Sleep and rest in PICU. Paediatric Nurse, 15(1):3–6.

Beyer J, Wells N. 1989. The assessment of pain in children. Pediatric Clinics of North America, 36(4):837–54.

British National Formulary for Children. 2008. London: BMJ Publishing Group.

Bruce E, Franck L. 2000. Self-administered nitrous oxide (entonox) for the management of procedural pain. Paediatric Nursing, 12(7):15–19.

Butcher D (2004) Pharmacological techniques for managing acute pain in emergency departments. Emergency Nurse, 12(1):26–35.

Coles L, Glasper A et al. 2007. Measuring compliance to the NSF for Children and Young People in one English Strategic Health Authority. Journal of Children's and Young People's Nursing, 1(1):7–15.

Collins M, Phillips S et al. 2006. A structured learning programme for venepuncture and cannulation. Nursing Standard, 20(26):34–9.

Cropper J. 2003. Postoperative urine retention in children. Paediatric Nurse, 15(7):15–18.

de Lima J, Lloyd-Thomas A et al. 1996. Infant and neonatal pain, anaesthetists' perceptions and prescribing patterns. British Medical Journal, 313(7060):787.

Dowling M. 2004. Pain assessment in children with neurological impairment. Paediatric Nurse, 16(3):37–40.

Fitzgerald M. 1995. Foetal Pain: an update of current scientific knowledge. London: Department of Health.

Garland L, Kenny G. 2006. Family nursing and the management of pain in children. Paediatric Nursing, 18(6):18–20.

Glover V, Fisk N. 1996. Do foetuses feel pain? British Medical Journal, 313(7060):796.

Grap M, Pickler R, Munro C. 2006. Observation of behavior in sedated, mechanically ventilated children, Pediatric Nurse, 21(5):216–20.

Gray J. 2002. Conscious sedation of children in A&E. Emergency Nurse, 9(8):26–31.

Griffiths H, Gallimore D. 2005. Positioning critically ill patients in hospital. Nursing Standard, 19(42):56–64.

Grunau R, Craig K. 1990. Facial activity as a measure of neonatal pain expression. In DC Tyler and EJ Krane (Eds). Advances in Pain Research and Therapy (Volume 15, pp. 147–55). New York: Raven Press.

Hall J. 2002. Paediatric pain assessment. Emergency Nurse, 10(6):31–3.

Hamilton H. 2006a. Complications associated with venous access devices part 1. Nursing Standard, 20(26):43–9.

Hamilton H. 2006b. Complications associated with venous access devices part 2. Nursing Standard, 20(27):59–65.

Harrison M. 1996. Foetal surgery. American Journal of Obstetrics and Gynaecology, 174(4):1225–64.

Health Care Commission. 2007. Commission for Healthcare Audit and Inspection: improving services for children in hospital. London: Health Care Commission.

Hicks C, Von Baeyer C et al. 2001. The faces pain scale revised, towards a common metric in paediatric pain measurement. Pain, 93(2):173–83.

James D. 1998. Foetal medicine. British Medical Journal, 316(7144):1580–3.

Jenkins G, Kemnitz C, Tortora G. 2006. Anatomy and Physiology from Science to Life (1st edition). New York: Wiley.

Johnston C, Stevens B. 1996. Experience in a neonatal intensive care unit affects pain response. Pediatrics, 98(5):925–30.

Khan M, Younger G. 2007. Promoting safe administration of subcutaneous infusions. Nursing Standard, 21(31):50–6.

Lee S, Ralston H et al. 2005. Foetal pain: a systemic and multidisciplinary review of the evidence. JAMA, 294(8):947–54.

Llewellyn N, Moriarty A. 2007. The National Paediatric Epidural Audit. Paediatric Anaesthesia, 17(6):520–33.

MacGregor R, Evans D et al. 1998. Outcome at 5–6 years of prematurely born children who received morphine as neonates. Archives of Disease in Children. Foetal and neonatal edition, 79(1):40–3.

Marieb E. 2004. Human Anatomy and Physiology (6th edition). San Francisco: Benjamin Cummings.

Mathews, J, McGrath, P, Pigeon H. 1993. Assessment and measurement of pain in children. In NL Schechter, CB Berde, M Yaster (Eds) Pain in Infants, Children and Adolescents (chapter 8). Philadelphia: Williams and Wilkins.

McCaffery M. 1980. Understanding your patient's pain. Nursing, 10(9):26–31.

McCance K, Huether S. 2006. Pathophysiology, the biologic basis for disease in adults and children (5th edition). St Louis, MO: Elsevier Mosby.

Melhuish S, Payne H. 2006. Nurses' attitude to pain management during routine venepuncture in young children. Paediatric Nursing, 18(2):20–3.

Melzack R, Wall P. 1965. Pain mechanisms a new theory. Science, 150(699):971–8.

Merkel S, Voepel-Lewis T, Shayevitz S. 1997. The FLACC: a behavioural scale for scoring postoperative pain in young children. Pediatric Nursing, 23(3):293–7.

Nursing and Midwifery Council (NMC) 2007. Standards for Medicines Management. London: NMC. www.nmc-uk.org.

Nursing and Midwifery Council (NMC) 2008. The Code. Standards of xconduct, performance and ethics for nurses and midwives. www.nmc-uk.org/Nurses-and-midwives/The-code/The-code-in-full.

Proudfoot C, Gamble C. 2006. Site-specific skin reactions to amethocaine. Paediatric Nurse, 19(5):26–8.

Razmus I, Wilson D. 2006. Current trends in the development of sedation/analgesia scales for the pediatric critical care patient. Pediatric Nursing, 32(5):435–41.

Royal College of Anaesthetists. 2004. Good Practice in the Management of Continuous Epidural Analgesia in the Hospital Setting. www.britishpainsociety.org.

Ruddle T. 2003. Sedation, an overview. Paediatric Nursing, 15(1):38–41.

Shaw S. 2006. Nursing and supporting patients with chronic pain. Nursing Standard, 20(19):60–5.

Slater R, Cantarella A et al. 2006. Cortical pain responses in human and infants. Journal of Neuroscience, 26(14):3662–6.

Steggal M. 2007. Acute urinary retention: causes clinical features and patient care. Nursing Standard, 21(29):42–6.

Taddio A, Katz J. 2005. The effects of early pain experience in neonates on pain responses in infancy and children. Paediatric Drugs, 7(4):245–57.

Thompson I. 2004. The management of nausea and vomiting in palliative care. Nursing Standard, 3(19):46–53.

Thurgate C, Heppell S. 2005. Needle phobia – changing venepuncture practice in ambulatory care. Paediatric Nursing, 17(9):15–18.

Tortora GJ, Derrickson BH. 2009. Principles of Anatomy and Physiology, 12th edition. Asia: John Wiley and Sons.

Twycross A. 1997. Nurses' perception of pain in children. Paediatric Nursing, 9(1):17–19.

Watt S. 2003. Safe administration of medicines. Paediatric Nurse, 15(5):40–4.

Waugh A, Grant A. 2006. In Ross and Wilson Anatomy and Physiology in Health and Illness (10th edition). Edinburgh: Churchill Livingstone Elsevier.

Weetman C, Allison W. 2006. Use of epidural analgesia in postoperative management. Nursing Standard, 20(44):54–64.

Williams V, Riley A et al. 2006. Inhaled nitrous oxide during a painful procedure: a satisfaction survey. Paediatric Nursing, 18(8):31–3.

Wolf A. 1999. Pain nociception and the developing infant. Paediatric Anaesthesia, 9(1):7–17.

Young S. 2000. Comparing the use of ketamine and midazolam in emergency settings. Emergency Nurse, 7(8):27–30.

Further reading

National Service Frameworks for Children and Young People. 2003–4. Standards for Children in Hospital. London: Department of Health.

RCN Guidelines. www.rcn.org.uk/publications/pdf/guidelines/cpg_pain_assessment.

Stevens B, Yamada J, Ohlsson A. 2003. *Sucrose for analgesia in newborn infants undergoing painful procedures.* Cochrane Database. Apps.who.int/rhl/reviews/cd0011069.pdf.

Wong D, Barker C. 1988. Pain in children: comparison of assessment scales. Pediatric Nursing, 14(1):9–17.

Chapter 14
MANAGING SKIN INTEGRITY, WOUND HEALING AND CARE

Doreen Crawford

School of Nursing and Midwifery, Faculty of Health and Life Sciences, De Montfort University, Leicester, UK

Introduction

This chapter reviews the normal anatomy of the skin and describes how to prevent iatrogenic damage when a child is in intensive care. Embryological development of the skin and briefly its anatomy and physiology are considered (Table 14.1). The chapter describes the process of healing when the integrity of the skin is breached and provides an overview of what the children's intensive care nurse can do to protect the skin and promote the best wound environment for healing. Finally, a summary of dressings which may be used with children and is currently contained in the BNF (2011–12) is presented.

Skin is much more than a surface. Its colour, texture and condition are accurate indicators of a child's health and wellbeing. The way young people manage and modify their skin can depict their level of self-esteem for skin is central to body image. Many of the conditions children come into ITU with result in scarring which will have lifelong ramifications for them.

Anatomy and physiology of the skin

The skin is a highly complex structure and only a brief overview is given here.

The skin is the largest organ in the body, covering the entire surface. By adulthood it weighs 2.5–3 kg. It serves as a protective barrier against heat, light, injury and infection, and skin also:

- thermoregulates;
- has a role in the fluid balance of the body;
- acts as a repository for fat and vitamin D, which has an important role in calcium homeostasis;
- has a role in sensory perception.

The skin is innervated with approximately 1 million afferent nerve fibres. The majority supply the face; relatively few populate the back. The cutaneous nerves contain axons with cell bodies in the dorsal root ganglia. The main nerve trunks entering the subdermal tissue and divide into smaller branches to form a network which usually follows the blood vessel pattern and forms a mesh of nerves in the dermis where they terminate as most do not extend into the epidermis. The skin is not uniform over the surface of the body, for example the head contains the most hair follicles, the palms of the hand and the soles of the feet contain none; areas which are modelled to endure high friction, such as the palms and soles, have thick layers.

Paediatric Intensive Care Nursing, First Edition. Edited by Michaela Dixon and Doreen Crawford.
© 2012 John Wiley & Sons, Ltd. Published 2012 by John Wiley & Sons, Ltd.

Table 14.1 Embryological overview

Developmental timeline	Skin status
Up to week 4	Early differentiation, skin cells arise from ectodermal and mesodermal origin cells. Elementary layering of simple ectoderm epithelium over mesenchyme. Differentiation of angioblasts forms a primitive vascular network.
Up to week 12	Prolific ectodermal activity, where germinative basal cells repeatedly divide and form stratified epithelium. Under this layer the mesoderm differentiates into connective tissue and models into extensive blood vessel networks. Clusters of cells which will form tooth buds appear in the jaws. Eyelids form and fuse.
From week 16	The proliferation of basal cells generates folds in the basement membrane. The connective tissue differentiates into dermis; a loose, continuous layer over a dense continuous layer; further differentiation will result in the subcutaneous layer. Adipose cells accumulate. The neural crest cells, melanocytes, which will eventually pigment the skin, migrate into the epithelium (the infant is not fully pigmented at birth). The ectoderm supports the development of nails, hair follicles (early hair growth is called lanugo) and sebaceous glands. Nails begin to form as small thickenings of ectodermal epidermis near the tips of the digits; finger nails precede toe nails.
20 weeks+	Downy hair lengthens; eyelashes and eyebrows appear. No more hair follicles form after birth. The specialism of glands and the waxy secretions from sebaceous glands results in vernix caseosa, which covers foetal skin and protects it from maceration from exposure to amniotic fluid. Keratinisation of epidermis begins at 22–24 weeks commencing at the head then progressing to the face, palms and soles of feet. Infants are not fully keratinised until several weeks after birth. The eyes can open from weeks 24–25, although layered; the skin is so thin it appears transparent. Fingerprints are forming.

Source: collated from Chamley 2005; Dixon et al. 2009; MacGregor 1999.

The epidermis is the outermost layer and is a multi-layered structure. Stratified epithelium is renewed continuously by cellular division from the basal layer. The cells produced by mitosis in the basal layer ascend towards the surface and undergo keratinisation and denucleation. By the time they reach the surface they are waterproof and dead.

The dermis varies in thickness and contains the lymphatic vessels, hair follicles, sweat glands, blood vessels, nerves, etc. The dermis also hosts mast cells which release histamine and play a central role in hypersensitivity reactions, and phagocytic macrophages which have a key role in the immune response.

The subcutaneous layer consists of adipose tissue lobules separated by dense fibrous walls and blood vessels.

The rate of skin cell production must be balanced by the rate of cell loss at the surface. The control mechanism of epidermopoiesis consists of a balance of stimulatory and inhibitory signals. Wound healing is one example. A wound results in a wave of epidermal mitotic activity as a result of trigger factors, which include cytokines and growth hormones.

Managing a child's skin in ITU

Early assessment of the child's skin will avoid confusion regarding when and how the damage occurred. This is particularly important if the damage to the child's skin becomes the subject of a complaint or clinical incident. There is some evidence to suggest that the prevention and treatment of pressure ulcers and maintenance of skin integrity in the critically ill child are not viewed as a high priority (Butler 2007). Benchmarking for one's unit can be difficult as the prevalence of pressure ulcers in PICUs in some studies is as high as 27% (Curley et al. 2003), but has been considered to be low in other literature (McLane et al. 2004). However, the incidence of other forms of skin breakdown, such as nappy rash and IV extravasation, was higher (McLane et al. 2004). Preventing any breaches in skin integrity is preferable to managing them when they occur.

Children in the ITU are uniquely vulnerable; their dermal capillary pressure may be compromised by impaired cardiac function and peripheral shutdown. A chronically ill child may have significantly reduced dermal capillary pressure compared to a usually healthy child who is suddenly ill or admitted because of trauma. Children in ITU are at particular risk of skin damage as they are usually sedated and cannot move freely. They may have multiple and invasive lines which influence the position in which they can be nursed. They may have fitted appliances such as traction, external fixators, plasters, splits, braces, etc., and secured probes, catheters, ventilator, tubing, etc. The fit of these appliances and the means of securing lines must be frequently revised (Willock et al. 1999).

Children who destabilise when being handled may not have probes changed frequently enough for their needs. They may have impaired circulation, reducing the level of oxygen and nutrients available for the maintenance of tissues. They may be in a hypercatabolic state and not have the nutrients available to support tissue regeneration. Decubitus ulcers or pressure sores are areas of localised skin damage, which once established can extend to under-lying structures such as muscle and bone (Allman et al. 1995). This may be as a result of a combination of factors, including prolonged exposure to pressure, the shearing force of friction and maceration of the skin from moisture. Pressure ulcers can develop in any area of the body (Rycroft-Malone and McInnes 2000) but generally occur over bony prominences (Jones et al. 2001; Murdoch 2002; Willock et al. 1999).

In young children nursed supine the back of the head and the ears are particularly at risk due to the size and shape of the head. Hair braids may need to be taken down to prevent hidden damage from occurring (Dixon and Ratliff 2011). The child's sacrum and heels are also at risk. Prone infants and children may have knees, elbows, shoulders and the side of the face on the mattress more at risk, so when children are nursed prone the position of the dependent ear should be checked.

Assessment of risk

Most units use skin assessment tools and a range is available. Many children's units use the Braden Q, although there is some evidence to suggest that the Glamorgan scale is more sensitive (Willock et al. 2009). Table 14.2 and Table 14.3 are examples of neonatal and children's skin assessment (McGurk et al. 2004) currently in use in an area where there are minimal critical incident reports generated.

Scores are totalled and 2 added for each of the following: intravenous cannula in situ; arterial line in situ; site of extravasation; wound; apparent birth trauma; nappy rash; electrolyte imbalance; cord clamp in situ.

Table 14.2 Northampton neonatal skin tool

Category	0	1	2
Gestation	Term	>32 weeks	<32 weeks
Weight	>2 kg	1–2 kg	<1 kg
Age	>14 days	7–14 days	<7 days
Skin integrity	No damage	Small amount of damage	Extensive damage
Temperature control	Normal support	Unstable when exposed	Highly unstable
Mobility	Normal	Restricted	Immobile
Nutritional status	Normal fluids/feeding for gestation	Restricted fluids/tolerance for gestation	Severely restricted/poor tolerance
Visual access	Unimpeded	Impeded in small areas	Impaired extensively
Level of care	Normal	Special	Intensive

Source: reproduced by kind permission of the lead author and the *Journal of Nursing Children and Young People*.

Table 14.3 Northampton Children's Skin Tool

Category	1	2	3
Weight	Average	Overweight	Underweight
Nutrition	Normal diet/fluids	TPN/NGT/PEG feeds	NBM/IV fluids only
Activity	Normal developmental age	Restricted	Immobile
Continence	Continent	Occasionally incontinent, wears pads/ nappies under 5	Incontinent of urine and faeces over 5
Pain	Pain-free	Intermittent pain on movement	Needs extensive pain management
Skin state	Intact	Superficial breaks	Extensive damage

Source: reproduced by kind permission of the lead author and the *Journal of Nursing Children and Young People*.

Final score:

- 0–8 Low risk: Recommend daily assessment.
- 8–15 Moderate risk: Recommend 6–8 hourly assessment and repositioning.
- 16–24 High risk: Recommend 4–6 hourly assessment and repositioning.
- >24 Extreme risk: Recommend 2–4 hourly assessment and repositioning.

Add 2 for each of the following: radiotherapy, chemotherapy, steroid therapy, diabetes, >2 hours on the operating table, splints/plaster cast, anaemia (Hb <8), sensation deficit.

Final score:

- 0–4 Low risk: Daily assessment.
- 5–8 Medium risk: Twice daily assessment.
- 9+ High risk: 4–6 hourly assessment or as condition dictates.

However, a tool is only as good as the nurses who use it. A child's skin should not be assessed in isolation but in conjunction with their clinical condition and their clinical needs and requirements taken into account. Whenever possible the child's parent/carer should be involved in the assessment process and the comfort, privacy and dignity of the child should be a high priority. The baseline assessment of the condition of the child's skin should be done soon after admission with the caveat that children transferred from a referring unit or having had long surgical procedures may already have suffered some pressure damage so may need immediate intervention. Children in ITU need to be assessed with every change of shift. If a child is at particular risk their skin should be assessed every time they have a change of position. Each assessment must be documented, signed and dated by the assessor.

Early signs of pressure ulcer development include erythema, particularly non-blanching erythema. There may be a discoloured area on the skin, localised heat, oedema or induration. The assessment should pay particular attention to the skin over bony prominences.

More advanced tissue damage may include an area which feels a different temperature or texture from the surrounding skin.

Planning skin management

Children at significant risk of pressure ulcer development should be identified and assessed at each shift change. The child's at-risk status must be clearly documented if the child is transferred out or moved to another ward for step-down care.

The assessment should involve the child's parents as they are often the first to notice any skin changes given their level of interaction with their child and their familiarity with the skin through dressing, changing nappies and bathing, etc. The assessment should involve the use of a tool (e.g. the Braden Q, where a score of 10 or below constitutes the child being at risk). If the child is identified as being at risk of developing a pressure ulcer a plan of care must be provided. For a child scoring 10 or lower this should include:

- An at least daily inspection of skin and bony prominences. The prophylactic use of a barrier film (e.g. Cavilon®) for children in nappies or pads, or the child could be nursed on top of the nappy/pad and discreetly covered with a light sheet.
- A plan for repositioning every 2–3 hours, using enough staff to perform the position change safely and eliminate

the risk of friction and shear without overhandling the child. Devices to assist manual handling (e.g. sliding sheets, hoists) should be used where possible to reduce the potential of skin damage to the child and injury to carers. Where this is not possible because the child cannot physiologically tolerate position changes a senior member of the team should explain the reason for this to the family and document this is the child's medical record.

- All episodes of repositioning should be recorded on the child's chart.
- The use of a pressure-relieving mattress and support where possible. The latter includes surfaces such as mattresses or cushions and pillows to support or separate limbs. There are two main forms of pressure-relieving support surface: the continuous low-pressure surface and the alternating-pressure surface. The continuously low-pressure surface contours to the shape of the child and spreads the pressure over a larger surface area; this reduces pressure over their bony prominences. Different types are available using a variety of substances (e.g. air, gel, foam, fluid, or a combination of these). The alternating-pressure devices consist of air cells which are time-cycled. They inflate and deflate. The inflated cells support the child's weight while the deflated cells provide pressure relief. These devices can cause some movement so are not suitable for some children; lines, catheters, etc. need to be secured. Pressure-relieving mattresses should be covered by appropriate bedding, which should be checked for creases and wrinkles when the child is moved. Pillows, foam wedges and rolls of Gamgee can be used to support and maintain position.
- Work with the multidisciplinary team to ensure that the child is adequately hydrated and their nutritional needs considered.

These actions should minimise pressure on bony prominences and avoid positioning on pressure ulcer if present (NICE 2005).

Essential skincare

The normal pH of the skin is acidic (pH 4.9) and skin oils keep the skin moist and supple. This surface environment provides a degree of antibacterial protection. As soaps and detergents can dry the skin and alter the pH they should be avoided, as should the routine use of baby wipes, as these can also cause the skin pH to be depressed (Priestley et al. 1996). In addition, many products contain dyes, preservatives and perfumes that can cause irritation and sensitisa-

tion. Where anything other than warm water is required, the use of aqueous cream should be considered.

In very young children nappy rash is a significant cause of skin breakdown. The presence of faeces and urine, combined with the mechanical friction and occlusion which the wearing of a nappy creates, increases the risk of nappy rash. Besides being a source of discomfort, these skin irritations pose a risk of secondary infections (Stamatas et al. 2011). There is a close correlation between skin wetness and altered skin pH with nappy rash/diaper dermatitis (Berg et al. 1994). Children who have loose stools (e.g. because of antibiotics) are particularly at risk. Where swabs have not identified fungal or bacterial causes first-line management should be more changes and exposure. Other strands of management can be discussed with tissue viability specialists. Gupta and Skinner (2004) reviewed the management of intractable 'diaper dermatitis'.

Management of pressure ulcers (Table 14.4)

Pressure ulcers are graded according to severity (ENPUA 2009). They are serious incidents and should be reported as Clinical Incidents to allow for auditing prevalence.

GRADING OF PRESSURE ULCERS

- Grade 1: Non-blanching erythema of intact skin: Discolouration of the skin, warmth, oedema, induration or hardness can also be used as indicators, particularly in individuals with darker skin.
- Grade 2: Partial thickness skin loss involving epidermis, dermis, or both: The ulcer is superficial and presents clinically as an abrasion or blister.
- Grade 3: Full thickness skin loss involving damage to or necrosis of subcutaneous tissue that may extend down to, but not through, underlying fascia.
- Grade 4: Extensive destruction, tissue necrosis, or damage to muscle, bone or supporting structures with/without full thickness skin loss.

Healing

This is an intricate process in which the skin undertakes self-repair. A brief summary of the process is offered here and some key issues with wounds are considered. There are some excellent journals and online resources to support the children's nurse in their care of the child's skin such as Gabriel et al. (2009) and Mercandetti and Cohen (2008). Wound care technology is a fast-moving speciality and new products are being developed all the time, so the professional nurse needs to keep abreast of new products.

Table 14.4 Management: pressure ulcers

Assessment of pressure ulcer	Suggested actions to be taken
Grade 1: Non-blanching erythema of intact skin/discolouration of the skin.	Document in the child's clinical records and in the nursing notes, inform the nurse in charge, institute an action plan and ensure that the incident is handed over to each shift.
	Review the Pressure Risk Assessment. If the child is sufficiently stable, increase the repositioning and turning frequency. Involve parents/carers if possible. Time on parent's lap can be considered as a position change but the pressure areas can still be at risk as the bony prominence over the buttocks may be exposed to more weight in this position.
	Consider specialist pressure-relieving mattress.
	Monitor and observe progress or improvement, complete clinical incident form.
Grade 2: Partial thickness skin loss involving epidermis, dermis, or both. The ulcer is superficial and presents clinically as an abrasion or blister.	As above.
	Gain consent from child/parents to photograph.
	Make urgent referral to tissue viability specialist.
	Use specialist pressure-relieving mattress or review effectiveness of the one in use.
	With the MDT review the fluid and nutritional status of the child. Make a referral to the dietician if not already involved.
Grade 3: Full thickness skin loss involving damage to or necrosis of subcutaneous tissue. Grade 4: Extensive destruction damage to muscle, bone or supporting structures.	As above and liaise with the child's consultant to see if a referral to the plastic surgery team is appropriate. Infection may have led to the deterioration of previously minor lesions, particularly if the immune system is compromised.

Intact skin helps the child to maintain homeostasis. The epidermis and dermis exist in equilibrium and form a protective barrier against the external environment on which microbiological flora flourish. Once the protective barrier is breached, homeostatic integrity is at risk and the process of wound healing is immediately triggered. For convenience, wound healing is divided into phases or stages although the process is continuous (Mercandetti and Cohen 2008):

- Haemostasis.
- Inflammation.
- Proliferation.
- Remodelling.

On injury in well-perfused skin, a set of complex biochemical events takes place immediately in a closely orchestrated cascade to repair the damage. Severed blood vessels results in bleeding and within seconds thrombocytes begin to aggregate at the site to form a fibrin clot. This clot will achieve haemostasis.

The breach in skin integrity may have allowed microbiological flora to enter the tissues so during the inflammatory phase, bacteria and debris are phagocytosed and removed. The aim of the inflammatory response is to create a clean wound bed on which to grow new tissue so any damaged tissue will have to be removed, proteases are released and these help debride damaged tissue. The inflammatory stage can be counterproductive if prolonged. This is more likely in heavily contaminated wounds and a prolonged inflammatory stage can delay healing.

Towards the end of the inflammatory stage factors are released that cause the migration and division of cells involved in the proliferative phase.

The proliferative phase is characterised by angiogenesis, collagen deposition, granulation tissue formation, epithelialisation and wound contraction. In angiogenesis, new blood vessels are formed by vascular endothelial cells. In fibroplasia and granulation tissue formation, fibroblasts grow and form a new, provisional extracellular matrix (ECM) by excreting collagen and fibronectin. Re-epithelialisation of the epidermis occurs, in which epithelial cells proliferate and migrate over the wound bed providing optimal conditions for new tissue growth.

In contraction, the wound is made smaller by the action of myofibroblasts, which establish a grip on the wound edges and contract themselves using a mechanism similar to that in smooth muscle cells. Any unneeded cells undergo apoptosis during the late remodelling phase. Collagen is remodelled and aligned along tension lines and excess cells are removed by apoptosis.

The medical literature and e-medicine have an abundance of materials on wound healing (Gabriel et al. 2009; Mercandetti and Cohen 2008) and use the following terms to describe types of wound management:

- Primary intention.
- Secondary intention.
- Tertiary intention – delayed closure.

Primary intention is when the wound edges are in a position where they are directly next to one another and there has been minimal tissue loss. Most surgical wounds heal by primary intention and the wound is supported by a closure technique which employs sutures, staples or adhesive tape. Primary intention results in wounds where there is minimal scarring.

Secondary intention is where the wound bed is allowed to granulate and surface superficial healing can be prevented by the use of a pack. The healing process can be slow due to the presence of a drain or healing compromised because of infection. With some systems of management wound care has to be performed daily to remove wound debris and allow for granulation tissue formation. Secondary intention wounds may result in a broader scar.

Tertiary intention is where the wound is initially cleaned, debrided and then observed for a period of time. The wound is purposely left open. Cosmetic results can be poor.

It is important to understand the normal process associated with acute wound healing and be familiar with the concept of moist wound healing as this enhances the nurse's range of interactive wound management and ensures that the most appropriate products are selected.

In wound care several algorithms can be used where modes of management and styles of dressing materials are utilised according to the character of the wound, location of the wound and patient compliance. Examples of a wound care algorithm based on evidence can be seen using the links in the resources list at the end of this chapter and

many of these algorithms have been validated (Beitz and van Rijswijk 1999).

Cleansing skin prior to surgical interventions or invasive procedures

The BNF for Children (2011–12) states that antiseptics such as chlorhexidine or povidone–iodine can be used on a child's intact skin before surgical procedures. Because their antiseptic effects are enhanced by an alcoholic solvent the area must be dry before an incision is made. Antiseptic solutions containing cetrimide can be used if a detergent effect is also required. Any preparations containing alcohol should not be used on neonatal skin and regular use of povidone iodine should be avoided.

Dressings

Much more research to identify the optimal wound dressings for children's wounds is needed as much of the evidence comes from adult studies and these are not necessarily transferable. The concept of a moist wound environment for optimal healing has been promoted since the early 1960s. Arguments for this include faster healing, less painful dressing changes (Benbow 2010) and a better cosmetic result (Benbow 2008). Non-necrotic wounds are frequently managed with moist wound dressings as these require fewer changes and this is likely to be less traumatic for children who are conscious or semi-conscious. Vogt et al. (2007) found that moist wound healing using a hydrofibre dressing in primary closed wounds after surgery did not lead to a significant difference in patient comfort, infection rates or length of hospital stay when compared to a standard dry dressing. Despite the need for fewer dressing changes the traditional dry dressing was significantly less expensive and, given the need to make economies, this is likely to influence the choice of dressing. However, the costs and risks have to be balanced when selecting a dressing material. Although analgesia and anaesthesia can be used to help reduce pain during dressing changes, these can be expensive for healthcare providers and carers, and some analgesic and anaesthetic agents are associated with undesirable side-effects (Soon and Acton 2006). Second, because of the small size of paediatric wounds and the difficulties associated with dressing unusually shaped wounds in awkward locations, such as wounds resulting from digit and limb injuries, the children's nurse needs access to highly flexible and conformable dressings (Morris et al. 2009) and not just the cheapest.

Table 14.5 Wound dressings

Dressing type	Wound characteristics and indicators
Hydrogel dressings	Hydrogel dressings are usually supplied as an amorphous, cohesive topical application that can take up the shape of a child's wound. A secondary, non-absorbent dressing is needed to cover these. The hydrogel dressings are used to donate liquid to dry sloughy wounds and facilitate autolytic debridement of necrotic tissue. A few also have the ability to absorb small amounts of exudate. Hydrogel sheets are best avoided in the presence of infection and are unsuitable for heavily exuding wounds. Hydrogel products that do not contain propylene glycol should be used if the wound is to be treated with larval therapy.
Vapour-permeable films and membranes	Allow the passage of water vapour and oxygen but are impermeable to water and micro-organisms. They are suitable for lightly exuding wounds. They are conformable and provide protection and a moist healing environment. The transparent dressing allows constant observation of the wound (this may cause some parents and children anxiety). Most are unsuitable for heavily exuding wounds as water vapour loss occurs at a slower rate than exudate and generated fluid accumulates under the dressing, which can lead to tissue maceration and wrinkling which can breach dressing integrity and risk microbial entry. They may be prescribed to protect fragile skin at risk of developing minor skin damage caused by friction or pressure. Some are combined with absorbent pads which makes them an ideal first-line postoperative dressing for simple surgical incision wounds.
Soft polymer dressings	Soft polymer/silicone polymer, in a non-adherent or gently adherent layer, is used for lightly to moderately exuding wounds. For more heavily exuding wounds, an absorbent secondary dressing can be added, or a combination of soft polymer dressing with an absorbent pad can be used. Soft silicone has gentle adhesive properties and can be used on fragile skin or where it is beneficial to reduce the frequency of primary dressing changes. These dressing should not be used on heavily bleeding wounds as drying blood clots can cause the dressing to adhere to the wound surface.
Hydrocolloid dressings	These dressings are made from modified carmellose fibres and resemble alginate dressings. Hydrocolloid-fibrous dressings are more absorptive and suitable for moderately to heavily exuding wounds. Hydrocolloid dressings are usually presented as a hydrocolloid layer on a vapour-permeable film or foam pad. They are semi-permeable to water vapour and oxygen. They form a gel in the presence of exudate to facilitate rehydration in lightly to moderately exuding wounds and promote autolytic debridement of dry, sloughy or necrotic wounds. They promote granulation.
Foam dressings	Dressings containing hydrophilic polyurethane foam (adhesive or non-adhesive), with or without plastic film backing, are suitable for all types of exuding wounds, but not for dry wounds. Some foam dressings have a moisture-sensitive film backing with variable permeability dependent on the level of exudate. Foam dressings vary in their ability to absorb exudate: some are suitable only for lightly to moderately exuding wounds; others have greater fluid-handling capacity and are suitable for heavily exuding wounds. Saturated foam dressings can cause maceration of healthy skin if left in contact with the wound so need frequent inspection even if not changed. Foam dressings can be used in combination with other primary wound contact dressings. If used under compression bandaging or compression garments, the fluid-handling capacity of the foam dressing may be reduced. Foam dressings can also be used to provide a protective cushion for fragile skin. A foam dressing containing ibuprofen is available and may be useful for treating painful exuding wounds.

(Continued)

Table 14.5 (*Continued*)

Dressing type	Wound characteristics and indicators
Alginate dressings	Non-woven or fibrous, non-occlusive, alginate dressings, made from calcium alginate, or calcium sodium alginate which is derived from brown seaweed, forms a soft gel in contact with wound exudate. Alginate dressings are highly absorbent and suitable for use on exuding wounds and for the promotion of autolytic debridement of debris in very moist wounds. Alginate dressings also act as a haemostatic, but caution is needed because drying blood clots can cause the dressing to adhere to the wound surface. Alginate dressings should not be used if bleeding is heavy, and extreme caution is needed if used for tumours with friable tissue. Alginate sheets are suitable for use as a wound contact dressing for moderately to heavily exuding wounds and can be layered into deep wounds. Alginate rope can be used in sinus and cavity wounds to improve absorption of exudate and prevent maceration. If the dressing does not have an adhesive border or integral adhesive plastic film backing, a secondary dressing will be required.
Capillary-action dressings	Capillary-action dressings consist of an absorbent core of hydrophilic fibres sandwiched between two low-adherent wound-contact layers to ensure that no fibres are shed onto the wound surface. Wound exudate is taken up by the dressing and retained within the highly absorbent central layer. The dressing may be applied intact to relatively superficial areas, but for deeper wounds or cavities it may be cut to shape to ensure good contact with the wound base. Multiple layers may be applied to heavily exuding wounds to further increase the fluid-absorbing capacity of the dressing. A secondary adhesive dressing is necessary. Capillary-action dressings are suitable for use on all types of exuding wounds, but particularly on sloughy wounds where removal of fluid from the wound aids debridement. Capillary-action dressings are contra-indicated for heavily bleeding wounds or arterial bleeding.
Odour-absorbent dressings	Dressings containing activated charcoal are used to absorb odour from wounds. The underlying cause of wound odour should be identified. Wound odour is most effectively reduced by debridement of slough, reduction in bacterial levels and frequent dressing changes. Fungating wounds and chronic infected wounds produce high volumes of exudate which can reduce the effectiveness of odour-absorbent dressings. Many odour-absorbent dressings are intended for use in combination with other dressings. Odour-absorbent dressings with a suitable wound contact layer can be used as a primary dressing.

Source: compiled from BNF for Children 2011–12.

The BNF for Children (2011–12) provides information on a range of advanced wound dressings which can be used for both acute and chronic wounds. These are divided into categories based of absorbency and components (Table 14.5).

Conclusion

This chapter has reviewed the normal anatomy of the skin and how to prevent iatrogenic damage when a child is in intensive care by using the appropriate tools. The chapter has considered the process of healing when the integrity of the skin is breached. The chapter has provided an over-view of what dressings can be used with children and that are currently contained in the BNF (2011–12).

References

Allman RM, Goode PS, et al. (1995) Pressure ulcer risk factors among hospitalized patients with activity limitation. JAMA, 273(11):865–70.

Beitz J, van Rijswijk L (1999) Using wound care algorithms: a content validation study. Journal of Wound, Ostomy and Continence Nursing, 26(5):238–9.

Benbow M. 2008. Exploring the concept of moist wound healing and its application in practice. British Journal of Nursing, 17(15):S4, S6, S8 passim.

Benbow M. 2010. Managing wound pain: is there an 'ideal dressing'? British Journal of Nursing, 19(20): 1273–4.

Berg R, Milligan M, Sarbaugh F. 1994. Association of skin wetness and pH with diaper. Dermatitis, 11(1):18–20.

British National Formulary for Children. 2011–12. bnfc. org/ bnfc/bnfc/current/106494. htm.

Butler C. 2007. Pediatric skin care: guidelines for assessment, prevention, and treatment. Dermatology Nursing, 19(5): 471–7.

Chamley C. 2005. Developmental Anatomy and Physiology of Children: A practical approach. Edinburgh: Churchill Livingstone.

Curley M, Quigley S, Lin M. 2003. Pressure areas in pediatric intensive care: incidence and associated factors. Pediatric Critical Care Medicine, 4(3):284–90.

Dixon M, Crawford D et al. 2009. Nursing the Highly Dependent Child or Infant: A manual of care. Singapore: Wiley-Blackwell.

Dixon M, Ratliff C. 2011. Hair braids as a risk factor for occipital pressure ulcer development: a case study. Ostomy Wound Management, 57(9):48–53.

European and US National Pressure Ulcer Advisory Panels Pressure Ulcer Prevention (ENPUA) 2009. www.epuap.org/ guidelines/Final_Quick_Prevention.pdf and grading guide www.epuap.org/pressure-ulcer-research/pressure-ulcer-grading-guide.

Gabriel A, Mussman J, Rosenberg L. 2009. Wound Healing, Growth Factors. emedicine.medscape.com/article/1298196-overview.

Gupta AK, Skinner AR. 2004. Management of diaper dermatitis. International Journal of Dermatology, 43(11):830–4.

Jones I, Tweed C, Marron M. 2001. Pressure area care in infants and children: Nimbus Paediatric System. British Journal of Nursing, 10(12):789–95.

MacGregor J. 1999. An Introduction to the Anatomy and Physiology of Children. London: Routledge.

McGurk V, Holloway B et al. 2004. Skin integrity assessment in neonates and children. Paediatric Nurse, 16(3):16–18.

McLane KM, Bookout K et al. 2004. The 2003 national pediatric pressure ulcer and skin breakdown prevalence survey: a multisite study. Journal of Wound and Ostomy Continence Nursing, 31(4):168–8.

Mercandetti M, Cohen A. 2008. Wound Healing and Repair. emedicine.medscape.com/article/1298129-overview.

Morris C, Emsley P et al. 2009. Use of wound dressings with soft silicone adhesive technology. Paediatric Nurse, 21(3):38–43.

Murdoch V. 2002. Pressure care in the paediatric intensive care unit. Nursing Standard, 17(6):71–6.

National Institute for Clinical Excellence (NICE). 2005. The Prevention and Management of Pressure Ulcers – Clinical Guideline. guidance.nice.org.uk/CG29/quickrefguide/pdf/ English.

Priestley GC, McVitie E, Aldridge RD. 1996. Changes in skin pH after the use of baby wipes. Pediatric Dermatology, 13(1):14–17.

Rycroft-Malone J, McInnes E. 2000. Pressure Ulcer Risk Assessment and Prevention. Technical report. London: RCN.

Soon K, Acton C. 2006. Pain-induced stress: a barrier to wound healing. Wounds UK, 2(4):92–101.

Stamatas GN, Zerweck C et al. 2011. Documentation of impaired epidermal barrier in mild and moderate diaper dermatitis in vivo using noninvasive methods. Pediatric Dermatology, 28(2):99–107.

Vogt K, Uhlyarik M, Schroeder T. 2007. Moist wound healing compared with standard care of treatment of primary closed vascular surgical wounds: a prospective randomized controlled study. Wound Repair and Regeneration, 15(5): 624–7.

Willock J, Baharestani M, Anthony D. 2009. The development of the Glamorgan paediatric pressure ulcer risk assessment scale. Wound Care, 18(1):17–21.

Further reading

Bridel J. 1993. The aetiology of pressure sores. Journal of Wound Care, 2(4):230–8.

Buckingham KW, Berg RW. 1986. Etiologic factors in diaper dermatitis: the role of feces. Pediatric Dermatology, 3(2):107–12.

Collins F, Shipperley T. 1995. Assessing the seated patient for the risk of pressure damage. Journal of Wound Care, 8(3):123–6.

Cullum N, Deeks J et al. 2000. Beds, mattresses and cushions for preventing and treating pressure sores. Cochrane Review, 1.

Flanagan M. 1993. Predicting pressure sore risk: a guide to the risk factors identified in the most common risk assessment scales in use. Journal of Wound Care, 2:215–18.

Gray M. 2004. Which pressure ulcer risk scales are valid and reliable in a paediatric population? Journal of Wound, Ostomy and Continence Nursing, 31(4):157–63.

Irving V. 2001. Caring for and protecting the skin of pre-term neonates. Journal of Wound Care, 10(7):253–6.

Loman D. 2000. Assessment of skin breakdown risk in children. Journal of Child and Family Nursing, 3(3):234–8.

Quigley S, Curley M. 1996. Skin integrity in the paediatric population: preventing and managing pressure ulcers. Journal of the Society of Paediatric Nurses, 1(1):7–17.

Solis I, Krouskop T et al. 1988. Supine interface pressure in children. Archives of Physical Medicine and Rehabilitation, 69(7):524–6.

Williams C. 1997. 3M Cavilon® no sting barrier film in the protection of vulnerable skin. British Journal of Nursing, 10:613–15.

Willock J, Hughes J, Tickle S. 1999. Pressure sores in children – the acute hospital setting. Journal of Tissue Viability, 10(2):59–65.

Resources

Skin barrier products solutions. 3m.co.uk/wps/portal/3M/
en_GB/Cavilon/skin-care/professionals/stoma last accessed
August 2009

Wound care. www.medscape.com/resource/wound-
management.

Wound care algorithm. National Guideline Clearinghouse
(NGC). 2006. www.guideline.gov/summary/summary.aspx?
ss=15&doc_id=8534&nbr=4749.

Wound care algorithms. www.hollister.com/us/wound/
resource/algorithms.html.

Chapter 15
TRANSPORTATION OF THE CRITICALLY ILL INFANT OR CHILD

Alison Oliver[1] and Michaela Dixon[2]

[1] Paediatric Intensive Care, University Hospital of Wales, Cardiff, UK
[2] Paediatric Intensive Care Unit, Bristol Royal Hospital for Children, University Hospitals Bristol NHS Foundation Trust, Bristol, UK

Introduction

There are essentially three elements to the initial care of critically ill children: recognition, effective resuscitation and comprehensive stabilisation. Critically ill children are usually cared for in specialist paediatric intensive care units and require transportation to these. This chapter considers some of the principles of transportation of the critically ill child, strategies used to asses, stabilise and ensure the safety of the child being transferred and the documentation required. As patient pathways change with the decreasing numbers of small children's units offering this level of support, it is likely that there will be a rise in the number of transports required and it is important that the child is not compromised as a result of being moved.

Types of transportation

There are three types of transportation: intra-hospital, inter-hospital and retrieval. No matter what method used, the same principles apply.

Retrieval is the transfer of a critically ill patient by a specialist team to a specialist service for an advanced level of care. *A Framework for the Future* (Department of Health 1997) recommended that all lead centres should have a fully equipped and resourced retrieval service available at all times. Retrieval services differ from transportation in that it is provided by specialist teams, who have standards for the delivery of that care (PICS 2001) and there are recognised benefits in reducing risk associated with transportation (Britto et al. 1995; Edge et al. 1994). Transportation of critically ill children increases the risk of morbidity and mortality. However, the benefits of being transferred to a lead centre for critical care outweigh the risks. In addition, adherence to the standards reduces these risks as specialist staff are trained in recognition, stabilisation, the equipment used and the transportation process.

Retrieval teams are not responsible for initial resuscitation. This is the responsibility of the referring hospital and it is essential that the local staff are trained in paediatric resuscitation in order to meet this standard. If hospitals are in close proximity to the lead centre, the retrieval team may arrive while the child is being resuscitated. Some cases require prolonged resuscitation and may not progress to stabilisation before the arrival of the retrieval team. However, depending on the geographical area covered, retrieval may take some time. Therefore the role of the district general hospital/referring hospital staff in caring for critically ill children cannot be underestimated. Their

Paediatric Intensive Care Nursing, First Edition. Edited by Michaela Dixon and Doreen Crawford.
© 2012 John Wiley & Sons, Ltd. Published 2012 by John Wiley & Sons, Ltd.

teamwork and clinical management can influence the success of resuscitation and the outcome of these cases.

Emergency transfer

Ideally, specialist retrieval teams should transfer all critically ill children. However, some cases (e.g. burns and closed head trauma) are time-critical and it is necessary to deliver these children to specialist centres for treatment as quickly as possible.

These emergency transfer cases are often the most unstable children, so it is critical that district general hospitals (DGHs) prepare for management of these cases through scenario training as recommended in the Tanner Report (Department of Health 2006). Emergency transfer teams should consist primarily of a doctor who can manage the child's airway. Both the nurse and doctor must be able to recognise any deterioration in the child's condition promptly and be able to treat changes appropriately. Therefore, some experience in the care of critically ill children is advantageous. Knowledge of equipment used for transfer is also desirable as functions and battery life vary. Electrical equipment should be charged and ready to use, which not always the case in these unanticipated situations.

Communication is critical during the referral process to ensure the correct information is given. Some teams have a policy of consultant-to-consultant referral to ensure that experienced personnel are giving and receiving this information. Lead centres should allocate a dedicated line for the retrieval service to try to ensure telephone line availability for advice and referrals. Telephone advice given by lead centres should be followed, as this could be critical to the outcome of the child. Some services record the information given during these calls for training and audit purposes.

The internet is a vital communication system and a useful resource in providing staff with a wealth of information regarding the care of the critically ill child. Policies can be quickly and easily located and accessed by all staff and care pathways followed. Referral forms should be available on these websites so that local staff can anticipate the information the lead centre will request during the initial referral.

Once retrieval is decided upon the ambulance team will need to be contacted. Processes for this will vary depending on the set-up of local services. Clarity in what type of transfer you are providing (e.g. a neonate requiring an incubator; retrieval of a critically ill child) needs to be specified as this can determine which vehicle is used. Con-figurations of ambulance teams vary depending on local arrangements.

During the journey to the referring hospital, a mobile telephone is essential so that the referring team can contact the retrieval team for further information and advice, or vice versa. This is especially important if going to collect a child outside the usual referral area and if the child is being moved locally from one location to another in the DGH. It also ensures that the lead centre can maintain contact should further referral calls be received during the journey.

Preparation of equipment

Equipment for retrieval should be kept separately from the paediatric intensive care unit in a secure area so that it cannot be used for inpatients. This reduces the risk of staff taking equipment from these areas and forgetting to replace it. This could delay the team's departure.

Equipment needs to be kept electrically charged and available for use at all times. Backpacks and integrated bag and trolley systems are used and there are a number of locking devices on the market to ensure bags are sealed prior to departure so no equipment should be missing from the kit if thoroughly checked and items used replaced by the previous team.

Checks on a large amount of equipment are required before departure take time but can be streamlined with practice and using a standard process. For this reason safety checklists should be developed so that not only is all equipment remembered but also safety checks are carried out on some items prior to departure. No matter how experienced the team, equipment can easily be forgotten, which could be difficult to manage without, especially if providing a service to a hospital with no paediatric inpatients. This is more likely to occur in the future, with developments in the health service possibly leading to further centralisation of paediatric services.

Staff employing the equipment need to be knowledgeable in its use so that they recognise alarms and battery warnings. They also need knowledge in alternative equipment that may need to be used should the equipment fail (e.g. using defibrillators as monitors only). Some modes (e.g. non-invasive blood pressure (NIBP) on the Propaq Encore monitor) use up battery life quickly.

Ideally, staff need to be familiar with the environment they will be using the equipment in and what resources are available in the ambulance. Although ambulances vary from service to service the vehicles in one region usually have an identical set-up. Many ambulances now have paediatric harnesses, transport ventilators, suction devices and defibrillators as standard. All equipment should be stored safely and securely in the back of a vehicle. Most vehicles now have purpose-built brackets for electrical and other equipment and these should always be used.

Some ambulances have generator systems, which enable staff to plug equipment into to maintain electrical function. This is especially useful on long journeys. If this is not the case, spare battery packs should to be carried.

A member of staff needs to be responsible for the maintenance of this equipment. This staff member will vary from service to service. The equipment will need a regular service record, be kept clean, well maintained and trouble-shooting promptly addressed if issues arise with it when in use.

Medical gases are essential to safe transportation and a member of the team also needs to ensure that adequate gases are available for the duration of the journey; the calculation for the amount of gas required is as follows:

tidal volume (litres) × frequency (rate) × duration (min)

for example:

tidal volume = 100 ml (0.1 l) × 20 bpm × 1.5 hr = 180 l

For safety, the litres calculated should be doubled as ventilation requirement may change during the journey.

Purpose-built vehicles and transport trolleys enable staff to house adequate supplies of oxygen and air for long journeys without the risk of error or a gas leak on route. Air-only adapters should be stored on vehicles or taken for use when ventilating neonates with congenital cardiac conditions.

Dedicated vehicles also enable additional equipment to be stored on vehicles to lighten backpacks. Safety equipment, such as torches and reflector jackets, can also be stored on vehicles in case of accidents.

Arrival at the referring hospital

Assessment and stabilisation

On arrival at the DGH the child will be resuscitated and/or stabilised in an identified place of safety. These areas are usually identified by the referring DGH, which makes it easier for local teams to set up paediatric equipment in a permanent place. Identified places of safety also enable retrieval staff to locate the child easily. It also benefits the local team as they become familiar with the location of paediatric equipment. These areas are typically:

- Recovery.
- Operating theatres.

- General intensive care.
- Paediatric high dependency.
- Emergency units (if the child is too unstable to be moved).

Introductions to staff should occur at this stage. This is not only polite, it also makes clear who is in which role in an often frenetic environment. Resuscitation and stabilisation of a critically ill child are extremely stressful in an unfamiliar situation. The approach of the retrieval team should be calm and measured. This not only gives confidence to the family, if present, but can help to reduce the anxiety levels of the whole team.

A review of the history and an assessment of the child on arrival are essential. This confirms whether the referral information has been correctly conveyed and understood. The condition of a critically ill child can change rapidly and the differential diagnosis may need revision. The child needs to be reviewed using the ABC approach no matter what the provisional diagnosis.

The assessment process will identify anything that needs to be addressed immediately, and using the ABC approach ensures this is done methodically.

Once assessment is complete the retrieval team need to agree on a plan. This will include when it is safe to transfer the child to the transport trolley. This will vary depending on the severity of the illness and the extent of stabilisation the local team have been able to achieve prior to the retrieval team's arrival. Some cases will have been comprehensively stabilised, while others will still be in the early stages of resuscitation. Experience in transportation has demonstrated that the more that is attached to the child once on the transport trolley, rather than before, the less likely the risk of displacement and entanglement of lines and equipment when the team is ready for departure.

However, retrieval should never be rushed, and eagerness to get the child on the trolley should not take priority over any stage in the assessment process. Securing of tubes and lines is critical before the transfer to trolley takes place.

Airway

The airway of a child being retrieved will usually be maintained with a endotracheal tube (ETT) as most retrieval services are commissioned to collect children of sickness levels 2 and 3 (DH 1997). DGH anaesthetists are responsible for the intubation of the critically ill child. Intubation may be reviewed by the retrieval team but should never be delayed awaiting their arrival.

The ETT maintaining the airway needs to be secured according to local policy. If the airway is not well secured at this time it needs to be taped again, as loss of the airway during transportation could be catastrophic. A chest X-ray should have been performed and should be reviewed prior to re-taping a tube. An ETT that is too short is vulnerable when moving critically ill patients so it should not be cut until the transport team reviews the chest X-ray.

Maintenance of the airway also depends on the sedation being continuously administered to the child during the stabilisation process. Transportation teams frequently use paralysing agents (see Chapters 4 and 13) so that the child will not lose their artificial airway during the transport process. For this reason the practitioner responsible for the security and functioning of the ET tube must ensure that placement is correct.

Breathing

The child that is intubated will be artificially ventilated using an ambu bag, Ayre's T-piece, Water's circuit or mechanical ventilator.

Chest movement should be assessed and should be easily viewed as equal and bilateral. The child should be breathing at a developmentally appropriate and comfortable rate. The chest needs to be auscultated to assess air entry, which should be equal and bilateral depending on aetiology and diagnosis.

The child that is agitated and breathing against the ventilator will be very evident as they will be causing the alarm on the ventilator to activate. These children are very difficult to manage. A child that is not compliant with ventilation will usually:

- Not be intubated correctly – ETT in oesophagus, too short or in one lung.
- Inadequately ventilated – low rate, low peak pressure levels or lack of PEEP (positive end expiratory pressure).
- Have a blocked airway – kinked tube or secretions.
- Be inadequately sedated.

Other items that may cause difficulty in ventilating the critically ill child in an environment that usually caters for adult patients are bacterial filters used to protect the patients and the machinery. Filters used in adults have large volumes. When used in infants these can result in the accumulation of carbon dioxide. Used together with a catheter mount, especially disposable-concertinaed brands, this can result in increased dead space and rebreathing of carbon dioxide.

Filters used in paediatrics have small volumes and maintain humidity. This is extremely important in the small diameter artificial airway as the moisture will prevent encrusting and potential blockage of the tube.

Transport ventilators can be used at this stage to stabilise the child while waiting for the retrieval team. However, some teams choose the ventilators that are used in their adult patients as staff are more confident in their use. Most of these have paediatric modes and may be the safest option.

Few transport ventilators are available in the United Kingdom. Two types are commonly used: for under 10 kg and for over 10 kg. The under 10 kg Smiths babyPAC ventilators are flow-dependent and very simple to use. Older children are ventilated using either a Smiths ventiPAC or the Drager Oxylog ventilator. There are multiple models of the latter in use. Newer models are electrically dependent.

Blood gases should be recorded once ventilation is established and when changing methods of ventilation. Handheld gas monitors are available for use during transportation. All blood samples, including cultures, should be taken for analysis at the referring hospital to establish the baselines and ensure any abnormalities are treated as promptly as possible.

Circulation

On the arrival of the retrieval team the child will be attached to the local monitoring systems. These usually have universal parameters, which can be assessed immediately by an experienced intensive care team. Vital signs, along with a central capillary refill time, will give staff the information required to assess current circulatory status.

The minimum acceptable access for transportation is two functioning venous cannula. Ideally, these will be 22 gauge as the 24 gauge will not provide adequate access to the circulation of the critically ill child should the child deteriorate.

Inotropic dependent children and those that will require multiple interventions will require central access, and for safety reasons this should be obtained prior to transporting this type of case. These lines offer multiple lumens so that numerous infusions can be administered.

Arterial access monitoring blood pressure is also desirable as it gives the team an immediate indication of changes in the child's cardiovascular status.

All of these devices will need to be well secured with time taken for comprehensive strapping to ensure that they do not become dislodged during any bed-to-bed manoeuvres. Sutures are frequently used to retain these lines in addition to tape dressings. Easy visibility of these lines is still desirable so bandages should be discouraged.

It is usually evident quite quickly if a child has high fluid requirement to resuscitate them. These cases will need urgent cross-match of blood products in their local hospital to avoid over-dilution of their circulatory system.

Drug infusion dosages should be checked at this time to ensure that the child is getting the correct dosages of inotropes and other infusions. PICUs tend to calculate infusions as mg/mcg/kg/hr/min. This method of calculation is not always used in other clinical areas and can be miscalculated in stressful scenarios.

Disability

Assessment of the critically ill child should always include assessment of the neurological system. The administration of sedatives and paralysing agents for intubation make this difficult. Therefore the child's pupil status should always be assessed. This gives the team a baseline and any changes in neurological status can be quickly identified.

Glucose levels should also be checked at this stage and any abnormality treated.

Due to the extremely stressful nature of resuscitating critically ill children there may be a point where a review of what has been done is needed. At this point a medication review can take place to ensure antibiotics, etc., have been given. Even experienced staff can find it difficult to remember all of these aspects of treatment because of the pace of the activity.

Prior to departure

Equipment required for duration of the journey needs to be well planned so that the team are prepared for most eventualities.

Airway

Airway replacement equipment needs to be prepared and placed in an accessible place in the transport vehicle. This tray should contain:

- Stethoscope.
- ET tube (the size in the child's airway and one size below).
- Laryngoscope (age appropriate).
- Guedel airway (age-appropriate).
- Ambu bag.
- Clear mask.

The size of all emergency equipment prepared needs to be checked at this stage and not in the ambulance. Suction catheters used in children also vary in size depending on the size of the ET tube. Size required and available should be checked and prepared. Teams that work in intensive care tend to prefer Ayre's T-piece or Water's circuits to ventilate. These are good items of equipment in the hospital environment but they are gas-dependent and for this reason the team must always remember to take ambu bags when leaving clinical areas. As teams have to enter lifts which are prone to stopping between floors or altogether, suction should always be available with the patient when transferring to the ambulance.

Breathing

Ventilation is dependent on a gas supply, therefore the oxygen supply cannot be checked too often, as this is one of the most important items. A baseline blood gas should be checked on the transport ventilator prior to departure and alterations made as necessary. End tidal carbon dioxide ($EtCO_2$) monitoring is essential in monitoring in the ventilated patient as it gives a continuous indication of this level and a prompt indication of ventilation problems arising or a dislodged ET tube.

Mainstream $EtCO_2$ monitoring is relatively cumbersome but most monitors can use side-stream $EtCO_2$ monitoring, which are lightweight and can be directly connected to the bacterial filter or ET tube.

Blood gases can be monitored during transportation using handheld blood gas monitors. Cartridges can be purchased depending on what the team preference for blood results are, but they are extremely useful not only for on-going blood gases but also other biochemistry.

Circulation

Continuous ECG monitoring is essential, along with blood pressure, temperature control, oxygen saturations and $EtCO_2$ monitoring.

The two venous cannulas should always be checked with a 0.9% saline flush prior to departure, as the line that was once functional may not be when you require it n in an emergency. Spare central access lines will need to be checked in the same way.

Clear labelling of multiple drug lines should be done prior to departure so that should the child require a bolus of medication during transport the team are clear about which line to use for access. This is especially important in the child that has multiple infusions and high fluid requirement, as resuscitation fluids may need to be given continuously. The end of this line should be kept exposed and easily accessible for the duration of the journey.

If using arterial blood pressure monitoring non-invasive blood pressure (NIBP) monitoring should also be set up to monitor cardiovascular status as failing arterial pressure mechanisms can result in inaccurate measurements. The NIBP can be checked to ensure that the reading is accurate without the team having to leave their seat. This will aid in detecting deterioration quickly.

All infusion volume status should be checked prior to departure as during the stabilisation process these may have been overlooked. Long journey times and more dilute mixes of infusions will make inadequate volume more likely. As few changes of infusions as possible during the transportation should be the aim.

Disability

The child who has seizures may present with further seizures during transportation although the use of paralysing agents may make this impossible to assess. Pupil changes and vital sign changes may indicate that this is happening so be prepared with medications to hand that may need to be given, especially during a prolonged transfer. This also applies in the case of head-injured children who may require a follow-up dose of mannitol.

Maintenance fluids containing dextrose will need to be prepared for paediatric patients to maintain blood sugar, the exception being head-injured children. They will require 0.9% saline. However, younger children will need frequent blood glucose assessment to avoid hypoglycaemia.

Normothermia

The transport process usually involves exposure of the child to changes in temperature. Infants have difficulty in maintaining normothermia when exposed. The critically ill child has usually been exposed for some time to access the limbs to insert lines. This, together with shock and peripheral shutdown, often results in a very cold child no matter what the extent of circulatory resuscitation. This usually requires some form of external warming. Chemical mattresses are commonly used as well as space blankets. Modern ambulances have the facility to heat the vehicle to high temperatures, which can also be beneficial if the retrieval team can tolerate it. Children should be covered for the duration of the transport process and adequate monitoring attached to ensure that early indication of changes in clinical condition are evident.

Neonates will often be transferred in incubators, which are made to create an ambient temperature in the pre-term infant. Some teams may use a purpose-built pod for transferring neonates, while others prefer the access that harnessing and chemical mattresses alone provide. As long as the temperature is continuously monitored and maintained, all methods are acceptable and will be influenced by the team leader's and clinician's preference.

During the journey

En route the minimum should need to be done to the patient due to the extensive preparation of the team prior to departure. The continuous monitoring and documentation of the patient's vital signs should be all that is required.

Alarm setting is critical when preparing the patient so that early indications of changes are given. In addition, an alarm set incorrectly may alarm continuously and result in the monitor being ignored. Due to the nature of their illness the child may require unexpected interventions, which cannot be prepared for. This is when the training and thorough knowledge of the vehicle and kit are invaluable.

Safety

Safety is of utmost importance in both the setting up and delivery of a retrieval service.

Safety belts should be worn by all staff for the entire journey. If the child requires any interventions during transportation the vehicle should be stopped at an appropriate place. The team should not stand in the vehicle while it is moving. Ambulances are not built for travelling at high speed as they have a poor centre of gravity. This, together with the large quantity of equipment that teams take out on retrieval, can result in accidents if travelling at high speed. For these reasons it is essential that all members of specialist teams have additional life insurance. This is usually arranged by retrieval coordinators for each service. The Paediatric Intensive Care Society (PICS) also provides additional cover in provision of transportation with membership of the society.

Preparation is critical prior to departure from the referring hospital. Infusions and other medications, including resuscitation drugs, should be prepared to reduce the need to do anything during the journey. This is particularly important when travelling for long distances so that infusions or changes in clinical condition can be acted on without having to stop, remove safety belt or stand up while the vehicle is in motion.

All children should be harnessed with either a purpose-built five-piece harness attached to the transport trolley or in older children using the harness on the trolley, including over the shoulder straps. Security of pre-term infants and neonates is difficult to achieve in incubators. Incubators do provide strapping, which should be used.

All equipment that may need to be used should be secured or in easy to reach cupboards in the ambulance so that no loose equipment can act as a missile while travelling. No equipment should be stored or hung above the child as this adds risk to their journey and the team. Manufacturers are working with specialist teams to provide purpose-built systems to secure bulky items such as monitors and ventilators as these constitute a huge risk if left unsecured. A number of companies are now constructing purpose-built trolleys with these fixtures made to local specification. These all need to be compliant with the European Standardisation Organisation standards (CEN) for transportation so that the risk is reduced.

Lifting is inevitable on retrieval, as the patient needs to be moved from bed to trolley and onto bed again. The child needs to be transferred into the ambulance. Many ambulances have now been modified so that winch and lifting systems are used to reduce the risk of back injuries to members of the team. Additional equipment should be moved using trolleys, and carrying large backpacks should be discouraged.

All staff will require training in the use of these systems to ensure they are used safely as well as the usual mandatory manual handling training.

The use of blue lights is something that needs to be agreed upon locally, according to local policy and the locality of the lead centre. Few retrieved children require the use of blue lights as the majority will have been stabilised and should only require monitoring for the retrieval back to base. They will have a senior doctor and nurse in attendance and the use of blue lights may add to the risk of the journey. However, inner city areas, peak traffic times and extreme instability may increase the requirement for use of blue lights in some cases.

Accidents in paediatric retrieval are rare and when they do occur the PICS national group share lessons learnt. Teams should devise a safety policy for local use so that all members of the team are aware of what should be done to maintain their safety. High-visibility jackets should be available as well as torches if an accident should occur. Staff should wear appropriate footwear to protect the feet and remain secure. Clogs without backstraps are not appropriate and can contribute to falls or injury.

Immobilising the trauma patient

Trauma patients have usually been immobilised for neck and spinal safety by the first-response ambulance team or the receiving emergency department. If this has not been done, it will need to be done by the retrieval team. However,

what usually needs to be done is a transfer to suitable equipment to transfer the child safely for the retrieval journey. Small spinal boards are available for infants and small children that have potential neck or spinal injuries but are too small for a standard spinal board. Standard spinal boards for the older child will have fixings for safety belts to secure the board to the transport trolley. These require over-the-shoulder harnessing.

Purpose-made hard neck collars and head blocks should be used for the transportation and not modifications which could cause more trauma.

Land versus air

Alternative modes of transfer are used by some services, as they are essential in more remote areas (e.g. the Scottish highlands and islands). Some services choose to use them as they wish to reduce time of transfer. However, additional considerations need to be taken into account when transferring using these methods. Air transport has increased risks and requires additional insurance for team members. Additional training in the care of critically ill patients at altitude is also essential. Specialist services are currently being developed to provide these as part of a national service as the numbers of paediatric patients requiring this type of transport in England and Wales is so small.

Parents

Parents have reported that separation from their child during the retrieval process was the worst part of their child's intensive care admission (Colville et al. 2003). For this reason some services do transport parents with their critically ill child. However, there is still much debate around this subject and many services do not transport parents with their child. If parents do travel in the ambulance, they must wear seat belt for the duration of the journey and remain seated should any procedure be necessary with their child during the journey.

Resuscitation literature argues that parents should be permitted to stay during resuscitation as long as they are adequately supported and have an ongoing explanation during the process (Clift 2006). This may not always be possible during the transport process depending on the number of members in the team.

Parents will be suffering extreme stress and this may affect their thinking and make their behaviour unpredictable. For these reasons it is imperative that retrieval teams know the parents' methods of transport. Local teams may need to contact other members of the family to transport them or provide transport for the family. It needs to be made clear that parents must not to chase the ambulance and or overtake if the ambulance is using blue lights. This may seem fundamental but both have been witnessed during this stressful time. Parents should also be asked to remain with their child until the retrieval team departs for the lead centre. Families have gone on ahead without the knowledge of the local team and their child has not survived.

Consent

Much debate continues around the issue of consent for the process of retrieval. Most teams do not request written consent at this time. Most parents are relieved that all is being done for their child and will not refuse permission for transfer even when told the risks. However, it is a procedure not without risk and one of the few that still does not require written permission. The debate will continue.

On return to the lead centre

Handover of the patient needs to be thorough and detailed. Documentation needs to be completed and checked. Prompt restocking and checking of equipment is essential, as the team may need to go out again at short notice. Recharge all battery-powered equipment as soon as possible.

Staff training

Staff training in transportation is essential. Transport teams usually consist of one medic and one nurse and if either is not experienced in caring for critically ill children or the transportation of them, the risk increases. There are few specialist courses currently available in transportation skills and the ones that are available tend to focus on neonatal transportation. In the absence of a nationally recognised certificate of education and competency lead centres have developed their own courses and competency programmes. These vary in duration and delivery but most nursing teams provide a comprehensive in service competency programme delivered through experiential learning with experienced mentors. Together with reflection on development through experience competent practitioners evolve.

Nurses that join the retrieval service not only require the experience and competence of caring for level 3 children independently; they also need to demonstrate the skills of being a team player. Retrieval services depend on the team working well together and increased dependence on each other's skills and knowledge.

One course currently exists in the UK to develop retrieval nurse practitioners. This is modular in format and consists of lectures and experiential learning. The PICS national retrieval group have developed multi professional competencies for use in developing both medical and nursing competence. These can be modified for the use of ODAs and ambulance technicians depending on the composition of your team.

Networking with the district general hospital

The relationship with the DGH is important to the success of an effective retrieval service for the critically ill child. Each hospital should establish a lead clinician and nurse who are the link to the lead centre. It is preferable to have links from each clinical area that the critically ill child may be admitted to – emergency units, intensive care and paediatrics. These staff have the responsibility for disseminating new information and are a central link to the lead centre. The more effective this communication is the better, as the link personnel will not hesitate to telephone regarding process or equipment queries. Any issues which then arise can be addressed promptly.

Outreach education is another essential element of the network and paediatric intensive care delivery. It ensures all staff have access to education resources to increase their knowledge and confidence when caring for the most critically ill children. This amounts to a small numbers of cases per hospital each year. In more remote areas this educational input can be even more essential as time of travel of the retrieval team will take longer and local teams are often required to stabilise the child for a number of hours.

Governance

All transport services require a thorough governance process. This ensures that all cases are reviewed to ensure that a safe and effective equitable service is maintained. Multidisciplinary feedback should also occur on patients to the referring hospital. This ensures both process there and the retrieval service are reviewed and if necessary, improvements made. This may have to take place more regularly if there are many patients. Immediate feedback should be given to the local link clinician or nurse depending on severity if an untoward incident occurs. Frequently, internal governance procedures have already addressed serious incidents. However this is not always the case. Communication between centres after such events is beneficial and helps to develop strong networking relationships.

The Tanner Report

Anyone involved in the delivery of care to critically ill children throughout their care pathway (in emergency units, district general hospital and transport teams) should read this report. It identifies six generic skills that can be expected of all personnel involved with the care of acutely or critically sick or injured children in the DGH. These are:

- To recognise the critically sick or injured child.
- To initiate appropriate immediate treatment.
- To work as part of a team.
- To maintain and enhance skills.
- To be aware of issues around safeguarding children.
- To communicate effectively with children and carers.

It also provides a wealth of guidance in process and procedures that should be adhered to throughout the pathway of the critically ill child.

Withdrawal in the futile case

There will be occasions when children have been fatally injured or referred to health care too late. These cases present difficult decisions and it is often in the child's and family's best interests to withdraw care locally. This ensures that family support is immediately available. In addition, it does not give the family false hope that their child will survive. These cases will be discussed individually and withdrawal management will vary depending on circumstances. Some teams are experienced and confident in providing withdrawal of care; others have little experience. Retrieval teams often provide this help and support, they provide the additional reassurance to the family that everything has been done for their child and survival is impossible. Some of these children may be suitable for organ donation and intensive care consultants are often more experienced in these discussions with families.

Debriefings

Reflection on events is a method commonly used in nursing. There is much discussion as to how beneficial this is. Debriefings do appear to be beneficial in cases of withdrawal of care, unsuccessful or prolonged resuscitation in children. They can be beneficial when conflict has arisen or the care pathway for the child has not functioned well. Ideally, they should be coordinated by staff not directly involved in the care of the child being discussed or a member of the local team. However, lessons learned and educational needs and updating requirements need to be reported back as appropriate.

The PICS National Retrieval Group

This is a subgroup that meets every year in the National Paediatric Intensive Care Society (PICS) meeting. It evolved as a result of the developing retrieval services throughout the United Kingdom. It shares information relevant to paediatric retrieval services and is a good resource to staff developing services or new to the service.

Conclusion

This chapter has reviewed key components of the retrieval and transfer process. It is not intended as an exhaustive review of the complex requirements of the critically ill child. The services are likely to change significantly in the future as children's care pathways are restructured, possibly in a similar configuration to the neonatal services. Independent providers are likely to make inroads and tender for NHS business and the retrieval and transportation of children between hospitals is one foreseeable business case.

References

Britto J, Nadel S et al. 1995. Morbidity and severity of illness during inter-hospital transfer: impact of a specialised paediatric retrieval team. British Medical Journal, 311 (709):836–9.

Clift L. 2006. Relatives in the resuscitation room: a review of benefits and risks. Paediatric Nursing, 18(5):14–18.

Colville G, Orr F, Gracey D. 2003. 'The worst journey of our lives': parents' experiences of a specialised paediatric retrieval service. Intensive and Critical Care Nursing, 19(2):103–8.

Department of Health. 1997. A Framework for the Future. London: DH.

Department of Health. 2006. The Acutely or Critically Sick or Injured Child in the District General Hospital: a team response. London: DH.

Edge WE, Kanter RK et al. 1994. Reduction of morbidity in interhospital transport by specialised pediatric staff. Critical Care Medicine, 22(7):1186–91.

European Standardisation Organisation standards (CEN) National Co-ordinating Group on Paediatric Intensive Care. 1997. Paediatric Intensive Care: a framework for the future. Report from the National Coordinating Group on Paediatric Intensive Care to the Chief Executive of the NHS Executive. London: DH.

Paediatric Intensive Care Society (PICS). 2001. Standards of Care (2nd edition). London: PICS.

Further reading

Department of Health. 2006. The acutely or critically sick or injured child in the district general hospital – a team response. http://www.dh.gov.uk/en/Publicationsandstatistics/Publications/PublicationsPolicyAndGuidance/DH_062668

Section 4
HOLISTIC CARE

Chapter 16
CARE OF THE FAMILY

Doreen Crawford[1] and Peter McNee[2]

[1] School of Nursing and Midwifery, Faculty of Health and Life Sciences, De Montfort University, Leicester, UK
[2] Cardiff School of Nursing and Midwifery Studies, Cardiff University, Cardiff, UK

Introduction

This chapter considers the impact on the family of a child's admission to an intensive care environment. It provides practical and supportive measures the children's nurse can take to make this experience less daunting. It also sets boundaries and realistic expectations about what is possible and, for nurses who sometimes feel considerable disquiet over clinical cases, provides a framework of thinking based on philosophical principles to guide them through what can sometimes be seen as an ethical minefield.

The family of a child in PICU are uniquely vulnerable and they require support on emotional and practical issues. Generally, emergency admissions are more fraught than elective admissions because of the lack of preparation for the admission and the shocked state of the family. In an emergency, admission information and explanations should be offered several times, with the expectation that only a fraction of what is said initially will be understood.

Because of the location of the services, many of these families do not live nearby and could be distant from their usual family and friend support networks. Some will have seen their child transferred over a considerable distance depending on bed availability and the speciality. Like the child, each family is unique and as a result will have indi-

vidual needs and requirements. Not all of these can be met by the healthcare professionals and there should be no expectation that the bedside nurse has total responsibility for the family's support so the expectation levels which are set should be realistic. Good communication is vital as effective relationships have to be forged quickly and the nurse needs to appreciate that what is said and done may continue to have an impact long after the child has been discharged. This chapter considers factors that have been recognised as having a major bearing on families, provides guidance and suggests some coping strategies and follow-up for families following the discharge.

Important factors in the family's journey

- Seeing the child in the PICU for the first time.
- Suspension of the normal parenting role and responsibility and family routines.
- Dealing with emotional highs and lows.
- Uncertainty.
- The impact on any siblings.

Seeing the child in PICU for the first time

Nurses are ideally placed to prepare the family for the sight of their child and should take a few moments to provide

Paediatric Intensive Care Nursing, First Edition. Edited by Michaela Dixon and Doreen Crawford.
© 2012 John Wiley & Sons, Ltd. Published 2012 by John Wiley & Sons, Ltd.

information about the sights and sounds and the amount of machinery at the bedside before the family are admitted to the unit for the first time. Despite this the first impression can still come as a severe shock to parents and families. In addition, even though the admission might have been planned and the parents thoughtfully prepared, there may still be an impact as the reality of the situation sets in. The fact that the child has been admitted to an ICU because their illness or injury is life-threatening and they need intensive support and 24-hour nursing observation while they are managed is a concept that some families struggle with as the environment is so alien. The level of supportive technology can frighten some parents, but serves to reassure others.

The appearance of the child can be distressing, with parents of intubated children more likely to be upset than parents of non-intubated children (Haines and Perger 2006) who have obvious injuries, bleeding, bruises and oedema distorting their normal appearance. Parents may remark about the colour of their child if they are excessively pale. Above all, the need for sedation resulting in a total lack of responsiveness and lack of recognition needs explanation. Photographs should be taken with sensitivity and the dignity of a child maintained. Most units have a welcome pack and leaflet explaining some of these concerns and providing reassurance, but as each child is different a total review of the child explaining all the equipment and setting the need for this in context is recommended. More research needs to be done on the impact of a child's admissions and how the family cope and make sense of the situation (Noyes 1999).

Suspension of the normal parenting role and responsibility, and family routines

Depending on the age of the child the parents are central to their life and the child is dependent on the decisions they make and for many of their routine needs. Although parenting authority and rights are not usually affected by their child's admission to PICU their confidence and ability to assert themselves as parents in providing care can be undermined. Parents need the reassurance that they are still central to their child, that their decisions are pivotal and that they can participate in supporting the staff in the essential care that their child requires. Expectations about what is required from parents should be clear (Palmer 1993). Many of these needs may be temporarily altered and some may seem unduly strange to the family (e.g. providing pressure area care to their toddler who under normal circumstances cannot sit still). Parents may need to be invited and encouraged to help provide mouth and eye care and

combing their child's hair. This has to be done with tact and sensitivity as in some cases the child will have gained independence. However, many parents like to participate, being aware that the body image was important to their now unconscious teenager who was accustomed to spending a lot of their time in front of a mirror.

Parents' opinions need to be respected and valued and their consent and permission obtained. Parents can be asked to keep a diary for the child to act as a resource about the illness, details of treatments and how they progress. Visitors and staff can write messages for the child, which will add a human touch to what may seem a difficult time, particularly where the child seems to have been maintained by machines.

Diaries have a therapeutic role as the concept of time in the PICU can be lost in the unreality of the situation. Minutes may seem like hours, and day and night merge. In addition, it is quite common for children and parents not to remember all that happened. On recovery the child may not know where they are or how sick they have been. Where a child retains elements of memory these can be frightening or delusional. Generally, young children are clinging and demanding for a period until life feels more normal again. However, such extreme life-changing experiences in adolescents and young people in some cases result in psychological difficulties such as flashbacks and elements of post-traumatic stress disorder.

The everyday life of family and the friends of the child are significantly altered by the child's admission to PICU. Local facilities can differ but most PICUs will offer a bedroom for parents of children who are very sick and for those who live considerable distances from the hospital. Most units have a fund which will provide basic refreshments for families and some provide some simple cooking and heating facilities. Eating three meals a day in the hospital facilities can be expensive and emergency funds and meal vouchers for families can sometimes be accessed to provide temporary support. Many families rely on their own resources, and friends can bring in meals and snacks; however, pungent foods such as pizza being eaten by a child's bedside needs to be discouraged as the children are mainly nil by mouth or may feel nausea and the sensory exposure is unwelcome. In addition, the aromas linger and may distress resident children and their families and present a less than professional image of the unit.

Generally, a PICU employs an open visiting policy so families can spend as much time as they want with the child. Most PICUs have a quiet period for a couple of hours in the afternoon for sleep and rest where interventions are restricted and monitors muted. There is good evidence that this is beneficial and most staff and parents welcome and respect it (Bennet 2003). Usually, because of lack of space, the number of visitors at the bedside at any one time is restricted. Open visiting can be confusing for families who may need guidance and reassurance that frequent short visits are better than unbroken bedside vigils which will be exhausting, particularly if the visits go on into the night and the small hours of the morning. Guilt at leaving the child for a rest period or some sleep can be assuaged by the diligent use of the mobile phone to update parents if there are changes in the child's condition. Other visitors also need somewhere to sit and wait as the PICU entrance needs to be kept clear for emergency and health and safety reasons and can quickly get congested.

Parents frequently feel torn between the need to stay at the hospital and the perceived needs of their other children. Some families divide up their day or week to try to accommodate both. Apportioning activities of family living such as care of pets, homes, shopping, cooking, laundry and the care and transport of other children to family members and friends who are keen to help and support, may be a solution. Parents may need to be aware that when they allocate other people to pick up their children from nurseries and schools these organisations may need written authority to allow them to release children into a 'stranger's' care. Such strategies work in the short term but may not be sustainable in the longer term as parents themselves need each other's support and relationships can get tense, particularly when exhaustion sets in.

Working parents can experience some distress and find themselves in a dilemma if their child has a lengthy admission. Most people depend on a salary and while some employers can be flexible in the short term, others might find it hard to accommodate requests for leave. Parents with particularly responsible jobs may feel guilty when they rank their priorities. Generally, it is the parents who have the lowest income who have fewer reserves to cope with the crisis. An early referral to supportive services or charities may help these families.

Some sources of distress may seem trivial and disproportionate to others but there can be a real sense of frustration when families are subjected to additional sources of stress. Not being able to park, parking in areas that are deemed to be unsafe, the worry of over-staying a ticket and being wheel-clamped can be real concerns to parents. Like so many aspects of management in hospitals and intensive care units, some problems are easier to solve than others.

Because the PICU experience can seem so unreal when admissions are prolonged there is a need for the family to take some time out together and resume normal life, even if only for a short period to attain a sense of balance.

Dealing with emotional highs and lows

When people are stressed and anxious information is poorly retained. What is more, people want information on different things at different stages. For example, when the child is first admitted the main question may be focused on the child's chance of survival. Later, once stable and making progress, the priority may shift towards the chance of the child being left disabled, brain-damaged, scarred or paralysed. Between these two points there may be days or even weeks of uncertainty.

Confidence in the medical staff can be damaged because in some cases the staff are also experiencing uncertainty and although information as to the general outcome expectation and the child's current condition can be given, this may not be enough to satisfy the family. False reassurance should never be given.

Some families consult the internet, books, journals or other sources for information or turn to support groups and speak to other families. Most support groups offer sound information, but the quality of information available on the internet is very variable and some families have been frightened by it. Some families are very open and supportive of each other, however the experience of families differs and the nurse may have to be diplomatic in rebalancing advice given from such sources without breaching confidentiality.

Not saying what they want to hear

In an intensive care environment it is inevitable that not all news is going to be good. This can lead to some testing ethical dilemmas which the children's nurse may have to work hard to resolve for their own peace of mind. There are a few current guidelines which inform practice although these are in considerable need of review and updating as society moves forward. The guidelines which support the practice of withholding or withdrawing life-sustaining treatment come from the Royal College of Paediatrics and Child Health (RCPCH 2004) and are framed against the Children Act and the Human Rights Act to which the United Kingdom is a signatory (Crawford and Way 2009; RCPCH 2004).

Withdrawing or withholding life-sustaining managements

There are five situations where it is ethically valid and currently legal to withdraw or withhold life-sustaining managements.

Brain death

Aggressive and extreme therapy can be withdrawn when the child is brain dead, although this criterion currently excludes neonates on the basis that it is more difficult to elicit cranial nerve responses in the premature and the immature. The diagnosis of brain death can be made following a series of cranial nerve tests which indicate that independent survival is no longer possible and that further intervention or continued support is futile. These criteria are adopted to assess beating heart donors who under current legalisation are on the donor register or who have expressed a wish to donate tissue and the parents have no objection (Crawford and Way 2009; RCPCH 2004).

Permanent vegetative state

The permanent vegetative state refers to a child who deteriorates to or develops a persistent condition resulting in the need for complex support. The child is unaware of their surroundings and it is not possible for the child to sustain any sort of reciprocal relationship with their familiar and loved ones. The vital centres are intact and the cardiac sinus rhythm is maintained, but although the child may survive and growth may be possible (providing management is sufficiently supportive and sustained) there will be no developmental progress. These children require continuous intervention to prevent a range of complications and deformities which will occur as a direct result of their condition (e.g. pneumonia, postural and orthopaedic abnormalities) (Crawford and Way 2009; RCPCH 2004).

No chance situations

The no chance situation refers to a child who has suffered such severe trauma or has such extensive disease that life-sustaining management merely delays death and prolongs suffering. These are very clear-cut cases. There could be religious and philosophical debate as to the rights of the child and parents in these situations, which could create tension between the family and the staff (Crawford and Way 2009; RCPCH 2004).

No purpose

Where survival may be in doubt, it is possible that what is in question is the quality of the survival. This criterion can be applied to cases where the mental and/or physical impairment is so great that that it would be unreasonable to expect the child to tolerate such a life, or the family or the healthcare professions to impose it. Examples include the asphyxiated infant who has suffered a catastrophic lack of oxygen but was successfully resuscitated and is now maintained by technology (Crawford and Way 2009; RCPCH 2004).

Unbearable illness

In the unbearable situation, the illness is progressive and irreversible and further treatment is more than can reasonably be borne. The family and sometimes the child may wish to refuse further treatment or have some withdrawn as in a severe case of spinal-muscular atrophy, where it may be decided not to intubate and ventilate or to withdraw conventional ventilation.

In all cases, the decision to withdraw life-sustaining management does not mean that the decision to remove all form of treatment has been taken. Palliative, holistic and comforting medical and nursing care continues. Whatever can be provided for the child and family should be until no longer required (Crawford and Way 2009; RCPCH 2004).

Withdrawing life-sustaining treatment often involves taking actions knowing that the likely outcome is the demise of the child. Having time to consider the child and the family, and having time for the luxury of negotiation and reflection on agreed care strategies, may make the decision harder for some and easier for others. There are no scripts to follow and it would be foolish to imagine that a protocol could ever be developed for the range of scenarios which can be encountered (Crawford and Way 2009). To help the children's nurse work though these difficult times and enable them to take part in the decision-making process an awareness of ethics can be useful.

A working ethical framework to support practice in a PICU

An ethical stance is an individually held viewpoint and perspective, often formed by experience and exposure to difficult circumstances. These views are unlikely to remain static through the children's nurse's working life. An ethical conflict or dilemma can frequently be the source of friction and disquiet and there is limited training available to support the health care professional (Sokol et al. 2011). The children's nurse may choose to rationalise why they adopt one stance in preference to another and to do this they may opt to use a framework. There are a range of frameworks available and this section focuses on two. It is important to remember when considering ethics that there is no correct answer. Ethics need to be set against the laws and governance of the country in which the healthcare professional works and usually do not infringe a child's human rights.

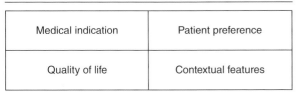

Medical indication	Patient preference
Quality of life	Contextual features

Figure 16.1 The four quadrants.

The four quadrants

The four quadrants is a practical method which can be used to analyse a case and is used to inform decision-making in a number of specialities. The approach consists of four quadrants (Figure 16.1).

The first is perhaps the most straightforward and weighs up how the child can be benefited with the minimum of harm. To do this the goals of the proposed treatment are measured against the probabilities of success. This is quite straightforward if the case is an acute asthma attack or a chest infection in an otherwise well child, but is less clear-cut if the team are struggling with the ventilation of an infant with borderline viability who has suffered intracranial bleeds.

The consideration of patient preference can be clear-cut if the case is a young person with end-stage cystic fibrosis or a neuromuscular disease who has completed a Wishes Document. In the UK a competent patient is legally entitled to refuse medical treatment, even if it will result in their death. However, for the children's nurse many of the patients are not mature enough to be deemed 'competent', and in any case the assessment of competency is not straightforward. Many children when well and rational can make a reasoned, informed decision, but as children can regress under pressure and when sick, would such a decision still reflect their views? To make matters more complex parents can overturn their child's stated wish and although the NMC desires every children's nurse to have the ability to advocate on behalf of the child (Crawford and Clarke 2010) it is probable that very few nurses would venture an opinion contrary to the strongly held views of the parents.

The quality of life quadrant has the potential to be emotive. The purpose of treating a child is not solely to prolong life but to maintain, improve or maintain the potential to enhance its quality. Most practitioners have a view as to what would be acceptable to them, and working with children who may have profound learning difficulties and poor mobility because of cerebral palsy, catastrophic spinal damage of massive neurological insult can help

clarify these views. When these children then become ill with a treatable condition a dilemma can arise. However, ethics is not about imposing a (perhaps biased) view, but informing a view, and where a child with intervention has good prospects of returning to a state similar to the one they were in before and that was deemed to be acceptable, then contrary to stated preference treatment is indicated.

The final consideration of the quadrant matrix takes into account religious, socioeconomic and cultural factors which were not considered in the other sections. The child's parents and spiritual advisers are best placed to advise the healthcare team on these aspects and although in future there may be some cap on state funding for radical forms of technological support which brings no perceivable and apparent benefit to the child, all that can be reasonably done to rescue the child should be done even if the best interest are unclear. Guidance from the courts have been mixed, in some cases compelling the medical team to continue therapy and in others providing guidance as to what can be done and withheld in the event of a deterioration. It is lawful to resuscitate without consent if it is deemed to be in the child's best interests, equally there is no obligation to take extreme action where it is doubtful that there would be a positive outcome.

Another more sophisticated framework, first developed by Beauchamp and Childress (1989), also focuses on four principles and provided a simple, accessible and culturally neutral approach to thinking about ethical issues in child health care. The approach is based on four moral commitments and although the language is unfriendly the headings categorise the underpinning philosophical paradigms well:

- Respect for autonomy.
- Beneficence.
- Non-maleficence.
- Justice.

The four principles are sufficiently flexible to be used to support the development of a personal philosophy and views on politics, religion, moral theory, and crucially when working in an intensive care environment a stance on the quality and value of life. The four principles approach can be used to deconstruct most of the moral issues that arise in paediatric healthcare, although the individual children's nurse/healthcare worker may have to apply these four principles to the individual problem themselves to support the decision-making process or when reflecting on moral issues that arise at work.

The four principles are regarded as prima facie. In the care of conflict the children's nurse would have to choose between them. The four principles approach confers no rank or value among the principles and this is a source of dissatisfaction to people who would prefer fixed rules and a clear answer.

Respect for autonomy

Autonomy (deliberate self-rule) is a special attribute of all reasoning and able individuals. If an individual has autonomy they can make their own difficult decisions on the basis of analysis and deliberation.

To have respect for autonomy is the moral obligation to respect the autonomy of others in so far as such respect is compatible with equal respect for the autonomy of all those potentially affected. Respect for autonomy has a deep base in ethical philosophy and was central in the deontological theory of Kant. In Kantian terms, respecting the autonomy of others means treating others as ends in themselves and never merely as means – one of Kant's formulations of his categorical imperative. This is something children's nurses understand quite well as they are familiar with the developmental stages in the perception of self.

In healthcare respecting people's autonomy has implications for consent and confidentiality, and of course this is enshrined in the registered nurse's professional code (NMC 2008). Respect for the autonomy of others also reduces the risk of deceit. Transparency and the absence of deceit are part of the implicit agreement among moral agents when they communicate with each other. Professionals organise their activity on the assumption that the family of the child will not deceive them.

Beneficence and non-maleficence

This is a balance between net benefit over possible harm and even when the child is unlikely to benefit the professional still needs to take steps not to harm and set in the perspective of a PICU there is an honest obligation to be clear about risk of intervention and the probability of harm.

Justice

Justice is often regarded as synonymous with being fair and providing equally. However people can be treated unjustly even if they are treated equally, for example, in the context of the allocation of resources a conflict can exist between providing basic health care to meet the needs of the majority and providing extraordinary resources for a few.

Outcomes

Some of the more difficult dilemmas result from the child surviving and becoming complex technology-dependent.

There is a range of strategies to help these families cope with life in the community. However, this has to be a decision which is right for them and the right one for them might not be a local option. Other outcomes do not involve the survival of the child and the dilemma is how to get the best possible outcome for the family.

Organ donation

Organ donation is a sensitive and emotive issue which nursing and medical staff sometimes have great difficulty in discussing with families. The discussion should be initiated by medical staff supported by nurses, though sometimes parents themselves will raise the possibility with staff. It is particularly sad when parents ask about the possibility of organ donation only to be told that their child is an unsuitable donor due to systemic infection or multi-organ failure.

Some children will die on the transplant waiting list before a suitable organ becomes available. For older children and young people they may have already expressed the view that they would want to donate their organs should anything happen to them. This can be particularly the case for children and young people with chronic illness or life-limiting conditions or for those who have experienced the death of close family members and friends and have subsequently considered their own mortality. Many parents experience great comfort in the knowledge that the death of their child has helped another child to live. Parents should be given the opportunity to discuss donation with the transplant coordinator who can talk them through the process in order for them to make an informed decision. Cook and colleagues (2002) note that some parents cannot make the final decision to donate their child's organs and this decision should be respected.

The child being prepared for organ harvest is treated like any other surgical candidate although sometimes the emphasis in care shifts away from protecting the head for example, by fluid restricting, to full perfusion. Some families feel in limbo at this point. They have been assured that there is no chance of recovery and BSD tests (see Chapter 7) will have been carried out to confirm this bleak diagnosis. Yet the child is pink and looks asleep. Some families continue with their bedside vigil and may need reminding that they need breaks and the child they knew is no longer there. It may be that they find it hard to let go, however it is equally likely that they need the continuity of the routine and the people they have come to depend on. The organ donation team have seen all this before and should be fully integrated into communication with the parents.

Following the harvesting of organs parents may ask to see and be with their child. It is important to have discussed this with them prior to donation so that they are aware that their child will return to the unit not breathing, cold, with surgical incision marks and weighing much less following a major harvest of organs. This is often difficult for parents to comprehend as following the confirmation of brain stem death and the consent to donate, their child will have left the unit for theatre breathing with the aid of a ventilator, warm, well perfused and with a heartbeat.

Before organs can be removed, stored or used for transplantation, appropriate consent must be obtained. The Human Tissue Act 2004 covers this. The Act came into force in 2006 in England, Wales and Northern Ireland. In Scotland there is the Human Tissue (Scotland) Act 2006. The Act makes it lawful for donation from the deceased to take place as long as consent was given by the person prior to their death or that consent has been obtained from a family member (usually a parent or guardian with parental responsibility) after death. The Human Tissue Authority (HTA) is the official body that oversees the Act. It provides guidance on consent and donation.

Natural end of life

Following discontinuation of aggressive but futile life-supporting technology there is frequently a natural and peaceful end of life. However, sometimes the child will need continuing and palliative support for a time. The speciality of palliative care for children has expanded in recent years and there is now a range of good practice guidelines (McNamara-Goodger and Cooke 2008) and increasing expertise in managing the emotional aspects of end of life care for children and young people (Mackenzie and MacCallam 2009; Pearson 2010).

For the parents of children who die in an ICU the cause of death is probably known and anticipated; however in some cases getting answers for the family becomes important and the medical team may request a postmortem.

Postmortem

Redfern (2001) defines a postmortem as 'a careful examination of a body after death by a pathologist'. There are two types of postmortem: a hospital postmortem and a coroner's postmortem. There are a number of reasons why a coroner's postmortem may be required, these include:

- After an accident or injury.
- Death during a surgical operation.
- Before recovery from an anaesthetic.
- If the death is linked to a medical intervention or procedure.
- If the cause of death is unknown.
- If the death was violent or unnatural (e.g. suicide, accident or drug or alcohol overdose).
- If the death was sudden and unexplained (e.g. a sudden infant death).

The postmortem is intended to establish the cause of a death, however an explicit cause is not always found and this will impact on the parents' grieving process. Following on from the Redfern Report (2001) consent for hospital postmortem and the retention of tissue samples is now

Table 16.1 The differences between a hospital and coroner's postmortem

	Hospital postmortem	Coroner's postmortem
Consent	Informed consent needed from parents before procedure.	The coroner gives the legal consent for the procedure not the parents.
The procedure	Can be limited to a specific body cavity related to the child's illness, e.g. cardiac disease; examination of the chest cavity.	No restrictions on the extent of the procedure.
Report	Feedback from the postmortem should be provided to parents at the follow-up meeting. The pathologist may also be present at this meeting if requested.	The report is forwarded from the pathologist to the coroner and clinician who would discuss the findings with the family.
Tissues and samples	Consent required from parents for the storage and future use of samples.	Consent required from parents for the storage and future use of samples after the coroner has identified a cause of death.

carefully explored with families to ensure that fully informed consent is given. The differences between a hospital and coroner's postmortem are included in Table 16.1.

Henderson (2006) identifies the benefits of a postmortem as being the information gained which will enable the family, clinicians and coroner to identify a cause of death; information about genetic disease which might influence future decisions around conception; the improvement of care management and the development and enhancement of clinical research and training. For the majority of families it is purely about knowing why their child died and whether they could they have done anything to prevent it. Sadly, the answers to these questions are not always provided by postmortem.

Acknowledgement

This section draws heavily from Singer 'Medical Ethics a Companion' and Gillon R (2003) 'Medical Ethics' published in H Kuhse and P Singer 2001 *A Companion to Bioethics*. Oxford: Blackwell. The chapter is informed by personal experience and by discussion with Kevin Power who is due to defend his PhD thesis on medical ethics and children's nurses' decision-making early in 2012.

References

Beauchamp TL, Childress JF. 1989. Principles of Biomedical Ethics (3rd edition). Oxford: Oxford University Press.

Bennet M. 2003. Sleep and rest in the PICU. Paediatric Nurse, 15(1):3–6.

Cook P, White DK, Ross-Russell RI. 2002. Bereavement support following sudden and unexpected death: guidelines for care. Archives of Disease in Childhood, 87(1):36–9.

Crawford D, Clarke D. 2010. Advocacy is a complex concept. Paediatric Nurse, 22(10):13.

Crawford D, Way C. 2009. Just because we can, should we? A discussion of treatment withdrawal. Paediatric Nursing, 21(1):22–5.

Haines C, Perger C. 2006. A comparison of the stressors experienced by parents of intubated and non-intubated children. Journal of Advanced Nursing, 21(2):350–5.

Henderson N. 2006. Communicating with families about postmortems: practice guidance. Paediatric Nursing, 118(1): 38–41.

Mackenzie J, MacCallam J. 2009. Preparing staff to provide bereavement support. Paediatric Nursing, 21(3):22–4.

McNamara-Goodger K, Cooke R. 2008. Children's and young people's palliative care: good practice guidelines. Primary Health Care, 19(2):40–7.

Noyes J. 1999. The impact of knowing your child is critically ill: a qualitative study of mothers' experiences. Journal of Advanced Nursing, 29(2):427–35.

Nursing and Midwifery Council (NMC). 2008. The Code: Standards of conduct, performance and ethics for nurses and midwives. www.nmc-uk.org/Nurses-and-midwives/The-code/The-code-in-full.

Palmer S. 1993. Care of sick children by parents: a meaningful role. Journal of Advanced Nursing, 18(2):185–91.

Pearson H. 2010. Managing the emotional aspects of end of life care for children and young people. Paediatric Nursing, 22(7):32–5.

Redfern M. 2001. The Report of the Royal Liverpool Children's Inquiry. London: Stationery Office.

Royal College of Paediatrics and Child Health. 2004. Withholding or Withdrawing Life Sustaining Treatment in Children (2nd edition). London: RCPCH. www.rcpch.ac.uk/sites/default/files/Witholding.pdf.

Further reading

Arcus KD, Kessel AS. 2002. Are ethical principles relative to time and place? A Star Wars perspective on the Alder Hey affair. British Medical Journal, 325:1493–5.

Aristotle. Nichomachean Ethics. Book 5. In R McKeon (Ed.) The Basic Works of Aristotle. New York: Random House, 1941.

Aristotle. Politics. Book 3, chapter 9. In R McKeon (Ed.). The Basic Works of Aristotle. New York: Random House, 1941.

Cox D. 1995. Ethics of rationing health care services. British Medical Journal, 310: 261–2.

Gardiner P. 2003. A virtue ethics approach to moral dilemmas in medicine. Journal of Medical Ethics, 29:297–302.

Gillon R. 1986. Philosophical Medical Ethics. Chichester: Wiley, 1986.

Gillon, R 2003. Four scenarios. Journal of Medical Ethics, 29: 267–8.

Gillon R, Lloyd A (Eds). 1994. Principles of Health Care Ethics. Chichester: Wiley.

Griffiths P. 2008. Ethical conduct and the nurse ethnographer: consideration of an ethic of care. Journal of Research in Nursing, 13:350–61.

Heaton J, Noyes J, Sloper P, Shah R. 2005. The experiences of sleep disruption in families of technology-dependent children living at home. Children and Society. DOI:10.1002/chi.881.

Hunter DJ. 1993. Rationing Dilemmas in Health Care. Research paper 8. Birmingham: National Association of Health Authorities and Trusts.

Klein R. 1991. On the Oregon trail: rationing health care – more politics than science. British Medical Journal, 302:1–2.

Lewis, W. 1995. A paper that changed my practice. British Medical Journal, 311:994.

Long-term ventilation. www.longtermventilation.nhs.uk/default.aspx.

Macklin R. 2003. Applying the four principles. Journal of Medical Ethics, 29:275–80.

Meddings F, Haith-Cooper M. 2008. Culture and communication in ethically appropriate care. Nursing Ethics, 15: 52–61.

Nilstun T, Cuttini M, Saracci R. 2001. Teaching medical ethics to experienced staff: participants, teachers and method. Journal of Medical Ethics, 27:409–12.

Noyes J. 2006. Health and quality of life of ventilator-dependent children. Journal of Advanced Nursing, 56(4): 392–403.

Noyes J. 2007. Comparison of ventilator-dependent child reports of health-related quality of life with parent reports and normative populations. Journal of Advanced Nursing, 58(1):1–10.

Noyes, J, Lewis M. 2005. Care pathway for the discharge and support of children requiring long-term ventilation in the community. National Service Framework for Children, Young People and Maternity Services. London: DfES and DH. www.dh.gov.uk.

Sokol DK, McFadzean WA, Dickson WA, Whitaker ISl. 2011. Ethical dilemmas in the acute setting: a framework for clinicians. British Medical Journal, 343(5528):d5528.

Vickers, DW, Maynard LC. 2006. Balancing biomedical, care, and support needs in the technology dependent child. Archives of Disease in Childhood, 91:458–60.

Wang K, Barnard A. 2004. Technology-dependent children and their families: a review. Journal of Advanced Nursing, 45(1):36–46.

Williams A. 1994. Economics, society and health care ethics. In R Gillon R, A Lloyd (Eds). Principles of Health Care Ethics (pp. 829–42). Chichester: Wiley.

Chapter 17
SPIRITUAL CARE AND BEREAVEMENT IN PAEDIATRIC INTENSIVE CARE

Peter McNee

Faculty of Health and Life Sciences, De Montfort University, Leicester, UK

Introduction

This chapter discusses spiritual and bereavement care within the paediatric intensive care environment. The death of a child in PICU is a challenge to the nursing staff and wider multidisciplinary team alike. We live in a society where it is assumed that children will and should outlive their parents. The pain, loss and grief experienced when a parent loses a child is immeasurable, however Davies (2009) identifies that the experiences and memories that parents have of the care delivered to their child will be long lasting. The concept of a 'good death' (Ellershaw et al. 2003), one that is dignified and pain-free, is something which should drive care and challenge nurses and other professionals to ensure that the care given is holistic, based on the child's and family's physical, psychological, cultural and spiritual needs. Nurses require a good level of understanding of spiritual care, cultural and religious practices, legal issues and the physical and psychological care that is delivered to the child and family until death and immediately after.

Death in PICU

A sudden death can be defined as one that 'occurs without any warning or period of known illness' (Kent and McDowell 2004). This definition includes children admitted to Accident and Emergency Departments following road traffic accidents and children nursed in a PICU environment where the death was preceded by several days of care. Due to the suddenness of the death the traumatic impact on the family can be extreme. When an illness has been chronic or life-limiting the family may have started the grieving process either at prognosis or following deterioration. Families will experience a rapid period of adjustment as they experience the complexity of care management within a PICU, which often involves children being cared for in an environment far from home and the family's usual support networks (Nussbaumer and Ross-Russell 2003). Stack (2003) estimates that 5–8 per cent of children admitted to PICU will die. The PICANet report (2009) has a follow-up mortality at discharge figure of 1.4 per cent, although it is acknowledged that these data are incomplete so the death rate is likely to be much higher.

Spiritual care

Spiritual care has been an overlooked aspect of nursing practice for some time. The Nursing and Midwifery Council (2004) identified the need for pre-registration nursing programmes to prepare student nurses to provide holistic care. Within the Nursing and Midwifery Council Code of Conduct (2008) a key message is to treat individuals with respect while recognising their individual needs. The Code identifies that there is a need to respond to the concerns and preferences of the individual, ensuring that they are not discriminated against. There is also a commitment to demonstrate a personal and professional commitment to equality and diversity. This could be related to treatment preferences on the grounds of culture, ethnicity, religion and spirituality. A holistic approach is one that envelops the whole person, providing for their physical, psychological, social, emotional and spiritual need. A holistic approach recognises the unique nature of the individual. Children and adults alike draw on previous experiences and beliefs in order to make some sense of their current situation. Culture, spirituality and religious beliefs will inform this process (Elkins and Cavendish 2004). Holism recognises the uniqueness of the individual child, young person and their family while moving away from the medical model of care with its focus on the presenting physical needs of the patient (Smith and McSherry 2004). Children's nurses have recognised the need to provide spiritual care, but it has been recognised that there is a gap in the knowledge and skills of the individual nurse in order to provide such care (Kenny 1999).

Defining spirituality

Individuals will often say they are not religious, but rarely claim they are not spiritual. This implies that spirituality is more widespread than religion. Offering a clear and concise definition of spirituality is fraught with difficulties. Spirituality has been aligned with organised religion specifically in the Judeo-Christian tradition. Yet Mallon (2008) defines spirituality as 'something that every person possesses and is not dependent on religious belief. It relates to the meaning and purpose of our existence.' This recognises the universal nature of spirituality regardless of a focused belief on a deity (Smith and McSherry 2004). The Scottish Executive (2002) offers a broad definition: 'spiritual care is usually given in a one to one relationship, is completely person centred and makes no assumptions about personal conviction or life orientation.' Hart and Schneider (1997) discuss spirituality in terms of the child's ability 'to derive personal value and empowerment' through a variety of relationships. The individual nature of one's own spirituality is what makes gaining consensus on a definition so difficult. What is important is to recognise that spirituality is personal and multifaceted. Recognising that the child or young person is as likely as an adult to have spiritual needs is paramount.

Children and spiritual needs

PICUs can seem alien environments for they are sometimes very clinical and impersonal due to the nature of the care provided. The machinery and noise can be stressful to new staff and visitors alike. For the parents of a child admitted to PICU this can be overwhelming (Haines and Perger 2006). But what is it like for the child? Due to ventilation, sedation and age or stage of development they may not be able to make any sense of the world around them. The care focus is the child's presenting condition and physical needs (this is not unique to PICU but typical of a range of clinical environments). Spiritual care can be consciously overlooked as staff find it difficult or are unprepared to offer such care (Hufton 2006). Nurses need to have a good understanding of children's development in order to appreciate how their spiritual needs might be expressed. Children will draw on their past experience in order to gain some understanding of their current illness and environment. Nurses need to consider how spirituality will be expressed, how they will recognise it in a ventilated child and how it can be facilitated in this care environment. To understand the expression of spirituality we first need to consider the child's cognitive development.

The child's understanding of spiritual needs

A number of developmental theorists have examined the child's ability to learn and understand the world around them. The cognitive theories that have subsequently been developed can be applied to spiritual care and the needs of the individual child. Piaget (1952) identified a number of stages that a child passes through in terms of their cognitive development. In the sensory–motor stage the child progresses from reflex activity through to repetitive behaviours to imitation. Early in this stage there is no concept of spirituality, however as children develop they discover a sense of self and object permanence. This should be remembered particularly for siblings of those admitted to PICU and twins. At the pre-operational stage children are egocentric and view the world from their own perspective. At this stage religious practice might be a regular part of the family's beliefs. It would be difficult with this group to separate spiritual belief or expression from religion (Kenny 1999). Spirituality is hard to assess in this group, but belief in a deity or other spiritual figure may be apparent; however children at this age may have some understanding of death due to personal loss and experience. Yet the permanency of death is not always apparent to them. At the concrete operational stage children children's thoughts become less self-centred and they have the capacity to consider other people's views.

However, they often associate action with reaction. Therefore illness can be seen as a punishment, particularly at the beginning of this stage. At the formal operational stage young people can think in abstract terms. Pehler (1997) notes that this group of children are best able to express feelings and concerns, which enables the nurse to broach less tangible subjects such as spirituality.

Erikson developed the Theory of Personality Development (1963). Like Piaget's this is a staged approach to development. (Staged theories have been criticised as being too rigid. A child with a chronic illness may appear more advanced in terms of their development due to repeated periods of hospitalisation and their understanding of their illness, but in other ways may regress and appear immature at times, particularly when complying with treatment or undergoing procedures.) Erikson's theory has eight stages, five of which extend from birth to around 18 years. The first – trust vs. mistrust – extends to the first year of life; basic trust is established in the primary care giver. Autonomy vs. shame follows and lasts up to the age of 3 years. Children gain greater understanding of themselves and their environment. They also learn to imitate and conform to social norms. At this stage the child might be aware of a 'god'-like or spiritual figure. Initiative vs. guilt follows. Here the child develops a conscience and feels guilt for wrongdoing. The key socialising institution is the family, and religious and spiritual values will start to be internalised. Industry vs. inferiority is the next stage; children build relationships and are fully able to cooperate with others. They develop self-assurance and a sense of mastery. The key socialising institution is still the family, but schools and teachers provide strong roles. In most schoolchildren are exposed to different cultures and religions and start to think of the world and their place in it. Spiritual awareness is increasing at this stage. Identity vs. role confusion occurs between 12 and 18 years of age. Children continue to explore the world around them but think at a much deeper level about their beliefs and attitudes across a range of subjects. The key socialising factor at this age is peer groups. Children now comprehend illness, death and dying and are also likely to have developed spiritual beliefs or religious affiliations. To facilitate spiritual expression in the ventilated child various communication strategies should be considered, including drawing, writing, picture boards and computer use.

Breaking bad news

Informing parents that their child is going to die is by far the hardest role that nurses undertake. For both nursing and medical staff this is often made more challenging due to the nature of the PICU environment where a child may be admitted, deteriorate and die in the course of a clinical shift. This limits the time available to build relationships with the parents. In breaking bad news the first consideration is who should do it. Ideally, the person delivering the information should be known to the parents and have good interpersonal skills. Commonly this will be the intensivist accompanied by the nurse who is caring for the child. It is important to consider the environment where the discussion will take place. This should be in a quiet room away from the unit where there will not be disturbed. The information should be relayed slowly at a pace that will enable the family to absorb what is being said. Opportunities should be given to enable the family to clarify any points that concern them or that they do not understand. It is essential to tell parents what is known about the child's condition and prognosis; what is not known (e.g. outstanding scan results) and what else can be done for the child. Parents will then need some time to absorb the information that has been given. It is at this stage that parents may start to come to terms with the impending death of their child and the grieving process starts. Parents may start to ask questions about future care, such as how treatment will be withdrawn if that is appropriate, how care will be managed; whether their child will be aware of their surroundings or feel pain. It is important that all questions are answered honestly and directly. Withholding information can lead to a breakdown in professional relationships, mistrust, anger and increased suffering in parents.

Case study 1

A 5-year-old girl was admitted to PICU following cardiac surgery. Her condition deteriorated over a number of days despite maximum ventilatory, fluid and inotropic support. During the course of a shift she had a cardiac arrest and requiredongoing resuscitation attempts. Her parents had left the hospital for a short time and were urgently called back. They were put in a sideroom by the unit receptionist. During the resuscitation it was decided that a member of staff should speak to the parents. As everyone was busy with the resuscitation it fell to a nurse who had never experienced breaking such bad news to parents to speak to them alone.

When the nurse enters the room she is greeted by the parents who are both crying and trying to console each other.

This case study demonstrates the enormous difficulty staff can face when breaking bad news. It highlights the importance of education and training to develop the knowledge and skills needed to fulfil this role.

Bereavement

To support parents nurses need to gain an understanding of grief and the bereavement process. Nurses are the one group of healthcare professionals who are likely to care for the child and family during the period prior to and immediately after death (Greenstreet 2004). Hindmarch (2009) defines bereavement as what happens at the time of death, grief is the reaction to that death, and mourning is how we express our loss. Loss is a recurring experience from birth to death and can be experienced in a number of ways:

- Illness.
- Diagnosis.
- Prognosis.
- Bereavement.
- Disability.
- Family breakdown.
- Unemployment.

Each individual will develop their own coping strategies in order to deal with loss. Child bereavement is the greatest loss that a parent can experience. It should be remembered that loss is a normal experience and that people demonstrate resilience. How that resilience is expressed in the bereaved will depend on cultural, social and spiritual experiences (Field and Payne 2003). The response to loss may be significantly different from that which the nurse expects. A failure to show emotion does not mean that the parent is not distressed; it may be that the individual is so overwhelmed by what they are experiencing that they cannot make a response. Culturally, the British both hide and deny their emotions and tend not to be expressive, with the goal of maintaining 'a stiff upper lip' (Read 2002). Often this is a façade that cannot be maintained and when the cracks appear emotions will be expressed.

Case study 2

A month old baby was admitted to PICU following a near cot death. The baby's mother was very young, lived alone and had very little family support. The baby was resuscitated in A&E then transferred to PICU. The baby's mother refused to enter the unit. It quickly became apparent that the baby had suffered brain stem death and following the appropriate tests treatment was withdrawn. During this period the mother who was resident within the hospital met medical and nursing staff away from the unit to discuss the baby's care management and subsequent withdrawal of treatment. Staff tried to encourage her to come onto the unit to spend time with her baby. The mother responded by saying that her baby had died on admission and once treatment had been withdrawn she would take her baby home. Once treatment was withdrawn the mother spent hours with her baby in a quiet room away from the unit.

This is an unusual but not a unique response and it is possible that the mother experienced more distress by staff repeatedly encouraging her to enter the unit. Although the staff believed they were acting in the best interests of the baby and mother, to some degree they were responding to what was perceived as an abnormal response to loss and impending bereavement. Parents will often withdraw from the PICU environment so that they do not have to face the death of their child. Avoidance could be supported, but it is important to be honest with the parents and continue to reinforce the facts around the deterioration and subsequent loss of the child.

It is an expectation that children will outlive their parents but this is not true for all children and the loss of a child will have a profound effect on the length and intensity of the grief experienced. Worden (1991) identifies a number of phases to the grieving process. First, the individual will accept the reality of loss, they will experience pain and grief, they will need to adjust to a new environment and emotionally relocate the deceased person, allowing them to move on. It is questionable how many parents will manage to move on. There will be a period of adjustment, but some parents will experience pathological grief which will be long-lasting. Grief is not a static process but evolves over time. A number of grief theories have been developed and are summarised in Table 17.1.

Theories of grief

It is important to have some knowledge of these theories, however it must be appreciated that individuals will

Table 17.1   Grief theories

Kübler-Ross (1969)	Bowlby (1980)	Worden (1991)
Denial	Numbness	Accepting the reality of loss
Anger	Yearning and searching	Working through the pain and grief
Bargaining	Disorganisation and despair	Adjusting to life without the deceased
Depression	Reorganisation of behaviour and adjustment	Emotionally relocating the deceased and
Acceptance		moving on

Table 17.2   Grief responses

Emotional	Physical	Behavioural	Psychological
Sadness	Hollowness in the stomach	Sleep disturbance	Disbelief
Anger	Tightness in the chest	Appetite disturbance	Confusion
Guilt	Tightness in the throat	Absentmindedness	Preoccupation
Self-reproach	Over-sensitivity to noise	Social withdrawal	Sense of presence
Anxiety	Sense of depersonalisation	Dreaming	Hallucination
Loneliness	Breathlessness	Searching	
Fatigue	Muscle weakness	Crying	
Helplessness	Lack of energy	Sighing	
Shock	Dry mouth	Restless over activity	
Yearning		Visiting old haunts	
Relief			
Numbness			

Source: adapted from Worden 1991.

progress through the stages at their own pace. Anger may be the prevailing emotion for some time. Parents will grieve at different times. One parent may make an adjustment to life without their child, while another may continue to work through the pain and grief without coming to a period of resolution. Stroebe and Schut (1999) have developed a dual-process model of coping with bereavement in which the individual will engage in a range of loss-oriented and restoration-oriented behaviour. This can be applied to families when they are given a prognosis for their child or following the death of a child. In loss-oriented activities the individual focuses on the loss and grief, whereas restoration-oriented activities are based on moving forward. The individual is distracted from grief, doing new things and developing new roles and identities. Thomas and Chalmers (2009) note that this behaviour can be gender-specific. Women may need more help to engage in restoration activities,whereas men may need help to face their grief and loss and express it so that emotions can be

explored. Worden (1991) identifies a range of grief responses (Table 17.2).

The grieving process can commence at diagnosis, prognosis or following the death of the child. It is important for nursing staff to look for these responses in the families that they are caring for and facilitate the appropriate support.

Caring for the child after death

Once a child has died in PICU it is incumbent on the staff to continue to provide appropriate care. It is important to establish any religious or cultural rituals which should be adhered to before handling the body. Once it has been established that the body may be handled by staff, the body may be washed. It is important to offer parents the chance to assist in this care. Any drains or tubes can be removed at this point unless there is a possibility of a coroner's postmortem. The removal of indwelling equipment can be proceeded with once the coroner's officer agrees to it. If any lines or drains have to be kept insitu they can be covered by gauze or other appropriate dressings. If the child is older, parents will usually have numerous mementos and photographs at home. However, it is still important to ask if they would like a lock of hair or hand- and footprints taken for babies and small children. For neonates parents may wish to have photographs taken. Photographs in which the baby is dressed will be better received than photographs of them taken naked. Clothing will also cover marks left from lines and surgical incisions. Most units will have access to a digital camera, alternatively hospital photographers can take the photograph. If staff have to use an instant camera it is important to make a family member aware that these pictures can fade over time so should be digitised to preserve the image. Mementos such as photographs can provide lasting comfort to bereaved parents (Osborne 2000).

Families should be given the time and space in which to grieve with their child. Kübler-Ross (1983) identified that the long-term outcomes of bereavement are improved if those who are bereaved can see and spend time with their loved one's body. PICUs are set up for acute, intense care. Where possible a side-room or quiet room should be made available for the family to spend time with their child. It is important that nurses negotiate with the family whether they want a nurse to stay with them or to come in periodically. Davies (2005), following interviews with bereaved mothers, found that they need time, space and privacy to be with their dying child and with the child's body after death.

Case study 3

The baby of a single mother died on PICU following a severe case of bronchiolitis. The father had left during pregnancy and the mother was estranged from her wider family. Following the baby's death, the mother and baby where taken to a quiet room off the hospital chapel where they wouldn't be disturbed. The mother asked the staff nurse to stay with them for a little while. During this time very few words were spoken. After a couple of hours the mother said that the nurse could leave but would they call back every hour or so. The nurse did this until the mother was ready to leave the hospital.

This case study emphasises the need that a parent may have for someone to be present to offer them comfort. Nurses will often feel that they should say something, but parents will find solace in just having someone there.

Once the parents are ready to leave they will want to know what happens next. Most clinical areas have bereavement packs which outline matters such as obtaining a death certificate, registering a death and arranging a funeral. The parents can take the child home with them, although this is not commonly done. Parents have rights to and ownership of the child's body (Kennedy 2001). The only reason why a body cannot be removed from a hospital once death has occurred is if a postmortem is likely to be legally required. Whittle and Cutts (2002) looked at parents' ability to take children home. The nurse must ensure that the parents write in the medical notes that they are taking the child home. As well as a death certificate, a hospital letter should be provided explaining to any authorities that this has been agreed and that a suitable form of transport is available. The contact details of the unit should also be provided in case any issues arise. As parents are often unaware of the option to take their child home, nurses should inform them. One year on from the death of her child one mother in Davies' study (2005) was very angry that she had not known that she could have taken her child home.

Most children will be taken to the mortuary. Parents will often want a comforter of some sort to accompany the child, possibly a teddy bear or blanket, so that they are not alone. In the author's experience mortuary technicians are very accommodating of and sensitive to parents' wishes. Some parents will also ask to return and see their child a day or two later before transfer to the funeral directors. It is good practice for a nurse who knows the family to accompany them to the mortuary chapel or viewing room. If possible check the body prior to allowing the parents to see the child in case bodily fluids have leaked. If they have, the body can be cleaned and redressed before the parents handle it. It is important to tell parents that the child will look and feel different from when they last saw them. The body has been in a refrigeration unit and will therefore be cold, blood will have pooled and the body will appear pale and waxy. Sometimes it is the coldness rather than the appearance that surprises parents.

Religious observance

Religious and cultural practices vary. Some families will strictly observe their religious practice; other families may observe aspects of that teaching. In order to avoid causing offence, it is better to ask first than proceed. Always ask if the body should be touched, cleaned and placed in any specific position. Enquire if a religious leader (rabbi, minister or imam) is to attend the body. Table 17.3 outlines common religious practices. However, there may be significant differences in the religious practices of groups within the same faith.

Siblings

Siblings are often overlooked when providing care for the dying child and family. It should be recognised that parents may experience grief and cope differently from children. Honesty is of the utmost importance and parents should be encouraged to keep siblings informed about the deterioration in their brother's or sister's condition. Siblings may be excluded from the PICU environment. This is often at the parents' discretion to protect the child from what is happening. But after the death of a child the sibling may feel guilty that they did not spend time with the dying child. Thomas and Chalmers (2009) recognise that siblings may experience a sense of isolation as their parents are immersed in their grief. To try to resolve some of the issues identified with bereaved children Winston's Wish (2009) have produced a charter for bereaved children. This identifies the need for children to have support from their family, school and people around them and be given time to express their thoughts and feelings. There is also an emphasis on involvement in key decisions, such as arranging the funeral. The charter makes clear the need for children's voices to be heard and to recognise the importance of children having the same access to support and counselling. When nurses provide help and support to families they should consider the following:

- Encourage the child to express their thoughts, feelings and emotions about their deceased sibling.
- The sibling will experience grief and have thoughts and feelings including anxiety, sadness, anger guilt and behavioural problems.
- Try to maintain normal activities so that the child has routine within their lives and their friends and support networks.
- The child may become more aware of their own and others' mortality so may want to keep close to parents as they fear further loss.
- Ensure that they know that they are not to blame for their sibling's death and encourage them to share both happy and sad memories of the deceased sibling.

Factors affecting sibling grief include the child's age and cognitive development; and their previous experience of

death (this may be that of a family member such as a grandparent or of a family pet which may have been replaced). It is important to consider whether the child understands the permanency of death in the current situation that they find themselves in. The stability of their life will impact on the child's ability to deal with the grief and to develop effective coping strategies. It is also important to communicate effectively with siblings and encourage the parents not to use euphemisms when talking about the dead child such as 'they passed away' or 'they fell asleep' (Nussbaumer and Ross-Russell 2003). This could have long-term connotations as the child may think that when they fall asleep they won't wake up again. There is also the potential risk that siblings will hide their feelings in order to protect their parents as they will not want to add to parents' distress.

Case study 4

Carys aged 5 years had a brother called Tom aged 3 months who was admitted to PICU with cardiomyopathy. Tom's cardiac function was very poor and his condition was deteriorating. Carys came into PICU to see Tom. During the visit Tom's heart rate and saturations dropped. Both the monitor and ventilator alarms went off. The nursing staff intervened and resolved the problem. This episode scared Carys and she never visited Tom in PICU again. Two weeks later Tom died. Following the funeral Carys expressed the view that it was her fault that he died because of the episode that she witnessed during the visit.

This case study illustrates how children will internalise their experiences. It is important for siblings to be encouraged to visit PICU, but they should be adequately prepared for how their sibling will look, and the sights, sounds and environment of a PICU.

Parents' emotional wellbeing and parenting after a child's death

Despite the loss of a child parents continue to parent after death. However, they need to create new meaning for the world that they find themselves in (De Jong-Berg and de Vlaming 2005).

Religion	Practices at death	Attitudes to postmortem	Attitudes to organ donation
Buddhism	Buddhists believe that it may take several days for the consciousness to leave the body and so prefer not to have the body disturbed. Solutions to this should be sensitively negotiated; however Buddhists are recognised for their tolerant attitudes.	Unlikely to consent, unless legally required due to disturbing the consciousness.	May be agreed to due to the good karma that will come from this act; however the issue around the consciousness leaving the body may prohibit this.
Christianity	Routine last offices are appropriate.	No objection on religious grounds.	No objection on religious grounds.
Christian Science	Routine last offices are appropriate. If the child is a girl female staff are preferred when handling the body.	Families are unlikely to consent unless legally obliged to do so.	Unlikely to donate or receive organs.
Hinduism	Do not wash the body; the family will do this. If the body needs to be touched by a non-Hindu, wear gloves and ask permission first. Cover the body with a white sheet. If the body has to be left alone, leave a light on as a mark of respect.	Families are unlikely to consent unless legally obliged to do so. The family will want any organs removed so that the body is buried intact.	No objections on religious grounds but should be explored sensitively.
Islam	Wear gloves to avoid directly touching the body. Straighten the legs and arms and close the eyes. Turn the person's head towards Mecca (usually south-east in the UK). Do not wash the body; the family will do this. Cover the body with a white sheet.	Families are unlikely to consent unless legally obliged to do so.	Muslims can donate and receive organs. However, there may be the proviso that organs can only be donated to another Muslim.
Jehovah's Witness	Routine last offices are appropriate.	No objection on religious grounds.	There may be objections due to someone else's blood flowing through their organs.
Judaism	Leave the arms at the side of the body and straighten the legs pointing towards the door. Close the mouth, secure with strapping if necessary. Cover the body with a clean white sheet.	Families are unlikely to consent unless legally obliged to do so.	An organ may be donated for immediate transplant only.
Rastafarianism	Routine last offices are appropriate.	Families are unlikely to consent unless legally obliged to do so.	The family are unlikely to agree to organ donation but should be asked.
Sikhism	Wear gloves when touching the body. Do not wash the body; the family may wish to do it. Do not remove the five Ks if the child is wearing them. Do not undress the body. Cover the body with a plain white sheet.	No objection on religious grounds.	No objection on religious grounds.

Case study 5

Paul's daughter Amy, aged 3 years, died 10 years ago after contracting meningococcal septicaemia. When he introduces his family he states that he has three children: Daisy, James and Amy. Amy was the eldest but she died.

In this case we can see the importance of keeping the child's memory alive. Some parents do not include their deceased child in this way as it may be too painful or personal. For Paul it is a way of expressing the fact that he will always be Amy's father and that she will always be a part of the family.

Following the death of a child parents may experience isolation from other parents as they no longer have the routines that come with having a child – the school run, parents' activities, driving the child to various activities. Suddenly an entire part of the wider parenting role has gone. Other parents may actively avoid contact (Bucaro, Brown and Curry 2005), perhaps because they do not know what to say. Although supporting parents at this point is not within the remit of the PICU staff, they will encourage parents to access wider support from the Trust Bereavement Service (if one is in place) or the wider statutory or voluntary services which offer counselling and support.

Case study 6

Ahmed's son died on PICU having sustained multiple injuries in a road traffic accident. At the anniversary of his son's death Ahmed visits PICU and sits in a chair at the nurses' station opposite the bed space where his son died. Ahmed has done this for five years. As the years have gone by and staff have moved on fewer nurses knew Ahmed or cared for his son prior to his death. At the time of his final visit, no member of staff on duty knew Ahmed or his son and the unit was about to move into a new building.

This case study illustrates the need for bereaved families to be near the place where their loved one died. When travelling on busy roads you often see flowers or other memorials at the place where someone has died. This activity appears to fulfil a need in the bereaved. To try to meet such needs many Trusts hold an annual memorial service for the children who have died during the year.

Waters (1999) tells the story of Jenny, who died in 1988. The article reflects on Rose's experience of care in both an ICU and a paediatric ward. It affords some insight into the memories that parents keep after bereavement. On the ward Jenny's care was holistic and the needs of all family members were considered. Following deterioration Jenny was moved to ICU; the care was then perceived to be more based on physical needs. The music that was played to Jenny on the ward was often turned off, the environment was clinical and in Rose's opinion the nurses were preoccupied with physical tasks and procedures. Following a poor blood gas a doctor commented, 'She has got a death wish' – a callous observation, but probably not meant to be heard by the family.

Following Jenny's death she was dressed in a blue babygrow, and when her parents visited her in the mortuary the technician referred to her as 'he' due to the association with blue for a boy and pink for a girl. Finally, when the parents returned to ICU to collect Jenny's belongings they had been placed in a black plastic bin bag. This is not typical of current care but is a salutary reminder of how parents will carry memories of poor care with them and the need to facilitate a 'good death' where the care provided has been individualised and holistic.

Follow-up care

Once the funeral has taken place families start to adjust to life without their child. Cook, White and Ross-Russell (2002) identify the value of a follow-up bereavement programme. This will enable parents to ask specific questions about the care and death of their child. The key elements of the bereavement programme are that it should take place 8–12 weeks following the death of the child. This time span allows for any new information to be discussed asby then any postmortem report will have become available to the family. Any outstanding investigations, scans or genetic testing will have been reported on. If organ donation has occurred feedback from the transplant coordinators will be available. Parents may find some comfort in knowing that their child's organs have been successfully transplanted. However, if the transplant has failed, this can add significantly to the parents' bereavement. It is expected that the clinician responsible for the child's care is present and a nurse who has cared for the child and family. As well as having questions answered, the family may wish to visit the clinical area. This meeting allows staff to assess how the family is coping, recognise the signs of pathological grief and refer on to wider support services.

References

Bowlby J. 1980. Attachment and Loss. Vol. 3: Loss, Sadness and Depression. London: Hogarth.

Bucaro P, Brown L, Curry D. 2005. Bereavement care: one children's hospital's compassionate plan for parents and families. Journal of Emergency Nursing, 31(3):305–8.

Cook P, White DK, Ross-Russell RI. 2002. Bereavement support following sudden and unexpected death: guidelines for care. Archives of Disease in Childhood, 87:36–9.

Davies R. 2005. Mothers' stories of loss: their need to be with their dying child and their child's body after death. Journal of Child Health Care, 9(4):288–300.

Davies R. 2009. Caring for the child at the end of life. In J Price, P McNeilly (Eds). Palliative Care for Children and Families: an interdisciplinary approach (pp. 192–212). Basingstoke: Palgrave Macmillan.

De Jong-Berg MA, de Vlaming D. 2005. Bereavement care for families' part 1: a review of a paediatric follow-up programme. International Journal of Palliative Care, 11(10): 533–9.

Ellershaw J, Ward C, Neuberger, J. 2003. Care of the dying patients: the last hours or days of life. British Medical Journal, 326:30–4.

Elkins M, Cavendish, R. 2004. Developing a plan for pediatric spiritual care. Holistic Nurse Practitioner, 18(4):179–84.

Erikson EH. 1963. Childhood and Society (2nd edition). New York: WW Norton.

Field D, Payne S. 2003. Social aspects of bereavement. Cancer Nursing Practice, 2(8):21–5.

Greenstreet W. 2004. Why nurses need to understand the principles of bereavement theory. British Journal of Nursing, 13(10):590–3.

Haines C, Perger C. 2006. A comparison of the stressors experienced by parents of intubated and non-intubated children. Journal of Advanced Nursing, 21(2):350–5.

Hart D,Schneider D. 1997. Spiritual care for children with cancer. Seminars in Oncology Nursing, 13(4):263–70.

Hindmarch C. 2009. On the Death of a Child (3rd edition). Oxford: Radcliffe.

Hufton E. 2006. Parting gifts: the spiritual needs of children. Journal of Child Health Care, 10(3):240–50.

Kennedy I. 2001. Learning from Bristol: The report of the public inquiry into children's heart surgery at the Bristol Royal Infirmary 1984–1995. London: TSO.

Kenny G. 1999. Assessing children's spirituality: what is the way forward? Paediatric Nursing, 8(1):28–32.

Kent H, McDowell J. 2004. Sudden bereavement in acute care settings. Nursing Standard, 19(6):38–42.

Kübler-Ross E. 1969. On Death and Dying. New York: Macmillan.

Kübler-Ross E. 1983. On Children and Death. New York: Macmillan.

Mallon B. 2008. Dying, Death and Grief: working with adult bereavement. London: Sage.

Nursing and Midwifery Council. 2004. Requirements for Pre-registration Nursing Programmes. London: NMC.

Nursing and Midwifery Council. 2008. The Code: Standards of conduct, performance and ethics for nurses and midwives. London: NMC.

Nussbaumer A, Ross-Russell R. 2003. Bereavement support following sudden and unexpected death in children. Current Paediatrics, 13:555–9.

Osborne M. 2000. Photographs and mementos: the emergency nurse's role following sudden infant death. Emergency Nurse, 7(9):23–5.

Pehler SR. 1997. Children's spiritual response: validation of the nursing diagnosis in spiritual distress. Nursing Diagnosis, 8(2):55–66.

PICANet. 2009. Paediatric Intensive Care Audit Network: National report 2006–2008. Universities of Leeds and Leicester.

Read S. 2002. Loss and bereavement: a nursing response. Nursing Standard, 16(37):47–53.

Scottish Executive. 2002. Spiritual Care in NHS Scotland. HDL (76). Scottish Executive.

Smith J, McSherry W. 2004. Spirituality and child development: a concept analysis. Journal of Advanced Nursing, 45(3):307–15.

Stack C. 2003. Bereavement in paediatric intensive care. Paediatric Anaesthesia, 13:651–4.

Stroebe MS, Schut H. 1999. The dual process model of coping with bereavement: rationale and descriptions. Death Studies, 23(3):197–224.

Thomas J, Chalmers A. 2009. Bereavement care. In J Price, P McNeilly (Eds). Palliative Care for Children and Families: an interdisciplinary approach (pp. 192–212). Basingstoke: Palgrave Macmillan.

Waters LA. 1999. Rose's story: Understanding events in nursing. Paediatric Nursing, 11(2):40–3.

Whittle M, Cutts S. 2002. Time to go home: assisting families to take their child home following a planned hospital or hospice death. Paediatric Nursing, 14(10):24–8.

Winston's Wish. 2009. The Charter for Bereaved Children. Cheltenham: Winston's Wish.

Worden WJ. 1991. Grief Counselling and Grief Therapy: A handbook for the mental health practitioner. London: Routledge.

Further reading

ACT and RCPCH. 2003. A Guide to the Development of Children's Palliative Care Services (2nd edition). Bristol: ACT.

Department of Health 2008. Better Care: Better Lives. Improving outcomes and experiences for children, young people and their families living with life-limiting and life-threatening conditions. London: DH.

Resources

www.bbc.co.uk/religion/religions. BBC religious affairs website.

www.childbereavement.org.uk. Child Bereavement Charity (Trust)

www.dh.gov.uk/en/Healthcare/Secondarycare/Transplantation/Organdonation/index.htm – DOH website covering organ transplantation and consent.

www.ethnicityonline.net. Website containing the religious and cultural practices of the major religions.

www.mfghc.com. Multi-faith group for healthcare chaplaincy.

www.winstonswish.org.uk. A leading bereavement charity and provider of services to bereaved children, young people and their families.

Chapter 18
SAFEGUARDING CHILDREN IN THE INTENSIVE CARE UNIT

Gillian Earl

CCJJ, Child Protection Training and Consultancy Services, Lincolnshire, UK

Introduction

This chapter reviews the key issues for nurses safeguarding children in the ITU and offers a background reading to augment professional practice. The chapter also offers a practical approach to dealing with some of the dilemmas which a paediatric intensive care nurse can encounter. Safeguarding children and ethics are not mutually exclusive and frequently safeguarding issues can pose their own ethical issues which can be difficult to resolve.

It should be noted that safeguarding guidelines are evolving rapidly and the paediatric ITU nurse is strongly advised to keep up to date with current practice. In contrast, consideration of the ethical issues affecting children in ITU seems slower to develop and arguably has been outpaced by the advanced technological support which is now available in the units. See Chapter 16 for a consideration of care of the family and applied ethics.

Background to the current safeguarding child recommendations

Lord Laming (2009) expressed a simple but profoundly important hope which was the very minimum on which every child and young person should be able to depend. He included in this the unborn child. This ethos applies to infants, children and young people who are lying critically ill in intensive care units around the country. Safeguarding children is relevant up to the child's 18th birthday and children's nurses may meet and be involved with vulnerable children and young people in a variety of settings, including neonatal units, paediatric intensive care units, other intensive care units either in district general hospitals or in more specialised tertiary hospital settings which provide services to children and young people. In addition, the children and young people who visit siblings, parents or carers within such units may be at risk.

Hospitals are often involved with critically ill patients and their families who are under extreme stress. They have an important role to play in the identification, referral, assessment and provision of services to children who are in need of protection and also the support of their families. Recent years have seen a particularly intense time of change with several reports, such as the Laming Report on the death of Victoria Climbié (2003), and the government's response to the services' failure to safeguard children with the 10-year programme of change (Department for Education and Skills 2003). This has highlighted the need to build and develop capability and capacity in child protection. The focus has been on organising services and resources around children to ensure their safety and proper

Paediatric Intensive Care Nursing, First Edition. Edited by Michaela Dixon and Doreen Crawford.
© 2012 John Wiley & Sons, Ltd. Published 2012 by John Wiley & Sons, Ltd.

development, and improve their wellbeing (Laming 2009). Laming acknowledged the complexities inherent in safeguarding frontline staff and recommended the development of simplified guidance, resulting in the publication of 'What To Do If You Are Worried A Child Is Being Abused' (Her Majesty's Government 2003, revised 2006 and 2010).

Laming's *The Protection of Children in England: a progress report* (2009), following the death of Peter Connelly ('Baby P'), highlighted the importance of frontline staff in the protection of children and the promotion of their welfare. Laming (2009) clearly identifies that if safeguarding children is everybody's responsibility, then everyone should know how and whom to contact if they are concerned about a child or young person. In addition, all health staff should be able to recognise abuse and neglect and be familiar with their Trust's policies and procedures when they have concerns, including making enquiries to find out whether a child is subject to a child protection plan. In 2010 the government commissioned a further review of the current child protection framework (Department of Education 2011). Although the focus was predominantly on social work practice, significant proposals for professional accountability and serious case review (SCR) processes were made. It was recommended that the government work collaboratively with health organisations on the impact of health reorganisation on effective partnership arrangements and the ability to provide effective help for children who are suffering, or are likely to suffer, significant harm. At the time of writing the government have not yet fully implemented the changes in the light of this review but it is likely to place greater responsibility on professionals for safeguarding children assessments, a move to more streamlined SCR processes more in line with root cause analysis models used currently in the NHS, and an expectation that health service providers focus on children's views on how they are treated and engaged with in hospital.

Over the last 30 years there have been a number of SCRs and there has been considerable consternation that greater progress has not been made in preventing such occurrences. Reviews and enquiries across the United Kingdom have consistently identified similar issues which were again seen in the SCR of Peter Connelly. These are:

• Inadequate sharing of information.
• Poor assessment processes.
• Ineffective decision-making.
• Poor recording and/or documentation of information.
• Lack of information on significant males.
• Poor communication.
• No supervision or training.

• Lack of inter-agency working.
• Failure to listen to children.
    (Department of Health 2000a, 2000b, 2002a, 2002b; Department for Children, Schools and Families 2008).

The purpose of an SCR is to:

• Establish whether there were lessons to be learned from the case about the way in which local professionals and organisations worked together to safeguard and promote the welfare of children.
• Identify clearly what those lessons are, how they will be acted on and what is expected to change as a result.
• As a consequence, improve inter-agency working and better safeguard and promote the welfare of children.

They are not inquiries into how a child has died, sustained a potentially life-threatening injury or serious and permanent impairment of health and development through abuse or neglect or who is culpable. These will be addressed within standard child protection procedures, coroner's and criminal courts respectively. The criteria for holding an SCR are detailed in *Working Together to Safeguard Children* (Department for Children, Schools and Families 2010).

This government guidance has outlined the responsibilities of NHS Trusts for providing health services. These include safeguarding arrangements and the identification of named professionals. This model is further supported by the recent Munro Review, which will lead to a revised version of *Working Together* in 2012.

Trusts recognise that child protection can generate a great deal of staff anxiety and the need for the topic to be dealt with sensitivity. There also has to be continuity and consistency in approach. To achieve this each Trust has a named nurse and doctor usually within a Child Protection Team to support and advise all staff when they have concerns about a child's welfare or safety. Each health organisation should have a safeguarding supervision process that allows all staff to have access to advice and supervision when they have concerns about a child in their care, and the named professionals should sit at the hub of this process. 'Supervision helps practitioners to think, to explain and to understand. It also helps them to cope with the complex emotional demands of the work with children and families' (Department for Children, Schools and Families 2008). These demands can be particularly significant in the intensive care environment.

Named professionals

Named professionals have a key role in promoting good professional practice within the Trust and provide advice and expertise for fellow professionals. They have expertise in children's health and development, child maltreatment and local arrangements for safeguarding and promoting the welfare of all children who are patients, are visiting services or have parents receiving a service (Department for Children, Schools and Families 2010). In addition, the named professionals support the Trust in its clinical governance role by ensuring audits on safeguarding are undertaken and that safeguarding issues are part of the Trust's clinical governance system. They are also responsible for undertaking the Trust's internal management reviews and ensuring any action plan is followed up (Department for Children, Schools and Families 2010).

Named professionals play an important role in promoting, influencing and developing relevant training on both a single and inter-agency basis to ensure the training needs of health staff are addressed. They also provide skilled professional involvement in safeguarding processes in line with Local Safeguarding Children's Boards' (LSCB) procedures and in undertaking Individual Management Reviews with involvement in SCRs.

Named professionals are supported by designated professionals who undertake a strategic professional lead on all aspects of the health service contributions to safeguarding children across the PCT area (this includes all providers).

Staff education and training

Different staff groups will have different training needs to fulfil their duties, depending on their degree of contact with children and young people and their level of responsibility. All hospital staff, including intensive care staff, should access appropriate training relevant to their role and level of responsibility to develop core competencies, as identified by the Royal College of Paediatrics and Child Health (2010).

Safeguarding Competency: Level 2 is relevant to intensive care nurses working in general intensive care units with child, young people or adult patients, while Level 3 is more suitable to nurses working in neonatal units, high dependency units or paediatric intensive care units.

Level 2

Clinical and non-clinical staff who have infrequent contact with parents, children and young people.

Competency required:

- Uses professional and clinical knowledge.
- Understands what constitutes child maltreatment.
- Identifies any signs of child abuse or neglect.

- Acts as an effective advocate for the child and young person.
- Recognises the potential impact of a parent's or carer's physical and mental health on the wellbeing of a child or young person.
- Is clear about their own and colleagues' roles, responsibilities and professional boundaries.
- Can refer as appropriate if a safeguarding/child protection concern is identified.
- Documents concerns, maintaining appropriate record-keeping, which differentiates between fact and opinion.
- Shares appropriate and relevant information.
- Follows local policies and procedures.
- Acts in accordance with key statutory and non-statutory guidance and legislation, including the UN Convention on the Rights of the Child and Human Rights Act.

Level 3

All staff working predominantly with children, young people and parents.

Competency required:

- As Level 2.
- Will have professionally relevant core and case-specific clinical competencies.
- Contributes to inter-agency assessments, gathering and sharing of information and, where appropriate, risk analysis.
- Documents concerns in a manner that is appropriate for safeguarding/child protection and legal processes.
- Undertakes regular documented reviews of own (and/or team) safeguarding/child protection.
- Practises, as appropriate, the role in various ways (e.g. audit, case discussion, peer review, supervision and as a component of refresher training).
- Contributes to serious case reviews/case management reviews/significant case reviews and child death review processes.
- Works with other professionals and agencies, with children, young people and their families when there are safeguarding concerns.
- Advises other agencies about the health management of individual children in child protection cases.

Action to take when a child is admitted to the unit

When a child is admitted to the ICU who has sustained a potentially life-threatening injury or serious, possibly permanent impairment of health and development or who subsequently dies as a result of abuse or neglect it may be known or suspected to be a factor in the admission. Staff should immediately consider whether there are other children at risk of harm and who require safeguarding. In these circumstances local policies should be followed and an immediate referral made to local children's social care services for the child on the ICU, including the identification of any relevant siblings or children. In addition, a check should be made with local children's social care services for all relevant children to check if any child is currently subject to a child protection plan as detailed in Trust policy. Staff should always seek professional and managerial supervision when referring a child, but this should not be allowed to delay the referral.

Consequently when a child is identified in such circumstances in addition to any ongoing child protection investigation undertaken under the Children Act 1989, Section 47 (Department of Health 1991) the Local Safeguarding Children Board will decide as detailed in *Working Together to Safeguard Children* (Department for Children, Schools and Families 2010, Chapter 8) whether to hold a serious case review. The roles and responsibilities of local safeguarding children boards are defined in the intra-agency guidance (Department for Children, Schools and Families 2010).

Recognising and taking responsibility

Everyone who comes into contact with children and young people has a duty to safeguard and promote their welfare and should know what to do if they have any concerns. Any holistic assessment of a child should be reviewed on a regular basis by all staff involved with the child and their family.

In the case of a child who is critically ill, a holistic assessment using the CAF (Common Assessment Framework, Department for Children, Schools and Families 2008) will be undertaken. This is usually led by the child's consultant and aims to understand the nature of the child's illness or injury and to consider in every case if there are any concerns about the child's health or wellbeing from a safeguarding aspect. Where there are identified concerns of a safeguarding nature the Assessment Framework (Department of Health, Department for Education and Science and HMG 2000) ensures the family is treated with sensitivity, discretion and respect at all times. It is important that professionals should approach their enquiries with an open mind.

Children from all cultures are subject to abuse and neglect. All children have a right to grow up safe from harm. In order to make sensitive and informed professional judgements about a child's needs and the parents' capacity to respond to those needs in the emotionally charged environment of the ITU it is important that professionals are culturally sensitive to family patterns and lifestyles. Child rearing patterns also vary among racial, ethnic and cultural groups but at the same time intensive care nurses must be clear that child abuse cannot be condoned for religious or cultural reasons (Department for Children, Schools and Families 2010).

At times there may be a difference of opinion between intensive care staff as to whether a child's injuries are due to abuse or there are concerns about a child's (or a sibling visiting the unit) health, welfare or safety. In all such cases support, advice and guidance can be obtained from the named professionals within the Trust, including guidance on actions to be followed when a child is already subject to a child protection plan.

Information confirming a child is subject to a child protection plan may be obtained from a number of different sources:

- A formal check by the intensive care nurse as required by Trust or Local Safeguarding Children Board policy.
- Informed by a child's social worker or police officer.
- Informed by a member of the Trust Safeguarding Team (named or designated professional).
- By the child's parent(s) or relative.

When further advice, support or guidance is required or there is a difference of opinion outside normal working hours support may be available from the named professionals via an on-call system or other on-call senior managers within the Trust. Alternatively, the local Social Services emergency duty team or police can be contacted for advice and support. Their contact numbers can be located within the Trust's safeguarding policies and procedures.

Assessment of children

There is no truly reliable way to identify which children may be at risk of abuse. Any child may be abused and any adult may become an abuser (Department of Health 2006). However, some factors or indicators appear to increase the vulnerability of children and carers to abuse. These risk indicators include:

- Their level of education, knowledge base and awareness of the child's needs.
- Their maturity and parenting capacity.
- The family resources and the family's environment.

The presence of risk factors does not mean that a child will be abused; it may highlight vulnerability to abuse and indicate that the child requires additional support with an appropriate referral to Children's Social Care Services as detailed in Trust Child Protection Procedures. The CAF and Assessment Framework are assessment tools used by all staff from different agencies and are also useful for intensive care nurses.

In order to be able to undertake an assessment it is important for professionals to understand the signs and symptoms of abuse and to be able to recognise when they have a concern in respect of a child's health or welfare. The following definitions and features are the ones currently used by all UK agencies and are detailed in the Children Act 1989, *Working Together to Safeguard Children* (2010) and the National Institute for Health and Clinical Excellence (2009). Intensive care nurses working in Scotland, Wales or Ireland may find local guidance definitions vary but not significantly.

Recognition of abuse or neglect

The local authority has a duty to make enquiries where it has reasonable cause to suspect a child is suffering significant harm or likely to suffer significant harm, but they can only do this when they have been alerted by a professional, family member or a member of the public that there are concerns about a child's welfare or safety. If an intensive care nurse identifies concerns about a child's health, welfare or safety then they have a duty to refer their concerns to children's social care services and/or the police following Trust policies and procedures.

What is abuse and neglect?

These are forms of maltreatment of a child. Somebody may abuse or neglect a child by inflicting harm or by failing to act to prevent harm. Children may be abused in a family or in an institutional or community setting by those known to them or, more rarely, by a stranger. They may be abused by an adult or adults, or another child or children (Department for Children, Schools and Families 2010).

> *actual or likely harm to the child, where harm includes both ill treatment (sexual abuse and non-physical ill-treatment such as emotional abuse) and the impairment of health and development, (physical or mental health) and physical, intellectual, emotional, social or behavioural development . . .*
> (Department for Children, Schools and Families 2010)

Physical abuse

Physical abuse may involve hitting, shaking, throwing, poisoning, burning or scalding, drowning, suffocating or otherwise causing physical harm to a child. Physical harm may also be caused when a parent or carer fabricates the symptoms of, or deliberately induces illness in a child (Department for Children, Schools and Families 2010).

Fabricated and induced illness

> *Fabrication or induction of illness in a child is a life endangering and sometimes fatal condition in which a parent, usually the mother, fabricates illness in a child either by inducing physical signs of illness or by deliberately misleading the doctor into believing that the child is ill.*
> (Department for Children, Schools and Families 2008)

There are three main ways the carer (usually the mother) can fabricate or induce illness in a child. These are not mutually exclusive and include:

- Fabrication of signs and symptoms. This may include fabrication of past medical history.
- Fabrication of signs and symptoms and falsification of hospital charts and records, and specimens of bodily fluids. This may also include falsification of letters and documents.
- Induction of illness by a variety of means.
  (Department for Children, Schools and Families 2008).

Foreman (2006) identified that the commonest methods for inducing illness appear to be poisoning, including misuse of prescription medicines, and suffocation, which may both be present in patients admitted to ICUs.

Features of physical abuse

These include abrasions, bites (human), bruises, burns, cold injuries, cuts, eye injuries, fractures, hypothermia, intra-abdominal injuries, intracranial injuries, intrathoracic injuries, lacerations, ligature marks, oral injuries, petechiae, retinal haemorrhage, scalds, scars, spinal injuries, strangulation, subdural haemorrhage (NICE 2009). It is also important to acknowledge that when nursing black or ethnic minority children with a dark skin colour it may be more difficult to identify bruising or easier to misdiagnose children with Mongolian blue spots (congenital dermal melanocytosis, a pigmented area which may look like a bruise) as having been abused when clearly they have not. Any health professional involved with a child who has a Mongolian blue spot(s) should fully document such findings in the child's record. As with any differential diagnosis it is important that the child is examined by a consultant or named doctor with expertise in this area for a careful and thorough assessment.

The evidence on the extent of abuse among disabled children in the United Kingdom suggests that disabled children are at increased risk of abuse and that the presence of multiple disabilities appears to increase the risk of both abuse and neglect (HMG 2010). As a result of these findings dedicated practice guidance was published (Department for Children, Schools and Families 2009).

Neglect

Neglect is the persistent failure to meet a child's basic physical and/or psychological needs, likely to result in the serious impairment of the child's health and development. Neglect may occur during pregnancy as a result of maternal substance abuse. Once a child is born, neglect may involve a parent or carer failing to:

- Provide adequate food, clothing and shelter (including exclusion from home or abandonment).
- Protect from physical and emotional harm or danger.
- Ensure adequate supervision, including the use of care-takers.
- Ensure access to appropriate medical care or treatment.

It may also include neglect of, or unresponsiveness to, a child's basic emotional needs (HMG 2010). Neglect may also occur as a discrete incident with serious life-threatening consequences, for example, leaving a very young child home alone, with inappropriate carers or allowing a young child to play on the road by themselves. Examples which might trigger an alert in the ITU nurse could be a child admitted with immersion near-drowning, a late-night traffic incident or ingestion of medicine such as methadone as a result of inadequate supervision.

Features of neglect

These include abandonment, bites (animal/insect), clothing, poor hygiene (e.g. dirty child, strong body odour), failure to thrive (centile position), faltering growth, poor state of footwear or wearing too small/large shoes, head lice, lack of engagement in health promotion programmes, health reviews, home conditions, persistent infestations, incomplete immunisation or developmental screening programme, absence of basic necessities, lack of supervision, poor adherence to prescribed medication, poor parental interaction with medical services, scabies, sunburn (care or sunblock not applied) or untreated tooth decay (NICE 2009).

Sexual abuse

This involves forcing or enticing a child or young person to take part in sexual activities, including prostitution,

whether or not the child is aware of what is happening. The activities may involve physical contact, including penetrative (e.g. rape or buggery) or non-penetrative acts. They may include non-activities, such as involving children in looking at, or producing, pornographic material or watching sexual activities or encouraging children to behave in sexually inappropriate ways (Department for Children, Schools and Families 2010).

Features of sexual abuse

Anal symptoms and signs (anogenital injuries, dysuria, foreign bodies), genital symptoms and signs (pregnancy, sexual exploitation, sexualised behaviour (see Emotional, behavioural, interpersonal and social functioning), sexually transmitted infections, vaginal discharge) (NICE 2009). The child in ITU admitted for other reasons may have a history of having suffered abuse of this nature if found to have an unusual anal/genital discharge or have unusual anal/genital features. Although a deeply uncomfortable suspicion, it is preferable to raise concerns and be subsequently reassured than to recover a child who is subsequently discharged into the same abusive circumstances.

Emotional abuse

This is the persistent emotional maltreatment of a child such as to cause severe and persistent adverse effects on the child's emotional development. It may involve conveying to children that they are worthless or unloved, inadequate or valued insofar as they meet the needs of another person. It may feature age or developmentally inappropriate expectations being imposed on children. These may include interactions that are beyond the child's development capability as well as overprotection and limitation of exploration and learning, or preventing the child from participating in normal social interaction. It may involve seeing or hearing the ill-treatment of another. It may involve serious bullying, causing children frequently to feel frightened or in danger, or the exploitation of children or corruption of children. Some level of emotional abuse is involved in all types of ill treatment of a child, though it may occur alone (Department for Children, Schools and Families 2010).

Features of emotional abuse

Age-inappropriate behaviour, aggression, body-rocking, changes in emotional or behavioural state, cutting, dissociation, drug-taking, eating and feeding behaviour, encopresis, fearfulness, runaway behaviour, low self-esteem, self-harm, sexual behaviour, smearing (of faeces), wetting (NICE 2009). The heavily sedated child in ITU cannot manifest many of these features but there may be evidence of self-harm and the features identified above may be seen in siblings.

Parent or carer–child interactions

The ICU is a stressful environment and people react in different ways to it. However, experienced children's nurses have experienced a range of reactions from parents and carers and some may seem to be unusual or inappropriate. The children's nurse needs to be aware of the possibility that these reactions may alert to cases of domestic abuse or be evidence of emotional unavailability and unresponsiveness. During bedside discussions the parents may provide evidence of age-inappropriate expectations or the child may be unusually defensive or openly hostile to the staff. A detailed history may indicate that the family are isolated or that there are marital disputes where the child is used as a bargaining tool. There is a range of indicators to suggest that the parent–child relationship may not be good; these also include rejection, scapegoating, inappropriate socialisation and response to wetting (NICE 2009). Given the circumstances, the quality of interaction between the sedated child and the parent may not be observed but the quality of interaction between family members and siblings may trigger alarm.

Domestic violence (DV)

This may be defined as any violence between current and former partners in an intimate relationship, wherever and whenever the violence occurs. The violence may include physical, sexual, emotional and financial abuse (Home Office 2009). Children living in homes where there is domestic violence are now generally recognised as being indirect victims of that violence even when it is not directed at them and is now included in emotional abuse definitions (Department for Children, Schools and Families 2010). In some cases children may be patients on the ICU as a result of either being direct victims of their carer's violence or as a result of attempting to protect their non-violent carer and having suffered physical harm. Other children may be admitted to the ICU through self-harming behaviours (overdose, cutting) or risky behaviours (joy-riding, binge-drinking) as a direct response to witnessing harm to their non-violent carer.

In other situations an adult patient may be admitted as a result of a domestic assault and their child or children are visitors. In all such cases safety planning must be undertaken in respect of the adult victim, any children involved and staff working on the unit. Named professionals and patient and staff safety teams will assist in action planning.

Impact of domestic violence

- Accounts for one quarter of all recorded violent crime.
- 1 in 4 women and 1 in 6 men will be victims.
- On average two women a week are killed by a current or former partner.
- Risks of DV do not differ significantly by ethnicity.
- Lesbian, gay, bisexual and transgender communities experience DV in similar proportions (1:4).
- A third of children know what is happening; this figure rises to 50% if the violence is repeated.
- Children may attempt to stop the DV and put themselves at risk.

Effects of DV on children

Growing up with DV can have a negative impact on school attainment and the likelihood of school exclusion. DV is not uniform; it has different consequences for victims according to culture, gender and community.

Impact of DV on the child

- DV features in 19% of child contact applications.
- Among children living in refuges 70% report being abused.
- Some men involve their children in abusing their mother.
- Children may feel powerless or guilty.
- Post-traumatic stress syndrome (PTSD).
- May affect school attendance and achievement.
- May interfere with social relationships.
- Often the child will use denial and silence to cope.

Signs and symptoms of DV

Babies under 1 year show distress characterised by poor health, poor sleeping habits and excessive crying as they may be caught up in the violence or physical abuse. Older children may exhibit PTSD – this has been identified in 80% of uninjured children witnesses and disturbing images and memories of the event are imprinted and return unbidden. The event may be re-experienced in full as a flashback in response to environmental triggers or memories.

Some boys copy behaviour or worry they will become an abuser, while girls are more likely to internalise their feelings. Some children will feel guilt that the abuse was their fault for 'being naughty'.

DV affects the way in which children behave; some become numb and detached, while others become highly compliant. Some children respond by becoming highly aroused, hyper-alert and jumpy with impaired concentration and memory. Many children exhibit disturbed sleep patterns.

Risk factors of DV

- Previous DV: 35% have a second incident within 5 weeks.
- Minor violence is a predictor of escalation to major violence.
- Separation: 22% are assaulted after separation.
- Substance misuse: 32% said their attacker had been drinking.
- Certain drugs (e.g. cocaine or crack cocaine) more likely to be associated with violence.
- Pregnancy: 33% of DV starts or escalates in pregnancy.
- Of all female homicides 45% are victims of DV (8% male victims).
- On average a woman will be assaulted 35 times before she tells a professional.

The common law duty of confidentiality; the Human Rights Act 1998 and the Data Protection Act 1998 may raise anxieties in staff in relation to concerns about patients or colleagues who may be exposed to domestic violence and they have been asked to keep this information confidential or are unsure whether this is child protection if the child appears unharmed. In all such cases, but in particular where there are children involved, support and advice can be obtained from the named nurse and where appropriate the Trust Child Protection Procedure and or Local Safeguarding Children Board domestic violence policy should be followed. Many areas now have multi-agency risk assessment conferences (MARAC) in which the management of perpetrators of DV and support for victims of DV are discussed, with multi-agency action plans agreed. It can also present as part of what is termed the toxic trio of concerns around mental health, substance misuse and DV. Recent research has also identified that DV, child protection and animal abuse may coexist, which staff should consider when assessing any risk to a child in the ICU (veterinary surgeons now receive child protection training with mandatory reporting in some areas such as Scotland when animal abuse has been identified and children live in the household).

Further information can be accessed in respect of domestic violence and its management, including a risk assessment matrix via the Safeguarding Children Abused Through Domestic Violence Procedure (March 2008, available from www.londonscb.gov.uk) or *Responding to Domestic Abuse: A Handbook For Health Professionals* (Department of Health 2005).

Identification of concerns

When an intensive care nurse or any professional has a concern in respect of a child's health, welfare or safety from a safeguarding aspect they are required to discuss their concerns with a more experienced colleague, manager or named professional and then alert their local children's social care services or police by a telephone referral as detailed in Trust policies and procedures followed by confirmation of their concerns by a written referral, usually within 24 hours.

It is important to be able to recognise when you have a concern about a child's welfare or safety. The following factors may raise your concerns:

- History changes.
- Delay in seeking help.
- History and injury not compatible with age/developmental stage (e.g. bruises in a non-mobile baby or a disabled child).
- Suspicious pattern of injury.
- Multiple injuries of different ages and sites.
- Other concerns such as failure to thrive, signs of neglect, emotional abuse.
- Behaviour of parent causes concern (alcohol or substance misuse, adult mental health problems, domestic violence).

Assessment and documentation

Taking into account the whole picture of the child, asking key questions, listening to and observing the child or young person (if appropriate) and family members including parents may raise your concern or clarify the circumstances of the child's current situation as acceptable. Examples of common questions to ask are:

- What actually happened?
- Where did it happen?
- When did it happen (including date and time)?
- Who was present?
- What did they see?
- How was the situation handled at the time?
- Who did what?
- Has this happened before?
- If yes, when and which hospital did the child attend?

As identified in the NICE Guidelines CG 89, seek an explanation for any injury or presentation from both the parent or carer and the child or young person in an open and non-judgemental manner. An unsuitable explanation would be one that is implausible, inadequate or inconsistent with how the child or young person has presented. This may be affected by normal activities, medical condition, age or developmental stage, or a difference in account compared with the parent's or given over a period of time, or cultural practice, although this should not justify causing harm to a child or young person no matter how well intentioned.

It is important that whenever a nurse has a concern about a child's welfare or safety their first action should be to discuss the nature of these concerns with a more experienced nurse, named nurse or medical staff within the unit. In particular, the concerns should be shared with the child's consultant and an action plan agreed, including referral to children's social care services or the police where appropriate following Trust procedures.

Where a member of staff feels that a child protection referral should be made and there is a failure to agree this course of action by more experienced staff for whatever reason, further advice, support and guidance can be obtained from the named nurse or senior manager on call out of hours. All such disagreements and their resolution should be detailed in the child's records.

Guidelines for recording concerns

It is important to record in the child or young person's clinical record exactly what is observed, what information is heard or shared with whom and when. If there are concerns in respect of a child's health or welfare the record should also detail the nature of those concerns and the actions taken, including discussions with other professionals.

It cannot be emphasised strongly enough the importance of record-keeping as required by the Trust and Nursing Midwifery Council (2007) Record keeping Guidance for nurses and midwives. In child protection cases in particular an intensive care nurse may not know that in the future they will be required to compile a child protection report, legal statement, attend court or be party to a serious case review process or audited within clinical governance framework. To ensure that record-keeping is of a high standard this art must be practised every time a patient's record is written, complies with Trust policies and meets professional standards (NMC 2007).

Purpose of recording

- Allows for a chronology of what happened and when.
- Shows a history of events and allows analysis of any patterns.
- Allows for continuity over time.

- Details actions taken by staff.
- Provides accountability.
- Provides a basis for evidence in court.
- Supplies information.
- Be specific – What is the exact nature of your concern?
- Show the evidence – What did you see, hear? Who said what, when?
- Be precise – What do you mean by frequent, always?
- State your professional judgement.
- Ensure your professional judgement is supported by evidence.

Signs and symptoms

In addition to the features already identified from the NICE CG 89 guidelines the following may alert you to consider that a child's welfare or safety may be of concern. It is important to be clear that your role is to identify that you have a concern in respect of a child's health, welfare or safety and not to diagnose whether this is a child protection issue. By following Trust policies and procedures you are alerting specialist agencies to your concerns and they will undertake to investigate your concerns within a child protection framework, undertaking a section 47 investigation, as defined in the Children Act 1989.

Clinical features

- Unusual or excessive bruising, or in the shape of a hand, ligature, stick, grip or implement.
- Any bruising in the non-mobile baby or child.
- Any serious or unusual injury with an absent or unlikely explanation.
- Head injuries in a child under 3 years; intracranial injury in a child if there is no major confirmed accidental trauma or known medical cause.
- Other inflicted injuries, retinal haemorrhages or rib or long bone fractures.
- Multiple subdural haemorrhages with or without subarachnoid haemorrhage with or without hypoxic ischaemic damage to the brain.
- Signs of spinal injury if there is no major confirmed accidental trauma.
- Cigarette burns, other burns or scalds in areas not expected to come into contact accidentally with hot objects or those indicating forced immersion.
- Bite marks – all human bites are abusive. A formal assessment by a forensic dentist may determine whether the bite is by an adult or child.

- Unusual injuries in inaccessible places (e.g. neck, ear, hands, feet or buttocks).
- Trauma or damage to intra-oral frena, or unexplained frenum injury in non-ambulant child.
- Genital/anal trauma (where no clear history or direct trauma is offered or part of the clinical presentation)
- Trauma without adequate history (e.g. intra-abdominal injury).
- Fractures in a child under 18 months with no predisposing medical condition or fractures of different ages.

(NICE 2009).

Due to the limited research on the identification of non-accidental injuries and the recent experience of paediatricians in the court system the National Society for the Prevention of Cruelty to Children (NSPCC), in association with Cardiff University, have undertaken systematic reviews on such injuries from a research aspect going back 10 years in the United Kingdom and other countries. Their research findings cover the following:

- Bruising.
- Fractures.
- Thermal injuries.
- Head and spinal injuries.
- Oral injuries.

(www.core-info.cf.ac.uk).

Using the intensive care nurse's professional judgement

Values, theoretical orientation, knowledge and research all influence the questions that are asked and how they are asked. Nurses are involved with a child and parents or carers at almost every level of engagement. This involves the analysis of past professional and personal experiences. It also involves reviewing and evaluating existing skills and knowledge which can cause professionals high levels of anxiety when deciding what to do. Help and support can be obtained from a number of sources (e.g. experienced colleagues, the named nurse or doctor). It may also be helpful to ask the following questions:

- What are the concerns?
- What is the evidence to support these concerns?
- What are the strengths of the family (e.g. appropriate attachment, response to the child)?
- What theoretical approaches are you drawing from?
- What is your professional judgement?
- Be specific – What is the exact nature of your concern?
- Show the evidence – What did you see, hear? Who said what, when?

- Be precise – What do you mean by frequent, always?
- State your professional judgement.
- Ensure your professional judgement is supported by evidence.

In addition, there are a number of good practice checklists available to support professionals in checking their actions and serve as a good practice prompt (e.g. London Child Protection Procedures, 2007; www.londonscb.gov.uk).

Making a referral

It is vital when an intensive care nurse decides to make a child protection referral that they have reflected on their concerns, discussed them with a more experienced colleague, child's consultant or manager, and made a holistic assessment of the child and family, including positives as well as concerns. The nurse must also be clear about the reason for making a referral, including:

- When they saw the child, pregnant woman or adult.
- Who was present.
- What they saw.
- What explanation was given, what the child and/or parent said.
- Assessment of the child, pregnant woman or adult, including details of any concerns.
- Information offered to parents or mature child (i.e. Fraser competent).
- Actions taken to protect the child (including the unborn child) and what you want Social Services or the police to do.
- Confirmation of telephone referrals in writing where relevant and a clear record of all actions taken in line with Trust policies and procedures.
- Information given to the child's consultant, manager, named nurse of all actions undertaken.
- A copy of the referral placed in the child's records (if the child is a patient). If the child is not a patient, then discuss and agree with your manager or named nurse where the referral copy will be filed.

Information sharing

Intensive care nurses recognise the importance of information sharing and there is evidence of good practice around the country. However, in some situations nurses may feel constrained from sharing information by uncertainty about when they can do so lawfully, especially in early intervention and preventative work where decisions may be less clear than in safeguarding or child protection situations.

For those who have to make decisions about information sharing on a case-by-case basis, government (HMG 2008) seeks to give clear practical guidance, drawing on experience and consultation from across a spectrum of adult and children's services. In addition, individual Trusts will have agreed information sharing protocols for work with other agencies in a number of different situations, including child protection.

If intensive care nurses have any concerns in relation to information sharing further support and advice can be obtained from the named nurse or Caldicott Guardian (a senior member of staff appointed to protect patient information).

Confidentiality

It is important that intensive care nurses respect people's right to confidentiality, but also to acknowledge that in child protection information can be shared without consent if there is concern that a child may be at risk (NMC 2008). It is important that you inform parents when you have a concern, and it is good practice to advise parents and mature children (where appropriate) that you are making a referral.

If you have a genuine concern that by informing the parent or mature child that you intend to make a referral you may place them at risk of further harm, yourself at risk of harm or lead to absconding or the destruction of forensic evidence, you should not tell them. In these cases you should advise the professional you are speaking to that you have not told the parent or mature (Fraser competent) child and the reasons why.

Emotional impact

When a child the nurse is caring for has life-threatening injuries or dies as a result of abuse or neglect this is likely to be more personally challenging and more emotionally charged than any other area. Nurses involved in such cases at almost every level of engagement with the child or family will find that it involves reflection on their past experiences, both professional and personal, which may trigger painful memories. In addition, such emotionally charged work involves reviewing and evaluating existing skills and knowledge and may result in nurses feeling inadequate, emotionally drained, distressed or even angry with colleagues or parents.

It is important that such feelings and identification of skill gaps are addressed within a supportive framework, such as debriefings, clinical or child protection supervision. In some cases referral to Trust counselling services

may be appropriate and should not be viewed as a weakness, but as a response to a traumatic event.

When a child dies

Each unexpected death of a child is a tragedy for the family, and subsequent enquiries and investigations should keep an appropriate balance between forensic and medical requirements and the family's need for support. Where there are concerns by any professional in relation to the Child Death Overview Process (CDOP) or the management of the child and family by another agency (police and forensic requirements) these should be shared with the designated doctor for child deaths, CDOP coordinator or named nurse for support, advice and resolution (Department for Children, Schools and Families 2010).

When a child dies in the ICU, two events may occur at the same time. First, since April 2008 all child deaths (i.e. deaths under the age of 18 years, including premature babies) are formally reviewed under the CDOP (Department for Children, Schools and Families 2010). This guidance, which is supported by local policies and procedures, sets out the steps to be taken when a child dies. There are two interrelated processes for reviewing child deaths, either of which can trigger child protection investigations and/or a Serious Case Review. These are:

- A rapid response by a group of key professionals who come together for the purpose of enquiring into and evaluating each unexpected or unexplained death of a child (guidance para. 7.48).
- An overview of all child deaths in the LSCB area(s) undertaken by a panel.

Second, where a child's death is unexpected or unexplained, it will be dealt with under the rapid-response procedures. In these cases the Trust procedures will detail who should be informed, together with relevant contact numbers on a 24-hour rota basis. All Trusts should have immediate access to the Designated Doctor for Child Deaths (or their deputy) for support and advice, together with the CDOP coordinator. In the majority of cases the police and coroner will be notified and the police usually visit the ICU to obtain further information in line with local CDOP procedure. The parents should be advised of the CDOP procedure, including the involvement of the police and coroner. In almost all cases of unexpected child death, the coroner will order a postmortem to be carried out as soon as possible by the most appropriate pathologist available. If the death, following collation of information by the police ·and Designated Doctor for Child Death, is found to be unnatural, or the cause of death has not been determined, the coroner will in due course hold an inquest.

LSCB (2007, 2008) offer examples of professional responsibility following unexpected child deaths (www. lscb-llr.gov.uk; www.londonscb.gov.uk).

In cases where there are concerns that the death may have been caused by abuse or neglect the Trust child protection policy will be followed with an immediate referral to Children's Social Care Services (Emergency Duty Team out of hours) and/or the police. Good practice should ensure that the named professionals (named doctor and named nurse) along with the Designated Doctor for Child Deaths are informed. Guidance will be offered by the police in respect of any forensic aspects of the case and the physical contact the parent or carer may have with the dead child.

When the process will not be invoked

When a child dies and that death was expected (e.g. a childhood disability or medical condition) and the consultant certifies the child's death, then this death will be reviewed by the child death panel and not be subject to a rapid response. In these cases the coroner will not be involved and the Trust bereavement policy will be followed. This will include the CDOP process for notifying the Trust CDOP coordinator, who will advise and support staff to ensure all relevant information required by the CDOP Panel is forwarded to him or her.

Where there are shared roles

In a number of Trusts the named professionals also undertake the role of the CDOP coordinator while in other Trusts this is a specialist post which may or may not be linked to the End of Life Care Pathway coordinator role. It is important for the children's intensive care nurse to ensure that they are fully aware of the policy and procedure of the CDOP protocol for their individual Trust.

In all cases information, usually in the form of a report, will be requested by the CDOP coordinator from the child's consultant and relevant staff, together with an invitation to attend panel meetings if required. Similar information will be ascertained from staff when child protection procedures are followed in line with Trust policies and procedures.

Conclusion

All intensive care nurses working with children and their parents or carers should understand that they are also working within the safeguarding continuum and not in a separate sphere (Brandon et al. 2008; Department for Children, Schools and Families 2008). Safeguarding is everyone's responsibility, so they should be clear as to their role and responsibility, including the role of other agencies when they have a concern about a child's health, welfare or safety.

Remember:

- Protect children and promote their safety and welfare – talk and listen to children.
- Read and understand local child protection procedures.
- Record keeping – keep it accurate, legible and contemporaneous.
- Don't investigate – remember that an allegation of child abuse or neglect may lead to a criminal investigation so do not do anything that may jeopardise a police investigation (e.g. asking a child leading question or attempting to investigate, justify or explain allegations of abuse).
- Safeguarding is a shared responsibility; you cannot act independently.
- Liaise with other agencies and professionals, including the Trust Safeguarding Team.
- Share information on a need to know basis.
- Do not delay your referral. If unsure, seek the advice of a more experienced colleague, your manager or a member of the Safeguarding Team.

References

Brandon M, Belderson P, Warren C, Howe D, Gardner R, Dodsworth J, Black J. 2008. Analysing Child Deaths and Serious Injury Through Abuse and Neglect: What Can We Learn? A biennial analysis of serious case reviews. London: DCSF.

Department for Children, Schools and Families. 2008. Safeguarding Children in Whom Illness is Fabricated or Induced. London: HMG.

Department for Children, Schools and Families. 2009. Safeguarding Disabled Children: practice guidance: Nottingham: HMSO.

Department for Children, Schools and Families. 2010. Working Together to Safeguard Children: a guide to inter-agency working to safeguard and promote the welfare of children. London: HMG. https://www.education.gov.uk/publications/eOrderingDownload/00305-2010DOM-EN-v3.pdf

Department of Education. 2011. The Munro Review of Child Protection: Final Report: a child centred system. London: DOE.

Department for Education and Skills. 2003. Every Child Matters. London: The Stationery Office.

Department of Health. 1991. The Children Act 1989: guidance and regulations. London: HMSO.

Department of Health. 2000a. Learning the Lessons. London: The Stationery Office.

Department of Health. 2000b. The Framework for the Assessment of Children in Need and Their Families. London: DH.

Department of Health. 2002a. Learning from Past Experience. London: DH.

Department of Health. 2002b. Safeguarding Children: a joint inspectors report on arrangements to safeguard children. London: DH.

Department of Health. 2005. Responding to Domestic Abuse: a handbook for health professionals. London: DH.

Department of Health. 2006. Responding to Domestic Violence: a handbook for health professionals. London: DH.

Foreman D. 2006. Detecting fabricated and induced illness in children. British Medical Journal, 7523:978–9.

Home Office. 2009. What is Domestic Violence? London: HMSO.

Her Majesty's Government (HMG). 2008. Information Sharing: guidance for practitioners and managers. London: HMSO. www.everychildmatters.gov.uk/information sharing.

Laming H. 2003. The Victoria Climbié Inquiry. London: Stationery Office.

Laming D. 2009. The Protection of Children in England: A progress report. London: Stationery Office.

Local Safeguarding Children Boards (LSCB). 2007. London Child Protection Procedures. Section 5: Children in Specific Circumstances (3rd edition). London: LSCB.

Local Safeguarding Children Boards (LSCB) 2008. Safeguarding Children Abused Through Domestic Violence. London: LSCB.

National Institute for Health and Clinical Excellence (NICE). 2009. When to Suspect Child Maltreatment, CG 89. London: NICE.

Nursing Midwifery Council. 2007. Record keeping: Guidance for nurses and midwives. London: NMC.

Nursing Midwifery Council. 2008. The Code: Standards of conduct, performance and ethics for nurses and midwives. London: NMC.

Royal College of Paediatrics and Child Health. 2010. Safeguarding Children and Young People: Roles and Competencies for Health Care Staff. RCPCH: London. http://www.rcpch.ac.uk/sites/default/files/asset_library/Education%20Department/Safeguarding/Safeguarding%20Children%20and%20Young%20people%202010G.pdf.

Further reading

Calder M. 2004. Children Living with Domestic Violence – towards a framework for assessment and intervention. Lyme Regis: Russell House.

Department for Education and Skills. 2006. What To Do If You Are Worried a Child is Being Abused. London: DfES.

Resources

Human Rights Act 1998. London: HMSO.
Data Protection Act 1998. London: HMSO.
Children Act 2004. London: HMSO.

INDEX